ANNUAL REVIEWS REPRINTS: IMMUNOLOGY, 1977-1979

ANNUAL REVIEWS REPRINTS: IMMUNOLOGY, 1977-1979

Compiled by Irving Weissman

Stanford University

ANNUAL REVIEWS INC.   4139 EL CAMINO WAY   PALO ALTO, CALIFORNIA 94306

Production Editor	S. HAWKES
Indexing Coordinator	M. A. GLASS
Subject Indexer	S. M. SORENSEN

INTRODUCTION

No longer are the major themes in immunology of interest only to immunologists. Now other biological scientists as well look to this discipline for tools of unparalleled specificity with which to study their own subjects more effectively. The concerns of immunologists have thus begun to converge upon those of cell biologists, biochemists, developmental biologists, pharmacologists, and others. Furthermore, immunological techniques are now of increasing usefulness in clinical medicine, where the description of phenomena has often outstripped our understanding of the mechanisms behind them.

Because the frontiers of many disciplines overlap those of immunology, review articles in immunology have appeared in various *Annual Review* series: Biochemistry, Biophysics & Bioengineering, Genetics, Medicine, Microbiology, and Pharmacology & Toxicology. A review volume in immunology has in fact lain hidden within these related publications. It has here been brought out of hiding. *Annual Reviews Reprints: Immunology, 1977-1979* has been designed to provide immunologists and other biologists with convenient and inexpensive access to current critical reviews in immunology, together with bibliographical guides to the developing interfaces between this and other disciplines. Here, too, the nonspecialist will find fundamental aspects of the art and science of immunology comprehensibly presented.

The volume contains a mixture of articles intended for the expert and the nonimmunologist. Both their selection and their arbitrary categorization reflect the biases of the compiler. However, I trust the reader will understand our objectives and appreciate the quality of the articles solicited originally by the Editors and Editorial Committees of the several *Annual Review* series from which materials have been drawn.

The publication of future collections, and perhaps of a new *Annual Review* series, depends upon your response to this volume. The editorial staff of Annual Reviews Inc. welcomes your comments and suggestions.

I. WEISSMAN

Annual Reviews Reprints:
Immunology, 1977–1979

CONTENTS

NOTE: These chapters have been repaged for this reprint collection and the new page number appears at the bottom of each page. The number and heading at the top of each page are as they appeared in the original publication.

ANNUAL REVIEWS INC. is a nonprofit corporation established to promote the advancement of the sciences. Beginning in 1932 with the *Annual Review of Biochemistry*, the Company has pursued as its principal function the publication of high quality, reasonably priced Annual Review volumes. The volumes are organized by Editors and Editorial Committees who invite qualified authors to contribute critical articles reviewing significant developments within each major discipline.

Annual Reviews are published in the following sciences: Anthropology, Astronomy and Astrophysics, Biochemistry, Biophysics and Bioengineering, Earth and Planetary Sciences, Ecology and Systematics, Energy, Entomology, Fluid Mechanics, Genetics, Materials Science, Medicine, Microbiology, Neuroscience, Nuclear and Particle Science, Pharmacology and Toxicology, Physical Chemistry, Physiology, Phytopathology, Plant Physiology, Psychology, Public Health, and Sociology. In addition, five special volumes have been published by Annual Reviews Inc.: *History of Entomology* (1973), *The Excitement and Fascination of Science* (1965), *The Excitement and Fascination of Science, Volume Two* (1978), *Annual Reviews Reprints: Cell Membranes, 1975–1977* (published 1978), and *Annual Reviews Reprints: Immunology, 1977–1979* (published 1980). For the convenience of readers, a detachable order form/envelope is bound into the back of this volume.

Ann. Rev. Biochem. 1979. 48:961–97

THREE-DIMENSIONAL STRUCTURE OF IMMUNOGLOBULINS

♦12030

L. Mario Amzel and Roberto J. Poljak

Department of Biophysics, Johns Hopkins University School of Medicine, 725 N. Wolfe Street, Baltimore, Maryland 21205

CONTENTS

PERSPECTIVES AND SUMMARY

Immunoglobulins are serum glycoproteins synthesized by vertebrates as antibodies against different antigens. They generally consist of two polypeptide chains called the light (L) chain and the heavy (H) chain (mol wts

0066-4154/79/0701-0961$01.00

961

25,000 and 50,000, respectively). The three-dimensional structure of several immunoglobulins and their fragments have been determined by single crystal x-ray diffraction methods. These studies have shown that immunoglobulins are multimeric proteins consisting of globular subunits arranged in pairs. These subunits of the L and H chains contain homologous amino acid sequences ("homology regions") about 110 amino acids long, and share a common pattern of three-dimensional chain folding ("immunoglobulin-fold").

The predominant secondary structure of the subunits is antiparallel β-pleated sheet. Each subunit contains two twisted, roughly parallel sheets formed by three and four antiparallel strands. The internal volume of the subunits is tightly packed with hydrophobic side chains enveloped by the two β-sheets. About 50% of the amino acid residues of the subunits form part of the β-sheets and have highly conserved sequences in different immunoglobulins.

The antigen-combining sites of immunoglobulins are formed by the two N-terminal subunits of the L and H chains and occur at the ends of the molecules, fully exposed to solvent. The conformation of the combining sites is determined by the amino acid sequence of segments of the H and L polypeptide chains ("complementarity-determining residues"). The amino acid sequences of these segments, unique to each different immunoglobulin, determine the specificities of antibody molecules. The structures of several ligand-immunoglobulin complexes determined by X-ray diffraction have provided useful models of antigen-antibody interactions.

The segments of polypeptide chain connecting the globular immonoglobulin domains show different degrees of flexibility. This flexibility of antibodies could be important for the mechanism of antigen binding and the ensuing activation of secondary or effector functions involving domains of the structure removed from the antigen-combining site.

Studies on the primary and tertiary structure of immunoglobulins substantiate the postulate that the different homology subunits arose during evolution by a mechanism of gene duplication and diversification. This mechanism provided the structural basis for the different functions of antibody molecules. The evolutionary mechanism did not alter the overall folding pattern of the subunits. However, within an immunoglobulin molecule the subunits pair in three different types of geometrical arrangement. These different pairing schemes are determined by amino acid substitutions in the β-sheets of the subunits. The major amino acid differences between immunoglobulin of the same class and of the same animal species occur in the loops connecting the β-pleated sheet strands.

Starting from the known structure of immunoglobulin fragments some attempts have been made to predict the conformation of the combining site of other immunoglobulins based solely on their amino acid sequences. Trial models have been derived by this general procedure but there is not yet enough information to evaluate their accuracy. The determination of three-dimensional structures of additional immunoglobulin-combining sites will be necessary to ascertain the ultimate potential of this approach.

The studies on the three-dimensional structures of immunoglobulins and their fragments, reviewed below, have provided invaluable information for the understanding of the structural basis of antibody function. Further studies will be needed, however, to complete our knowledge of the chemical basis of antibody specificity and to understand the triggering and the structural localization of effector functions.

INTRODUCTION

Several reviews on the function and the three-dimensional structure of immunoglobulins have been published (1–8) including one in this series (2). Consequently, we limit ourselves to a brief outline of the most recent results in the study of the structure of immunoglobulins by X-ray diffraction and a brief discussion of related topics.

Antibodies belong to the class of serum proteins called γ-globulins or immunoglobulins (Ig). Myeloma proteins, associated with the spontaneous occurrence of multiple myelomatosis and other pathological lympho-proliferative disorders in man, and with experimentally induced tumors in mice, are closely related to serum immunoglobulins and antibodies by a number of structural and functional properties. Human or murine myeloma proteins can be obtained in large, easily purified quantities that provide suitable material for structural studies. Immunoglobulins (Ig) are divided into major classes or isotypes characterized by their H-chain type. They all contain carbohydrates, largely hexose and hexosamine but also sialic acid and fucose, covalently attached to the protein moiety. The IgG class is the most abundant in normal serum and the most commonly observed class in human myeloma immunoglobulins. Its diagrammatic structure, including homology regions, is shown in Figure 1. The C_H1, C_H2, C_H3, and C_L regions are highly homologous to each other and less homologous to V_H and V_L. The N-terminal variable regions, V_H and V_L, are highly homologous to each other.

The L chains of IgG can be antigenically classified into two isotypes (or classes) called κ and λ, each characterized by a unique (or nearly unique) sequence in their C-terminal regions. IgM, IgA, IgD, and IgE possess similar κ and λ light chains but their H chains (called μ, α, δ, and ϵ, respectively) are different and are specific to each class. Amino acid sequence studies of human myeloma L chains have shown that in those of the same class (κ or λ) C_L's have constant amino acid sequences while V_L's have variable sequences. Because of the genetic and possible functional implications, the patterns of variability of L-chain sequences have been extensively analyzed. It is observed that within a given class of L chains there are sequences that are very similar to each other which define a "subgroup." Three or four such subgroups have been proposed for human κ-chains and five for human λ-chains. All chains within a subgroup are very similar in sequence except at certain positions within V_L, where extreme variability is observed. Kabat & Wu (9, 10) proposed that these hypervariable sequences constitute the regions of the L-chain structure that come in contact with antigen, so that the presence of different sequences in these regions will

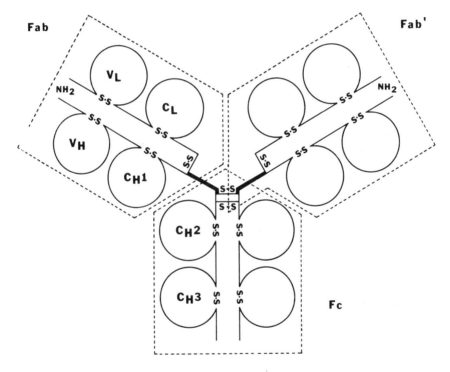

Figure 1   Diagram of a human immunoglobulin (IgG1) molecule. The light (L) chains (mol wt ~25,000) are divided into two homology regions, V_L and C_L. The heavy (H) chains (mol wt ~50,000) are divided into four homology regions, V_H, C_H1, C_H2, and C_H3. The C_H1 and C_H2 are joined by a "hinge" region indicated by a thicker line. Cleavage of the IgG1 molecule by papain generates Fab fragments (mol wt ~50,000) consisting of an L and an Fd polypeptide chain, and Fc fragments (mol wt ~50,000). Cleavage by pepsin followed by reduction of inter-H-chain disulfide bonds generates an Fab' fragment consisting of an L and an Fd' polypeptide chain. Interchain and intrachain disulfide bonds and the N termini of the L and H chains are indicated. [Reproduced from (52) with permission.]

result in different antibody specificities. Comparative studies on H chains of the same class have shown that the sequences of C_H1, C_H2, and C_H3 remain constant whereas those of V_H display variability. Just as in the L chain, the variable region of the H chain occurs at the N-terminal end of the molecule, is approximately 110 amino acid residues long, and also contains hypervariable regions (11).

Pepsin, papain, trypsin, and other enzymes split bonds in the "hinge" region which links Fab to Fc (see Figure 1) and which, by this criterion, appears openly accessible to solvent. In this review we use the term "region" (Fab region, Fc region) to denote that part of the immunoglobulin structure that corresponds to fragments such as Fab and Fc.

BASIC STRUCTURAL PATTERNS OF IMMUNOGLOBULINS

Homology Subunits

The homology regions of immunoglobulin chains fold into independent, compact units of three-dimensional structure (homology subunits). X-ray diffraction studies (12, 13) have shown that all homology subunits of immunoglobulins share a common pattern of three-dimensional chain folding ("immunoglobulin fold") shown in Figures 2 and 3. The immunoglobulin fold consists of two twisted, stacked β-pleated sheets that surround an internal volume tightly packed with hydrophobic side chains. These two β-sheets are covalently linked by an intrachain disulfide bridge in the inner volume, in a direction approximately perpendicular to the plane of the sheets. The V subunits have an extra length of polypeptide chain that forms the two-stranded loop represented by dotted lines in Figure 2. Stereo diagrams of the four homology subunits of the Fab fragment of human IgG New are shown in Figure 4. Comparison of these diagrams shows the structural homology of the subunits. The extra loop characteristic of the V subunits is clearly seen in V_H. The V_L subunit of Fab New has a deletion of seven amino acids in this region and therefore the extra loop is appreciably shorter. The structures of the different homology subunits of Fab New are also represented schematically in Figure 5 where the two β-pleated sheets are shown as two clusters of polypeptide chain, with hydrogen bonds between main chain atoms represented by dotted lines.

Several labelling systems (2, 3, 14) have been used to name the different segments of polypeptide chain according to their position in the immunoglobulin fold. For the purpose of this discussion we introduce the modified labelling represented in Figure 6 that includes many of the features of the previously proposed nomenclatures. The four-stranded β-pleated sheet, called 4β, contains strands $4\beta1$, $4\beta2$, $4\beta3$, and $4\beta4$. The three-stranded

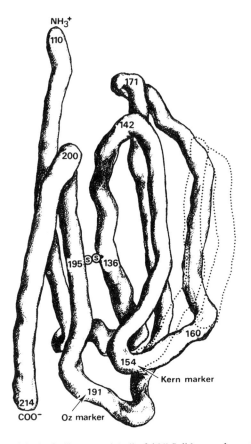

Figure 2   Diagram of the basic "immunoglobulin-fold." Solid trace shows the folding of the polypeptide chain in the constant subunits (C_L and C_H). Numbers designate L (λ) chain residues, beginning at NH_3^+ which corresponds to residue 110 for the L chain. Broken lines indicate the additional loop of polypeptide chain characteristic of the V_L and V_H subunits.

β-pleated sheet, called *3β,* contains strands *3β*1, *3β*2, and *3β*3. The two strands of the extra loop characteristic of the V homology subunits also occur in the *3β* sheet and are called *3β*4 and *3β*5 (dotted lines in Figure 6). The modified *3β* sheets of the V subunits are called *3β'*. The regions containing the segments (loops) that connect the β-sheet strands are labelled according to whether they occur at the same side as the N-terminal front loops, *fl',* or the C-terminal back loops, *bl,* of the immunoglobulin fold. The front end contains the connecting segments *fl*1, *fl*2, and *fl*3 while the back end contains segments *bl*1, *bl*2, and *bl*3. The connecting segments *fl*4 and *bl*4 are associated with the extra loop and occur only in V subunits (dotted lines in Figure 6). In some cases (e.g. some *fl*3's) these segments

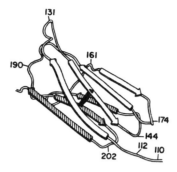

Figure 3   Schematic Diagram of the α-carbon backbone of the C_L homology subunit showing two planes of β-pleated sheet (one containing four hydrogen-bonded antiparallel chains shown by white arrows and another containing three hydrogen-bonded antiparallel chains shown by striated arrows). These two twisted and roughly parallel sheets surround the intrachain disulfide bond (shown in black) which links the two sheets in a direction approximately perpendicular to their planes. [Reproduced from Edmundson et al (32) with permission.]

form regular reverse turns (β-bends, etc) while in most cases they show no secondary structure. Several connecting segments sometimes contain short α-helical stretches (approximately one helical turn).

About 50% of the residues in each homology subunit are contained in the two β-pleated sheets (strands $4\beta1–4\beta4$ and $3\beta1–3\beta3$ or $3\beta5$). The expected pattern of alternating polar-apolar residues is observed in the β-sheets, especially in the sheets that are not involved in the intersubunit interactions. In this alternating pattern of the V subunits, serine and threonine are the most frequently observed amino acids at the surface, exposed to solvent. In contrast, there is a greater diversity of residues at the surface of C-domains (14). The three-dimensional structure of the β-sheet strands is highly conserved between the different homology subunits (15, 16), while most of the structural differences occur in the connecting segments. The hypervariable regions of the V subunits (V_L, V_H) form the connecting segments $f\!l1$, $f\!l2$, and $f\!l4$ which occur in spatial proximity in the three-dimensional structure. These segments contain the largest structural differences between different V homology subunits (17) and determine the conformation of the antigen-combining site.

Subunit Interactions

In immunoglobulin molecules a large number of noncovalent interactions stabilize the arrangement of the different homology subunits. These interactions occur between adjacent subunits of the same chain (*cis* interactions) and between subunits in different chains (*trans* interactions). *Trans* interactions are in general quite extensive and stabilize the structural domains

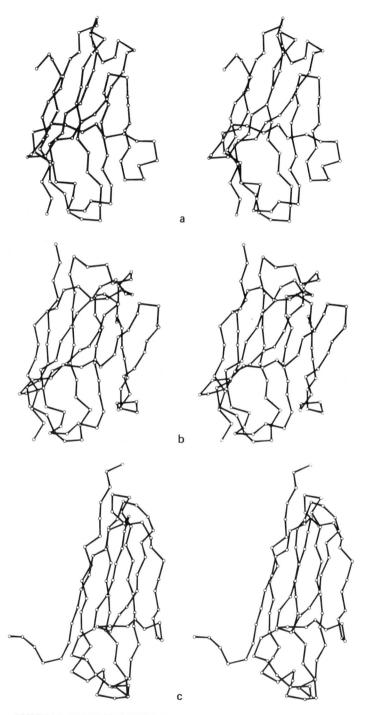

a

b

c

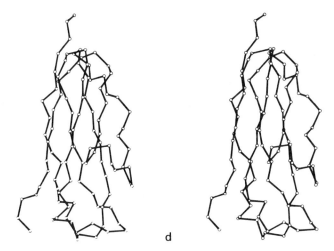

d

Figure 4   Stereo pair drawings of the α-carbon backbones of the four homology subunits of Fab New (V_L, V_H, C_L and C_H1) viewed in approximately the same orientation. The structural similarity is clearly shown in this drawing. The V_H homology subunit, *b*, shows the 'extra loop' characteristic of the V subunits. The V_L subunit of Fab New, *a*, has a much shorter 'extra loop.'

formed by pairs of homology subunits. Conversely, *cis* interactions involve a small number of contact residues and the subunit arrangements stabilized by these interactions are generally flexible (18, 19). These interactions can be seen for example in the structure of the Fab fragment of human IgG New (Figure 7).

SUBUNIT PAIRS AND STRUCTURAL DOMAINS: *TRANS* INTERAC- TIONS   In immunoglobulins the homology subunits are found associated in pairs (20, 21) through *trans* interactions. With the exception of the C_H2 region the structural association between subunits is very close and involves a large area of contact. Two types of close associations are ob- served in subunit pairs. The first (V-type pair) has been observed in the structures of V_κ dimers (22–24), and in the V regions of Fab fragments (13, 25, 26), whole immunoglobulins (19, 27), and an L chain (λ) dimer (12). In all these cases the contact area is formed by the modified *3β'* sheets of both subunits (strands *3β*1–*3β*5). The geometry of this type of pairs is such that the associated subunits are related by approximate (V_L-V_H pairs) or exact (V_L-V_L pairs) twofold axes of symmetry (Figure 7). The interactions between subunits are very extensive and in the case of V_L-V_H pairs the association constant was estimated to be larger than $10^8 M^{-1}$ (28). The arrangement of subunits in all V-type pairs studied is similar even when a V_L-V_L pair and a V_L-V_H pair are compared. Furthermore, this arrangement seems to be independent of L- and H-chain classes since κ- and λ-L chains and γ- and α-H chains associate in similar patterns in the structures that have been studied thus far. The expected alternating pattern of polar-apolar residues is clearly observed in the *4β* sheets of the V subunits while the residues at the outer face of the *3β'* sheets are less polar and participate in

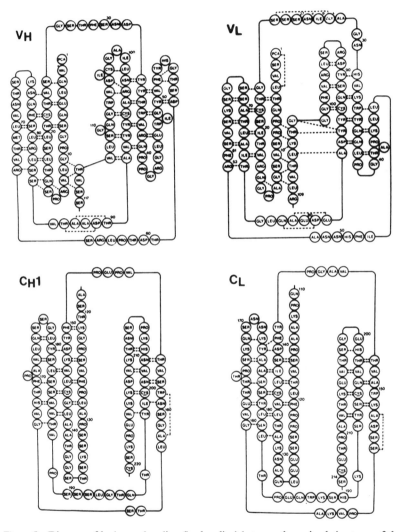

Figure 5   Diagram of hydrogen bonding (broken line) between the main chain atoms of the V$_H$, V$_L$, C$_H$1, and C$_L$ homology region of Fab New. The hydrogen bonded clusters correspond to the two β-sheet structures of each subunit. Cysteine residues that participate in intrachain disulfide bonds are underlined.

the *trans* interactions. The *fl* segments containing the hypervariable regions occur in close spatial proximity defining a large cavity in V_L-V_L pairs and the antibody-combining site in V_L-V_H pairs.

The second type of close association (C-type pairs) is observed in the structures of an L-chain dimer (12), the C regions of three Fab fragments (13, 25, 26), and two immunoglobulins (19, 27) and an Fc fragment (21). In this type of association the contact area is formed by the 4β sheets of the homology subunits (strands 4β1–4β4). To this type belong the C_L-C_L, C_L-C_H1, and C_H3-C_H3 pairs. Again, the geometrical arrangement of subunits in these pairs is highly conserved and involves an exact or an approximate two fold axis of symmetry (Figure 7). In these C-type pairs the conservation of the structure extends to the geometrical arrangement of subunits in different structural domains of the same immunoglobulin (i.e. C_L-C_H1 and C_H3-C_H3).

A third type of association of homology subunits is that observed in C_H2 pairs. This association is observed in the structures of an Fc fragment (21) and a whole immunoglobulin (27) and is much weaker than those of the V- and C-type pairs, in agreement with the available physical chemical information (28, 29).

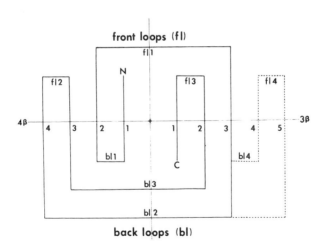

Figure 6   Diagrammatic representation of the β-sheet structure of the homology subunits. The antiparallel strands *1, 2, 3,* and *4* of the 4β sheet begin at N (the "N terminus" of each homology subunit). The 3β sheet consists of strands *1, 2,* and *3,* and in the V_H and V_L subunits only, of additional strands (dotted line) *4* and *5.* The strands are connected by "front" loops (*fl*) which in the case of V_H and V_L are exposed to solvent, and by "back" loops (*bl*). C denotes the "C terminus" of each homology subunit. See Figure 5 to correlate the features of this diagram with actual sequences.

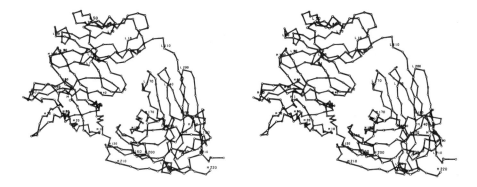

Figure 7 Stereo pair drawing of the β-carbon backbone of Fab New. The interactions between subunits can be clearly seen in this diagram. The interactions between subunits of different chains (*trans*) are much more extensive than those between subunits of the same chain (*cis*).

CIS INTERACTIONS   The interactions between consecutive subunits of the same chain in immunoglobulin molecules are very limited and involve a small number of contacts. These contacts are made between some of the *bl* segments of one subunit and *fl* segments of the next subunit of the same chain. At least three different arrangements involving C_H1-V_H and three involving C_L-V_L were observed in the structures studied so far. Apart from indicating the presence of flexibility in the "switch regions" connecting V to C, no other common characteristic of these V-C *cis* interactions has emerged from these studies. We discuss *cis* interactions in more detail in our review of the structures studied by X-ray diffraction methods.

X-RAY DIFFRACTION STUDIES OF IMMUNOGLOBULIN L CHAINS

Three-Dimensional Structures of V_κ Fragments

The three-dimensional structures of three dimeric V_κ fragments (Rei, Au, and Roy) have been reported (22–24, 30). These fragments show the same overall three-dimensional structure of the V-type dimers described in the previous section. An interesting observation was made concerning Tyr 49, a constant residue in the three V_κ dimers which could therefore be expected to adopt the same conformation in the three structures. However, Tyr 49 occurs in close spatial proximity to residue 96 which is a Leu in Roy, a Tyr in Rei, and a Trp in Au. The proximity of these residues at position 96 imposes different conformations on the side chain of Tyr 49 in the three dimers. Thus, amino acid substitutions in the hypervariable regions are shown to have an effect not only in the character of the position at which they occur but also at neighboring positions of the antigen-combining site.

Although there is now a general understanding about the relationship between molecular structure and antigen binding, and in particular about hypervariability and the antigen-combining site, the specific details about the effect of amino acid substitutions, and the extent of the antigen-antibody interactions are not known. Studies such as those reported above for closely related κ-chains are of great interest to our understanding of this topic.

The Mcg Dimer

The crystal structure of the Bence-Jones protein (L-chain dimer) Mcg has been analyzed to 2.3 Å resolution and partially refined (14). The complete amino acid sequence of the λ-chain Mcg has also been determined (31) and correlated with the electron density map. The structure of the Mcg L-chain dimer is similar to that of Fab fragments. The cavity determined by the hypervariable regions is also similar to that observed in Fabs but contains a solvent channel not observed in V_L-V_H pairs. The fact that the contact residues between V_L-V_L and those between C_L-C_L are nonhomologous has been described as arising from "rotational allomerism" (14). Edmundson et al (14) suggest that the genetic changes necessary to bring about suitable amino acid contacts leading to rotational allomerism of V and C domains are key steps in the evolution of immunoglobulins.

The cavity and also the solvent channel of the Mcg dimer were found to provide binding sites (located by difference-Fourier maps) for a number of ligands (32). These included an iodinated derivative of 1-fluoro-2,4 dinitrobenzene, DNP derivatives of lysine and leucine, 5-acetyluracil, menadione, caffeine, theophylline, ϵ-dansyl lysine, phenantroline, and colchicine. Edmundson et al (32) suggest that the L-chain dimer behaves as a primitive antibody. However it is difficult to ascertain the physiological significance of this binding activity since the complete Mcg myeloma IgG protein (which occurs in the Mcg serum) does not appear to bind the same ligands.

A most interesting aspect of the Mcg structure is that although the L chains of the dimer have identical amino acid sequence their quaternary structures are different. This difference can be described as one in the angle made by the major axes of V_L and C_L in one chain (70°) and the corresponding angle in the second L chain of the dimer (110°). In this respect the L-chain dimer resembles the Fab M603 and New structures (described below).

STRUCTURE OF FAB FRAGMENTS

The Three-Dimensional Structure of Fab M603

The structure of Fab-M603 [(mouse IgA, κ; (25)] is very similar to that of the previously reported Fab New (human IgG, λ) which shows that the structures of immunoglobulins are conserved across species and H- and L-chain classes. The pseudo twofold axes relating V_H to V_L and C_H1 to C_L make an angle of 135° (Figure 8). The long axes of the subunits of the L chain make an angle of approximately 100° while the corresponding angle for the H chain is approximately 80°. Segal et al (25) postulate that the close approach of the two H-chain subunits is facilitated by the presence at the interface of amino acids with small side chains, such as Gly 8-Gly 9-Gly 10 of strand $4\beta1$ and Gly 109-Ala 110-Gly 111 of strand $3\beta1$. The equivalent residues in Fab New are Gly 8-Pro 9-Gly 10 and Gly 108-Gln 109-Gly 110. In Fab New, however, only Gly 10 is in a position such that a bulkier side chain could interfere with the observed contacts between V_H and C_H1. Furthermore the sequence Gly-Gln-Gly (positions 108–110) of V_H M603 is homologous to Gly-Gly-Gly (positions 100–102) of the λ-chain of IgG New which assumes, however, an open structure with fewer V_L-C_L

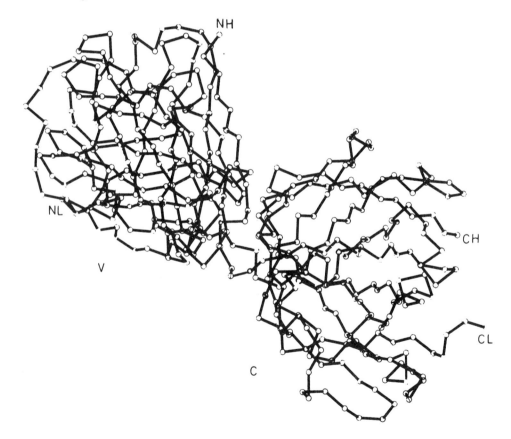

Figure 8   Drawing of the α-carbon positions of the Fab fragment of mouse myeloma M603, projected in a direction approximately perpendicular to the "switch regions." [Reproduced from Huber et al (53) with permission.]

contacts. This sequence was previously shown to participate in intrasub-
unit interactions (18).

The site of hapten binding of M603 was identified by diffusing phosphorylcholine into Fab crystals and calculating a difference-Fourier map.
It is located in a large wedge-shaped cavity approximately 12 Å deep, 15
Å wide, and 20 Å long which is lined with hypervariable residues. Only five
hypervariable regions, designated as L1, L3, H1, H2, and H3 contribute to
the formation of the cavity. L2 does not contribute to the lining of this
cavity because it is screened by the large *fl*1 loop of the first hypervariable
region. Phosphorylcholine occupies only a small part of the cavity and it
is bound mainly to the H chain. The choline group is buried in the interior
of the cavity while the phosphate group remains closer to the exterior. This
mode of binding is consistent with the occurrence of the choline moiety as
the most exposed determinant of natural phosphorylcholine antigens (33).
The phosphate group is hydrogen bonded through two of its oxygens to the
hydroxyl group of Tyr 33 (H chain) and to an amino group of the side chain
of Arg 52 (H chain) (Figure 9). The positive charge of the guanidinium

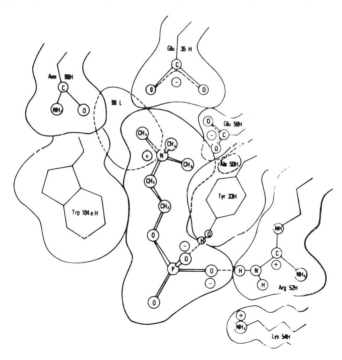

Figure 9 Schematic representation of the specific interactions between phosphorylcholine
and the protein side groups in M603. The binding cavity is located in the cleft between the
L and H chains. Choline binds in the interior while the phosphate group is towards the exterior
of the cavity. [Reproduced from Padlan et al (34) with permission.]

group also contributes to the binding of the negatively charged phosphate. In addition, the amino group of Lys 54 (H) is in close proximity with the phosphate and probably contributes to stabilize the complex. The positively charged trimethylammonium group interacts with the negatively charged side chains of Glu 35(H) and Glu 59(H). Furthermore, there are extensive van der Waals interactions between atoms of the hapten and main chain atoms of residues 102 and 103 of the H chain and residues 91–94 of the L chain, and with the ring atoms of H-chain Tyr 33 and Trp 104a. In a recent paper Padlan et al (34) compare the sequences of the hypervariable regions of the H chain of the seven phosphorylcholine-binding mouse myeloma proteins (Table 1). They find that all residues identified as participating in phosphorylcholine binding in M603 (Tyr 33, Glu 35, Arg 52, Lys 54, and Glu 59) are conserved in all seven H chains. In addition, position 50 is Ala in all the chains and position 104a is Trp in all except M167. Based on this evidence the authors suggest that the binding site of these phosphorylcholine binding proteins is very similar. Moreover, they predict that the hapten will bind to them in essentially the same manner. The differences in affinity for phosphorylcholine (35) are attributed to amino acid substitutions in other residues.

The Structure of Fab New

The description of the immunoglobulin fold, and the characterization of the homology subunits and of subunit pairs (structural domains), were made on the bases of the structure of Fab New determined at 6.0 Å (20) and 2.8 Å (13) resolution. These studies showed that the Fab fragment can be divided into two structural domains, V and C, of approximate dimensions 40 × 50 × 40 Å. Each structural domain was shown to contain two homology subunits (V_H and V_L; C_H1 and C_L) related by an approximate twofold axis of symmetry (Figure 7). The V and C structural domains of Fab New are not colinear and their pseudo twofold axes of symmetry form an angle of approximately 137°. The L chain is more extended than the H chain so that the angle formed by the major axes of the V_L and C_L subunits is approximately 110° while that of V_H and C_H1 is approximately 80°. From the extensive sequence homologies of different classes of immunoglobulins, the sharing of a peptide chain folding pattern in V_H, V_L, C_H1, and C_L and the fact that different intrachain and interchain disulfide bonds of immunoglobulins could be explained on the basis of the Fab New model, it was concluded that the immunoglobulin fold and the association of subunits in globular domains are general features of all classes of immunoglobulins in all animal species (13).

Hypervariable regions of the L and H chain occur in close spatial proximity, surrounding a shallow groove that was identified as the binding site of

Table 1   Heavy chain complementarity region sequences of mouse phosphorylcholine-binding immunoglobulins[a]

	H1			H2					H3		
	31	35	50	55	58 a b	60	65	100 a		104 a b	
M167	D F Y M E		A A S R S K	A H D Y	R T E Y S	A S V K G	D	A D Y G (D) S Y		F G Y	
M511	B ———		——— D —	N ——	T ————	————	—	G ————— S —		— W —	
T15	———		————	N ——	T ————	————	—	Y- ———— S —		— W —	
S107	B ———		——— B —	N ——	T ————	————	—	Y- ———— S —		— W —	
H8	B ———		——— B —	N ——	T ————	————	—	Y- ———— B —		— W —	
M603	———		——— N – C	N K –	T ————	————	N	Y- ———— S –		– T W	
W3207	B ———		——— B —	N ——	T ————	————	—	Y ————————		— Y —	

[a] Reproduced from Padlan et al (34) with permission. The one letter code for amino acids is as used in Figure 11.

the Fab fragment (36). Fab New binds several haptens at this site with affinity constants ranging from 10^3M^{-1}–10^5M^{-1}. A schematic diagram of the binding of a γ-hydroxyl derivative of vitamin K_1 (K_1OH) to Fab New is shown in Figure 10.

The structure of Fab New has been partially refined and the improved model used to quantitatively compare the homology subunits (15) V_H, V_L, C_H1, and C_L using the method of Rao & Rossman (37). All the possible pairs of homology subunits were aligned and superimposed and the matching was optimized by minimizing the sum of the squares of the distances between equivalent $C\alpha$'s. Table 2 shows that the largest numbers of equivalenced $C\alpha$'s occurring at distances shorter than 1.5 Å and 3.0 Å are found when comparing V_H to V_L and C_H1 to C_L. The average minimum base change per codon for equivalenced amino acids is smallest for these pairs and, in general, seems to be in inverse relation to the number of $C\alpha$'s equivalenced. Moreover, the average minimum base change per codon is,

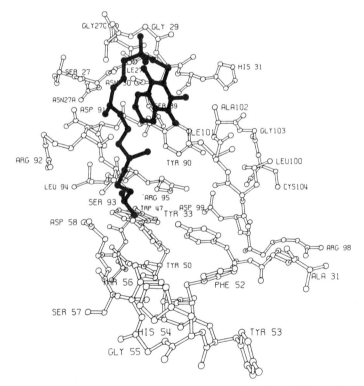

Figure 10   Schematic representation of vitamin K_1OH bound to the combining region of Fab New. Some of the amino acid residues in this figure correspond to a tentative sequence and are different from those of Figures 11 and 13 that contain the final sequence.

in all cases, smaller when the more stringent condition ($d_{C\alpha\text{-}C\alpha} \leqslant 1.5$ Å) is used for the scoring of equivalences. Thus, the conservation of fine structural details seems to be mainly a reflection of the conservation of sequence. The quantitative three-dimensional matching procedure leads to amino acid sequence alignments that clearly reflect the well-established homologies between V_H and V_L and between C_H1 and C_L (Figure 11). The closest sequence similarities are found between C_H1 and C_L and between V_H and V_L. In addition Table 2 and Figure 11 show that there is considerable homology between V and C regions. These results indicate that all homology subunits contain a basic core of amino acid residues with highly preserved three-dimensional structure. The chemical nature of these residues is also preserved as shown by the low values of the average minimum base change per codon. This basic core of residues forms part of the two β-sheets (3β and 4β) and includes the two cysteines of the intrachain disulfide bonds and a constant Trp occurring at 14 or 15 positions after the first Cys of the disulfide bond. These findings reinforce the postulate that the different homology regions of immunoglobulins appeared during evolution through a gene duplication mechanism.

The refined model of Fab New has been used to evaluate the chemical contacts between the different homology subunits (15). The results of this analysis are diagrammatically presented in Figure 12, and show that the *trans*-interactions between V_H and V_L and between C_H1 and C_L are far more extensive than the *cis*-interactions between V_L and C_L and between C_H1 and V_H. Also, most of the residues involved in *trans*-interactions in C subunits occur in the 4β sheets while in the V subunits they occur in the $3\beta'$ sheets. The *cis*-interactions occur in *bl* segments in the V subunits and in *fl* segments in C subunits. The smaller number of contacts between V_L and C_L than between V_H and C_H1 are a consequence of the more extended structure of the L chain. A more detailed description of the intersubunit contacts is given in Table 3. The contacts between V_H and V_L are of

Table 2 Alignment of α-carbon coordinates of four homology subunits of Fab (New)

Subunits	Number of C pairs equivalenced with $d_{C\alpha-C\alpha}$(Å) $\leqslant$ 1.5	Average minimum base change per codon for $d_{C\alpha-C\alpha}$(Å) $\leqslant$ 1.5	Number of C pairs equivalenced with $d_{C\alpha-C\alpha}$(Å) $\leqslant$ 3.0	Average minimum base change per codon for $d_{C\alpha-C\alpha}$(Å) $\leqslant$ 3.0
V_H-V_L	56	0.98	81	0.97
C_H1-C_L	60	0.71	82	0.80
C_L-V_L	40	1.03	66	1.23
C_L-V_H	29	1.04	59	1.28
C_H1-V_L	27	1.04	58	1.24
C_H1-V_H	25	1.29	49	1.40

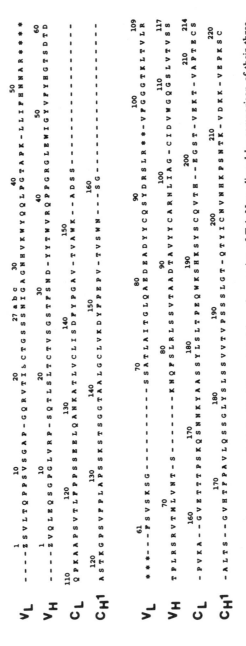

Figure 11 Amino acid sequences of the V_L, V_H, C_L, and C_H1 homology region of Fab New aligned by comparison of their three-dimensional structure. Dashes indicate gaps introduced to maximize alignment of the three-dimensional structures. Asterisks indicate a deletion in the V_L sequence. Abbreviations for amino acids are as given in *Atlas of Protein Sequence and Structure*, Vol. 5. 1972. ed. M. O. Dayhoff. Washington, DC: Natl. Biomed. Res. Found. [Reproduced from (15) with permission.]

particular interest in relation to the structural viability of different V_H- and V_L-chain pairs. Unrestricted pairing of different H and L chains would provide a simple mechanism for increasing antibody diversity from a given number of H- and L-chain genes. Three types of V_H-V_L contacts were discussed: 1. those at the core of the contacting region, which involves residues that are invariant or semi-invariant in V_H and V_L sequences; 2. those made by conserved residues with hypervariable residues; and 3. those made between hypervariable residues.

The first type of contact occurs at the core of the contacting region between V_H and V_L and involves equivalent residues from the two chains. These contacts include residues Val 37, Gln 39, Leu 45, Tyr 94, and Trp 107 in V_H and residues Tyr 35, Gln 37, Ala 42, Pro 43, Tyr 86, and Phe 99 in V_L. These residues are structurally homologous between both chains with the exception of Ala 42 of the L chain. The contacts between these homologous residues of V_H and V_L account for about 50% of all contacts listed in Table 3. All these residues are invariant or are replaced by homologous residues in V_L and V_H sequences from different classes and different animal species. The presence of these invariant or nearly invariant residues at the main V_H-V_L contact area together with the constant C_H1-C_L contacts, explains the property that different H and L chains can recombine to form new immunoglobulin molecules (38, 15).

The second and third types of contacts are more difficult to evaluate in general terms, since they are different for different immunoglobulins. These kinds of contacts could perhaps provide a structural explanation of the preferred reassociation sometimes observed between complementary H and L chains derived from a single immunoglobulin molecule (38).

The interactions between the constant domains C_H1 and C_L are very extensive (Figure 12 and Table 3). The core of the contact region is formed by residues which appear to be invariant or nearly invariant in the H- and L-chain sequences of different classes and of different animal species (15).

The refined structure of Fab New provided more precise information about the structural homology of the subunits, the interactions between L and H chains, and the conformation of the residues in the hypervariable regions (Figure 13). Further work in this system is being directed toward detailed studies of hapten-combining site complexes.

The Structure of Fab Kol

The study of Fab Kol (26) is of particular interest since the crystal structure of the parent IgG molecule has also been determined (see below). IgG Kol and Fab Kol can thus be used to examine the possible influences that the Fc region may have on the tertiary and quaternary structure of the Fab region.

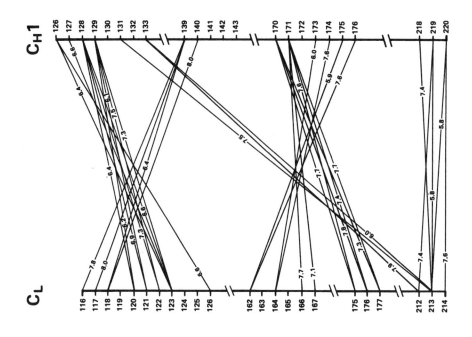

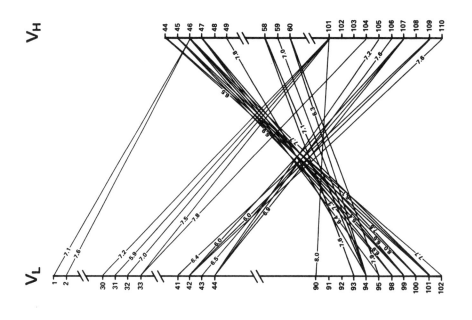

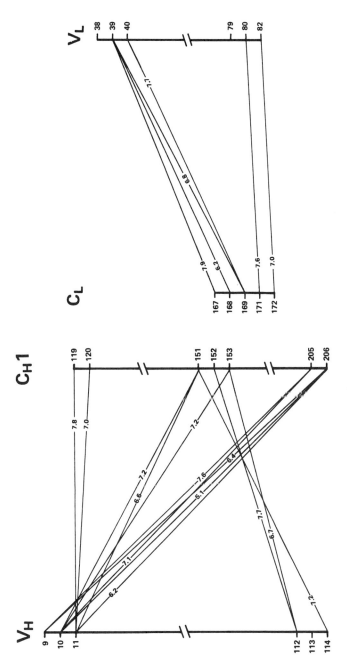

Figure 12 Intersubunit α-carbon contacts at distances of 8 Å or less. Contacts are indicated by lines joining the corresponding amino acid residue numbers. Numbers on the lines indicate the Cα-Cα distance in Angstroms. [Reproduced from (15) with permission.]

Table 3 Intersubunit contacts[a]

V_H	V_L	No. of contacts	C_H1	C_L	No. of contacts
Val 37	Phe 99	1	Phe 126	Glu 126	14
Gln 39	Gln 37	5	Phe 126	Glu 125	1
Arg 43	Asp 84	14	Phe 126	Ser 123	3
Arg 43	Tyr 86	7	Leu 128	Phe 120	20
Arg 43	Gln 37	3	Leu 128	Val 135	2
Leu 45	Tyr 86	4	Leu 128	Pro 121	1
Leu 45	Phe 99	2	Ala 129	Phe 120	8
Glu 46	Phe 99	3	Ala 129	Pro 121	2
Trp 47	Arg 95	19	Lys 133	Glu 212	1
Trp 47	Leu 94	8	Thr 139	Thr 118	3
Trp 47	Ser 93	1	Thr 139	Lys 206	2
Asp 58	Ser 93	2	Ala 141	Phe 120	6
Asp 60	Leu 94	3	Leu 142	Phe 120	4
Thr 61	Leu 94	1	Gly 143	Phe 120	5
Tyr 94	Ala 42	6	Leu 145	Tyr 179	1
Asn 98	Arg 95	8	Leu 145	Val 135	1
Leu 99	Arg 95	3	Lys 147	Glu 126	1
Ala 101	Tyr 90	6	Lys 147	Lys 131	3
Ala 101	His 31	7	Lys 147	Thr 133	2
Ala 101	Lys 33	2	Phe 170	Leu 137	10
Gly 102	Lys 33	6	Phe 170	Ile 138	4
Ile 104	Tyr 35	3	Phe 170	Ser 177	4
Ile 104	Gln 88	3	Pro 171	Ser 167	2
Ile 104	Leu 45	2	Pro 171	Ala 175	1
Trp 107	Pro 43	21	Val 173	Tyr 179	6
Trp 107	Ala 42	2	Gln 175	Glu 162	7
Trp 107	Phe 99	4	Ser 176	Glu 162	8
Trp 107	Tyr 35	2	Leu 182	Tyr 179	2
			Ser 183	Tyr 179	6
C_H1	V_H		Ser 183	Val 135	1
			Ser 183	Leu 137	1
Ala 118	Leu 11	2	Val 185	Leu 137	3
Ser 119	Leu 11	2	Val 185	Phe 120	3
Thr 120	Leu 11	3	Lys 218	Cys 213	2
Phe 150	Leu 11	3	Ser 219	Glu 212	2
Phe 150	Thr 114	1	Ser 219	Cys 213	6
Pro 151	Leu 11	2	Cys 220	Cys 213	7
Pro 151	Thr 114	2			
Glu 152	Leu 112	4			
Pro 153	Leu 112	7			
C_L	V_L				
Gln 110	Glu 82	1			
Lys 168	Pro 39	5			
Asn 172	Glu 82	7			

[a] The number of interatomic distances not larger than 1.2 times the sum of the Van der Waals radii (C–C = 4.32 Å; O–O ≤ 3.65 Å; N–N ≤ 3.72 Å; C–O ≤ 3.98 Å; and C–N ≤ 4.02 Å) are listed. [Reproduced from (15) with permission.]

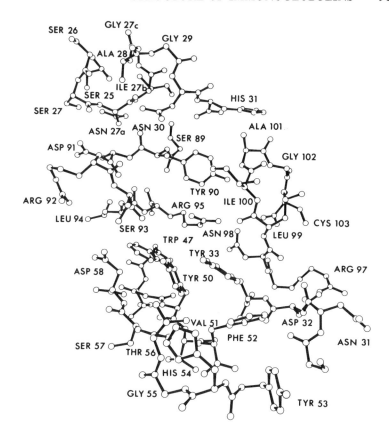

Figure 13   View of some of the amino acid residues at the combining site of IgG New.

The crystal structure of Fab Kol was determined by the multiple isomorphous heavy atom substitution method to a resolution of 3.0 Å. The Cα coordinates of the V_κ Rei dimer (22) were fitted to the electron density map of the V domain. The Cα coordinates of C_H1 and C_L from M603 and from Fab New were fitted to the electron density of the C domains. The fitting of these different coordinates to the electron density map of Fab Kol helped distinguish its H and L chains. Since the amino acid sequences of V_H and V_L of Kol have not yet been obtained, the model is based on tentative assignments of amino acid side chains, in particular in the segments corresponding to the hypervariable regions. From the crystallographic model the L chain was identified as a λ-chain. The tentative model was subjected to constrained crystallographic refinement.

As expected, the tertiary structure of the Fab Kol homology subunits is essentially the same as that reported before for other immunoglobulins. The quaternary structure of Fab Kol (Figure 14) differs, however, from that found in Fab M603 (Figure 9) and Fab New (Figure 7). This difference can be described as a change in the relative orientations of the V and C homology subunits or as a change in the angle made by the approximate twofold axes of symmetry relating V_H to V_L and C_H1 to C_L. The changed angular relationship between the V and C domains is due to a change in

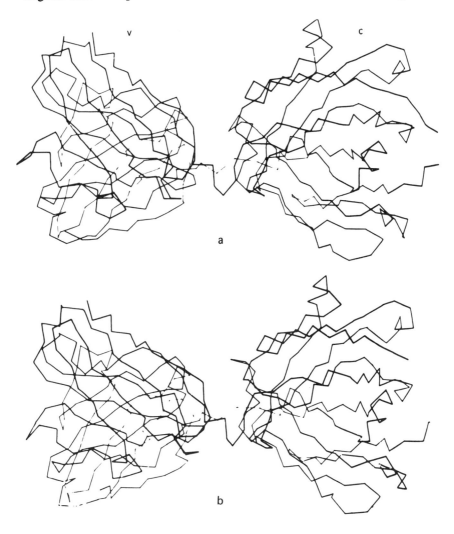

Figure 14 Cα drawing of *a* Fab Kol and of *b* the Fab portion of IgG Kol viewed along an axis through the switch peptides. [Reproduced from Matsushima et al (26) with permission.]

conformation at the switch regions ("elbow bending") such that the V and C domains are more nearly colinear in Fab Kol. As a result of the change in quaternary structure there are fewer V-C contacts in Fab Kol than in Fab New. Matsushima et al postulate (26) that the intermolecular contacts (crystal packing) rather than the V-C cis-contacts may be the factor influencing the bending of the switch regions.

In Fab Kol the crystal packing is a result of contacts between hypervariable regions and C_H1-C_L residues. The same contacts are observed in the crystalline IgG Kol, which is a cryoglobulin. The authors suggest that these contacts may explain the phenomenon of cold precipitation. This suggestion is in line with that presented in a recent biochemical study on cryoglobulins (39). The structure of Fab Kol will be discussed further in connection with that of the parent protein, IgG Kol.

STRUCTURE OF Fc FRAGMENTS

The Structure of the Human Fc Fragment

The structure of a human Fc fragment has been determined to 3.5 Å resolution using a combination of multiple isomorphous heavy atom replacement and molecular replacement techniques (21). The Fc structure has been described as having the approximate shape of a "mickey mouse" with the C_H2 domains forming the ears and the C_H3 subunits forming a globular head (see Figure 15). The overall tertiary structure of C_H2 and C_H3 is as described for the immunoglobulin fold. A loosely folded segment of polypeptide chain extending from Ser 337 to Gln 342 connects the two domains. This segment of polypeptide chain is exposed to solvent, a feature that explains its susceptibility to proteolytic attack by enzymes. The C_H3 subunits interact very closely in a pattern which is similar to the C_H1-C_L interactions described above for Fab fragments. The C_H2 subunits show no close interaction with each other. The N terminus, including the sequence -Cys-Pro-Pro-Cys- appears to be disordered since it cannot be traced in the electron density map; the segment that follows it in the N-terminal sequence (to Pro 238) may be in close contact with part of the carbohydrate chains attached to Asn 297. This sequence and the carbohydrate chains lie in between the C_H2 subunits (see Figure 15). The structure of the carbohydrate chains is somewhat tentative but their general location and overall conformation are clear. The electron density assigned to carbohydrate is compatible with a branched chain of the general type:

$$\begin{array}{c} \text{H} \qquad\qquad \text{H–H} \\ | \qquad\qquad / \\ \text{Asn 297–H–H–H–H–H} \\ \qquad\qquad\qquad \backslash \\ \qquad\qquad\qquad \text{H–H} \end{array}$$

R

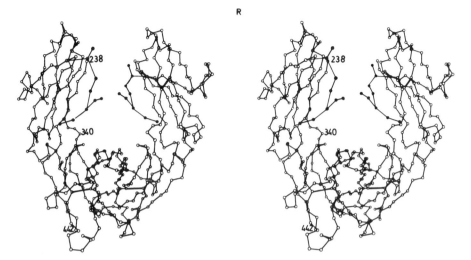

Figure 15   Stereo drawing of the Cα carbon positions and the centers of the carbohydrate hexose units of the Fc fragment. The black dots represent the approximate centers of carbohydrate hexose units. The carbohydrate attachment site is Asn 297. The positions of the α carbons are indicated by the open circles. The disulfide bonds are indicated. [Reproduced from Huber et al (53) with permission.]

where H is a hexose unit. This chain appears to be longer than those that have been observed in myeloma proteins. The attachment site (Asn 297) is at an accessible turn of the polypeptide chain, in agreement with a posttranslational attachment of the sugar moiety by specific transferase enzymes.

STRUCTURE OF IgG MOLECULES

The crystalline human myeloma IgGl Kol has been studied by X-ray diffraction techniques to a resolution of 5 Å (19), 4.0 Å, and 3.5 Å (26), and subsequently refined by constrained crystallographic procedures (40). This study is of particular interest due to the fact that the crystals diffract to a resolution of 3.5 Å, and also, that IgG Kol appears to contain a normal hinge region, unlike other crystalline immunoglobulins that have been studied (41–43). However, the structural analysis of IgG Kol revealed that no electron density could be assigned to the Fc region. This part of the molecule seems to be disordered in the crystal, probably due to the presence of an intact hinge region which is capable of motion even in the crystal lattice. The electron density corresponding to the Fab regions of the molecule could be traced to residues 213 (H chain) and 209 (L chain) and beyond these points, in a tentative way, down to the hinge region sequence -Cys-Pro-Pro-

R

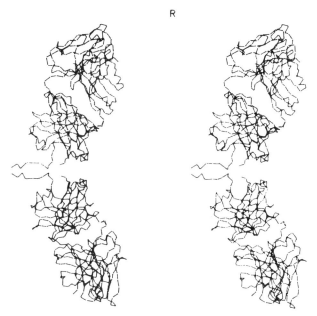

Figure 16   Stereo pair of the Cα positions of IgG Kol. The Fc portion of the molecule was disordered in these crystals and is not represented in the diagram. [Reproduced from Matsushima et al (26) with permission.]

Cys-Pro- (residues 226–230, see Figure 16). The Fc part cannot be traced or even be assigned to a general area in the unit cell of the crystal without overlap problems. However, the tight packing around the hinge peptide in the crystal structure requires that this peptide be rather extended. From this interpretation the authors conclude that the C_H2 domains do not come close to the Fab region, that is to say, that there are no contacts between C_H1 and C_H2 except for those resulting from the continuity of the peptide chain.

An interesting feature of the IgG Kol is the quaternary structure of its Fab regions. As described above for Fab Kol, the V_H-V_L domain is more linear with the C_H1-C_L domain than in the crystal structures of the Fab fragments M603 and New (Figures 7, 9, and 17). Although an 8° difference in the relative orientations of the V and C domains was detected, the Fab model still provided a suitable description of the IgG structure.

The three-dimensional structure of human IgG1 (κ) Dob, a cryoglobulin, has been determined to a nominal resolution of 6 Å (41) using the multiple isomorphous heavy atom replacement technique. Recently, this structure has been reinvestigated (27) by fitting the coordinates of the Fc fragment (21) and those of the Fab M603 fragment (25) to the electron density map. This analysis provides a reasonably accurate description of the relative

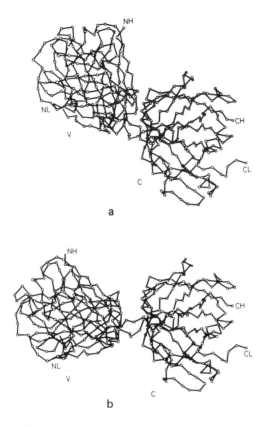

Figure 17 Drawing of α-carbon atoms of the structures of *a* Fab M603 (McPC 603) and of *b* the Fab part of IgG Ko*l*. Both molecules are shown in the same orientation to facilitate their comparison. The N and C termini of all chains are labelled. The constant regions of both molecules on exactly the same orientation showing a different position for the variable regions. [Reproduced from Huber et al (53) with permission.]

positions and orientations of the domains of the molecule although it does not extend to finer details of secondary or tertiary structure (Figure 18). The resulting model shows several interesting features. The structure of the Dob Fc part corresponds closely to that of the Fc fragment within the limits of the resolution and the fitting procedure mentioned above. The C_H2 domains are separated by the carbohydrate chains and make no contact with each other (see Figure 18). The carbohydrate moiety is wedged between C_H1 and C_H2 which prevents close contacts between them (see Figure 19). In the Fab part, a distinction could be made between the H and L chains based on the fact that the L chains are linked to each other by a disulfide bond at their C termini. The angle made by the pseudo twofold axes relating V_H to V_L and C_H1 to C_L is 147°.

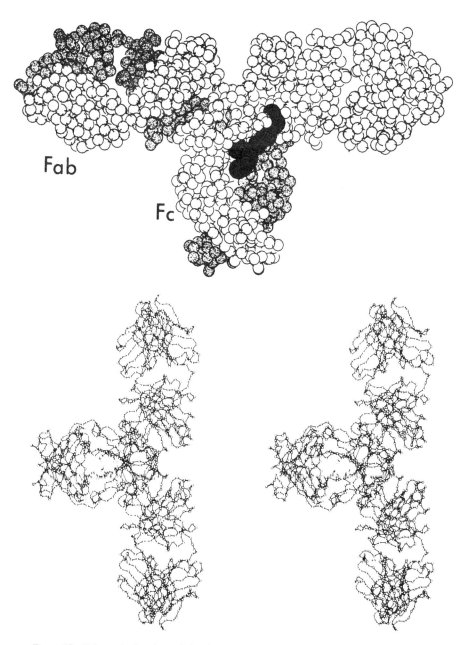

Figure 18 Schematic drawings of the three-dimensional structure of IgG Dob. The lower panel contains stereo pairs of the α-carbon position (small circles) and the positions of the carbohydrate hexose unites (large circles). The twofold axis of symmetry relating the two halves of the molecule is horizontal. One complete H chain is white while the other is dark gray. The two L chains are lightly shaded and the hexose units are represented as large black spheres. The upper panel contains a space-filling view of the same molecule rotated 90° in the plane of the drawing. [Reproduced from Silverton et al (27) with permission.]

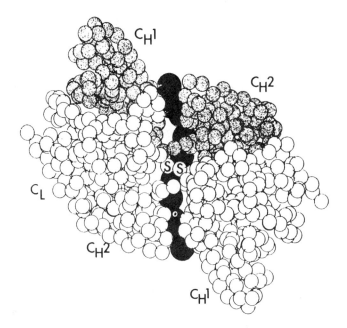

Figure 19 Space-filling view of the constant regions of IgG Dob looking down the twofold axis of symmetry. The shading is as described for Figure 18. The carbohydrate chains seem to provide most of the contacts between C_H2 subunits. [Reproduced from Silverton et al (27) with permission.]

A third crystalline human IgG protein, Mcg, is under crystallographic study. Its hinge region is also affected by a deletion of fifteen residues (42). Only preliminary results have so far been reported (43).

Based mainly on the results of the crystallographic studies of the Fab fragments M603 and New, and those of the human Fc and of IgG Kol, Huber et al (44) proposed an attractive structural model to explain a putative conformational change that could be transmitted from the antigen-combining site. The transmission of such a conformational signal to the $C\gamma2$ domain could be essential for a secondary function such as complement fixation. This model was partly based on the observation that isolated Fab fragments have different quaternary structures from that of the complete immunoglobulin IgG Kol. The determination of the structure of Fab Kol however showed the same V-C arrangement as that of IgG Kol. In addition, in IgG Dob the angle between the pseudo twofold axes in the V_H, V_L, and C_H1, C_L domains is intermediate between those observed in the Fabs M603 and New and that observed in IgG Kol. Thus, the model is not sustained by the more recent structural analyses.

Perhaps the most striking feature that the crystallographic studies of immunoglobulins have revealed is that of molecular flexibility. Segmental flexibility had been well-established before the crystallographic studies; the major structural site of this property is the hinge region. Taken together, the crystallographic studies of immunoglobulins and their fragments indicate that flexibility is also present in the switch regions connecting V_H to C_H1, V_L to C_L, and, possibly, the segment connecting C_H2 to C_H3. Segmental flexibility (hinge region) and intrasegmental flexibility (switch regions) may facilitate antigen-binding by allowing an optimal fit of the combining site to antigenic determinants occurring at varying distances and angles.

MODEL BUILDING OF ANTIGEN-BINDING SITES

The specificity and the affinity of antigen-combining sites of immunoglobulins are determined by the sequence of their hypervariable regions. These regions can be considered as attached to the highly conserved rigid framework of the V homology subunits formed by the 4β and $3\beta'$ sheets and by the bl-connecting segments. The hypervariable regions, on the other hand, are contained in the connecting loops $fl1$, $fl3$, and $fl4$ and are highly variable in both amino acid sequence and structure. The larger structural differences are those arising from the existence of deletions and insertions in these regions. However, the number of amino acids contained in these loops is not very large and in many cases, different immunoglobulins have loops of the same length. Therefore, starting from the known three-dimensional structures and the amino acid sequences of different immunoglobulins, attempts could be made at predicting the conformation of their antigen-combining sites. The simplest approach consists of building a model with the desired sequence following the framework and loop structures of other immunoglobulins that have been determined by crystallographic studies. The description of the phosphorylcholine-binding site of several mouse myeloma proteins based on the structure of M603 (discussed in a previous section) is a good example of model building using highly homologous sequences (34). Another example is that of the analysis of the effects of amino acid substitutions at specified positions in mouse λ chains, based on the structure of Fab (λ) New (45). The conformation of the combining site of mouse myeloma protein MOPC315 has also been described on the basis of the structures of other immunoglobulins (18, 46).

The future availability of a larger number of known three-dimensional structures of immunoglobulins and other proteins will help make predictive schemes more accurate. The use of more elaborate techniques as described for other systems (energy minimization, resonance methods, etc) will be necessary for constructing detailed models of antigen-combining sites based solely on sequence data. Any predictive scheme should be tested by its ability to predict a known structure that has not been included in the data base of the scheme. Clearly, this condition is not met by the attempts described above. Unfortunately the number of immunoglobulin-combining sites with known three-dimensional structure available so far is insufficient to propose and test more elaborate predictive schemes.

SIMILARITIES IN THE POLYPEPTIDE CHAIN FOLDING OF IMMUNOGLOBULINS AND OTHER PROTEINS

Although no amino acids sequence homology can be detected between the bovine Cu,Zn superoxide dismutase enzyme and immunoglobulins, there is a striking similarity in their three-dimensional structures (16). Superoxide dismutases are not related to immunoglobulins by their function since they are intracellular metalloenzymes that process superoxide radicals into O_2 and H_2O. Figure 20 gives a diagrammatic representation of the polypeptide chain folding in both proteins. As can be seen from the figure, superoxide dismutase contains an additional N-terminal strand that contributes to the β-pleated sheet structure. The remaining strands of superoxide dismutase are topologically equivalent to those of an immunoglobulin C region. The packing of subunits is different in the two proteins, since the two superoxide dismutase subunits that constitute a dimer make contacts that are not similar to those made by the V or C domains in immunoglobulins.

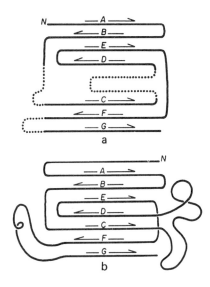

Figure 20   Schematic representation of the folding of the polypeptide chains of *a* the variable region of an immunoglobulin and *b* of bovine Cu,Zn superoxide dismutase. Strands common to both structures are labeled A to G. Dotted lines indicate the hypervariable regions of the immunoglobulin V subunit. [Reproduced from Richardson et al (16) with permission.]

The folding of the polypeptide chain in the blue Cu protein azurin from *Pseudomonas aeruginosa* (47) and in the Cu-containing protein plastocyanin from poplar leaves (48) is topologically equivalent to that of superoxide dismutase, and consequently, to the immunoglobulin fold. Adman et al (47) postulate that similar chain folding in proteins of widely different function may arise from a folding process by which strands having short connecting loops (A and the N-terminal strand; E and D; F and G, Figure 18) assume their secondary structure first. The process is then completed by a "super folding" into the final structure. However, as pointed out by Richardson et al (16) the process of protein folding is not yet sufficiently understood to judge the merits of this proposal. A second alternative, a common evolutionary origin followed by gene duplication and amino acid sequence divergence favoring new functional requirements remains an appealing explanation of the observed similarity in three-dimensional structure.

The amino acid sequence of β_2 microglobulin, a polypeptide chain associated with the heavy chains of histocompatibility antigens, is highly homologous to those of the C regions of immunoglobulins (49). This and other facts have led to speculation that the heavier chain (mol wt 45,000) of histocompatibility antigens may share sequence homologies with immunoglobulins, which would indicate a common evolutionary origin. It has recently been shown (50) that indeed the heavy chain of a human histocompatibility antigen (HLA-B7) has a segment of polypeptide chain with an amino acid sequence highly homologous to that of a human V_H sequence. More complete sequence data is awaited to ascertain the extent of homology, the possible existence of similar domains in both structures, etc. Haptoglobins (50) and the C-reactive protein (51) also show sequence homology with immunoglobulins which leads to the expectation of topological similarity in their three-dimensional folding.

ACKNOWLEDGMENTS

The authors are grateful to Mrs. Arleen Skaist for her devoted and patient secretarial work in preparing this review. The research work in this laboratory has been supported by Research Grant AI 08202 from the National Institutes of Health. During the preparation of this paper R. J. Poljak was a Faculty Scholar of the Josiah Macy Jr. Foundation.

Literature Cited

1. Nisonoff, A., Hopper, J. E., Spring, S. B. 1975. *The Antibody Molecule,* New York: Academic pp. 542
2. Davies, D. R., Padlan, E. A., Segal, D. M. 1975. *Ann. Rev. Biochem.* 44:639–67
3. Beale, D., Feinstein, A. 1976. *Q. Rev. Biophys.* 9:135–71
4. Poljak, R. J. 1975. *Adv. Immunol.* 21:1–33
5. Poljak, R. J. 1975. *Nature* 256:373–76
6. Poljak, R. J., Amzel, L. M., Phizackerley, R. P. 1976. *Prog. Biophys. Mol. Biol.* 31:67–93
7. Padlan, E. A. 1977. *Q. Rev. Biophys.* 10:35–65
8. Poljak, R. J. 1978. *CRC Crit. Rev. Biochem.* 5:45–84
9. Wu, T. T., Kabat, E. A. 1970. *J. Exp. Med.* 132:211–50
10. Kabat, E. A., Wu, T. T. 1971. *Ann. NY Acad. Sci.* 190:382–91
11. Kehoe, J. M., Capra, J. D. 1971. *Proc. Natl. Acad. Sci. USA* 68:2019–21
12. Schiffer, M., Girling, R. L., Ely, K. R., Edmundson, A. B. 1973. *Biochemistry* 12:4620–31
13. Poljak, R. J., Amzel, L. M., Avey, H. P., Chen, B. L., Phizackerley, R. P., Saul, F. 1973. *Proc. Natl. Acad. Sci. USA* 70:3305–10
14. Edmundson, A. B., Ely, K. R., Abola, E. E., Schiffer, M., Panagiotopoulos, N. 1975. *Biochemistry* 18:3953–61
15. Saul, F., Amzel, L. M., Poljak, R. J. 1978. *J. Biol. Chem.* 253:585–97
16. Richardson, J. S., Richardson, D. C., Thomas, K. A., Silverton, E. W., Davies, D. R. 1976. *J. Mol. Biol.* 102:221–35
17. Segal, O. M., Padlan, E. A., Cohen, G. H., Silverton, E. W., Davies, D. R., Rudikoff, S., Potter, M. 1974. *Progress in Immunology-II.Immunochemical Aspects,* ed. L. Breat, J. Holborow, 1:93–101. Amsterdam: North-Holland. 337 pp.
18. Poljak, R. J., Amzel, L. M., Chen, B. L., Phizackerley, R. P., Saul, F. 1974. *Proc. Natl. Acad. Sci. USA* 71:3440–44
19. Colman, P. M., Deisenhofer, J., Huber, R., Palm, W. 1976. *J. Mol. Biol.* 100:257–82
20. Poljak, R. J., Amzel, L. M., Avey, H. P., Becka, L. N., Nisonoff, A. 1972. *Nature New Biol.* 235:137–40
21. Deisenhofer, J., Colman, P. M., Epp, O., Huber, R. 1976. *Hoppe-Seylers Z. Physiol. Chem.* 357:1421–34
22. Epp, O., Coleman, P. M., Fehlhammer, H., Bode, W., Schiffer, M., Huber, R.,

Palm, W. 1974. *Eur. J. Biochem.* 45:513–24
23. Fehlhammer, H., Schiffer, M., Epp, O., Colman, P. M., Lattman, E. E., Schwager, P., Steigemann, W., Schramm, H. J. 1975. *Biophys. Struct. Mech.* 1:139–46
24. Colman, P. M., Schramm, H. J., Guss, J. M. 1977. *J. Mol. Biol.* 116:73–79
25. Segal, D. M., Padlan, E. A., Cohen, G. H., Rudikoff, S., Potter, M., Davies, D. R. 1974. *Proc. Natl. Acad. Sci. USA* 71:4298–302
26. Matsushima, M., Marquart, M., Jones, T. A., Colman, P. M., Bartels, K., Huber, R., Palm, W. 1977. *J. Mol. Biol.* 121:441–59
27. Silverton, E. W., Navia, M. A., Davies, D. R. 1977. *Proc. Natl. Acad. Sci. USA* 74:5140–44
28. Hochman, J., Garish, M., Inbar, D., Givol, D. 1976. *Biochemistry* 15:2706–10
29. Ellerson, J. R., Yasmeen, D., Painter, R. H., Dorrington, K. J. 1976. *J. Immunol.* 116:510–17
30. Hilschmann, N. 1967. *Hoppe-Seylers Z. Physiol. Chem.* 348:1077–80
31. Fett, J. W., Deutsch, H. F. 1974. *Biochemistry* 13:4102–14
32. Edmundson, A. B., Ely, K. R., Girling, R. L., Abola, E. E., Schiffer, M., Westholm, F. A., Fausch, M. D., Deutsch, H. F. 1974. *Biochemistry* 13:3816–27
33. Watson, M. J., Baddiley, J. 1974. *Biochem. J.* 137:399–404
34. Padlan, E. A., Davies, D. R., Rudikoff, S., Potter, M. 1976. *Immunochemistry* 13:945–49
35. Leon, M. A., Young, N. M. 1971. *Biochemistry* 10:1424–29
36. Amzel, L. M., Poljak, R. J., Saul, F., Varga, J. M., Richards, F. F. 1974. *Proc. Natl. Acad. Sci. USA* 71:1427–30
37. Rao, S. T., Rossmann, M. G. 1973. *J. Mol. Biol.* 76:241–56
38. DePreval, C., Fougereau, M. 1976. *J. Mol. Biol.* 102:657–78
39. Middaugh, C. R., Gerber-Jenson, B., Hurvitz, A., Paluszek, A., Scheffel, C., Litman, G. W. 1978. *Proc. Natl. Acad. Sci. USA* 75:3440–44
40. Deisenhofer, J., Steigemann, W. 1975. *Acta Crystallogr. Sect. B* 31:238–50
41. Sarma, V. R., Silverton, E. W., Davies, D. R., Terry, W. D. 1971. *J. Biol. Chem.* 246:3753–59
42. Deutsch, H. F., Susuki, T. 1971. *Ann. NY Acad. Sci.* 190:472–85
43. Edmundson, A. B., Schiffer, M., Wood, M. K., Hardman, K. D., Ely, K. R.,

Ainsworth, C. F. 1971. *Cold Spring Harbor Symp. Quant. Biol.* 36:427–32

44. Huber, R., Deisenhofer, J., Colman, P. M., Matsushima, M., Palm, W. 1976. *Nature* 264:415–20

45. Poljak, R. J., Amzel, L. M., Chen, B. L., Chiu, Y. Y., Phizackerley, R. P., Saul, F., Ysern, X. 1977. *Cold Spring Harbor Symp. Quant. Biol.* 41:639–45

46. Padlan, E. A., Davies, D. R., Pecht, I., Givol, D., Wright, C. 1977. *Cold Spring Harbor Symp. Quant. Biol.* 41:627–37

47. Adman, E. T., Stenkamp, R. E., Sieker, L. C., Jensen, L. H. 1978. *J. Mol. Biol.* 123:35–47

48. Colman, P. M., Freeman, H. C., Guss, J. M., Murata, M., Norris, V. A., Ramshaw, J. A. M., Venkatappa, M. P.

1978. *Nature* 272:319–24

49. Peterson, P. A., Cunningham, B. A., Berggard, I., Edelman, G. M. 1972. *Proc. Natl. Acad. Sci. USA* 72:1612–16

50. Terhorst, C., Robb, R., Jones, C., Strominger, J. L. 1977. *Proc. Natl. Acad. Sci. USA* 74:4002–6

51. Osmand, A. P., Gewurz, H., Friedenson, B. 1977. *Proc. Natl. Acad. Sci. USA* 74:1214–18

52. Poljak, R. J. 1973. In *Contemporary Topics in Molecular Immunology,* ed. R. A. Reisfeld, W. J. Mandy, 2:1–26. New York: Plenum

53. Huber, R., Deisenhofer, J., Colman, P. M., Matsushima, M., Palm, W. 1976. *The Immune System,* 27th Mosbach Colloquium, pp. 26–40. Berlin: Springer

Ann. Rev. Pharmacol. Toxicol. 1979. 19:427–45
Copyright © 1979 by Annual Reviews Inc. All rights reserved

EARLY MOLECULAR EVENTS ✦6748
IN ANTIGEN-ANTIBODY
CELL ACTIVATION

Henry Metzger

Section on Chemical Immunology, Arthritis and Rheumatism Branch,
National Institute of Arthritis, Metabolism & Digestive Diseases,
National Institutes of Health, Bethesda, Maryland 20014

INTRODUCTION

Immunoglobulins are multichained glycoproteins synthesized by all vertebrate species, which serve as the fundamental recognition units in immune
reactions. In such reactions they serve a dual role. One role is to serve as
receptors, stimulation of which initiates the immune response to a particular antigen. This stimulation can result in both a proliferation of antigen-
specific lymphocytes and differentiation of lymphocytes into plasma cells
that secrete antigen-specific immunoglobulins ("antibodies").

A second role of immunoglobulins is to serve as the effector substances
which, upon interaction with the antigen, ultimately lead to disposal of the
latter. Antibodies have no capacity to degrade or alter irreversibly the
offending antigen. A variety of indirect mechanisms are utilized instead. For
example, antibodies directed to surface antigens on a cell may destroy the
cell by initiating a complex interaction involving the set of proteins collectively called *complement* (1). Complement activation can directly damage
cell plasma membranes leading to cytolysis. In other instances, particles
coated with antibodies may become phagocytosed with subsequent degradation occurring in the phagocyte's lysozomes (2, 3). Still another mechanism
(with which I deal in greater detail) involves adherence of antibodies to
cells, exposure of which to the antigen initiates exocytosis of granules from
the cells (4). The contents of these granules stimulate a variety of reactions
that can be loosely grouped as inflammatory. These reactions are apparently
directed to the removal of the antigen by nonspecific means.

0362-1642/79/0415-0427$01.00 427

In this review, I describe what is known about how immunoglobulin molecules interact with antigens and how this interaction leads to the consequences discussed above. Much more is known about the former than about the latter. Several of the topics discussed have been the subjects of separate recent reviews. The literature cited is therefore meant to be illustrative rather than exhaustive.

GROSS STRUCTURE OF ANTIBODIES

Almost all the information we have about the structure of antibodies is derived from analyses of immunoglobulins secreted by cells. Historically the first molecules studied were those whose production was stimulated by immunization with specific antigens (5). The ability to perform detailed analyses was considerably enhanced as it became recognized that the products of neoplastic plasma cells—or plasma-like cells—were antibody-like (6). In diseases such as multiple myeloma or Waldenström's macroglobulinemia the serum may contain vast amounts of homogeneous immunoglobulins, which can be isolated readily, sequenced, and even subjected to crystallographic analysis (7–9). In this section I summarize those aspects of immunoglobulin structure necessary to understand how these proteins function. Detailed descriptions are available (e.g. 10, 11).

Chain Structure

As already mentioned, immunoglobulins are multichained. They can be described by the formula $(HL)_{2n}$. In most instances $n = 1$; that is, there are four chains. In two "classes" of immunoglobulins, higher polymers are formed: $n = 2$ or 3 in some IgA and $n = 5$ in most IgM proteins. As suggested by the formula, an individual immunoglobulin shows $2n$-fold symmetry.

LIGHT CHAINS   L in the formula signifies light chains. These have a molecular weight of approximately 23,000. Two major classes are found in many species: κ and λ. There are no known functional correlates that can be assigned to these two classes. Moreover, since in several species one of the classes is practically absent (12) without an apparent deficiency of immune responsiveness, it is unlikely that the classes have contemporary significance. Light chains have an internal repeat structure consisting of two globular units ["domains" (13)] each about 110 amino acids long. While the amino acid sequences of the two units show only a distant relationship, the three-dimensional structure exhibits a fundamental similarity (14) referred to as the immunoglobulin fold. The 110-amino acid unit at the amino terminal end shows great sequence diversity and is termed the variable domain of the light chain (V_L). The variability in V_L is not random; several short "hypervariable" stretches are interspersed among more invariant "framework" sequences (15, 16). While linearly separated in the primary sequence, the hypervariable stretches are brought together spatially by the three-dimensional folding of the V_L domain. The carboxy-terminal unit (C_L) is almost invariant among chains of the same class.

HEAVY CHAINS The H chains of immunoglobulins have a structure reminiscent of that of L chains. There is an internal repeating structure of four or five globular domains, each again about 110 amino acids in length. The unit at the amino-terminal end shows a distinctive sequence variability much like that of V_L and is termed V_H. The remaining domains show more obvious sequence homology to each other. Each is folded into the characteristic immunoglobulin fold pattern. These domains are referred to as C_H1, C_H2, C_H3, and where present C_H4.

In humans there are nine classes of heavy chains; seven ($\gamma1,\gamma2,\gamma3,\gamma4$, $\alpha1,\alpha2$, and δ) have three C_H domains, while two (μ and ϵ) have four. Other differences among heavy chain classes include class-specific constant region sequence differences and carbohydrate side chains. In addition, all except the μ and ϵ chains have an additional stretch of amino acids which is interposed between two C domains. The sequences of these extra segments bear no obvious relationship to the sequences in the domains. These segments are referred to as the "hinge" regions (17) because there is a variety of evidence suggesting that they serve as the principal site of flexibility in the immunoglobulin (18). The hinge regions of the different classes of immunoglobulins are distinctive (Table 1). There are no known functional correlates to these variations.

Table 1 Comparison of hinge regions of human immunoglobulins

Immunoglobulin class	Length of amino acid residues[a]	Number of cysteines	Number of prolines	Location of hinge or flexible interface
IgG1	18	3[b]	5	$C_H1:C_H2$
IgG2	15	4	4	$C_H1:C_H2$
IgG3	65	11	22	$C_H1:C_H2$
IgG4	15	2	5	$C_H1:C_H2$
IgA	25	3	11	$C_H1:C_H2$
IgM	0[c]	1	—	$C_H2:C_H3$[d]
IgE	0[c]	2	—	$C_H2:C_H3$

[a] See Reference (19). Residue 216 (20) was used as the starting point. Data on IgG2 and IgG3 from References (21, 22) respectively.
[b] One of these contributes to the heavy-light chain disulfide.
[c] No apparent hinge sequence.
[d] There is also evidence for flexibility at the $C_H1:C_H2$ interface (23).

Topology of Domains

Most immunoglobulins have at least one disulfide bond that links each light chain to a heavy chain and one disulfide that links the two heavy chains to each other. The exact sequence position and number of these interchain disulfides vary for the different classes. Nevertheless, the available information suggests that they are similarly arranged in space. While undoubtedly stabilizing the overall structure of the molecule, in many instances mild reduction, which selectively cleaves these interchain disulfide bonds (leaving the intrachain disulfides intact), causes no gross chain dissociation. The domains are topologically arranged as follows (proceeding from the amino terminal ends): $V_L : V_H$, $C_L : C_H1$, $C_H2 : C_H2$, $C_H3 : C_H3$, and when present $C_H4 : C_H4$. The structure is Y-shaped with the arms formed by the two "Fab" regions ($V_L : V_H$, $C_L : C_H1$) and the leg (Fc region) formed by the remaining heavy chain constant region domains (24).

Combining Sites

Since antibodies have no known intrinsic capacity to irreversibly affect the antigens to which they bind, it is clear that they must interact with two classes of substances: antigens and effector substances. The latter I refer to by the general term *receptors*. I discuss the justification of this term below.

COMBINING SITES FOR ANTIGENS   The combining sites for antigens on antibodies have been defined in considerable detail (9). The stoichiometry is one site per heavy chain–light chain pair. In IgG, $(HL)_2$, there are two such identical sites; in IgM, $(HL)_{10}$, there are ten. Each site forms a depression at the tip of a Fab region. The walls of the cavity are largely formed by the hypervariable regions of V_L and V_H. It is the spatial arrangement and chemical nature of the side chains of the amino acid residues in the hypervariable regions that account for antibody specificity. Though in some instances charge-charge interactions may play a role, mostly cooperative weak interactions account for the free energy of binding (25, 26). In several instances, there is evidence that small conformational changes in either the antigen (27) or the combining site (28) enhance complementarity (induced fit). In favorable circumstances the ΔG of binding can be < -9 kcal though ~ -7 kcal is more commonly observed. The combining sites vary in size encompassing, e.g. 2–6 monosaccharide or amino acid residues (10). The kinetics of binding are unremarkable; the first-order dissociation rate constant usually determines the relative magnitude of the equilibrium constant (29, 30). To the extent that information is available there is nothing unique about antibody-combining sites for antigens compared to the combining sites for ligands on other proteins.

COMBINING SITES FOR RECEPTORS   Immunoglobulins are known to interact physiologically with three substances other than those required for the biosynthesis, physiological transport, and degradation of the polypeptide chains. One of the three is J chain, an $\sim$15,000 molecular weight polypeptide associated with the polymeric forms IgM and IgA (31). It is likely that J chain contributes to the polymerization process; other functions for it are more speculative (31). A second substance is secretory component—a 70,000 dalton glycoprotein which is associated with immunoglobulins found in secretions (32). Its likely role is to protect the immunoglobulin from premature degradation. Both J-chain and secretory component are associated with the Fc regions. Finally there is the class of substances referred to here as *receptors*. By this term I mean those entities that upon interaction with antigen-antibody complexes stimulate some form of effector system. The extent to which these receptors have been defined and characterized is quite variable. In one instance, the classical complement system, the receptor (Clq) has been visualized by electronmicroscopy (33, 34) and detailed structural analysis is proceeding rapidly (35). At the other extreme, e.g. the receptor *for* endogenous immunoglobulin on B-lymphocytes, the existence of a receptor can only be inferred and even that inference is not accepted by some (see section on B lymphocytes).

With only one well-documented exception, the evidence suggests that the receptors of various effector systems interact with the Fc region of immunoglobulins. The one documented exception is the "alternate" complement pathway, activation of which can be mediated by Fab regions (36).

The sites of interaction between receptors and the Fc regions of antibodies are as yet only poorly defined. There is considerable evidence that Clq interacts principally with the C_H2 regions on IgG molecules (37–39), and a 62 amino acid peptide from this region shows substantial Clq binding activity (40). Tryptophans have been implicated in the interaction (39, 41, 42). Active peptides derived from the C_H4 domain of IgM have been described (43). As discussed elsewhere (44), the significance of this finding is uncertain.

Mast cells have receptors for IgE and there is indirect evidence that the penultimate C_H3 domains of the ϵ-chains are involved (45). The evidence for a combining site on a pentapeptide sequence from the C_H2 region of the ϵ-chains (46) is very doubtful (47).

A variety of cells contain so-called Fc receptors, that is, plasma-membrane components that bind antigen-antibody complexes via the Fc of the antibodies. There is evidence for C_H2, C_H3, or both C_H2 and C_H3 being involved (48). The apparent discrepancies remain unresolved.

The cells (B-cells) from which the antibody secreting cells (plasma cells) are derived have immunoglobulins on their surfaces whose specificity is identical with that of the antibody which the daughter cell(s) will produce. There is evidence that most of the Fc region of the surface immunoglobulin on B-cells is exposed [reviewed in reference (49)]. This suggests that only the carboxy-terminal region of the surface immunoglobulin reacts with the putative cell receptor.

COMBINING SITE INTERACTIONS

Structural Studies

DOMAIN INTERACTIONS   It is clear from the previous discussion that the combining sites on antibodies for antigens are spatially removed from the combining sites for the receptors of effector systems. It is therefore appropriate to consider how these combining sites and the domains in which they reside may interact.

Trans interactions   *Trans* interactions are the interfaces between domains lying on alternate sides of the axes of pseudosymmetry between the heavy and light chains and the axis of symmetry between the carboxy-terminal halves of the heavy chains. These interactions are with one exception strong; however, direct studies are still limited.

The V_L and V_H domains interact so strongly that noncovalently bound "F_V" fragments consisting of one V_L and one V_H can be isolated (50). The antigen-binding properties of such fragments are little different from those of the intact antibodies. This suggests that the three-dimensional structure of the two domains is well maintained.

The C_H1 and C_L domains face each other over a broad interface. There are numerous close interactions as determined directly in several X-ray analyses (7, 8). The interface between C_H3 domains is very similar to that between C_H1 and C_L (24, 51). Selective cleavage of the heavy chains amino-terminal to the C_H3 domains yields a dimeric fragment $(C_H3)_2$ whose non-covalently bound domains cannot be dissociated from one another without denaturants (52).

The only domains that are known to have weak or even mildly repulsive interactions are the C_H2 domains. There is evidence that in the absence of interchain disulfides these domains can, and perhaps prefer to, spread apart (52–54); however, the disulfide bond(s) can be reformed by deliberate oxidation.

Cis interactions   While there is ample evidence for significant interactions between domains normal to the long axis of the molecule, longitudinal or *cis* interactions are much fewer. The X-ray data indicate few interactions between V_L and C_L or V_H and C_H1 in the Fab regions (7, 8). Furthermore, the angle formed by the axes of pseudosymmetry between V_L and V_H and C_L and C_H1 is quite variable (24).

There is a striking lack of evidence for *cis* interactions between the carboxy-terminal domains of Fab (C_L and C_H1 and the amino terminal domains of Fc (C_H2). In the most intensively studied immunoglobulins— IgG—a hinge region separates these domains (Table 1). It is here that the well known ready cleavage of immunoglobulins by proteases occurs. By a variety of criteria the fine structure of the resulting fragments is unchanged by this cleavage. Moreover, the fragments produced, Fab and Fc, show no tendency to associate.

Some data suggest that C_H2 and C_H3 interact strongly (55); however, other data do not support this (56, 57). In any case, such interactions do not appear to perturb the basic structure of the individual domains substantially.

ANTIGEN-INDUCED CHANGES   While the study of domain interactions in immunoglobulins can provide valuable clues about the likelihood of combining site interactions, the results are usually too imprecise to permit one to predict accurately whether such interactions actually occur. A more reliable approach is to search for ligand-induced changes directly. In this section I consider changes in the structure of immunoglobulins induced by ligands; in the following sections, I consider changes in the functional properties of the combining sites themselves. The older data as well as the results of more recent studies have been reviewed in detail (44, 58) and I limit my discussion here to a description of the methods used and a summary of the principal findings.

Direct studies, e.g. by X-ray diffraction analyses of myeloma proteins in the presence and absence of antigen-like ligands, have failed to detect changes in conformation (9). These studies have so far been limited to an investigation of Fab fragments. Nonetheless, if the Fab regions do not change it is hard to imagine that the Fc regions in the intact molecule would change *unless cleavage of the molecule into its Fab and Fc regions itself would produce a liganded conformation.* This was in fact proposed by Huber et al (59). These workers raised the possibility that antigen-induced changes in the Fab regions would lead to altered Fab:Fc interactions through a shortening of the hinge regions. The failure to observe the antigen-induced changes in the isolated Fab regions was explained by postulating that they were already in the liganded form as a result of the proteolytic cleavage used to produce the fragments. The authors made two predictions that posed critical tests of their theory. One was that the Fab (and the Fc regions) would be different in the intact versus the cleaved molecule. The second prediction was that antigen should induce a change in the rate with which the hinge region can be cleaved by proteases or the rate at which hinge region disulfides can be cleaved by reducing agents. Both predictions appear to have been wrong (24, 60), and there is really no direct evidence for this theory. This theory potentially explained the unusual findings of Pilz et al (61, 62). These workers, using low angle X-ray scattering, described antigen-induced changes in the calculated radius of gyration of antibody but not in the radius of gyration of the isolated Fab fragments. The failure to find support for the theory of Huber et al leaves the results of the scattering studies unexplained.

Other indirect studies by a wide variety of physicochemical techniques (optical rotatory dispersion, circular dichroism, circular polarization of luminescence, depolarization of fluorescence, fluorescence, electron spin and nuclear magnetic resonance, neutron scattering, hydrogen exchange, immunochemical analysis) have failed to detect changes in Fc due to antigen binding, have detected changes that cannot be clearly assigned to the Fc regions, or have failed to document that the observed changes are stoichiometrically correlated with antigen combining site saturation (44, 58).

Functional Studies

ACTIVATION BY ANTIGENS   The most direct way to study the effect of antigen binding on the interaction of antibody with receptors is to look for functional correlates. It has long been known that a variety of effector systems are optimally stimulated by antigen-antibody complexes consisting of more than one antibody molecule. What has been uncertain is whether the aggregation of antibody molecules (a) provides the critical signal per se, (b) is important only indirectly (aggregation being required to initiate or enhance conformational changes), or (c) is incidental.

An apparent exception to the rule that antibody aggregates are required for optimal responses is the observation that single molecules of IgM appear to be capable of initiating the classical complement cascade upon interaction with antigen (63). This is more of a semantic exception than a real one. Since effector system receptors interact with the Fc regions it is aggregation of the Fc regions with which we are concerned. IgM contains five Fc regions per molecule and in this case Fc aggregation may still be of importance. In this instance the aggregation would be an *intra-* rather than *inter*-molecular.

All of the older and much of the recent data are consistent with a failure of antibodies to activate effector systems unless the Fc regions of two or more antibody molecules are aggregated. The results of two recent investigations appear to be exceptions. In the first, an apparently monofunctional antigen stimulated complement interaction with IgM antibodies (64). There are two unusual aspects to these and related experiments. First though the antigen may be monovalent it must be large—much larger than conceivably necessary to fill the antigen-combining site. Second, the stoichiometry does not seem appropriate. Optimal interaction with complement occurred under conditions where apparently only a minute fraction of the antigen-combining sites should have been saturated (44).

In the second study a bivalent antigen was used—an artificial dimer of the "loop" sequence of chicken lysozyme (65). Upon interaction with IgG antibodies several phenomena occurred that led to the proposal that a circular complex between the bivalent antigen and single bivalent antibodies occurred. Substantial additions of antigen did not appear to disrupt the postulated circular complexes. Nevertheless, the interaction with complement observed with such complexes was remarkably sensitive to excess antigen. Thus, in its functional properties this system behaves just like other systems where aggregation of antibodies appears to be critical. I can only conclude that the exceptional findings of Brown and Koshland (64) and Pecht et al (65) need further clarification before their more general significance can be evaluated.

ACTIVATION WITHOUT ANTIGENS   The importance of aggregation is suggested by the finding that aggregation of antibody Fc regions by whatever means can stimulate effector systems. Aggregation induced by heating, cross-linking reagents, and antibodies to antibodies have all been found effective (66–68). Moreover, the same results can be obtained with isolated Fc regions. Thus neither antigens nor the antigen-combining sites of antibodies are required.

The principle of parsimony leads me to conclude that the aggregation is the critical event per se. I think it unlikely that in all the procedures used to aggregate the antibody, a similar specific conformational change occurs in the Fc regions. Others conclude differently (reviewed in 69).

MECHANISM OF ANTIBODY-MEDIATED ACTIVATION

In some systems (e.g. complement), receptor binding is promoted by complexing of antigen with antibody. In others (e.g. the IgE-mast cell system) the receptor interacts with the antibody in the absence of antigen, but the system is not activated unless the antibody becomes aggregated.

Regardless of whether the antibody is simply aggregated or aggregated and conformationally changed, several possibilities can be envisioned with regard to the role of the antibody in the subsequent events.

Alternative Mechanisms

One possibility is that the antibody is directly involved. It may be, for example, that the aggregated or aggregated and altered Fc regions become enzymatically active. Alternatively, the altered Fc regions might interact with a new component and changes in the latter might generate the signal.

A second possibility is that the antibody is only very indirectly involved, that it is the receptor that binds to the antibody which plays the critical role. A clear choice between these major alternatives can now be made in one antibody-mediated system: the IgE-mast cell system.

IgE-Mast Cell System

IgE is a four-chained immunoglobulin whose epsilon (ϵ) heavy chains have four constant region domains (70). Like all other immunoglobulins it is secreted by plasma cells. Its unique property is its ability to bind with exceedingly high affinity to mast cells or the related peripheral blood basophils (71). The binding is via the Fc region, and by itself is not known to perturb the cell to which it is bound. Since the Fc regions of IgE are the same regardless of the specificity of the antigen-combining sites in the Fab regions, a single mast cell may bind antibodies of a variety of specificities. As many as 10^6 IgE can bind specifically to the surface membrane (72). Any manipulation that leads to surface aggregation of the IgE Fc regions [cross-linking by antigens (73), bifunctional reagents (74), anti-IgE (75), and lectins (76)] stimulates the cells to undergo degranulation. Other, nonantibody reagents can also trigger the cells (77). In some of these studies it has been shown that the cells are compartmentalized in that local, partial, degranulation can occur (78, 79). It appears likely that IgE-mediated stimulation is similarly compartmentalized so that multiple stimulatory events over the cell surface may be necessary to achieve maximal release. It has recently been demonstrated unambiguously that dimers of IgE (prepared with bifunctional cross-linking reagents) are fully capable of initiating individual stimulatory events ("unit signals") (73). The cell component that binds IgE to the cell surface is being studied by several groups. It is a glycoprotein $5–10 \times 10^4$ daltons in mass and behaves like an integral membrane protein (reviewed in 80). Importantly, it is functionally univalent; one molecule of receptor binds only one molecule of IgE. Thus when IgE is aggregated, there is a stoichiometric aggregation of the receptors. Using antibodies directed to the receptor, it has recently been shown that mastocytoma cells *grown in the total absence of IgE can be triggered by (bivalent) antireceptor antibodies* (81). IgE blocks the antireceptor-induced release. Similar studies on normal cells have yielded similar results (82, 83). While the latter cells contain some IgE on their surfaces, control studies suggested no role for the IgE in the antireceptor-stimulated degranulation.

Thus in this system, the antibody appears to function exclusively as a mechanism by which specific antigens can aggregate (dimerize) receptors. No other role for the IgE must be invoked.

Complement

The importance of aggregation of antibodies in antibody-mediated complement activation has already been referred to. In the classical pathway, this involves the interaction of Clq with antibody. By unknown mechanisms Clr and Cls, components attached to Clq, are activated leading to proteolytic conversion of inactive Cls to active Cls by Clr. Activated Cls is itself a protease that reacts with subsequent components. It is uncertain whether the initial activation requires the participation of specific regions on the immunoglobulin other than those directly involved in binding Clq. There are some data that suggest that simple interaction of Clq is inadequate (42); however, in those experimental manipulations it is possible that changes in the topology of the combining sites were affected. These changes may have been responsible for the failure to observe complement activation in the face of unaltered Clq binding. It would be interesting to test whether cross-linking of the combining sites for antibody on Clq (e.g. with antibodies directed to those regions) would result in Cl activation.

B Lymphocyte

Another system of paramount interest to immunologists is the B-lymphocyte. As indicated previously these cells have surface-bound immunoglobulin which they themselves produce. (This is in contrast to the mast cells referred to above, in the section on the IgE-mast cell system, which do not synthesize the IgE bound to their surface membranes.) The surface immunoglobulin on the ontogenetically most primitive B-cells is IgMs—the four-chained subunit of IgM. Later, IgD may appear and still later other classes of antibody (84). On any particular cell all the surface immunoglobulins have identical combining sites for antigens (85).

The surface immunoglobulins have the properties of integral membrane proteins. The structures involved in the integration of the immunoglobulins in the membrane have not been identified. There is conflicting evidence for a hydrophobic "tail" or other constituent on the surface immunoglobulin that would explain its capacity to bind to the membrane of B-cells (86–89; see also 49). Consequently it is possible that a still unidentified immunoglobulin-binding component exists. It would be interesting to explore this possibility by the use of cross-linking reagents.

There is still considerable controversy about the role of the immunoglobulin of B lymphocytes. At one extreme is the proposal that the role of the antibody is exclusively to bind antigens (90). It is suggested that structures on the antigen itself or structures that have become attached to the antigen (e.g. by prior interaction of antigen with other cells or cell products) provide the stimulatory signal. Others have postulated a direct role for the immunoglobulin with or without invoking "second" signals (91).

Nevertheless, a variety of studies have shown that antibodies directed to this surface immunoglobulin are stimulatory (92–97). Bivalent antibody is required. Even in those cases where the signal appears to have been inhibitory (98), more than a passive role for the surface immunoglobulin (or the component that binds it to the cell surface) is implied.

Other Systems

IMMUNOLOGICAL SYSTEMS   Recent results suggest that thymus-derived (T) lymphocytes have intrinsic antibodies on their surface membranes (99). The precise nature of these antibodies, and even their presence, has been in much dispute (100). Too little is known about this system to allow one to compare it to the others referred to above.

A variety of other cells have the capacity to bind extrinsic antibody to their surface membranes with or without the presence of complement [see Chapters 8, 10–13 in reference (101)]. In all of these, cell activation appears to require aggregated antibody (Fc regions). Undoubtedly the requirement for aggregated antibody is partially explained by the enhanced binding achieved by multivalent interactions. Whether in addition the aggregation is required to activate is uncertain. Experiments with antibodies directed to the Fc receptors on such cells would be of interest. Since bivalent fragments of antibodies can be prepared that lack Fc regions, the effect of aggregating the Fc receptors per se could be assessed.

NONIMMUNOLOGICAL SYSTEMS   It has recently been observed that bivalent (i.e. cross-linking) antibodies directed to hormone receptors can in certain instances mimic the activity of the hormone [see Chapters 25–27 in reference (101)]. I mention these not as other examples of antibody-mediated cell activation; they are, but in a different sense than used in this review. The results with antibody-mediated triggering of hormone receptors do, however, raise the possibility that in other systems aggregation of receptors may be significant. In at least one of these systems—the insulin system —there is new evidence that the hormone is self-aggregating when bound to the surface membrane (102).

SEQUELAE OF ACTIVATION

Surface Phenomena

It is by now well known that many cell membrane components are more or less freely mobile in the plane of the membrane. It is not surprising therefore that cross-linking of surface antibody, if extensive enough, can lead to substantial surface redistribution (reviewed in 49, 103).

In one well defined system, the IgE-mast cell system (see section on IgE-mast cell system), it has been possible to investigate directly the role of gross surface redistribution in the IgE-mediated cell activation (104, 105). There is good evidence that redistribution, though it can occur, does not contribute to cell stimulation. In studies in which IgE-coated cells were reacted with anti-IgE the dose of the latter could be titrated such that various amounts of IgE redistribution occurred. No correlation between exocytosis and gross redistribution was observed. Indeed, doses of anti-IgE that were high enough to induce gross redistribution during the time period in which exocytosis was anticipated were inhibitory (104). The mechanism of this inhibition is unknown.

Comparable studies on systems such as B-lymphocytes are difficult to perform. The problem is that most of the criteria used to study activation occur long after the addition of the stimulant. Discussions on the role of redistribution in the variety of B-lymphocyte responses are not conclusive (49, 10).

In addition to causing surface rearrangements, cross-linking reagents can induce endocytosis of membrane components. The possible role of internalization in antibody-mediated cell activation is uncertain (49, 103).

Metabolic Changes

In no instance are there data that define the immediate sequelae of antigen-antibody reactions on the surfaces of cells. In the IgE-mast cell system, receptor aggregation appears to provide the initial signal. What the signal consists of is unknown. In that system the only extrinsic substance required is free Ca^{2+} (106). Several studies suggest that a change in Ca^{2+} permeability occurs at an early stage but whether this is step two or twenty-two is unknown (107, 108). Recent discussions of other metabolic events in this system can be found in reference (77). In the IgE-mast cell system it is possible to isolate the receptor. Studies are proceeding in several laboratories to see whether isolated receptors (a) can produce detectable changes or (b) are altered during triggering.

There is a vast literature on metabolic changes in lymphocytes stimulated by antigen and other substances. There are recent reviews by Gomperts (107) dealing with the role of calcium, by Ferber & Resch (109) on changes in membrane lipids, by Kaplan (110) on Na+/K+ transport, and by Wedner & Parker (111) on cyclic nucleotides and other changes. The interested reader may, however, first want to read the review by Waksman & Wagshal (112). These authors while focusing on the role of "cytokines"—soluble mediators produced by or acting upon lymphocytes—emphasize the complexities that must be dealt with. There is enormous heterogeneity of cell types and cell cycle stages in the usual systems studied. The frequent use of lectins that can react with a vast number of different cell-surface components complicates the interpretation of findings even more. It seems likely that definitive information will require the use of more well defined systems than are commonly used at present.

SUMMARY AND CONCLUSIONS

The importance of aggregation in antibody-mediated reactions has been widely accepted for decades. What has eluded definition are the reasons aggregation is so necessary. One simple possibility, that by permitting multiple cooperative interactions it enhances antigen binding to antibody, undoubtedly is part of the answer. The weight of the evidence suggests that this explanation is insufficient, however. Rather, aggregation per se is necessary and in particular, aggregation of those regions of the antibody molecule that react with the receptors of effector systems. Again one might postulate that this simply enhances the binding of antibody to receptors but again while this is undoubtedly true it is only a partial explanation. It could be that aggregation of the antibody creates changes in the latter that are required for activation of the receptor. To the extent that the changes are postulated to be topological, i.e. that they involve changes in the arrangement in space of the combining sites on antibodies for receptors, there is considerable evidence in support of this notion. There is little or no evidence in favor of the postulate that aggregation produces meaningful changes in the structure of the combining sites for receptors per se, and there is at least one system where this can be pretty well ruled out. In IgE-mediated stimulation of mast cells it is possible to eliminate the IgE altogether; aggregating the receptor itself is sufficient.

My own conclusion is that the receptors of the effector systems should now receive the intensive experimental attention that has heretofore been directed toward the antibody molecules. We need to understand the role of aggregation in triggering the receptors. In the case of the classical pathway of complement activation this means understanding how intramolecular changes in Clq activate Clr. In the case of the cell receptor for IgE this means understanding how dimerization of the surface receptor produces changes. Such knowledge could provide the basis for new approaches to therapeutic intervention.

Literature Cited

1. Müller-Eberhard, H. J. 1975. Complement. *Ann. Rev. Biochem.* 44:697–724
2. Nelson, D. S., ed. 1969. *Macrophages and Immunity.* Amsterdam: North-Holland. 336 pp.
3. Weismann, G., Dukar, P. 1970. The role of lysozomes in immune resposes. *Adv. Immunol.* 12:283–331
4. Becker, E. L., Henson, P. M. 1973. In vitro studies of immunologically induced secretion of mediators from cells and related phenomena. *Adv. Immunol.* 17:94–193
5. Kabat, E. A. 1939. The molecular weight of antibodies. *J. Exp. Med.* 69:103–18
6. Putnam, F. W. 1953. Proteins in multiple myeloma: Physicochemical study of serum proteins. *J. Biol. Chem.* 202:727–43
7. Poljak, R. J. 1975. X-ray diffraction studies of immunoglobulins. *Adv. Immunol.* 21:1–33
8. Davies, D. R., Padlan, E. A., Segal, D. M. 1975. Three dimensional structure of immunoglobulins. *Ann. Rev. Biochem.* 44:639–67
9. Padlan, E. A. 1977. Structural basis for the specificity of antibody-antigen reactions and structural mechanisms for diversification of antigen-binding specificities. *Q. Rev. Biophys.* 10:35–65
10. Nisonoff, A., Hopper, J. E., Spring, S. B. 1975. *The Antibody Molecule.* New York: Academic. 542 pp.
11. Kabat, E. A. 1976. *Structural Concepts in Immunology and Immunochemistry.* New York: Holt, Rinehart and Winston. 547 pp. 2nd ed.
12. Hood, L., Gray, W. R., Sanders, B. G., Dreyer, W. J. 1967. Light chain evolution. *Cold Spring Harbor Symp. Quant. Biol.* 32:133–45
13. Edelman, G. M., Gall, W. E. 1969. The antibody problem. *Ann. Rev. Biochem.* 38:415–66
14. Schiffer, M., Girling, R. L., Ely, K. R., Edmundson, A. B. 1973. Structure of a λ-type Bence-Jones protein at 3.5 Å resolution. *Biochemistry* 12:4233–4631
15. Franek, F. 1969. In *Developmental Aspects of Antibody Formation and Structure,* ed. J. Sterzl, I. Riha. New York: Academic
16. Wu, T. T., Kabat, E. 1970. An analysis of the sequences of the variable regions of Bence-Jones proteins and myeloma light chains and their implications for antibody complementarity. *J. Exp. Med.* 132:211–50

17. Feinstein, A., Rowe, A. J. 1965. Molecular mechanism of an antigen-antibody complex. *Nature* 205:147–49
18. Noelken, M. E., Nelson, C. A., Buckley, C. E. III., Tanford, C. 1965. Gross conformation of rabbit 7S γ-immunoglobulin and its papain-cleaved fragments. *J. Biol. Chem.* 240:218–24
19. Beal, D., Feinstein, A. 1976. Structure and function of the constant regions of immunoglobulins. *Q. Rev. Biophys.* 9:135–80
20. Edelman, G. M., Cunningham, B. A., Gall, W. E., Gottlieb, P. D., Rutishauser, U., Waxdal, M. J. 1969. The covalent structure of an entire γG immunoglobulin molecule. *Proc. Natl. Acad. Sci. USA* 63:78–85
21. Milstein, C., Frangione, B. 1971. Disulphide bridges of heavy chain of human IgG2. *Biochem. J.* 121:217–25
22. Michaelson, T. E., Frangione, B., Franklin, E. C. 1977. Primary structure of the "hinge" region of human IgG3. *J. Biol. Chem.* 252:883–89
23. Holowka, D. A., Cathou, R. E. 1976. Conformation of immunoglobulin M: Nanosecond fluorescence depolarization analysis of segmental flexibility in anti-ε-1 dimethylamino-s-naphalene-sulfonyl-L-lysine IgM from horse, pig and shark. *Biochemistry* 15:3379–90
24. Silverton, E. W., Navia, M. A., Davies, D. R. 1977. Three dimensional structure of an intact human immunoglobulin. *Proc. Natl. Acad. Sci. USA* 74:5140–44
25. Pauling, L. 1962. In *The Specificity of Serological Reactions,* ed. K. Landsteiner, pp. 275–93. New York: Dover. 330 pp.
26. Karush, F. 1962. Immunologic specificity and molecular structure. *Adv. Immunol.* 2:1–40
27. Samuels, A. 1963. Immunoenzymology-reaction processes, kinetics and the role of conformational alteration. *Ann. NY Acad. Sci.* 103:858–89
28. Lancet, D., Pecht, I. 1976. Kinetic evidence for hapten-induced conformational transitions in immunoglobulin MOPC 460. *Proc. Natl. Acad. Sci. USA* 73:3549–53
29. Day, L. A., Sturtevant, J. M., Singer, S. J. 1963. The kinetics of the reactions between antibody to the 2,4-dinitrophenyl group and specific hapten. *Ann. NY Acad. Sci.* 103:611–25
30. Pecht, I., Lancet, D. 1977. In *Chemical Relaxation in Molecular Biology,* ed. I.

Pecht, R. Rigler, pp. 306–38. Heidelberg: Springer. 418 pp.

31. Koshland, M. E. 1975. Structure and function of the J-chain. *Adv. Immunol.* 20:41–69

32. Frangione, B. 1975. In *Immunodeficiency and Immunogenetics*, ed. B. Benacerraf, pp. 2–53. Lancaster: Med. Tech. Publ. Co.

33. Shelton, E., Yonemasu, K. and Stroud, R. M. 1972. Ultrastructure of the human complement component, Clq. *Proc. Natl. Acad. Sci. USA* 69:65–68

34. Svehag, S. E., Manheim, L., Bloth, B. 1972. Ultrastructure of human Clq protein. *Nature* 238:117–18

35. Reid, K. B. M., Sim, R. B., Faiers, A. B. 1977. Inhibition of the reconstitution of the haemolytic activity of the first component of human complement by a pepsin-derived fragment of subcomponent Clq. *Biochem. J.* 161:239–45

36. Götze, O., Müller-Eberhard, H. J. 1976. The alternative pathway of complement activation. *Adv. Immunol.* 24:1–35

37. Colomb, M. G., Porter, R. R. 1975. Characterization of a plasmin-digest fragment of rabbit IgG that binds antigen and complement. *Biochem. J.* 145:177–83

38. Yasmeen, D., Ellerson, J. R., Dorrington, K. J., Painter, R. H. 1976. Structure and function of immunoglobulin domains. IV. Distribution of some effector functions among Cγ2 and Cγ3 homology regions of human IgG. *J. Immunol.* 116:518–26

39. Isenman, D. E., Ellerson, J. R., Painter, R. H., Dorrington, K. J. 1977. Correlation between the exposure of aromatic chromophores at the surface of the Fc domains of immunoglobulin G and their ability to bind complement. *Biochemistry* 16:233–40

40. Kehoe, J. M., Bourgois, A., Capra, J. D., Fougereau, M. 1974. Amino acid sequence of a murine immunoglobulin fragment that possesses complement fixing activity. *Biochemistry* 13:2499–2504

41. Cohen, S., Becker, L. A. 1968. The effect of benzylation or sequential amidination and benzylation on the ability of rabbit γG antibody to fix complement. *J. Immunol.* 100:403–6

42. Allen, R., Isliker, H. 1974. Studies on the complement-binding site of rabbit immunoglobulin G. I. Modification of tryphophan residues and their role in anti-complementary activity of rabbit IgG. *Immunochemistry* 11:175–80

43. Hurst, M. M., Volanakis, J., Hester, R. B., Stroud, R. M., Bennett, J. C. 1975. The structural basis for binding of complement by IgM. *J. Exp. Med.* 140:1117–21

44. Metzger, H. 1978. The effect of antigen on antibodies: Recent studies. *Contemp. Top. Mol. Immunol.* 7:119–52

45. Dorrington, K. J., Bennich, H. 1973. Thermally induced structural changes in immunoglobulin E. *J. Biol. Chem.* 248:8378–84

46. Hamburger, R. N. 1975. Peptide inhibition of the Prausnitz Kustner reaction. *Science* 189:389–90

47. Bennich, H., Ragnarsson, U., Johansson, S. G. O., Ishizaka, K., Ishizaka, T., Levy, D. A., Lichtenstein, L. M. 1977. Failure of the putative IgE pentapeptide to compete with IgE for receptors on basophils and mast cells. *Int. Arch. Allergy Appl. Immunol.* 53:459–68

48. Ovary, Z., Saluk, P. H., Quijada, L., Laurin, M. E. 1976. Biologic activities of rabbit immunoglobulin G in relation to domains of the Fc region. *J. Immunol.* 116:1265–71

49. Loor, F. 1977. Structure and dynamics of the lymphocyte surface in relation to differentiation and activation. *Prog. Allergy* 23:1–153

50. Inbar, D., Hochman, H., Givol, D. 1972. Localization of antibody-combining sites within the variable portions of heavy and light chains. *Proc. Natl. Acad. Sci. USA* 69:2659–62

51. Deisenhofer, J., Colman, P. M., Epp, O., Huber, R. 1976. Crystallographic structural studies of a human Fc fragment. II. A complete model based on a fourier map at 3.5 Å resolution. *Hoppe-Seyler's Z. Physiol. Chem.* 351:1421–34

52. Charlwood, P. A., Utsumi, S. 1969. Conformation changes and dissociation of Fc fragments of rabbit immunoglobulin G as a function of pH. *Biochem. J.* 112:357–65

53. Romans, D. G., Tilley, C. A., Crookston, M. C., Falk, R. E., Dorrington, K. J. 1977. Conversion of incomplete antibodies to direct agglutinins by mild reduction: Evidence for segmental flexibility within the Fc fragment of immunoglobulin G. *Proc. Natl. Acad. Sci. USA* 74:2531–35

54. Chan, L. M., Cathou, R. E. 1977. The role of the inter-heavy chain disulfide bond in modulating the flexibility of immunoglobulin G antibody. *J. Mol. Biol.* 112:653–56

55. Michaelson, T. E. 1976. Indications that the Cγ2 homology region is not a regular domain. *Scand. J. Immunol.* 5:1123-27

56. Burton, D. R., Forsén, S., Karlström, G., Dwek, R. A., McLaughlin, A. C., Uain-Hobson, S. 1977. The determination of molecular-motion parameters from proton-relaxation enhancement measurements in a number of Gd(III) antibody fragment complexes. *Eur. J. Biochem.* 75:445-54

57. Burton, D. R., Dwek, R. A., Forsén, S., Karlström, G. 1977. A novel approach to water proton relaxation in paramagnetic ion macromolecular complexes. *Biochemistry* 16:250-54

58. Metzger, H. 1974. Effect of antigen binding on antibody properties. *Adv. Immunol.* 18:169-207

59. Huber, R., Deisenhofer, J., Colman, P. M., Matsushima, M., Palm, W. 1976. Crystallographic structure studies of an IgG molecule and an Fc fragment. *Nature* 264:415-20

60. Wright, J. K., Engel, J., Jaton, J-C. 1978. Selective reduction and proteolysis in the hinge region of liganded and unliganded antibodies. Identical kinetics suggest lack of conformational change in the hinge region. *Eur. J. Immunol.* 8:309-14

61. Pilz, I., Kratky, O., Licht, A., Sela, M. 1973. Shape and volume of anti-polyalanine antibodies in the presence and absence of tetra-D-alanine as followed by small-angle x-ray scattering. *Biochemistry* 12:4998-5005

62. Pilz, I., Kratky, O., Karush, F. 1974. Changes of the conformation of rabbit IgG antibody caused by the specific binding of a hapten. *Eur. J. Biochem.* 41:91-96

63. Borsos, T., Rapp, H. J. 1965. Hemolysin titration based on fixation of the activated first component of complement: Evidence that one molecule of hemolysin suffices to sensitize an erythrocyte. *J. Immunol.* 95:559-66

64. Brown, J. C., Koshland, M. E. 1975. Activation of antibody Fc function by antigen-induced conformational changes. *Proc. Natl. Acad. Sci. USA* 72:5111-15

65. Pecht, I., Ehrenberg, E., Calif, E., Arnon, R. 1977. Conformational changes and complement activation induced upon antigen binding to antibodies. *Biochem. Biophys. Res. Commun.* 74: 1302-9

66. Ishizaka, K., Ishizaka, T. 1960. Biologic activity of aggregated γ-globu-

lin. II. A study of various methods for aggregation and species differences. *J. Immunol.* 85:163-71

67. Ishizaka, K., Ishizaka, T., Banovitz, J. 1965. Biologic activity of aggregated γ-globulin. VII. Minimum size of aggregated γ-globulin or its piece III required for the induction of skin reactivity and complement fixation. *J. Immunol.* 94:824-32

68. Augener, W., Grey, H. M., Cooper, N. R., Müller-Eberhard, H. J. 1971. The reaction of monomeric and aggregated immunoglobulin with Cl. *Immunochemistry* 8:1011-20

69. Hoffmann, L. G. 1976. Antibodies as allosteric proteins. III. An alternative model, and some predictions. *Immunochemistry* 13:737-42

70. Bennich, H. H., Johansson, S. G. O., von Bahr-Lindstöm, H. 1978. In *Immediate Hypersensitivity,* ed. M. Bach, pp. 1-36. New York: Dekker

71. Ishizaka, T., Ishizaka, K. 1975. Biology of immunoglobulin E. *Prog. Allergy* 19:60-121

72. Metzger, H. 1977. In *Receptors and Recognition,* ed. P. Cuatrecasas, M. F. Greaves, 4:7-102 London: Chapman & Hall Ser. A

73. Siraganian, R. P., Hook, W. A., Levine, B. B. 1975. Specific in vitro histamine release from basophils by divalent haptens: Evidence for activation by simple bridging of membrane bound antibody. *Immunochemistry* 12: 149-57

74. Segal, D. M., Taurog, J. D., Metzger, H. 1977. Dimeric immunoglobulin E serves as a unit signal for mast cell degranulation. *Proc. Natl. Acad. Sci. USA* 74:2993-97

75. Ishizaka, K., Ishizaka, T. 1969. Immune mechanisms of reversed type reaginic hypersensitivity. *J. Immunol.* 103:588-95

76. Magro, A. M. 1974. Involvement of IgE in Con A-induced histamine release from human basophils in vitro. *Nature* 249:572-73

77. Morrison, D. C., Henson, P. M. 1978. See Ref. 70, pp. 431-502

78. Diamant, B., Kruger, P. G., Uvnas, B. 1970. Local degranulation of individual rat peritoneal mast cells induced by compound 48/80. *Acta Physiol. Scand.* 79:1-5

79. Tasaka, K., Yamasaki, H. 1973. Local degranulation and histamine release from a single rat mast cell by microelectrophoretic application of basic hista-

mine releasers and antigen. *Acta Dermatol. Venereol. Suppl.* 73:167–74
80. Metzger, H. 1978. The IgE-mast cell system as a paradigm for the study of antibody mechanisms. *Immunol. Rev.* 41:186–99
81. Isersky, C., Taurog, J. D., Poy, G., Metzger, H. 1978. Triggering of cultured mastocytoma cells by antibodies to the receptor for IgE. *J. Immunol.* 121:549–58
82. Ishizaka, T., Chang, T. H., Taggart, M., Ishizaka, K. 1977. Histamine release from rat mast cells by antibodies against rat basophilic leukemia cell membrane. *J. Immunol.* 119:1589–96
83. Ishizaka, T., Ishizaka, K. 1978. Triggering of histamine release from rat mast cells by divalent antibodies against IgE-receptors. *J. Immunol.* 120:800–5
84. Parkhouse, R. M. E., Cooper, M. D. 1977. A model for the differentiation of B-lymphocytes with implications for the biological role of IgD. *Immunol. Rev.* 37:105–26
85. Pernis, B., Brovet, J. C., Seligmann, M. 1974. IgD and IgM on the membrane of lymphoid cells in macroglobulinemia: Evidence for identity of membrane IgD and IgM antibody activity in a case with anti-IgG receptors. *Eur. J. Immunol.* 4:776–82
86. Melcher, U., Eidels, L., Uhr, J. W. 1975. Are immunoglobulins integral membrane proteins? *Nature* 258:434–35
87. Melcher, U., Uhr, J. W. 1976. Cell surface Ig. XVI. Polypeptide chain structures of mouse IgM and IgD-like molecules. *J. Immunol.* 116:409–15
88. Melcher, U., Uhr, J. W. 1977. Density differences between membrane and secreted immunoglobulins of murine splenocytes. *Biochemistry* 16:145–52
89. McIlhinney, R. A. J., Richardson, N. E., Feinstein, A. 1978. Evidence for a C-terminal tyrosine residue in human and mouse B-lymphocyte membrane μ chains. *Nature* 272:555–57
90. Coutinho, A., Gronowicz, E., Möller, G. 1975. In *Immune Recognition*, ed. A. Rosenthal, pp. 63–83. New York: Academic. 855 pp.
91. Cohen, M. 1971. The take home lesson. *Ann. NY Acad. Sci.* 190:529–84
92. Sell, S., Gell, P. G. H. 1965. Studies on rabbit lymphocytes in vitro. I. Stimulation of blast transformation with an anti allotype serum. *J. Exp. Med.* 122:423–40
93. Kishimoto, T., Miyake, T., Nishizawa, Y., Watanabe, T., Yamamura, Y.

1975. Triggering mechanism of B-lymphocytes. I. Effect of anti-Ig and immunoglobulin enhancing soluble factor on differentiation and proliferation of B-cells. *J. Immunol.* 115:1179–84
94. Kishimoto, T., Ishizaka, K. 1975. Regulation of antibody response in vitro. IX. Induction of secondary anti-hapten IgG antibody response by anti-immunoglobulin and enhancing soluble factor. *J. Immunol.* 114:585–91
95. Weiner, H. L., Moorhead, J. W., Yamaga, K., Kubo, R. T. 1976. Anti-immunoglobulin stimulation of murine lymphocytes. II. Identification of cell surface target molecules and requirements for cross-linkage. *J. Immunol.* 117:1527–31
96. Weiner, H. L., Scribner, D. J., Moorhead, J. W. 1978. Anti-immunoglobulin stimulation of murine lymphocytes. IV. Re-expression and fate of cell surface receptors during stimulation. *J. Immunol.* 120:1907–12
97. Sieckmann, D. G., Asofsky, R., Mosier, D. E., Zitron, I. M., Paul, W. E. 1978. Activation of mouse lymphocytes by anti-immunoglobulin. I. Parameters of the proliferative response. *J. Exp. Med.* 147:814–29
98. Andersson, J., Bullock, W. W., Melchers, F. 1974. Inhibition of mitogenic stimulation of mouse lymphocytes by anti-mouse Ig antibodies. I. Mode of action. *Eur. J. Immunol.* 4:715–22
99. Sercarz, E. E., Herzenberg, L. A., Fox, C. F., eds. 1977. *Immune System: Genetics and Regulation.* New York: Academic. 761 pp.
100. Warner, N. L. 1974. Membrane immunoglobulins and antigen receptors on B and T lymphocytes. *Adv. Immunol.* 19:67–216
101. Cinader, B., ed. 1977. *Immunology of Receptors.* New York: Dekker. 524 pp.
102. Schlessinger, J., Shechter, Y., Willingham, M. C. and Pastan, I. 1978. Direct visualization of binding, aggregation and internalization of insulin and epidermal growth factor on living fibroblastic cells. *Proc. Natl. Acad. Sci. USA* 75:2659–63
103. Schreiner, G. F., Unanue, E. R. 1976. Membrane and cytoplasmic changes in B lymphocytes induced by ligand-surface immunoglobulin interaction. *Adv. Immunol.* 24:37–165
104. Becker, K. E., Ishizaka, T., Metzger, H., Ishizaka, K., Grimley, P. 1973. Surface IgE on human basophils during histamine release. *J. Exp. Med.* 108:394–409

105. Lawson, D., Fewtrell, C., Gomperts, B., Raff, M. C. 1975. Antiimmunoglobulin induced histamine secretion by rat peritoneal mast cells studied by immuno-ferritin electron-microscopy. *J. Exp. Med.* 142:391–402

106. Uvnas, B. 1974. Histamine storage and release. *Fed. Proc.* 33:2172–76

107. Gomperts, B. D. 1976. See Ref. 72, Vol. 2, pp. 43–102

108. Foreman, J. C., Hallet, M. B., Mongar, J. L. 1977. The relationship between histamine secretion and ^{45}Ca uptake by mast cells. *J. Physiol.* 271:193–214

109. Ferber, E., Resch, K. 1977. In *The Lymphocyte,* ed. J. J. Marchalonis, pp. 593–618. New York: Dekker. 704 pp.

110. Kaplan, J. G. 1978. Membrane cation transport and the control of proliferation of mammalian cells. *Ann. Rev. Physiol.* 40:19–41

111. Wedner, H. J., Parker, C. W. 1976. Lymphocyte activation. *Prog. Allergy* 20:195–300

112. Waksman, B. H., Wagshal, A. B. 1978. Lymphocyte functions acted on by immunoregulatory cytokines. Significance of the cell cycle. *Cell. Immunol.* 36:180–96

Ann. Rev. Med. 1978. 29:593–603

RECENT MEMBRANE RESEARCH AND ITS IMPLICATIONS FOR CLINICAL MEDICINE

◆7301

Vincent T. Marchesi, M.D., Ph.D.
Department of Pathology, Yale University School of Medicine, New Haven, Connecticut 06510

LIPIDS ARE ARRANGED AS A DYNAMIC ASYMMETRIC BILAYER

One of the most remarkable structural features of biological membranes was first clearly described in the mid 1920s when Gorter & Grendel (38) suggested that the lipids of the red cell membrane might be arranged in the form of a double layer of phospholipid molecules. This remarkably simple idea was based on the fact that the surface area of red cell ghosts contained approximately twice as many lipid molecules as were needed to make a monomolecular film surrounding the cell. This lipid-bilayer hypothesis received a certain amount of support from early X-ray diffraction studies carried out on model membrane systems and on myelin membranes, and lately it has been supported by studies using more modern physical techniques. The development of freeze-etching techniques was a significant step forward in the analysis of membranes by electron microscopy. With this approach it was discovered that cell membranes cleaved roughly in half along planes that corresponded to the middle of the hydrocarbon regions of the lipid bilayers (1).

Studies with some of the newer physical techniques also revealed that lipid molecules in bilayers appeared to be in very active motion. By placing probes on different segments of phospholipid molecules and sampling different layers of the hydrocarbon matrix, it has been shown that the hydrocarbon chains of fatty acids of the phospholipids are rapidly flexing. Individual phospholipid molecules also move at significant rates within the lateral plane of the lipid bilayer. Hence, it is now recognized that the individual phospholipid molecules are in a dynamic state within the intact membrane (2).

These new discoveries resulted in the concept of membrane fluidity. In general terms, fluidity refers to the degree of viscosity objects would encounter if they were able to float freely within the interior of the bilayer. The fluidity of a

0066-4219/78/0401-0593$01.00

593

membrane is determined by the types of lipids and fatty acids that make up the bilayer and by the temperature of the system. As rough generalizations, it may be stated that fatty acids with greater degrees of unsaturation are more fluid at lower temperatures than fatty acids that are more fully saturated. Also, shorter-chain fatty acids are more fluid than longer-chain fatty acids. Recent studies on the role of sterols and their effects on membrane fluidity are interesting in that sterols have a somewhat paradoxical effect: They can either increase or decrease the relative fluidity of membranes, depending upon the types of phospholipids and the concentrations of sterols in the preparations.

One additional recent modification of the bilayer hypothesis is the fact that the individual classes of lipid molecules appear to be arranged asymmetrically within the bilayers of intact cells. In the case of red blood cells, phosphatidylcholine and sphingomyelin, which are choline-containing phospholipids, seem to be concentrated in the external leaflet of the bilayer, while phosphatidylserine and phosphatidylethanolamine are concentrated in the cytoplasmic half (3). Now that the concepts of membrane fluidity and lipid asymmetry are more or less established, investigators are actively pursuing the biological meaning of these remarkable properties.

INTEGRAL PROTEINS INTERACT WITH LIPIDS VIA HYDROPHOBIC ASSOCIATIONS; EXTRINSIC PROTEINS (MAY) INTERACT ELECTROSTATICALLY

Approximately one half of the mass of most mammalian cell membrane fractions is made up of proteins, and the number of types of different polypeptide chains seems to vary with the cell type. Human red blood cells have at least seven major polypeptide chains, as determined by sodium dodecyl sulfate (SDS) gel electrophoresis (Figure 1), and in addition there are an indeterminate number of minor protein species.

As a result of the initial attempts to extract proteins from cell membrane fractions, it became evident that some of the polypeptide chains were easily detached from membrane elements, while others seemed resistant to all but the most disruptive solubilizing agents. On the basis of such experiences from many different laboratories, Singer (5) suggested that polypeptide chains of red cell membranes might be operationally classified into two types, based on the apparent mode by which they associate with the membrane lipids. He suggested that the polypeptide chains that are relatively loosely bound to the membrane and can be removed by manipulating the pH or ionic strength of solubilizing media be called extrinsic membrane proteins. One of the most characteristic of the extrinsic membrane proteins of the red cell membrane is the set of polypeptide chains called spectrin, which appears as bands one and two on SDS gels.

Many investigators discovered that the spectrin polypeptides could be rapidly and quantitatively eluted from red cell ghosts by simply immersing the membranes in low-ionic-strength media that contained a dilute chelating agent (6). Although red cell membranes treated this way fragment into small vesicles as a

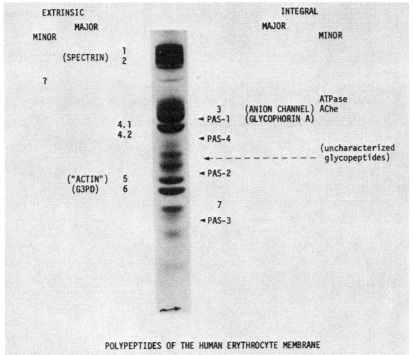

POLYPEPTIDES OF THE HUMAN ERYTHROCYTE MEMBRANE

Figure 1   Electropherogram of the proteins of human red cell membranes in SDS poly-acrylamide gels detected by staining with Coomassie brilliant blue. The numerical designation for the major polypeptides is adopted from Fairbanks et al (4). The bands indicated as 4.1 and 4.2 are not separated under the conditions used (1% SDS). For the sake of simplicity, designations for minor components are not included. The positions where the four sialoglycopeptides migrate on appropriately stained gels (PAS) are indicated by arrows.

result of the spectrin released from the membrane, it is generally thought that the spectrin polypeptides probably do not intercalate within the lipid bilayer, but instead associate electrostatically either with other proteins of the membrane or, possibly, with the polar groups of the phospholipids.

In contrast to extrinsic membrane proteins, the polypeptide chains that resist solubilization from membranes by simple buffer washings represent an entirely different class of macromolecules. These proteins are called integral proteins, largely because they cannot be dissociated from the lipid elements of the membrane without the use of detergents or harsh denaturing agents. Hence, it is considered likely that these proteins form an integral part of the membrane structure. One of the most characteristic of the integral membrane proteins is the major sialoglycoprotein of the human red cell membrane called glycophorin A.

Glycophorin A has been isolated by a number of different laboratories using a wide variety of protein solvents (see 7–9), and as the result of an intensive amount of study, it is now possible to construct a provisional model of its primary structure and offer some ideas of how and where it is oriented in the intact red cell membrane. The complete amino acid sequence and the sites of oligosaccharide attachment were recently determined (10), and are shown in Figure 2.

The polypeptide portion of glycophorin A, which comprises approximately 40% of the total dry weight, is made up of 131 amino acids. The distribution of different amino acids is rather interesting in that there is a very high concentration of threonine and serine residues located near the N-terminal end of the polypeptide chain. There is also a striking concentration of nonpolar amino acids located approximately midway between the N-terminal third of the polypeptide and the C-terminal third. In the diagram shown in Figure 2, the segment starting from amino acid 71 and extending through amino acid 90 is depicted between two vertical lines; this is thought to be the segment of polypeptide that is buried within the lipid bilayer.

It is also evident from this diagram that there are 16 oligosaccharide chains attached to the polypeptide chain, and their positions are assigned to the threonine and serine residues shown. It is significant that the glycosylated residues start from the N-terminal end of the molecule and extend to residue 50, but no additional sugar residues have been detected in amino acids beyond residue 50. One of the oligosaccharide chains linked to asparagine is of the complex variety (11), while the remaining 15 seem to be of the tetrasaccharide type originally described by Winzler & Thomas (12).

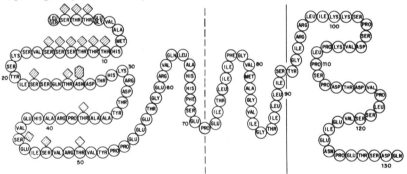

Figure 2   The amino acids of glycophorin A are arranged in this diagram to simulate, in a very general way, the positions they might have if the glycophorin molecule were arranged perpendicular to the lipid bilayer of the membrane. The limits of the bilayer are defined by the two vertical lines. The solid vertical line, which passes between residues 92 and 93, should be the approximate location of the polar groups of the inner half of the phospholipid bilayer. This assignment is based on the results of enzymatic iodination of tyrosine 93 and the distribution of ferritin-antibody conjugates directed against antigenic determinants defined by residues 102 to 118. Since we do not have comparable data with regard to the amount of the N-terminal end of glycophorin A that is buried with the lipid bilayer, we can only guess at the location of this outer lamella of the bilayer relative to the glycophorin molecule. Hence, the outer edge of the bilayer is defined by the dashed vertical line.

Since all of the glycosylated residues are concentrated at one end of the molecule, and some of these sugars probably represent receptor sites for lectins and perhaps for some blood groups antigens, this end of the molecule has been designated as the receptor domain.

The amino acid sequence of the 40 C-terminal amino acids is unusual in that this portion of the polypeptide chain contains a large number of charged amino acids with a peculiar clustering of acidic amino acids at the C-terminal segment of the chain. This portion of the polypeptide chain also contains a substantial number of prolines, which may play a major role in determining the conformation of this part of the molecule.

The peptide stretch of 22 amino acids, which connects the glycosylated receptor region with the C-terminal end (Figure 2), is composed solely of nonpolar residues, and it is logical to suggest that this segment is the part of glycophorin that interacts with the lipids of the membrane.

Some Integral Membrane Proteins Span the Lipid Bilayer

There is a considerable amount of experimental data in support of the idea that glycophorin A, and other integral membrane proteins of the red cell, are in a transmembrane configuration. This idea was originally based on the attempts to differentially label portions of the polypeptide chain in intact cell membranes and from the membrane preparations that resulted from osmotic lysis. Bretscher (13) originally showed that a segment of the polypeptide chain of glycophorin A was not accessible to labeling by a radioactive isotope introduced outside intact cells; however, this inaccessible segment could be labeled when the cell membranes were damaged or rendered permeable to the reagent. One interpretation of this experiment was that part of the polypeptide chain of the molecule extends outside the intact red cell, and another part is either buried within the membrane or situated in the cytoplasmic compartment of the cell. This experiment was repeated in several laboratories using a gentler labeling procedure, lactoperoxidase iodination.

In theory, lactoperoxidase iodination should be an effective probe for analyzing the orientation of glycophorin A, since this molecule has four tyrosines, three of which are located in the glycosylated portion of the polypeptide chain, while the fourth is close to the C-terminal end. Thus, three tyrosines should be labeled when intact cells are incubated with lactoperoxidase, while the fourth, located at position 93, should not be labeled unless the permeability of the membrane is broken. Several investigators have reported the expected results (14, 15), although other investigators were not able to reproduce these findings (16, 17).

In the light of the controversy surrounding the results of radiolabeling, we recently reinvestigated this problem and attempted to study the orientation of glycophorin A in intact red cells using ferritin-conjugated antibodies directed against specific polypeptide segments of glycophorin A.

Antibodies prepared against a 17-amino-acid peptide derived from the C-terminal end of this molecule localized uniformly along the inner surfaces of intact red blood cells (18). This was achieved by incubating frozen sections of glutaraldehyde-fixed red cells with ferritin-conjugated antibodies.

Comparable radiolabeling studies have shown that the band 3 protein also assumes a transmembrane orientation while in the red cell membrane. The fact that there are two major integral proteins of the red cell membrane and both have a transmembrane orientation suggests that perhaps all integral membrane proteins are transmembrane. This orientation might be the result of some special biosynthetic mechanisms responsible for membrane protein synthesis or it might be related to the functions of integral proteins. However, we cannot draw any conclusions until we find out whether integral membrane proteins of other cells are also transmembrane. It will also be important for us to have a better idea of how a transmembrane orientation contributes to the functional properties of these molecules.

Membrane Glycoproteins May Exist as Multimeric Complexes

Recent studies suggest that some membrane glycoproteins have a remarkable capacity to form multimeric complexes in the presence of sodium dodecyl sulfate (SDS) (19, 20). Almost all glycophorin preparations analyzed by SDS acrylamide gels contain multiple PAS-staining bands, usually designated PAS-1, -2, and -3. These bands correspond to molecular weights of 83,000, 45,000, and 25,000 when they are compared with the mobilities of standard proteins. However, we are not sure that these values represent the true molecular weights of the glycoproteins, since they are known to migrate anomalously on SDS gels (21). PAS-1 is the predominant form and represents approximately 75% of the total.

When this pattern was first obtained, it was not clear whether the multiple bands represented a series of chemically distinct polypeptide chains, or whether the smaller PAS-staining bands represented degradation products of the larger component. In a series of recent studies we showed that two of the PAS-staining bands (PAS-1 and PAS-2) were interconvertible, and their relative amounts depended on the conditions used to prepare the glycoproteins for SDS electrophoresis. Glycophorin A appears to exist as a dimeric form, which corresponds to PAS-1, and this dimeric form seems to be stabilized by noncovalent associations between hydrophobic segments of its polypeptide chains (20). This association can be disrupted by heating the glycoproteins in SDS or by modifying the methionine located in position 81 by specific alkylation in the presence of denaturing agents (22).

The conditions for the selective alkylation are extremely stringent: High concentrations of alkylating agents must be used in the presence of either urea or guanidine, and the glycoprotein must have been previously delipidated with organic solvents. Since the presence of either lipid or SDS interferes with the alkylation of methionine 81, and in so doing renders the molecular aggregate less susceptible to dissociation, it is conceivable that when the molecule is oriented in the intact cell membrane, the surrounding membrane lipids serve a similar function. On the basis of this, we might speculate that glycophorin A actually exists as dimeric, or possibly, even multimeric forms in situ. If this proves to be true, then it is possible for multimer-monomer association and dissociation reactions to take place in membranes, which could play a role in regulating the functions of these macromolecules. This hypothetical idea is consistent with recent studies on the apparent mobility of membrane components and the important role the lipid matrix may play in regulating this process.

Band 3 also seems to exist in the form of a dimer held together by noncovalent associations (29). Band 3 has a particularly reactive sulfhydryl group on its cytoplasmic segment, which can be oxidized to form band 3 dimers held together by a disulfide linkage (29). It is conceivable that the oligomeric state of band 3 can be influenced by the oxidation-reduction conditions inside the cytoplasm of the intact red cell.

The ability of membrane glycoproteins to aggregate reversibly could have great physiologic implications, if the molecules function as receptors for hormones and other ligands. The formation (or dissociation) of oligomers could serve as an on-off switching mechanism, if, for example, hormone activation required some specific multimeric form. Similarly, changes in the aggregation state of membrane glycoproteins must also have marked effects on the antigenic properties of the external position of such molecules. Neoantigens could be created by the close proximity of the receptor domains of glycoproteins brought together in the process of creating multimeric forms. The potential for creating a large number of antigenic forms exists, if different glycoproteins are able to form heteroaggregates. Clearly the factors that regulate the formation of glycoprotein complexes must be understood before we can begin to approach these questions.

MEMBRANE PROTEINS ARE DISTRIBUTED IN A MOSAIC: SOME MAY BE MORE MOBILE THAN OTHERS

One of the most intriguing and still largely unanswered questions in membrane biology concerns the three-dimensional arrangement of proteins at the cell surface. Do membrane proteins occupy fixed positions relative to some internal cytoplasmic structure, or are they in continuous motion, constantly changing their positions within the bilayer? One of the earliest suggestions concerning the arrangement of membrane proteins was that monomolecular sheets of polypeptide coated the phospholipid polar groups of the lipid bilayer. For many reasons, this idea now seems unlikely. Most of the evidence suggests that the bulk of the red cell membrane proteins exist as discrete macromolecular complexes, which are attached to the lipid bilayer by insertion of hydrophobic segments into the hydrocarbon interior (like glycophorin A) or are bound to polar groups of lipids electrostatically.

Our conceptions about the arrangement of proteins in membranes have also been heavily influenced by the spectacular experiments demonstrating membrane fluidity and phospholipid mobility described above. Since the lipid matrix in which the protein molecules must be inserted is in a constant state of flux, many have reasoned that protein molecules are probably also in a mobile state, although it is not clear whether they are simply floating passively in the lipid sea or are directed by some other agents independent of the surrounding lipids.

A vivid demonstration of the fact that some membrane proteins can be mobilized by external forces has been provided by the results of applying multivalent ligands to lymphocytes and other cells in suspension. Appropriately labeled ligands form patches and caps on such cells within minutes after their application. Other evidence for the mobility of surface components comes from cell fusion studies that show that surface antigens can freely intermix over the combined surfaces of hybrid cells at a remarkably rapid rate (23). Both sets of observations demonstrate rather unequivocally that certain types of surface macromolecules are capable of moving within the plane of the membrane. Unfortunately, the dramatic nature of these experiments may be over-emphasizing the potential importance of the mobility of membrane proteins. It is likely that only certain types of membrane proteins are completely mobile, while others may be more or less in a fixed position at the cell surface relative to some cytoplasmic structures. We still do not know whether any proteins in the human red cell membrane are potentially mobile, or whether all of the major integral membrane proteins are firmly fixed at their respective sites.

Two of the most prominent integral proteins of the red cell membrane, band 3 and glycophorin A, probably are associated with the intramembranous particles seen by freeze-etching (24, 25). Since these particles do not appear to move within the plane of the intact membrane (based on their inability to patch or cap by the usual techniques), it is reasonable to conclude that these proteins are not extremely mobile. The intramembranous particles are movable, however, when osmotically lysed membranes are incubated with protease (24) or pH-5.5 buffers (26).

Integral Membrane Protein Interaction with Other Membrane Components

There have been several recent provocative studies purporting to show that glycophorin A and band 3 may have specific interactions with other membrane proteins. In particular, it has been suggested that the buried or cytoplasmic segment of glycophorin A may have the capacity to interact with the spectrin polymers, and the resulting complex may have some important function in regulating the stability of the membrane or in determining the relative positions of different membrane proteins. This exciting idea is based on the capacity of antispectrin antibodies to modify the topographical distribution of glycophorin A molecules (27), and on recent attempts to modify the distribution of intramembranous complexes by manipulating the polymeric state of spectrin.

Branton and co-workers (26, 28, 30) confirmed that incubation of red blood cell ghost membranes at pH 5.5 caused the reversible aggregation of the intramembranous particles, but they also showed, that this effect only occurred if the ghost membranes were partially depleted of their spectrin. They reason that spectrin normally restrains particle mobility, and shifts occur in spectrin-depleted membranes at the isoelectric point of spectrin because the residual aggregated spectrin can rearrange the intramembranous particles without opposition.

Yu & Branton (31) also showed that artificial reconstituted liposomes containing band 3, spectrin, and band 5 (actin) could be formed, and intramembranous particles would aggregate when the liposomes were incubated at pH 5.5. This remarkable result is the first demonstration that the components involved in the formation and regulation of the intramembranous particles can be dissociated and reconstituted into chemically defined liposomes. The authors note, however, that the components used to prepare the reconstituted vesicles were not completely characterized, and thus they do not rule out the participation of other proteins in the binding of spectrin to the membranes. Bennett & Branton (32) recently described conditions for the binding of purified spectrin back onto the inner surfaces of red blood cell ghost membranes through use of inside-out vesicles, and they found that neither glycophorin A nor band 3 were essential for this process.

Many investigators have found that the shape and deformability of the red cell membrane is related in some as yet undefined way to the ATP and calcium content of the cell (33–35). Sheetz & Singer (36) found that red blood cell ghosts underwent a shape change in the presence of salt solutions. This change required ATP and was enhanced by antispectrin antibodies. They attribute this effect to the crosslinking or polymerization of spectrin that is coupled to the hydrolysis of ATP. The process is enhanced by antispectrin antibodies as the latter further promote spectrin-spectrin associations.

Birchmeier & Singer (37) also found that the ATP utilized during the shape change of the red blood cell membranes was involved in the phosphorylation of band 2 of spectrin rather than serving as a substrate for a myosin-like ATPase. These investigators showed that incorporation of phosphatases inside red blood cell ghost membranes during osmotic lysis caused a reversal of the shape change effected by incubating the membranes with ATP.

These recent studies provide convincing evidence that spectrin plays a major role in regulating the shape and macromolecular topography of the red cell membrane. It is also clear that further insight into the mechanisms behind these processes, and their physiological and pathological implications, will only be achieved when we have a much clearer idea of the molecular properties of each of the interacting units.

SUMMARY

Our understanding of the molecular organization of even the simplest mammalian cell membrane—that of the red blood cell—is still incomplete, yet we are reasonably sure of where and how the major components are arranged. The so-called integral membrane proteins are the most likely candidates to serve as receptors and transport sites of surface membranes, and these may be organized as macromolecular complexes with parts of their polypeptides in contact with both sides of the bilayer. These complexes may be either mobile or fixed, and if the latter, perhaps by specific interactions with other membrane proteins.

The exposed segments of such glycoproteins could have recognition sites that confer cell, tissue, and/or species specificity created by oligosaccharides attached to the peptide backbone, or by specific amino acid sequences, or a combination of both.

Literature Cited

1. Branton, D. 1969. Membrane structure. *Ann. Rev. Plant Physiol.* 20:209
2. Edidin, M. 1974. Rotational and translational diffusion in membranes. *Ann. Rev. Biophys. Bioeng.* 3:179–201
3. Zwaal, R. F. A., Roelofsen, B., Colley, C. M. 1973. Localization of red cell membrane constituents. *Biochim. Biophys. Acta. 300:159–82*
4. Fairbanks, B., Steck, T. L., Wallach, D. F. H. 1971. Electrophoretic analysis of the major polypeptides of the human erythrocyte membrane. *Biochemistry* 10:2606–17
5. Singer, S. J. 1974. The molecular organization of membranes. *Ann. Rev. Biochem.* 43:805–33
6. Marchesi, V. T., Steers, E. 1968. Selective solubilization of a protein component of the red cell membrane. *Science* 159:203–4
7. Juliano, R. L. 1973. The proteins of the erythrocyte membrane. *Biochim. Biophys. Acta.* 300:341–78
8. Steck, T. L. 1974. The organization of proteins in the human red blood cell membrane. *J. Cell Biol.* 62:1–19
9. Marchesi, V. T. 1975. Biochemistry of cell walls and membranes. In *MTP International Review of Science Biochemistry*, ed. C. F. Fox, Ser. 1. Vol. 2., p. 123. Baltimore: Univ. Park
10. Tomita, M., Marchesi, V. T. 1975. Amino-acid sequence and oligosaccharide attachment sites of human erythrocyte glycophorin. *Proc. Natl. Acad. Sci. USA* 72:2964–68
11. Kornfeld, R., Kornfeld, S. 1970. The structure of a phytohemagglutinin receptor site from human erythrocytes. *J. Biol. Chem.* 245:2536–45
12. Thomas, D. B., Winzler, R. J. 1971. Structure of glycoproteins of human erythrocytes. *Biochem. J.* 124:55–59
13. Bretscher, M. S. 1971. Major human erythrocyte glycoprotein spans the cell membrane. *Nature New Biol.* 231:229–32
14. Segrest, J. P., Kahane, I., Jackson, R. L., Marchesi, V. T. 1973. Major glycoprotein of the human erythrocyte membrane evidence for an amphipathic molecular structure. *Arch. Biochem. Biophys.* 155:167–83
15. Morrison, M., Mueller, T. J., Huber, C. T. 1974. Transmembrane orientation of the glycoproteins in normal human erythrocytes. *J. Biol. Chem.* 249:2658–60
16. Shin, B. C., Carraway, K. L. 1974. Lactoperoxidase labeling of erythrocyte membranes from the inside and outside. *Biochim. Biophys. Acta.* 345:141
17. Reichstein, E., Blostein, R. 1975. Arrangement of human erythrocyte membrane proteins. *J. Biol. Chem.* 250:6256–63
18. Cotmore, S., Furthmayr, H., Marchesi, V. T. 1977. Immunochemical evidence for the transmembrane orientation of glycophorin A: localization of ferritin-antibody conjugates in intact cells. *J. Mol. Biol.* 113:539–53
19. Marton, L. S. G., Garvin, J. E. 1973. Subunit structure of the major human erythrocyte glycoprotein: depolymerization by heating ghosts with sodium dodecyl sulfate. *Biochem. Biophys. Res. Commun.* 52:1457–62
20. Furthmayr, H., Marchesi, V. T. 1976. Subunit structure of human erythrocyte glycophorin A. *Biochemistry* 15:1137–44
21. Segrest, J. P., Jackson, R. L., Andrews, E. P., Marchesi, V. T. 1971. Human erythrocyte membrane glycoprotein: a re-evaluation of the molecular weight as determined by SDS polyacrylamide gel electrophoresis. *Biochem. Biophys. Res. Commun.* 44:390–95
22. Silverberg, M., Furthmayr, H., Marchesi, V. T. 1976. The effect of carboxymethylating a single methi-

onine residue on the subunit interaction of glycophorin A. *Biochemistry* 15: 1448–54

23. Frye, L. D., Edidin, M. 1970. The rapid intermixing of cell surface antigens after formation of mouse human heterakaryons. *J. Cell Sci.* 7: 319–35

24. Tillack, T. W., Scott, R. E., Marchesi, V. T. 1972. The structure of erythrocyte membranes studies by freeze etching. *J. Exp. Med.* 135: 1209–27

25. Nicolson, G. L., Singer, S. J. 1974. The distribution and asymmetry of mammalian cell surface saccharides utilizing ferritin-conjugated plant agglutinins as specific saccharide stains. *J. Cell Biol.* 60: 236–48

26. Elgsaeter, A., Branton, D. 1974. Intramembrane particle aggregation in erythrocyte ghosts. *J. Cell Biol.* 63: 1018–36

27. Nicolson, G. L., Painter, R. G. 1973. Anionic sites of human erythrocyte membranes. *J. Cell Biol.* 59: 395–406

28. Elgsaeter, A., Shotton, D. M., Branton, D. 1976. Intramembrane particle aggregation in erythrocyte. *Biochim. Biophys. Acta.* 426: 101–22

29. Steck, T. L. 1972. Cross-linking the major proteins of the isolated erythrocyte membrane. *J. Mol. Biol.* 66: 295–305

30. Shotton, D. M., Elgsaeter, A., Branton, D. 1975. The influence of spectrin on particle aggregation, surface protein distribution and lipid vesicle blebbing in erythrocyte

ghosts. *J. Cell Biol.* 67: 397a

31. Yu, J., Branton, D. 1976. Reconstitution of intramembrane particles in recombinants of erythrocyte protein band 3 and lipid: effects of spectrin-action association. *Proc. Natl. Acad. Sci. USA* 73: 3891–95

32. Bennett, V., Branton, D. 1977. Selective association of spectrin with the cytoplasmic surface of human erythrocyte plasma membranes. *J. Biol. Chem.* 252: 2753–63

33. Weed, R. I., Lacelle, P. L. 1969. *Red Cell Membrane: Structure and Function.* ed. G. A. Jamieson, T. J. Greenwalt, pp. 318–338. Philadelphia: Lippincott

34. Weed, R. I., Lacelle, P. L., Merrill, E. W. 1969. Metabolic dependence of red cell deformability. *J. Clin. Invest.* 48: 795–809

35. Kirkpatrick, F. H. 1976. Spectrin: Current understanding of its physical, biochemical, and functional properties. *Life Sci.* 19: 1–18

36. Sheetz, M. P., Singer, S. J. 1977. On the mechanism of ATP-induced shape changes in human erythrocyte membranes. I. The role of spectrin complex. *J. Cell Biol.* 73: 638–46

37. Birchmeier, W., Singer, S. J. 1977. On the mechanism of ATP-induced shape changes in human erythrocyte membranes. II. The role of ATP. *J. Cell Biol.* 73: 647–59

38. Gorter, E., Grendel, F. 1925. On bimolecular layers of lipoids on the chromocytes of the blood. *J. Exp. Med.* xli: 439–43

Ann. Rev. Biochem. 1977. 46:49–67

IMMUNOLOGICAL PROPERTIES OF MODEL MEMBRANES

❖939

Stephen C. Kinsky and Robert A. Nicolotti

Departments of Biological Chemistry and Pharmacology,
Washington University School of Medicine, St. Louis, Missouri 63110

CONTENTS

PERSPECTIVES AND SUMMARY

Since the original description of thin lipid bilayer films (1) and liposomes (2), these model membranes have been extensively exploited as experimental tools in a number of biological disciplines. This article is restricted to just two immunological applications. The first section is devoted to efferent responses—specifically, the ability of these model membranes to substitute for natural membranes in immune cytolytic phenomena, and the information derived from these studies regarding lytic mechanism. The second section considers afferent responses—in particular, the ability of liposomes

8243-2502/80/0310-0071$01.00

49

to induce antibody formation and delayed hypersensitivity reactions, and the unique features of liposomes that distinguish them from conventional immunogens.

EFFERENT RESPONSES

Cytolysis by immunologic agents is often designated as "humoral" if only soluble factors are involved and "cell mediated" if cells are obligatory participants. This classification is, therefore, employed here in regard to the efferent responses of model membranes.

Humoral (Complement-Mediated) Lysis

CLASSICAL PATHWAY   Traditionally, complement (C) is defined as a system of nine serum protein components that react in a specific order (C1, C4, C2, C3, C5, C6, C7, C8, C9) to produce lysis of target cells. The distinguishing feature of this classical pathway is the activation of the complement sequence by appropriate antigen-antibody complexes on the cell membrane surface. Although we shall have occasion to refer to certain aspects of the complement cascade, a detailed discussion is unnecessary because this topic has been recently reviewed in this series (3).

In 1968, two reports appeared documenting changes in model membrane permeability that mimic immune damage by the classical pathway. Barfort et al (4) generated thin lipid bilayers from a mixture of sphingomyelin and α-tocopherol and observed that electrical resistance rapidly decreased by approximately two orders of magnitude when protein antigens (e.g. lysozyme, insulin, ribonuclease) and the corresponding antisera were added to opposite sides of the film. Aging or heat treatment (56°C, 30 min) of the antisera abolished their ability to alter resistance; this capacity could be restored by the addition of unheated guinea pig serum (GPS) as source of complement. Haxby et al (5) prepared liposomes from a total lipid extract of sheep erythrocyte membranes and observed 65% release of trapped glucose marker in the presence of GPS and rabbit antisheep erythrocyte antiserum (RAS) as source of antibodies. Negligible glucose release occurred if GPS had been heated as above to destroy hemolytic complement activity, or if RAS was replaced by serum from unimmunized rabbits. Subsequent investigations have concentrated on liposomes [see (6) for a review of the earlier literature]; the effect of antibody-complement on thin lipid-bilayer films has lain dormant until only recently (see below).

   Sheep lipid liposomes, which had bound antisheep erythrocyte antibodies, fixed guinea pig or human complement as measured by either reduction of hemolytic titer (7) or protein absorption by the liposomes (8). Furthermore, using purified components of human complement and specific anti-component antibodies as inhibitors, Haxby et al showed that immune damage of the liposomes involved the same classical sequence responsible for the antibody-induced cytolysis of cells (9). Thus, glucose release was absolutely dependent on C2 and C8 and markedly stimulated by C9. Studies by a number of laboratories have since provided additional evidence that sheep lipid liposomes can release a variety of markers upon incubation with RAS and either whole guinea pig, human, or rabbit serum as source of complement (10, 11).

Sheep erythrocyte membrane lipids were initially employed for the generation of liposomes because the extract contains Forssman antigen [see (12) for structure], and RAS possesses antibodies directed against this glycolipid. It was anticipated that the nonpolar (ceramide) region of Forssman antigen would anchor this compound in the liposomal bilayers in a manner that leaves the polar portion (bearing the oligosaccharide antigenic determinants) accessible to anti-Forssman antibodies; immune complexes formed on the liposomal surface would, therefore, activate the classical complement sequence resulting in damage to the model membrane. This rationale was also validated by the demonstration (13) that immunologically sensitive liposomes could be prepared by addition of pure Forssman antigen to a mixture containing a phospholipid (either lecithin or sphingomyelin), a sterol (cholesterol), and a charged amphiphile (dicetylphosphate for negative liposomes, stearylamine for positive liposomes) in molar ratios of 2:1.5:0.2, respectively. These results constituted the first indication that lipids in bilayer configuration could alone serve as target for complement.

Subsequent experiments (14–16) showed that other mammalian ceramides besides Forssman antigen (e.g. globoside I, galactocerebroside), as well as bacterial lipopolysaccharides and lipid A (isolated from either S or R forms of *Salmonella*), could be incorporated into liposomes of defined composition; these model membranes also released up to 70% of their trapped glucose when incubated with antibodies of the appropriate specificity and a source of complement. The list of naturally occurring lipid antigens capable of rendering liposomes susceptible to antibody-complement has now been extended considerably to include, for example, gangliosides and mono- or digalactosyl diglycerides (17), and cardiolipin (18).

Synthetic amphipathic haptens can also be employed for this purpose as initially shown by a comparative study (19) of the 2,4-dinitrophenyl derivatives of phosphatidylethanolamine (Dnp-PE), lysophosphatidylethanolamine (Dnp-lysoPE), and glycerophosphorylethanolamine (Dnp-GPE). Dnp-PE and Dnp-lysoPE were equally effective in actively sensitizing liposomes to immune damage as evidenced by glucose release upon incubation with appropriate anti-Dnp antibodies (raised in rabbits immunized with either dinitrophenylated hemocyanin or ovalbumin; see below) and guinea pig complement. Active sensitization means that the derivatives were present at the time the lipids were dispersed in the swelling (marker) solution to generate the model membranes. In contrast, liposomes prepared in the presence of Dnp-GPE, which were also visibly yellow, did not release glucose under the same conditions. This could be attributed to the fact that Dnp-GPE is essentially nonamphipathic due to removal of both esterified fatty acids; hence, this completely water-soluble compound is not inserted in the bilayers, but is trapped in the aqueous liposomal compartments where it is inaccessible to anti-Dnp antibodies.

An additional property of Dnp-lysoPE was its ability to passively sensitize liposomes; that is, it could be added after formation of the model membranes from the basic lipid mixture containing lecithin (or sphingomyelin), cholesterol, and dicetylphosphate (19). Passive sensitization of liposomes to antibody-complement has not been obtained with mammalian ceramides (13) or bacterial lipopolysaccharides, with the notable exception of lipopolysaccharides that have been treated with dilute alkali to remove the esterified fatty acids attached to the lipid A moiety (15, 16). Because both Dnp-lysoPE and saponified lipopolysaccharide are more water-soluble than the parent compounds (i.e. Dnp-PE and untreated lipopolysaccharide), it seems likely that their ability to be incorporated into preformed lipid bilayers may reflect a higher critical micelle concentration.

Complement-dependent glucose release from liposomes sensitized by Dnp-PE occurred only if the reaction was initiated by high-affinity rabbit IgG anti-Dnp antibodies with an association constant (K_0) for ϵ-Dnp-lysine of 10^8 liters mole^{-1} (19). Accordingly, Six et al (20) synthesized dinitrophenyl-ϵ-amino-caproylphosphatidylethanolamine (Dnp-Cap-PE; see Figure 1) because the polar region of this compound has a greater structural similarity to the predominant antigenic determinants (ϵ-Dnp-lysine residues) in the proteins used for immunization. Dnp-Cap-PE proved far more effective than Dnp-PE in sensitizing liposomes to immune damage in the presence of high-affinity antibodies. For example, by using this derivative and a fluorometric assay, it was possible to demonstrate 100% release of trapped marker (umbelliferone phosphate) from unilamellar vesicles (21).

Moreover, liposomes sensitized by Dnp-Cap-PE released glucose in the presence of low-affinity rabbit IgG and IgM anti-Dnp antibodies (K_0 of 10^5 liters mole^{-1}) (20). Two observations merit particular emphasis: (a) less IgM than IgG (on either a weight or molar basis) was required to initiate marker release from liposomes containing a constant amount of Dnp-Cap-PE, and (b) liposomes could be prepared with a Dnp-Cap-PE content so low that only IgM antibodies promoted glucose release. It is now

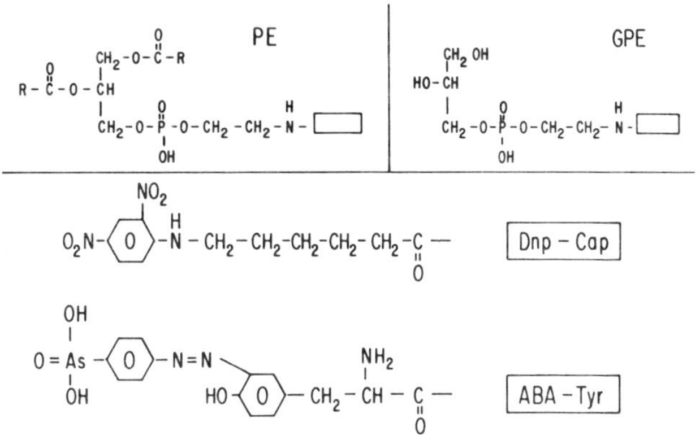

PE   GPE

$$R-\overset{O}{\overset{\|}{C}}-O-\overset{\overset{\displaystyle CH_2-O-\overset{O}{\overset{\|}{C}}-R}{|}}{\underset{\underset{\displaystyle OH}{|}}{CH}}-\overset{H}{O-CH_2-CH_2-N-\boxed{}}$$

$$HO-\overset{\overset{\displaystyle CH_2\,OH}{|}}{\underset{\underset{\displaystyle OH}{|}}{CH}}\quad CH_2-O-\overset{O}{\overset{\|}{P}}-O-CH_2-CH_2-\overset{H}{N}-\boxed{}$$

$$O_2N-\overset{\overset{\displaystyle NO_2}{|}}{\underset{}{\langle O\rangle}}-\overset{H}{N}-CH_2-CH_2-CH_2-CH_2-CH_2-\overset{O}{\overset{\|}{C}}-\qquad \boxed{Dnp-Cap}$$

$$O=\overset{\overset{\displaystyle OH}{|}}{\underset{\underset{\displaystyle OH}{|}}{As}}-\langle O\rangle-N=N \diagdown \quad HO\langle O\rangle-CH_2-\overset{\overset{\displaystyle NH_2}{|}}{CH}-\overset{O}{\overset{\|}{C}}-\qquad \boxed{ABA-Tyr}$$

Figure 1 Structures of phosphatidylethanolamine (PE) and glycerophosphoryl-ethanolamine (GPE) derivatives in which the amino (N) group is substituted with either a 2,4-dinitrophenyl-ε-aminocaproyl (Dnp-Cap) or a mono(p-azobenzenearsonic acid)tyrosyl (ABA-Tyr) residue. The corresponding N-substituted derivatives of lysophosphatidylethanolamine (lysoPE) lack the esterified fatty acid [RC(=O)O] at the 2 position of glycerol (not shown).

commonly believed that a single antigen-antibody complex is able to activate the complement sequence when formed with IgM antibodies, whereas a minimum of two antigen-antibody complexes in close proximity are necessary if the latter involves IgG antibodies. The above results appear to be the liposomal counterpart of this phenomenon.

In addition to immunoglobulin class and affinity for the determinant, the composition of the lipid bilayer is a significant factor. An influence of phospholipid was initially revealed by the observation that liposomes containing egg lecithin released more glucose than those prepared with beef sphingomyelin, regardless of whether they were actively sensitized with ceramide antigens (14), lipopolysaccharide (15), or lipid A (16), or passively sensitized with Dnp-lysoPE (19). This was originally attributed to a greater inherent stability of sphingomyelin-cholesterol-dicetylphosphate liposomes, although the possibility that the determinants in egg lecithin liposomes may be more accessible to antibodies could not be excluded (14). The second alternative is supported by the experiments of Alving et al (17) using galactocerebroside-sensitized liposomes prepared either with beef sphingomyelin (SM) or with synthetic dimyristoyl (DMPC), dipalmitoyl (DPPC), or distearoyl (DSPC) phosphatidylcholines. The extent of glucose release was in the order DMPC > DPPC > DSPC > SM, suggesting that the antibody-binding site was more deeply buried in bilayers with longer hydrocarbon chains. This would also be consistent with the observation that the influence of fatty acid chain length was less pronounced when the liposomes were sensitized with glycolipid antigens (e.g. ganglioside or Forssman) having a more extended hydrophylic determinant than galactocerebroside (17, 22).

However, steric hindrance per se may not be responsible since the transition temperatures of DMPC (23°C), DPPC (41°C), and DSPC (57°C) differ markedly. Furthermore, the general "fluidizing" and "condensing" effects of cholesterol below and above the transition temperature, respectively, play an important role. Kitagawa & Inoue (23) have shown that glucose release from Forssman-sensitized DPPC liposomes, which were prepared without cholesterol, increased with temperature over the range 15°C to 35°C. In contrast, when 50 mole % cholesterol was incorporated into the liposomes, little (if any) temperature dependence was apparent. These observations were interpreted as indicating that susceptibility to immune damage requires a certain degree of lipid fluidity and were consistent with a proposal that lysis involved penetration of a complement component(s) into the bilayer (see below).

Subsequent experiments by Humphries & McConnell (18), using cardiolipin-sensitized DMPC and DPPC liposomes, revealed another role for cholesterol. In the presence of human syphilitic serum as source of anticardiolipin antibodies (primarily IgM), complement was not fixed under a variety of conditions unless more than 35 mole % cholesterol was incorporated. A phase diagram was constructed showing that, at mole fractions greater than this value, the antigen may have become immobilized in a relatively pure solid region or may have formed concentrated patches with the sterol. The authors suggest that in this state cardiolipin may more readily bind several sites on the antibody molecule, i.e. the net result of cholesterol incorporation is an increase in the effective valency of the antigen. This conclusion is not at variance with the evidence that immune damage may be contingent on bilayer fluidity because complement activation (as measured by fixation) is not necessarily synonymous with complement attack. Conditions favoring the initiation of the classical sequence may differ from those conducive to lysis.

ALTERNATIVE PATHWAY; REACTIVE LYSIS   The classical pathway is not the sole means by which the complement components eventually exert a variety of effector functions including membrane damage. In recent years, an alternative pathway has been elucidated that has resurrected many of the factors implicated in the original properdin system (3, 24). The distinguishing feature of this alternative pathway is that it bypasses the requirement for antigen-antibody complexes and the early components in the classical sequence (C1, C4, C2) to activate C3 and subsequently C5 through C9.

The phenomenon of "reactive lysis," which has been extensively studied by Thompson & Lachmann (25), shares this property with the alternative pathway. They have been able to isolate a complex of activated C5 and C6 from sera; this complex is unable to produce lysis of erythrocytes when incubated with C7 alone. Lysis is, however, observed upon the addition of C8 and C9. Lachmann et al (26) have shown that reactive lysis can also be duplicated with egg lecithin liposomes that were either positively or negatively charged; maximal release of trapped markers (chromate or glucose) required the presence of the activated C5,6 complex plus C7, C8, and C9. Additional studies using this system are described in the following sections.

MECHANISM   Two theories have long prevailed in the literature on complement to explain how the terminal complement components (i.e. C8 and/or C9) may produce membrane damage. The first assumes that their activation stimulates a latent membrane-localized autolytic enzyme and seems plausible because such enzymes are ubiquitous in prokaryotic and eukaryotic cells. The second assumes that the terminal components acquire an enzymatic property resulting in degradation of some membrane constituent and is predicated on the massive evidence that activation of the early components (C1 through C5) in the classical sequence occurs via generation of proteolytic enzyme activities (3). As regards both of these hypotheses, it should again be emphasized that immunologically sensitive liposomes can be prepared from lipids alone. This fact not only argues against the involvement of an endogenous enzyme, but also precludes endogenous membrane proteins as substrates for the putative enzyme derived from the terminal complement components.

The only possible substrate is phospholipid because this is the sole liposomal constituent invariably present in the membranes of cells susceptible to immune damage by either the classical or the alternative pathway. Inoue & Kinsky (27) examined the fate of ^{32}P-labeled rat lecithin and sphingomyelin that were used separately to prepare liposomes sensitized with either Forssman antigen or globoside I. After incubation with antibody-complement (50–80% glucose release), all of the counts could be extracted with chloroform-methanol. Chromatographic analysis of the extracts showed that at least 98% of the recovered radioactivity was present in the form in which it had been originally incorporated into liposomes. The procedures employed were sufficiently sensitive to detect a 1% degradation of phospholipid, had any radioactive product been formed with mobilities similar to phosphatidic acid, lysolecithin, glycerophosphorylcholine, or sphingosylphosphorylcholine. These experiments suggested that complement-dependent marker release from liposomes and, by implication, immune cytolysis does not involve direct enzymatic attack. As an obvious alternative, it was proposed that activation of the terminal components results in the exposure of a hydrophobic region within these proteins (or liberation of a hydrophobic fragment) followed by insertion into the lipid bilayers so that the latter can no longer function as permeability barriers.

In the preceding investigation, control experiments were performed by incubation of liposomes containing radioactive lecithin with a commercial preparation of phospholipase C. Fifty percent glucose release (i.e. an amount comparable to that induced by antibody-complement) occurred when approximately 45% of the phospholipid had been degraded. Thus, measurable quantities of labeled phosphorylcholine should have been formed if activation of the terminal components had led to generation of enzymatic activity with properties analogous to exogenous phospholipase C. Moreover, it was observed that phospholipase C did not cause glucose release from liposomes prepared with sphingomyelin, although these liposomes were susceptible to damage by antibody-complement. Similar findings were subsequently reported by Hesketh et al (28). They also demonstrated that liposomes prepared with dipalmitoylphosphatidylcholine, which is not a substrate for phospholipase A, released glucose when incubated with anti-Forssman antibodies and guinea pig complement, or the components involved in reactive lysis.

The conclusion drawn from these experiments was nevertheless questionable for several reasons. Although pholpholipase A activity was originally excluded (5) because sphingomyelin contains fatty acids in amide linkage, the possibility remained that activation of the terminal components produced an enzyme with both esterolytic and amidolytic properites. As regards phospholipase C, the possibility existed that such activity generated in situ (i.e. on the membrane surface) may have better access to sphingomyelin than exogenous enzyme. Finally, the fact that phospholipase D has been exclusively isolated from plants did not rule out transient formation of this enzyme from the terminal components.

These alternatives were, however, eliminated by using synthetic phosphonyl and phosphinyl analogs of the naturally occurring phospholipids to prepare liposomes. In the initial experiments, the liposomes were sensitized with either Forssman antigen or lipopolysaccharide (29, 30); in a more recent study Dnp-Cap-PE was employed (31); in all cases, incubation with the appropriate antibodies and guinea pig complement resulted in glucose release comparable to that observed with lecithin or sphingomyelin liposomes. One of these analogs of lecithin possessed the following distinctive properties: (a) the aliphatic side chains were attached to the glycerol moiety via ether, instead of ester, linkages and hence were not susceptible to the action of either phospholipase A_1, A_2, or B; (b) the aliphatic side chains were saturated and, therefore, not liable to peroxidation; (c) the compound lacked the C–O–P bond cleaved by phospholipase C; and (d) it did not contain the P–O–C bond hydrolyzed by phospholipase D.

A discordant statement in a 1970 review (32) referred to a paper ("in press") showing that "C5–9, acting via a phospholipase C, disrupts liposomes;" we have not been able to locate this article. However, in 1973, Lachmann et al (33) described experiments on the reactive lysis of liposomes prepared with a mixture of ^{32}P-labeled yeast lecithin and rat liver lecithin esterified at the 2 position with ^{14}C-oleic acid. Experimental tubes contained liposomes incubated with the activated C5,6 complex plus C7, C8, and C9; control tubes contained liposomes incubated only with C8 and C9. In both cases, slightly more than 1% of the total radioactivity incorporated (^{32}P) remained in the aqueous phase, whereas greater than 99% (^{14}C) was recovered in the chloroform phase. In addition, the patterns of radioactivity distribution among water-soluble compounds (glycerophosphorylcholine, phosphorylcholine, glycerophosphate) and chloroform-soluble compounds (lecithin, lysolecithin, fatty acid) were the same in experimental and control situations. The authors concluded, therefore, that phospholipid hydrolysis is probably not responsible for lysis of liposomes and may be due to contamination of the complement components by phospholipases A and C.

ELECTRON MICROSCOPIC OBSERVATIONS; HOLE FORMATION   It is not yet known whether immune damage of liposomes involves the C5b–9 attack complex depicted by Müller-Eberhard (3), or the formation of "doughnuts" as suggested by Mayer and co-workers (34, 35), or an eclectic combination of these proposals. Both are compatible with, and in large measure based on, the preceding evidence that (a) lipids in bilayer configuration serve as the target for complement, and (b) complement-mediated lysis does not involve direct enzymatic action. Both also advocate insertion of one or more complement components into or through lipid bilayers leading to the production of transmembrane channels or holes.

One difference between these proposals is the greater emphasis that the doughnut hypothesis placed on the formation of rigid and stable holes to accommodate the electron microscopic observations of Humphrey & Dourmashkin (36). These investigators demonstrated the presence of negatively stained circular lesions (approximately 10 nm in diameter), surrounded by a light ring, in a variety of natural membranes after immune lysis. According to the doughnut model (34), the light ring was presumably composed of late-acting components embedded in the membrane with hydrophobic portions of these proteins on the exterior in contact with lipids, and hydrophilic portions in the interior forming a cylinder that permits passage of water-soluble substances.

However, comparable lesions have been also detected in cell membranes and liposomes after incubation with the polyene antibiotic, filipin, which is a nonprotein amphipathic lytic agent that interacts with cholesterol (37). Moreover, in regard to liposomes that have been treated with complement, there does not seem to be any reproducible correlation between the presence of these lesions and release of trapped marker. Thus, Lachmann et al (26, 33) have seen the lesions in lecithin liposomes subjected to reactive lysis, as have Hesketh et al (11) in sheep lipid liposomes incubated with RAS and either human or rabbit complement. In contrast, Knudson et al (10) were unable to demonstrate lesions in sheep lipid liposomes treated with RAS and guinea pig complement. This finding was essentially confirmed by Kataoka et al (38) using lecithin-cholesterol-dicetylphosphate liposomes sensitized with globoside I. In these experiments, the extremely rare appearance of rings (remotely resembling the lesions) could not be reconciled with the fact that antibody-complement consistently induced the parallel release of glucose and β-galactosidase (a protein of molecular weight 518,000 and dimensions similar to the lesions). Failure of some laboratories to find lesions has been attributed (11) to a possible reassembly of damaged liposomes into smaller fragments that do not attach to grids, but this would not explain why filipin-treated liposomes containing cholesterol invariably display the lesions (38). In addition, the lesions so far have not been detected in unilamellar vesicles incubated with antibody-complement under conditions leading to 100% marker release (H. R. Six, T. W. Tillack, S. C. Kinsky, unpublished observations).

Iles et al (39) have provided particularly convincing evidence that the lesions do not correspond to holes by freeze-etch and freeze-fracture examination of erythrocyte membranes. Their pictures clearly show that the lesions are raised rings on the external surface with a central depression parallel to the plane of the membrane; the cleavage face of the cytoplasmic leaflet appears normal. [Subsequent application (40) of the same techniques indicated that the lesions produced by filipin in erythrocytes and liposomes also cannot be equated with transverse holes.] They further demonstrated that, when erythrocytes were treated with antibody-complement in the presence of ferritin, this electron-dense protein could be detected in all of the lysed cells; however, if ferritin was added after completion of immune lysis, only 15% of the erythrocytes were permeated by the protein. These results suggest that the openings caused by complement are transient and/or can undergo rapid changes in size and shape.

Wobschall & McKeon (41) have recently described experiments that bear on this point using thin lipid-bilayer films exposed on opposite sides to whole bovine serum and rabbit anti-bovine serum as source of antigen and antibody plus complement, respectively. High concentrations of the immunologic reactants produced a rapid rise in conductance and eventual rupture of the film, whereas low concentrations induced either single or multiple step increases. A plot of mean step sizes as a function of salt concentration revealed proportionality to solution conductivity that was consistent with the formation of pores having an average diameter of 2.2 nm. The authors emphasize that this value is only a statistical approximation because the step sizes were not uniform and amplifier response time would not have detected opening and closing of pores faster than one step change per second.

This and an earlier investigation (4) are somewhat compromised because (a) the sources of antigen, antibody, and complement were extremely crude, and (b) unlike lipid antigens and synthetic amphipathic haptens that can be introduced as integral constituents of the model membrane, determinant density is difficult to control with protein antigens added after generation of the film. In spite of these limitations, subsequent experiments (42, 42a, 43), in which planar lipid bilayers were treated with purified complement components under conditions of reactive lysis, confirm the formation of channels.

ADDITIONAL APPLICATIONS   The efferent response of lipid-bilayer films potentially provides a means for detecting either antibodies or antigens (44, 45, 41), although this application so far has been primarily realized with liposomes. Marker release from appropriately sensitized liposomes has revealed (a) the formation of anti–lipid A antibodies in rabbits immunized with a lipid A–bovine serum albumin complex (16); (b) the formation of anti-cholesterol antibodies in rabbits immunized with human serum lipoproteins (46); (c) the existence of a Waldenstrom macroglobulin with anti-Forssman specificity (47, 22); and (d) the antigenicity, in rabbits, of sialoglycolipids isolated from sea urchin spermatozoa (48, 49) and, in monkeys of a lipid fraction from schistosomal worms (50). Two reports (51, 52) advocate the use of a spin-label marker (instead of glucose) to increase the sensitivity of such assays; at the moment, routine application of electron spin resonance is obviously limited by the expense of the spectrometer. A convenient radioimmunoprecipitation test for immunoglobulins against lipid antigens involves incubation of liposomes (containing ^{3}H-cholesterol and the appropriate antigen) with the putative source of antibodies; this is followed by precipitation of the liposome-immunoglobulin complex with heterologous polyvalent antiserum or class-specific antibodies (53).

Cell-Mediated Lysis

Henkart & Blumenthal (54) have recently demonstrated that the same strategy, which has exploited model membranes to study complement mechanism, may be applicable for investigating cell-mediated, antibody-dependent membrane damage. Marked increases in conductance were obtained after exposure of thin lipid-bilayer films (containing oxidized cholesterol and Dnp-PE) to purified rabbit IgG anti-trinitrophenyl antibodies followed by addition of human lymphocytes. Neither antibodies nor lymphocytes alone produced this effect. The lymphocytes apparently were attached to the Fc region of the antibodies on the surface of the bilayer because $F(ab)_2$ fragments and lymphocytes depleted of Fc receptor-bearing cells were inactive. Among several alternatives, Henkart & Blumenthal propose that the lymphocyte-induced increase in conductance probably reflects the formation of small channels, a conclusion analogous to that of Wobschall & McKeon regarding complement (41). These experiments are also particularly significant because they suggest the feasibility of preparing model membranes that might be targets for cell-mediated, antibody-independent damage.

AFFERENT RESPONSES

"Liposomal immunogenicity" is a field still in its infancy, yet there are already sufficient indications in the literature that this subject does not have the same meaning for all investigators. Interest in the immunogenicity of liposomes has developed in part because of the potential application of these model membranes as vehicles for the transport of therapeutic agents (e.g. drugs, enzymes) to specific target cells. However, the early anticipation (55, 56) that enclosure within the aqueous compartments of liposomes might, for example, minimize or prevent an immune response to a foreign protein has not fully materialized. Allison & Gregoriadis have shown that mice actually produced more antibodies against diphtheria toxoid after immunization with this antigen trapped inside negatively charged liposomes (57), although allergic manifestations (e.g. Arthus reaction, serum sickness) to subsequent challenges were mitigated by encapsulation of diphtheria toxoid in liposomes (58).

   At the risk of emphasizing the obvious, it should be stated that liposomes can be prepared without proteins or drugs, but not without lipids. Therefore, in the following sections, we have adopted a much narrower definition of liposomal immunogenicity as denoting the capacity of lipids to induce either a humoral or a cell-mediated response, and the effect that incorporation into liposomal bilayers has on these phenomena.

Humoral Immunity (Antibody Formation)

After purification, naturally occurring lipid antigens (e.g. glycolipids, cardiolipin, phosphatidylinositol) can function as haptens, but generally not as immunogens even when administered in complete Freund's adjuvant (CFA). Significant production of antibodies in response to these compounds usually requires immunization in CFA with either cell membranes, subcellular fractions, or a mixture of a micellar solution of the antigen with a heterologous protein carrier (59, 60). However, the common textbook generalization that pure lipids are not immunogenic is no longer valid. Ironically, this was first demonstrated with Dnp-Cap-PE which, as already mentioned, was originally designed solely as a synthetic amphipathic hapten that could replace natural antigens to render liposomes susceptible to damage by antibody-complement.

In the initial investigation (61), Dnp-Cap-PE (either free or incorporated into liposomes) was administered to guinea pigs in CFA via the footpads; antibody titer was determined 2–3 weeks later by hemagglutination assay. Dnp-Cap-PE per se (500 nmole) could induce some anti-Dnp antibodies, but a much greater response (titer of 2^9, equivalent to approximately 300 μg antibody per milliliter of serum) was obtained when the same amount was incorporated into sphingomyelin-cholesterol liposomes either negatively charged with dicetylphosphate or positively charged with stearylamine. Liposomes actively sensitized with Dnp-Cap-lysoPE were just as effective as those sensitized with Dnp-Cap-PE; however, no anti-Dnp antibodies were formed when the liposomes were prepared in the presence of Dnp-Cap-GPE. These results demonstrate that a humoral response to liposomes requires incorporation of an amphipathic derivative, i.e. the same structural features that are necessary to actively sensitize liposomes to lysis by antibody-complement [cf earlier discussion of (19)].

Liposomes made under passive sensitization conditions with Dnp-Cap-PE yielded the same titer as the free derivative when given in CFA (61). The enhanced immunogenicity of liposomes is, therefore, not simply due to the presence of sphingomyelin, cholesterol, and charged amphiphile (i.e. the basic liposomal constituents). Moreover, these results suggest that liposomal structure has largely survived emulsification with the adjuvant; if the sphingomyelin liposomes had been extensively disrupted, actively and passively sensitized liposomes should be equally potent immunogens. The ability to induce antibody formation was not a peculiar property of Dnp-Cap-Pe or Dnp-Cap-lysoPE because guinea pigs immunized with liposomes, which have been actively sensitized with the fluorescein isothiocyanate conjugate of PE, elaborated anti-fluorescein antibodies (61).

In a subsequent study (62), the response of guinea pigs to liposomes sensitized with Dnp-Cap-PE was characterized at both the cellular and serologic levels. At various times following primary immunization, the frequency of IgM (direct) and IgG (indirect) plaque-forming cells (PFC) paralleled the appearance of anti-Dnp antibodies in the serum. Plaque inhibition by ε-Dnp-lysine revealed that the PFC induced by liposomes encompassed a much narrower range of avidity groups than those obtained after immunization with dinitrophenylated proteins. In this regard, the PFC produced in response to liposomes resembled a mouse plasmacytoma (MOPC-315), which secretes a myeloma protein with affinity for dinitrophenyl groups. The restricted nature of the serum IgG anti-Dnp antibodies following liposomal immunization was also confirmed by isoelectric focusing.

Cell-Mediated Immunity (Delayed Hypersensitivity Reactions)

In the course of the preceding investigations, guinea pigs were challenged, at appropriate intervals after primary immunization, by intradermal injection into depilated back sites of Dnp-Cap-PE (either free or incorporated into liposomes), various dinitrophenylated proteins, or dinitrofluorobenzene. None of these substances elicited a delayed hypersensitivity reaction. Therefore, another N-substituted PE derivative was synthesized to determine whether liposomal immunogenicity was limited exclusively to antibody formation (63). This compound was mono-(p-azobenzenearsonic acid)tyrosylphosphatidylethanolamine (ABA-Tyr-PE; see Figure 1).

ABA-Tyr-PE was prepared because extensive studies by several laboratories have demonstrated that ABA-Tyr [i.e. mono-(p-azobenzenearsonic acid)tyrosine] conferred only cellular immunity when administered to guinea pigs in CFA (64–66). However, coupling of ABA-Tyr and PE produced an immunogen capable of inducing both a humoral and a cell-mediated response (63). More anti-azobenzenearsonate (anti-ABA) antibodies were formed when the animals were immunized with actively sensitized liposomes than free ABA-Tyr-PE, and none could be detected after immunization with liposomes prepared in the presence of ABA-Tyr-GPE. These results thus confirmed previous experiments with Dnp-Cap-PE and its analogs which indicated that a humoral response was only obtained with an amphipathic derivative and was maximal when the derivative had been inserted into liposomal bilayers. In contrast, free ABA-Tyr-PE and the sensitized liposomes were equally effective in conferring a cellular response; i.e. incorporation into bilayers was not required. This observation was consistent with the fact that ABA-Tyr-GPE resembled ABA-Tyr in its ability to produce pure cell-mediated immunity, i.e. no antibodies. In these experiments, delayed reactions were elicited by challenge with either azobenzenearsonate–bovine serum albumin or ABA-Tyr-PE–sensitized liposomes.

Liposomes with Multiple Determinants

The sphingomyelin-cholesterol-dicetylphosphate bilayers of liposomes apparently function as nonimmunogenic carriers for the N-substituted PE derivatives. This conclusion is based on the following observations: (a) sera from guinea pigs given unsensitized liposomes (i.e. not containing any N-substituted PE derivative) were unable to initiate complement-dependent glucose release from unsensitized liposomes (61); and (b) challenge with unsensitized liposomes did not produce a delayed reaction (63). Because ABA-Tyr-PE can induce the effector T (thymus derived) cells involved in delayed reactions, the question arose as to whether this derivative could transform the lipid bilayers into immunogenic carriers capable of stimulating helper T cells. Precedence for this phenomenon has been provided by the studies of Alkan et al (65, 67), which demonstrated that ABA-Tyr can function as a carrier for covalently attached haptens such as Dnp-Cap and poly-D-glutamate.

Accordingly, guinea pigs were immunized with four types of liposomes that differ in number and site of the determinants, as depicted schematically in Figure 2. (a) Homogeneous liposomes are those prepared in the presence of a single N-substituted PE derivative, which is localized within the bilayers. (b) Hybrid liposomes are those prepared in the presence of more than one N-substituted PE derivative so that each is localized within the bilayers of the same liposomes. (c) Heterogeneous liposomes are those prepared in the presence of one N-substituted PE derivative and one N-substituted GPE derivative; in this case, one derivative is localized in the aqueous compartments, and the other in the bilayers, of the same liposomes. (d) Mixed liposomes are simply combinations of homogeneous liposomes, each prepared with a different N-substituted PE derivative; in this case, the derivatives are localized within the bilayers but not in the same liposomes.

Hybrid liposomes containing different amounts of Dnp-Cap-PE and a constant quantity of ABA-Tyr-PE did induce a significantly greater anti-Dnp response than homogeneous liposomes (68). For example, after 3 weeks the hapten-binding capacity (nmole of Dnp-Cap bound per milliliter of serum) was 0.56 in animals receiving homogeneous liposomes (50 nmole Dnp-Cap-PE) and 5.0 in guinea pigs immunized with hybrid liposomes (50 nmole Dnp-Cap-PE and 250 nmole ABA-Tyr-PE). Neither mixed nor

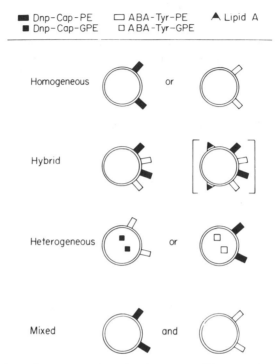

Figure 2 Schematic representation of various types of liposomal immunogens. For the sake of simplicity, only one bilayer (circular double track), which surrounds one aqueous compartment, is depicted. The PE derivatives are incorporated noncovalently in both halves of the bilayer (not just the exterior half as shown), whereas the GPE derivatives are trapped in the aqueous compartment. The bracketed hybrid liposome contains two different determinants and also the amphipathic B cell mitogen, lipid A, in the same bilayer [see (70) for structure of lipid A]. It should be emphasized that "homogeneous" and "heterogeneous" do not refer to the morphological appearance of liposomes, but rather to the number and site of the determinants (see text).

heterogeneous (Dnp-Cap-PE and ABA-Tyr-GPE) liposomes enhanced the humoral response, indicating that this phenomenon depends on the presence of ABA-Tyr determinants in the same lipid bilayers in which Dnp-Cap-PE is incorporated.

Conversely, incorporation of a sufficient amount of Dnp-Cap-PE into hybrid liposomes completely inhibited the guinea pig antibody response to ABA-Tyr-PE (68). This phenomenon also was uniquely characteristic of hybrid liposomes; anti-ABA antibody formation was not diminished in guinea pigs that had been immunized with mixed or heterogeneous (Dnp-Cap-GPE and ABA-Tyr-PE) liposomes. These results constitute additional evidence that lipid bilayers containing ABA-Tyr-PE can be regarded as immunogenic carriers, since Amkraut et al (69) have demonstrated similar intramolecular hapten competition when Dnp and ABA groups were simultaneously covalently linked to various T cell–dependent immunogens (e.g. keyhole limpet hemocyanin, sheep erythrocyte stroma, bovine serum albumin).

In addition to supporting the previous contention that sphingomyelin-cholesterol-dicetylphosphate liposomes essentially retain their structure after emulsification in CFA, the preceding observations also bear on the persistent question of whether liposomal immunogenicity proceeds indirectly, e.g. as a consequence of in vivo transpeptidation reactions by which Dnp-Cap and ABA-Tyr determinants are removed from N-substituted derivatives and become covalently attached to host protein. Although this possibility can not be rigorously excluded, it seems unlikely. Thus, transfer to endogenous carriers should occur in guinea pigs immunized with either hybrid, mixed, or heterogeneous liposomes, yet stimulation of the anti-Dnp response and inhibition of the anti-ABA response were only obtained in animals given hybrid liposomes.

Subsequent experiments have shown that liposomes are also immunogenic in mice, and that a humoral response can be enhanced by simultaneous incorporation of a N-substituted PE derivative and lipid A into the bilayers (cf Figure 2); lipid A is generally accepted as being a mitogenic signal for B (bone marrow–derived) cells. It is also noteworthy that, in both mice and guinea pigs (61), incorporation of Dnp-Cap-PE into liposomes prepared with egg lecithin instead of beef sphingomyelin did not significantly stimulate production of anti-Dnp antibodies over that obtained by immunization with the free derivative. Further investigation of this phenomenon, using a variety of synthetic phosphatidylcholines, has suggested a correlation between the potency of liposomal immunogens and the transition temperature of the phospholipid (T. Yasuda, G. F. Dancey, S. C. Kinsky, manuscript in preparation).

In summary, liposomal model membranes are novel immunogens in which B and T cell determinants, as well as appropriate mitogens, can be noncovalently inserted either individually or collectively within lipid bilayers. Therefore, liposomes differ from conventional immunogen preparations in which haptens are covalently bonded to carriers such as proteins or synthetic amino acid polymers. Because of this difference, preparation of liposomes provides an extremely convenient method for controlling epitope density, molecular complexity of the determinants, and their chemical environment, since these parameters can be simply regulated by varying the composition of the lipid mixture used to generate the model membranes.

ACKNOWLEDGMENTS

The senior author dedicates this paper to Professor Oliver H. Lowry, who, during his long tenure as chairman, not only tolerated—but actively encouraged—the pursuit of immunology in a pharmacology department. The authors are greatly indebted to Drs. George F. Dancey and Tatsuji Yasuda for their comments and assistance in the literature survey, which was concluded 15 August 1976. Mrs. Pat Fennell contributed the secretarial skills that enabled completion of this manuscript on time. Research in this laboratory has been supported by National Institutes of Health Grants AI-09319 and AI-13414.

Literature Cited

1. Mueller, P., Rudin, D. O., Tien, H. T., Wescott, W. C. 1962. *Circulation* 26:1167–71
2. Bangham, A. D., Standish, M. M., Watkins, J. C. 1965. *J. Mol. Biol.* 13:238–52
3. Müller-Eberhard, H. J. 1975. *Ann Rev. Biochem.* 44:697–724
4. Barfort, P., Arquilla, E. R., Vogelhut, P. O. 1968. *Science* 160:1119–21
5. Haxby, J. A., Kinsky, C. B., Kinsky, S. C. 1968. *Proc. Natl. Acad. Sci. USA* 61:300–7
6. Kinsky, S. C. 1972. *Biochim. Biophys. Acta* 265:1–23
7. Alving, C. R., Kinsky, S. C., Haxby, J. A., Kinsky, C. B. 1969. *Biochemistry* 8:1582–87
8. Alving, C. R., Kinsky, S. C. 1971. *Immunochemistry* 8:325–43
9. Haxby, J. A., Götze, O., Müller-Eberhard, H. J., Kinsky, S. C. 1969. *Proc. Natl. Acad. Sci. USA* 64:290–95
10. Knudson, K. C., Bing, D. H., Kater, L. 1971. *J. Immunol.* 106:258–65
11. Hesketh, T. R., Dourmashkin, R. R., Payne, S. N., Humphrey, J. H., Lachmann, P. J. 1971. *Nature* 233:620–23
12. Siddiqui, B., Hakomori, S. 1971. *J. Biol. Chem.* 246:5766–69
13. Kinsky, S. C., Haxby, J. A., Zopf, D. A., Alving, C. R., Kinsky, C. B. 1969. *Biochemistry* 8:4149–58
14. Inoue, K., Kataoka, T., Kinsky, S. C. 1971. *Biochemistry* 10:2574–81
15. Kataoka, T., Inoue, K., Lüderitz, O., Kinsky, S. C. 1971. *Eur. J. Biochem.* 21:80–85
16. Kataoka, T., Inoue, K., Galanos, C., Kinsky, S. C. 1971. *Eur. J. Biochem.* 24:123–27
17. Alving, C. R., Fowble, J. W., Joseph, K. C. 1974. *Immunochemistry* 11:475–81
18. Humphries, G. M. K., McConnell, H. M. 1975. *Proc. Natl. Acad. Sci. USA* 72:2483–87
19. Uemura, K., Kinsky, S. C. 1972. *Biochemistry* 11:4085–94
20. Six, H. R., Uemura, K., Kinsky, S. C. 1973. *Biochemistry* 12:4003–11
21. Six, H. R., Young, W. W., Uemura, K., Kinsky, S. C. 1974. *Biochemistry* 13:4050–58
22. Alving, C. R., Joseph, K. C., Wistar, R. 1974. *Biochemistry* 13:4818–24
23. Kitagawa, T., Inoue, K. 1975. *Nature* 254:254–56
24. Medicus, R. G., Schreiber, R. D., Götze, O., Müller-Eberhard, H. J. 1976. *Proc. Natl. Acad. Sci. USA* 73:612–16
25. Thompson, R. A., Lachmann, P. J. 1970. *J. Exp. Med.* 131:629–57
26. Lachmann, P. J., Munn, E. A., Weissmann, G. 1970. *Immunology* 19:983–86
27. Inoue, K., Kinsky, S. C. 1970. *Biochemistry* 9:4767–76
28. Hesketh, T. R., Payne, S. N., Humphrey, J. H. 1972. *Immunology* 23:705–11
29. Kinsky, S. C., Bonsen, P. P. M., Kinsky, C. B., van Deenen, L. L. M., Rosenthal, A. F. 1971. *Biochim. Biophys. Acta* 233:815–19
30. Kinsky, S. C. 1972. *Ann. NY Acad. Sci.* 195:429–38
31. Kinsky, S. C., Six, H. R. 1975. In *Proteases and Biological Control*, ed. E. Reich, D. B. Rifkin, E. Shaw, pp. 243–53. New York: Cold Spring Harbor Lab.
32. Weissmann, G., Dukor, P. 1970. *Adv. Immunol.* 12:283–331
33. Lachmann, P. J., Bowyer, D. E., Nicol, P., Dawson, R. M. C., Munn, E. A. 1973. *Immunology* 24:135–45

34. Mayer, M. M. 1972. *Proc. Natl. Acad. Sci. USA* 69:2954–58
35. Hammer, C. H., Nicholson, A., Mayer, M. M. 1975. *Proc. Natl. Acad. Sci. USA* 72:5076–80
36. Humphrey, J. H., Dourmashkin, R. R. 1969. *Adv. Immunol.* 11:75–115
37. Kinsky, S. C., Luse, S. A., Zopf, D., van Deenen, L. L. M., Haxby, J. 1967. *Biochim. Biophys. Acta* 135:844–61
38. Kataoka, T., Williamson, J. R., Kinsky, S. C. 1973. *Biochim. Biophys. Acta* 298:158–79
39. Iles, G. H., Seeman, P., Naylor, D., Cinader, B. 1973. *J. Cell. Biol.* 56:528–39
40. Tillack, T. W., Kinsky, S. C. 1973. *Biochim. Biophys. Acta* 323:43–54
41. Wobschall, D., McKeon, C. 1975. *Biochim. Biophys. Acta* 413:317–21
42. Abramovitz, A. S., Michaels, D. W., Mayer, M. M. 1976. *Fed. Proc.* 35(3): 493 (Abstr.)
42a. Michaels, D. W., Abramovitz, A. S., Hammer, C. H. 1976. *Fed. Proc.* 35(7): 1762 (Abstr.)
43. Michaels, D. W., Abramovitz, A. S., Hammer, C. H., Mayer, M. M. 1976. *Proc. Natl. Acad. Sci. USA* 73:2852–56
44. del Castillo, J., Rodriguez, A., Romero, C. A., Sanchez, V. 1966. *Science* 153:185–88
45. Toro-Goyco, E., Rodriguez, A., del Castillo, J. 1966. *Biochem. Biophys. Res. Commun.* 23:341–46
46. Sato, J., Hara, I. 1972. *Immunochemistry* 9:585–87
47. Joseph, K. C., Alving, C. R., Wistar, R. 1974. *J. Immunol.* 112:1949–51
48. Nagai, Y., Ohsawa, T. 1974. *Jpn. J. Exp. Med.* 44:451–64
49. Ohsawa, T., Nagai, Y. 1975. *Biochim. Biophys. Acta* 389:69–83
50. Alving, C. R., Joseph, K. C., Lindsley, H. B., Schoenbechler, M. J. 1974. *Proc. Soc. Exp. Biol. Med.* 146:458–61
51. Humphries, G. K., McConnell, H. M. 1974. *Proc. Natl. Acad. Sci. USA* 71:1691–94
52. Wei, R., Alving, C. R., Richards, R. A., Copeland, E. S. 1975. *J. Immunol. Methods* 9:165–70
53. Fry, J. M., Lisak, R. P., Manning, M. C., Silberberg, D. H. 1976. *J. Immunol. Methods* 11:185–93
54. Henkart, P., Blumenthal, R. 1975. *Proc. Natl. Acad. Sci. USA* 72:2789–93
55. Gregoriadis, G., Leathwood, P. D., Ryman, B. E. 1971. *FEBS Lett.* 14:95–99
56. Gregoriadis, G., Ryman, B. E. 1972. *Eur. J. Biochem.* 24:485–91
57. Allison, A. C., Gregoriadis, G. 1974. *Nature* 252:252
58. Gregoriadis, G., Allison, A. C. 1974. *FEBS Lett.* 45:71–74
59. Rapport, M. M., Graf, L. 1969. *Prog. Allergy* 13:273–331
60. Hakomori, S. 1972. *Methods Enzymol.* 28:232–36
61. Uemura, K., Nicolotti, R. A., Six, H. R., Kinsky, S. C. 1974. *Biochemistry* 13:1572–78
62. Uemura, K., Claflin, J. L., Davie, J. M., Kinsky, S. C. 1975. *J. Immunol.* 114:958–61
63. Nicolotti, R. A., Kinsky, S. C. 1975. *Biochemistry* 14:2331–37
64. Leskowitz, S., Jones, V. E., Zak, S. J., 1966. *J. Exp. Med.* 123:229–37
65. Alkan, S. S., Williams, E. B., Nitecki, D. E., Goodman, J. W. 1972. *J. Exp. Med.* 135:1228–46
66. Becker, M. J., Levin, H., Sela, M. 1973. *Eur. J. Immunol.* 3:131–35
67. Alkan, S. S., Nitecki, D. E., Goodman, J. W. 1971. *J. Immunol.* 107:353–58
68. Kochibe, N., Nicolotti, R. A., Davie, J. M., Kinsky, S. C. 1975. *Proc. Natl. Acad. Sci. USA* 72:4582–86
69. Amkraut, A. A., Garvey, J. S., Campbell, D. H. 1966. *J. Exp. Med.* 124:293–306
70. Rietschel, E. T., Lüderitz, O. 1975. *Z. Immunitaetsforsch.* 149:201–13

Ann. Rev. Biochem. 1979. 48:293–325
Copyright © 1979 by Annual Reviews Inc. All rights reserved

PHOTOAFFINITY LABELING ❖12011
OF BIOLOGICAL SYSTEMS[1]

Vinay Chowdhry[2]

Central Research & Development Department, E. I. du Pont de Nemours & Co., Experimental Station, Bldg. 328, Wilmington, Delaware 19898

F. H. Westheimer

Department of Chemistry, Harvard University, Cambridge, Massachusetts 02138

CONTENTS

[1]The following abbreviations are used: AChE, acetylcholine esterase; cAMP, cyclic 3',5' adenosine monophosphate; Chy, chymotrypsin; Chy–CH$_2$OH, chymotrypsin, showing hydroxymethyl group of "active site" serine; cGMP, cyclic 3',5' guanosine monophosphate; NAP, 4-azido-2-nitrophenyl; O–CM cysteine, O-carboxymethylcysteine; O–CM histidine, O-carboxymethylhistidine; O–CM serine, O-carboxymethylserine; O–CM tyrosine, O-carboxymethyltyrosine; RPRAd, adenosine diphosphoribosyl.

[2]Address correspondence to this author.

0066-4154/79/0701-0293$01.00 293

PERSPECTIVES AND SUMMARY

The elucidation of molecular interactions leading to biochemical processes is a major objective of chemical and biochemical research. Essential to an understanding of the interactions involved in biological processes at the molecular level is the identification and structural characterization of the components of the complex systems involved. Although a multitude of enzymes has been isolated, their biological substrates identified, and some understanding of their mechanism of action reached, the identification and isolation of hormone receptors, transport proteins, proteins regulating nucleic acid transcription and translation, and the topographical distribution and function of membrane proteins have not progressed as much. An understanding of the mechanism of action of enzyme-catalyzed reactions requires the identification of the amino acids in the active site involved in binding and those more directly involved in catalysis. The classical approach to acquiring such information has been the use of general and specific reagents for chemical modification of active site residues, commonly referred to as affinity labeling (1–3).

Other techniques are also widely used. Spectroscopy is not yet fully applicable to macromolecules. Determination of structures of crystalline proteins (4, 5) and nucleic acids (6, 7) by X-ray diffraction has provided, in many instances, molecular information in fascinating detail. Such structural information, although limited by the static picture it provides of these conformationally dynamic systems, complements that obtained by chemical studies conducted in solution. A promising new approach combining solution studies with X-ray crystallographic analysis has been recently introduced (8–10). NMR spectroscopy has provided valuable information on the dynamic structure of some macromolecules in solution but is as yet limited by macromolecular size and the need for relatively large quantities of material (11, 12). Other spectroscopic techniques, such as laser Raman spectroscopy (13), fluorescence spectroscopy (14, 15), ESR spectroscopy (16, 17), and neutron diffraction (18, 19), are being increasingly used.

More recently, another approach to chemical modification of active site residues has been introduced—suicide inhibition (20–24). This method makes use of the catalytic function of enzymes to generate a reactive molecule in the active site from an "inert" precursor. The reactive molecule, commonly an allenic moiety, then may function as a chemical trap for nucleophilic residues of the enzyme. Affinity labeling in general, and suicide inhibition in particular, however, require the presence of appropriately positioned reactive functional groups on the enzyme to bring about inactivation and labeling. Such a requirement, though generally satisfied in the active sites of enzymes (electrophilic and nucleophilic groups responsible for catalytic action are usually present in the active site of enzymes), does not necessarily obtain in proteins other than enzymes or indeed even in regions of enzymes, such as allosteric binding sites where the primary events of catalysis do not take place.

Ideal labeling reagents should react not only with nucleophiles but even with the significantly less reactive but ubiquitous hydrophobic regions (C–H bonds) of proteins. The high (indiscriminate) reactivity of such reagents should be "masked" but capable of activation in situ at the discretion of the experimentalist. Such reagents can provide valuable information on the constitution of binding and/or catalytic sites of isolated macromolecules in addition to tagging and therefore identifying different kinds of macromolecular receptors. Photogenerated reagents have the potential for satisfying both the requirement of high reactivity and that of activation in situ.

The use of photogenerated reagents to study biological macromolecules was introduced for the photolysis of diazoacetylchymotrypsin by Singh, Thornton & Westheimer (25) in 1962. Photoaffinity labeling has since evolved into a major technique for studying molecular interactions in biological systems (26–29). A photolabile reagent is anchored to the macromolecule, when possible by a covalent bond; photolysis of the complex then leads to the generation of a highly reactive species that, by reacting (by insertion) rapidly with the immediate environment, labels the macromolecule or specifically the active site. The technique has the potential for identifying complex biological receptors and providing information on their molecular structure. Since the initial experiment the method has been used to investigate receptors and transport proteins, membrane structure and function, protein-nucleic acid interaction, and antibodies, in addition to enzymes. These and other applications are discussed here to highlight the potential of the method, and its limitations; finally, the properties of various photolabile groups are evaluated. In the next section early experiments by different groups are presented to illustrate the basic approaches that have subsequently been amplified in the diverse uses presented in the section on recent applications.

HISTORICAL DEVELOPMENT

Diazoacetyl Chymotrypsin

Diazoacetylchymotrypsin was prepared by reacting p-nitrophenyl diazoacetate with chymotrypsin at pH 6.2, in analogy with the preparation of acetylchymotrypsin by Balls & Wood (30, 31). The inactivation of the enzyme by 10^{-3} M p-nitrophenyl diazoacetate is rapid, being 95% complete in 12 min at 25°C; the esterolytic activity was restored with 2 M hydroxylamine at pH 8. Reaction of chymotrypsin with p-nitrophenyl-[2-^{14}C]-diazoacetate yielded inactive enzyme having 0.98 mole of label per mole of enzyme, which suggests stoichiometric diazoacylation of the reactive serine residue in the active site (Equation 1).

$$\text{Chy}-\text{CH}_2\text{OH} + \overset{\text{N}_2}{\underset{}{\overset{\|}{\text{HC}}}}-\overset{\text{O}}{\overset{\|}{\text{C}}}-\text{O}-\!\!\!\bigcirc\!\!\!-\text{NO}_2 \xrightarrow{\text{pH 6.2}}$$

$$\text{Chy}-\text{CH}_2-\text{O}-\overset{\text{O}}{\overset{\|}{\text{C}}}-\text{CHN}_2 + \text{HO}-\!\!\!\bigcirc\!\!\!-\text{NO}_2$$

1.

Although acetylchymotrypsin was reactivated by hydrolysis in 10 min at pH 7, diazoacetylchymotrypsin remained unchanged on standing in the dark at pH 6.2 for 48 hr. Diazoacetylchymotrypsin, in contrast to acetylchymotrypsin, could therefore conveniently be isolated and stored as the stable acyl enzyme. Photolysis of ^{14}C-labeled diazoacetylchymotrypsin with long wavelength UV light for 3–4 hr led to 20–25% irreversible incorporation of the radioactive label into the protein with regeneration of 70–75% of the enzymatic activity (25, 32). Regeneration of activity proceeds at least in part according to the reactions shown in Equation 2; the asterisk denotes the position of the radiolabel.

$$\text{Chy-CH}_2-\text{O}-\overset{\text{O}}{\overset{\|}{\text{C}}}-\overset{*}{\text{CHN}_2} \longrightarrow \text{Chy-CH}_2-\text{O}-\overset{\text{O}}{\overset{\|}{\text{C}}}-\overset{..}{\underset{*}{\text{CH}}} + \text{N}_2 \xrightarrow{\text{H}_2\text{O}}$$

2.

$$\text{Chy-CH}_2-\text{O}-\overset{\text{O}}{\overset{\|}{\text{C}}}-\underset{*}{\text{CH}_2\text{OH}} \xrightarrow{\text{H}_2\text{O}} \text{Chy-CH}_2\text{OH} + \text{HO}-\text{CH}_2-\overset{*}{\text{CO}_2\text{H}}$$

active   glycolic
enzyme   acid

Isolation of 2-^{14}C-labeled glycolic acid accounted for 55% of the label bound to enzyme prior to photolysis. Acid hydrolysis of the photolyzed radiolabeled enzyme followed by amino acid analysis revealed two major radioactive products, O-carboxymethylserine and O-carboxymethyltyrosine in addition to glycolic acid (32, 33). N-Carboxymethylhistidine was also obtained together with three other minor and as yet unidentified products. Hexter has subsequently shown (34) that the material identified as O-carboxymethylserine (32) may have been contaminated with 7–8% of

S-carboxymethylcysteine. A brief discussion of the mode of formation of these four carboxymethylated amino acids will help illustrate the potential of and problems associated with the use of photogenerated reagents to obtain information at the molecular level.

O-Carboxymethylserine is produced by a photoreaction analogous to the Wolff rearrangement of α-diazoketones, which may proceed either via the carbene or the excited state of the diazo group. The mechanism written below is intended only as a formal representation, and not a statement of the precise sequence of events.

$$Chy\text{-}CH_2\text{---}O\text{---}\overset{\overset{O}{\|}}{C}\text{---}CHN_2 \xrightarrow{h\nu} Chy\text{-}CH_2\text{---}O\text{---}\overset{\overset{O}{\|}}{C}\text{---}\overset{..}{C}H \xrightarrow[\text{rearrangement}]{\text{Wolff}}$$

$$Chy\text{-}CH_2\text{---}O\text{---}\underset{\underset{H}{|}}{C}{=}C{=}O \xrightarrow{H_2O} Chy\text{-}CH_2\text{---}O\text{---}CH_2\text{---}CO_2H \qquad 3.$$

$$\xrightarrow{6NHCl/110^\circ C} O\text{-}Carboxymethylserine$$

O-Carboxymethyltyrosine is formed by "insertion" of the carbene, or of an equivalent species, into the hydroxyl group of tyrosine. The yield of O–CM tyrosine was found to be dependent on enzyme concentration (increasing with concentration of enzyme) and on pH (the yield was 33% at pH 4.0 but diminished to 21% at pH 6.0). Subsequent analysis of peptides (33) established that the labeled tyrosine was number 146 in the amino acid sequence, and was produced by insertion of the carbene, initially bound to the macromolecule, into the hydroxyl group of tyrosine 146 of another molecule of chymotrypsin. Proof that the chemical reaction occurs in a noncovalent dimer of trypsin is based not only on the dependence of the yield on concentration, but also on isolation of the "dimeric" product by gel chromatography. The dimeric product is believed to be linked from the glycolate ester of serine 195 of one molecule to tyrosine 146 of another:

$$\underset{\text{SERINE 195}}{Chy-CH_2-O-\overset{\overset{O}{\|}}{C}-CH_2-O-}\underset{\text{TYROSINE 146}}{\langle\bigcirc\rangle-CH_2-Chy}$$

The mode of formation of N-carboxymethylhistidine is however not as clear. Although some of it may be formed by an insertion mechanism via the carbene, control experiments suggest that most, if not all, of it may be formed by an acid-catalyzed light-independent process. Finally, the S-carboxymethylcysteine obtained is likely formed by insertion of the carbene into the disulfide bond, between cysteines 42 and 58. X-ray crystallographic analysis of chymotrypsin places this disulfide bond in the proximity of serine 195 which is presumed to carry the diazoacetyl moiety. Significantly, diazomalonylchymotrypsin on photolysis yields S-carboxymethylcysteine as one of the primary products (35).

The formation of O-CM serine suggested that α-diazoesters could undergo the Wolff rearrangement on photolysis, as do α-diazoketones. The Wolff rearrangement of diazoacetylchymotrypsin, which accounts for 40% of the irreversibly incorporated ^{14}C label, "wastes" the carbene produced because it labels the serine which had been known to be in the active site prior to the experiment. The objective of photoaffinity labeling, to map the active site by reaction of a carbene with amino acid residues other than the one used to anchor the bifunctional reagent in the active site, is therefore not fulfilled by this reaction. Although the ketene generated by the rearrangement may in other instances react with active site nucleophiles, thereby salvaging some of the carbene that would otherwise be wasted by the Wolff rearrangement pathway, trapping of such a ketene may suffer from some of the same difficulties as those encountered in conventional affinity labeling studies. The formation of O–CM tyrosine and S–CM cysteine, on the contrary, illustrates the potential of photoaffinity labeling. O-Carboxymethyltyrosine in particular, because it is formed in an intermacromolecular reaction, demonstrates the novelty and potential of photoaffinity labeling in providing information on dynamic structures in solution and on the nature of intermacromolecular contact. The rapid reaction of a photogenerated carbene could therefore, in principle, be used to trap short-lived macromolecular complexes, in addition to mapping stable macromolecular ensembles. The high percentage yield of the insertion of carboxymethylcarbene into water, leading to glycolic acid, though undesirable, will depend on the accessibility of the carbene to water in the system being studied. Chymotrypsin, a hydrolytic enzyme, is clearly expected to hold a substantial amount of water in the active site. The formation of N–CM histidine identifies another potential difficulty. Acid-catalyzed and copper ion-catalyzed decomposition of diazo groups leading to labeling of enzymes has been demonstrated (36). Such labeling does not however enjoy the advantages, elucidated before, of photoaffinity labeling, and may lead to nonspecific labeling.

Other Diazoacyl Enzymes

Subsequent investigations have dealt with the photolysis of diazomalonylchymotrypsin (35), diazomalonyltrypsin (35, 37) and diazoacetylsubtilisin

(38). The photolysis of both diazomalonylchymotrypsin and diazoacetyl-chymotrypsin produced the same products, although their relative yields were different. Photolysis of both diazomalonyltrypsin and diazomalo-nylchymotrypsin yielded the same products, but in the former case, 1–3% of ^{14}C-radiolabeled glutamic acid was also obtained (37). This product is presumably formed by insertion of the carbene into the C–H bond of the methyl group of an alanine residue found in the active site (Figure 1). This result is an important demonstration of the potential of photoaffinity labeling to tag the ubiquitous but difficult to label C–H bonds found in biological macromolecules.

Photolysis of diazoacetyl glyceraldehyde-3-phosphate dehydrogenase identified another important problem (L. J. Crane, unpublished results). The diazoacetyl group may be attached as a thioester to a reactive cysteine in the active site. The only product of photolysis observed was S-carboxymethylcysteine, formed by the Wolff rearrangement. This rearrangement, which wastes $\sim 30\%$ of the carbene on photolysis of the diazo moiety of an O-ester, thus leads to a complete waste of the reagent on photolysis of this thioester. Model studies suggest that diazomalonylthioesters also suffer exclusive Wolff rearrangement of the thioalkyl group on photolysis (39). By contrast, thioesters of the recently introduced 2-diazo-3,3,3-trifluoropropionyl chloride (40) undergo significant insertion on photolysis, and therefore hold promise for use in photoaffinity labeling as α-diazothio-esters of biological molecules.

Labeling of Enzyme-Photolabile Reagent Complexes

The majority of small molecules that interact with proteins (coenzymes, inhibitors, allosteric modulators, neurotransmitters, antigens, hormones) function primarily by forming a specific complex with the protein which either alters its conformational state or, as in the case of coenzymes, in-

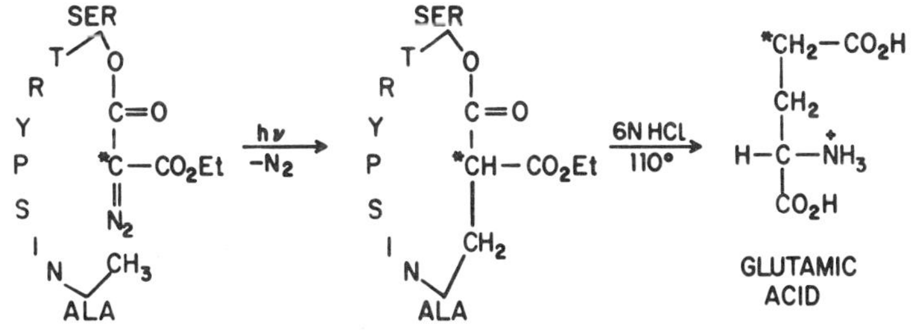

Figure 1   Insertion of diazomalonyl carbene into the C–H bond of the methyl group of alanine in the active site of trypsin. Acid hydrolysis followed by decarboxylation led to incorporation of a carboxymethyl moiety into the methyl group of alanine, thereby transforming it to glutamic acid.

creases greatly the effective concentration of the reactant, thereby leading to enhanced rate of chemical reaction. The potential for generation of a highly reactive reagent in situ by photoexcitation, and for labeling of sites not necessarily rich in reactive nucleophilic residues, in principle provides photoaffinity labeling with a special advantage in studying such binding sites. In a generally unsuccessful attempt to take advantage of this possibility, Browne, Hixon & Westheimer prepared a 3-diazoacetoxymethyl analogue of NAD (I) and investigated its use in photoaffinity labeling of yeast alcohol dehydrogenase (41).

$$
\underset{\substack{| \\ \text{RPRAd} \\ \mathbf{I}}}{\overset{}{\text{pyridinium}}}\!\!-CH_2-O-\overset{\overset{\displaystyle O}{\|}}{C}-CHN_2
\qquad\qquad
\underset{\substack{| \\ \text{RPRAd} \\ \mathbf{II}}}{\overset{}{\text{pyridinium}}}\!\!-N_3
$$

The dissociation constant for the enzyme-NAD analogue complex was 5×10^{-4} M; the analogue, then, does not bind tightly. Although 20% incorporation of the radiolabel was observed on photolysis, the reduction in the amount incorporated in the presence of saturating concentrations of NAD was far less than expected. The labeling result is therefore ambiguous. Subsequently an azido analogue of NAD (II) was prepared and used to photolabel yeast alcohol dehydrogenase. There was only 7% incorporation of the radiolabel, of which about half may have been due to nonspecific labeling (42). These examples illustrate the problems inherent in photoaffinity labeling of "loose" receptor ligand complexes. In principle, if the dissociation constant is low (10^{-5}–10^{-6} M), and binding of the analogue is competitive with that of the natural ligand, specific labeling of the receptor would be expected provided the lifetime of the reactive species generated in situ is short (10^{-5}sec or less).

The ketenes generated by Wolff rearrangement of the diazoacyl moiety and the nitrenes produced on photolysis of aryl azides may have lifetimes long compared to the times for the dissociation of loosely bound complexes; if so, labeling may be inefficient or nonspecific. The problem of low yield of incorporated radiolabel on photolysis of loose complexes may sometimes be avoided by continuous replacement of the reagent being used for photo-inactivation (43).

Labeling of Antibodies

The use of photoaffinity labeling to map the combining sites of antibodies was introduced by Knowles and co-workers (44), and simultaneously by

Richards et al (45), in 1969. Knowles and co-workers isolated antibodies to the antigenic determinant, 4-azido-2-nitrophenyl (NAP). The dissociation constant for purified anti-NAP antibody with NAP-^{3}H-lysine was 1.4×10^{-7} M at 4°C. This high association constant facilitated isolation of the complex by gel chromatography; two moles of NAP-^{3}H-lysine were complexed per mole of antibody. Photolysis of the isolated complex for 18 hr led to incorporation of about 1 mole of radiolabel per mole of antibody. This experiment not only illustrated the potential for successful specific labeling when "tight" complexes are photolyzed, but introduced the use of aromatic azides as reagents for photoaffinity labeling. They have since been widely used for this purpose (26–29).

Pseudophotoaffinity Labeling

Singer and co-workers, in an attempt to label the acetylcholine esterase of erythrocyte membranes (AChE), encountered problems due to nonspecific labeling that presumably arose from the relatively long lifetime of the reactive species generated on photolysis of an aromatic azide; they named such nonspecific incorporation pseudophotoaffinity labeling (46). Photolysis of AChE in the presence of 10^{-5} M [^{3}H]4-azido-2-nitrobenzyltrimethylammonium ion (III) caused 82% irreversible inactivation of the enzyme. Photolysis of the azide was needed for inactivation; the presence of good competitive inhibitors protected the enzyme from such photoinactivation. The amount of irreversibly incorporated radiolabel far exceeded the extent of inactivation both in the presence and in the absence of competitive inhibitor. Thus, photolysis is apparently accompanied by significant nonspecific incorporation. The latter was reduced tenfold upon photolysis in the presence of p-aminobenzoate, a scavenger that is believed to react with photoactivated reagent present in the solution rather than that at the binding site. More importantly, no photoinduced inactivation of AChE was observed in the presence of added scavenger. This result strongly suggests that inactivation did not occur by reaction of photogenerated nitrene before it diffused out of the active site, but that the reactive species diffused in and out of the active site several times before reacting. Such a labeling process is, of course, similar to conventional affinity labeling and does not enjoy the special advantages of photoaffinity labeling.

In an extension of their study cited earlier (45) Richards and co-workers (47–50) have conducted photoaffinity labeling studies on protein 460, a mouse IgA myeloma immunoglobulin (capable of binding the 2,4-dinitrophenyl group) with two different reagents 2,4-dinitrophenylalanyldiazoketone (IV), and 2,4-dinitrophenyl azide (V).

$$III \qquad IV \qquad V$$

$$K_d = 2 \times 10^{-5}\,M \qquad K_d = 5 \times 10^{-5}\,M$$

The dissociation constants of the myeloma protein complexes with compounds IV and V are shown with their structures. Photolysis with either reagent resulted in incorporation of radiolabel into protein and with IV there was an equivalent loss of binding sites for ϵ-2,4-dinitrophenyllysine. Although the diazoketone IV was found bonded primarily to the light chain, only 15% of the azido compound V that was incorporated was detected on this chain. Peptide analysis showed that the diazo compound reacted almost quantitatively with the ϵ-amino group of lysine 54 of the light chain to form an amide bond, but the azido reagent that bound to the light chain was found in three different peptides. However, the majority of the azide label (85%) was incorporated into tyrosines 33 and 88 in the variable region of the heavy chain. Assuming these residues to be homologous with residues in the human myeloma protein NEW [for which the crystal structure has been determined (51)], the two tyrosines are estimated to be too far apart (23 Å) to be contact residues at the same site.

Labeling by the azido reagent of residues 23 Å apart points to the possible ambiguities in interpretation of results when the labeling process and the diffusion of reactive species from the site of photogeneration proceed at comparable rates. Since lysine 54 was attached by an amide bond to the residue from photolysis of the diazo reagent, labeling must have proceeded via ketene obtained by Wolff rearrangement. As ketenes are expected to be less reactive than the corresponding carbenes, the exclusive reaction of the antibody with the ketene generated on photolysis of IV raises the possibility of nonspecific labeling. This result is not entirely unexpected as α-diazoketones such as IV are indeed more prone to undergo the Wolff rearrangement than α-diazoesters such as the α-diazoacyl enzymes discussed earlier.

Even when the dissociation constant is low, as in the case of the interaction of carbonic anhydrase and p-azidobenzene-sulfonamide ($K_i \sim 10^{-6}$M, with $\sim 99\%$ active site occupancy), photolysis leading to covalent labeling "occurs largely at a point removed from the active site" (52).

Photolabile Natural Ligands

Ideally, in studies of affinity labeling, the perturbation caused by the reactive group, or its precursor, to the molecular interaction being examined is kept to a minimum. If precise information about molecular interaction is desired, it is imperative to establish that the probe not only binds to the same site but also that it binds in a mode identical to that of the true substrate. If, however, the experiment is designed only to identify and tag binding sites or to identify specific receptors in a complex milieu, demonstration of competitive binding and true photoaffinity labeling will suffice even if the precise mode of binding is not known. The presence in a natural ligand of a functional group, such as an α,β-unsaturated system, might provide in some instances an advantage over reagents that incorporate synthetic photolabile groups, especially if the photochemical behavior is well understood. Martyr & Benisek have used photoexcited α,β-unsaturated ketosteroids to inactivate Δ^5-ketosteroid isomerase (53). Photolysis, although slow, leads to up to 90% inactivation. Reinvestigation, however, has shown that in contrast to the earlier report of covalent attachment of steroid to enzyme (53) the radiochemically labeled steroid, although tenaciously bound to the enzyme, is released on denaturing the enzyme (W. F. Benisek, private communication). Recently, amino acid analysis and sequence analysis (54) have shown that the photoinactivation is accompanied by the transformation of aspartic acid 38 to an alanine residue! No mechanism for this novel photochemical reductive decarboxylation has been proposed. Although the excited singlet states of α,β-unsaturated ketones are known to be short-lived, $\sim 10^{-5}$ 10^{-9} sec, an efficient process of intersystem crossing to the longer lived triplet state (10^{-3} sec) is also known, posing the potential for problems, discussed earlier, arising from long lifetimes of reactive species. The excited state generally reacts with C–H bonds by hydrogen abstraction but a high degree of selectivity is observed. Galardy and co-workers have similarly used aromatic ketones for photoaffinity labeling (55).

Several groups have shown that cyclic nucleotides undergo photoincorporation into different receptors. Cooperman and co-workers observed incorporation of N^6-butyryl cAMP into erythrocyte ghost membranes on photolysis (56). Kallos has used the same derivative of cAMP to photolabel a cytoplasmic receptor for cAMP (57). Ferguson and co-workers have used both cAMP and cGMP in photoaffinity labeling studies with cyclic nucleotide receptors in extracts from testis, adrenal cortex (58, 59), and in messenger ribonucleoprotein-like particles (60).

Many different groups have studied the photochemical cross-linking of proteins to nucleic acids, generally utilizing the photoreactivity of nucleic acids (61–64). The photochemical processes involved are not well understood and product analysis has rarely been achieved. A brief discussion of such studies is presented later.

The experiments discussed in this section have been presented to focus attention on the potential problems possible in photoaffinity labeling of biological macromolecules. Since 1972 the use of photogenerated reagents has proliferated in spite of these and other problems. The method has been limited however by these difficulties and definitive interpretation of results at a molecular level has often proven difficult. Use of the approach has been extended to widely different systems, and many new reagents, primarily incorporating the α-diazoacyl and p-azidonitrophenyl photolabile groups, have been prepared (26–29). However, as has been repeatedly stressed in recent years, the development of new photolabile groups free of the defects discussed here is expected to greatly enhance the general utility of photogenerated reagents (26–29). The experiments presented here fall into two principal groups: one in which the photolabile reagent is covalently bound to the macromolecule at a specific site prior to photolysis, and the other in which the reagent is associated with the macromolecule as a reversible complex, but where photoactivation leads to irreversible incorporation of the bound ligand. The binding of small molecules to proteins and intermacromolecular interaction have been studied by the use both of synthetic photolabile groups and of photoreactive natural ligands. The diverse uses of photoaffinity labeling presented in the next section extend the potential applicability of the method.

RECENT APPLICATIONS

Although the initial experiments presented above were conducted on purified proteins, the method has now been applied to complex ensembles such as macromolecular receptors, ribosomes, and membranes, wherein the use of photogenerated reagents has special and perhaps unique advantages compared to other methods. Emphasis in this discussion is on photoaffinity labeling studies of macromolecular assemblies, as these represent novel areas of application of the technique. As a consequence new photoaffinity labeling studies on purified proteins are discussed only briefly.

Receptors and Transport Proteins

The term receptors is used broadly to encompass both soluble and membrane-bound proteins that function as receptors for hormones, neurotransmitters, cyclic nucleotides, sugars, amino acids, peptides, and drugs. Most hormone and drug receptors are membrane-bound and are not easily solubilized from the membrane, nor do they always retain physiological function or specific binding capacity upon such solubilization (65–67). The isolation of functional receptors has generally not been feasible. Significant advances in the experimental detection of receptors, usually present only at low concentrations, have been made (68–71), facilitated in part by the availability of analogues of natural ligands with radiolabel of high specific activity. Affinity labeling of receptors has been utilized by several groups, but successful isolation of an intact, functional receptor has not yet been achieved.

ACETYLCHOLINE RECEPTOR   The first attempts to utilize photoaffinity labeling to study receptors were directed by Schwyzer, Waser, and co-workers (72, 73) at the acetylcholine receptor in mouse phrenic nerve diaphragm, and simultaneously by Singer and co-workers (74) at the receptor in whole-frog sartorius muscle. Schwyzer and co-workers synthesized diazoacetylcholine bromide and studied its chemical and photochemical properties. They found it was hydrolyzed by acetylcholine esterase 10^4 times more slowly than was acetylcholine iodide, a finding reminiscent of the hydrolytic stability of diazoacetylchymotrypsin noted earlier. Neuromuscular transmission in isolated mouse phrenic nerve diaphragm was blocked by III (p. 302) (10^{-5}M) through prolonged depolarization of post-synaptic membranes; photolysis at long wavelength caused an irreversible depolarizing block of neuromuscular transmission. Acetylcholine esterase activity was, however, inhibited only 20% by a 5×10^{-4}M solution of III, which suggests that the active enzyme and the cholinergic receptor are present at different locations. These experiments suggested the potential use of photogenerated reagents to switch on or off the physiological function of specific receptors in complex biological systems.

The arylazide III was used to label the peptide chains of detergent-solubilized purified acetylcholine receptor from the electric tissue of *Torpedo californica* (75). Four polypeptide chains of different molecular weight are found in the isolated protein, and all are labeled on photolysis and are protected against labeling by agonists and antagonists containing a quarternary ammonium group; the neurotoxin from *Naja naja siamensis,* however, protected only the α-chain. The authors conclude that the α-chain is the binding site of the neurotoxin but explain that the labeling of all four chains is observed because a "photo-activated intermediate of the label exists long enough to react with polypepdide chains in the neighborhood of the initial binding site." This result then, is similar to that obtained earlier by Singer (46) with the same arylazide, and suggests that the problem of nonspecific labeling may be caused by the apparently long lifetime of the species obtained on photolysis of this photolabile group. Raftery & Witzemann have synthesized and used 1,10-bis(3-azidopyridinium)-decane diiodide as a photoaffinity label for the acetylcholine receptor of the electric organ of *Torpedo californica* (76). The receptor is composed of four different polypeptides of molecular weight 40, 50, 60, and 65 thousand. In addition to labeling the 40K subunit (the specific ligand binding site), photoaffinity labeling led to incorporation of the radiolabel into the 50K subunit in the membrane-bound receptor preparation, but into the 60K subunit when the purified receptor was utilized. This difference in the labeling pattern may reflect changes in the structural arrangement of the subunits upon solubilization and purification. The authors further suggest that the labeling of the 50K and 60K subunits may be due to nonspecific labeling caused by diffusion of the long-lived nitrene from the specific site into a neighboring subunit where reaction could have occurred with appropriately positioned nucleophiles.

Since proteins associated with changes in conductivity during synaptic transmission show a high affinity for positively charged ligands (77), studies on such proteins are included in this section. Hucho, Kiefer, and co-workers have used the N-triethylammonium analogue of III to photolabel the potassium transport channel in myelinated nerve fibers (78). Prior to irradiation, the arylazide, at 4 mM, caused 50% reversible inhibition of the potassium current. Photolysis, however, led to an 80% decrease in potassium current but less than a 10% decrease in sodium current. Even after washing the nerve fiber with Ringer's solution, 65% inhibition of potassium conductance was irreversible. When reagent was applied to the internal side of the nodal membrane by diffusion from the cut ends of the nerve fiber and then photolyzed, a surprising increase in potassium conductance was observed. This was interpreted to mean that "the binding site for the quaternary ammonium group is situated close to the internal opening of the potassium channel, because the 'reactive tail' of the photoaffinity label can react only with sites outside the channel—for example with proteins from the axoplasm, the latter thereby being removed from the channel." Such detailed conclusions, derived in the absence of radiolabeled studies and in light of the problems of nonspecific labeling by III, (46, 74, 75) though fascinating, must be regarded as speculative. Recently, the triethylammonium binding sites of unmyelinated crayfish nerve fibers have also been photolabeled with the same N-triethylammonium analogue of III (79).

Guillory and co-workers have used an arylazido-β-alanine tetrodotoxin derivative to photolabel the receptor sites associated with the sodium pores of excitable membranes in amphibian skeletal muscle (80). Tetrodotoxin is known to inhibit the sodium-dependent depolarization of crayfish (81) and amphibian (82) muscle. The arylazido analogue, at 8.5×10^{-7} M, produced an inhibition of depolarization similar to that observed with unmodified tetrodotoxin.

Photolysis is believed to have led to irreversible incorporation of the tetrodotoxin moiety into the receptor, since repeated washings in the Ca-free medium after photolysis led to no detectable decrease in inhibition of the sodium ion-dependent depolarization. This experiment provides another demonstration of the potential of photoaffinity labeling to attach small effector molecules permanently onto their macromolecular receptors thereby enabling either isolation of the receptor or perhaps opening the way to a study of the complex system in vivo.

NUCLEOTIDE RECEPTORS   Since Sutherland's discovery of the action of cAMP as a second messenger (83, 84) this compound has been implicated in a vast array of biological functions such as regulation of enzyme and membrane function (85), growth and contact inhibition of mammalian cells (86, 87), synaptic transmission (88, 89), and modulation of inflammation and immunity (90). Photolabile cAMP derivatives could help study these diverse functions. Cooperman & Brunswick were the first to synthesize and use a variety of cAMP derivatives (VI), incorporating the diazomalonyl photolabile group into both the adenine and ribose moieties (91, 92). Haley and co-workers synthesized 8-azido cAMP VII (93) and an 8-azido ATP analogue (94).

i) $R^1 = COCN_2CO_2C_2H_5$,
   $R^2 = H$

ii) $R^1 = R^2 = COCN_2CO_2C_2H_5$

iii) $R^1 = H$,
    $R^2 = COCN_2CO_2C_2H_5$

VI   VII

Both the α-diazoacyl and azido derivatives have been used to study cAMP receptors on erythrocyte membranes. Rubin, in extending the results of Cooperman and co-workers (56), showed that the single protein that was labeled was a regulatory subunit of a membrane-bound protein kinase (95). The 8-azido analogue used by Haley (93, 96, 97) labeled two proteins on the membrane in slightly higher yield than did the α-diazo analogue; one of the two proteins appears to be identical to that labeled by VI while the other may be a glycoprotein. A small amount of radiolabel was found in four other proteins, a finding that may have been the result of nonspecific labeling or the presence of secondary cAMP binding sites of low affinity. The mechanism of ATP regulation of the membrane-bound protein kinase has been investigated through the use of the 8-azido analogues of cAMP and ATP (98). The enzyme (type I protein kinase) has a membrane-bound regulatory subunit that contains binding sites for cAMP and ATP; the binding of ATP at this site appears to inhibit both cAMP binding and the cAMP-induced release of the catalytic unit from the membrane bound regulatory subunit. Recently, cAMP receptors on porcine venal cortical plasma membranes have been labeled by utilizing the intrinsic photolability of cAMP (99). Greengard et al have used VII to examine differences in the cAMP receptors in the cytosol of various tissues of rats (100). Primarily, only two receptors of different molecular weight were labeled; these are believed to be the regulatory subunits of Types I and II protein kinases. This example illustrates the potential of photogenerated reagents to identify, and perhaps even estimate the concentration of, different receptors in cytosol from different tissues or animal species.

Haley and co-workers have used 8-azido cAMP to label and thus to help distinguish cyclic AMP binding sites in whole cells of the sarcoma 37 line (101). In principle, such labeling studies on whole cells followed by cell fractionation may lead to information on the distribution of such receptors in nuclei, mitochondria, etc. The 8-azido analogue may enjoy a special advantage in that it is expected to be more stable to hydrolysis in whole cells than are the acyl derivatives, VI. Both acyl and alkyl derivatives of cAMP similar to VI have, however, been shown to be more potent than cAMP in provoking hormonal responses in intact cells (102, 103). An 8-azido analogue of GTP has been used to label the GTP-binding site on tubulin dimers (104). Synthesis of 8-azido GTP and other 8-azido purine analogues has been reported (105). Two newly introduced fluorescent photoaffinity labels for nucleotides, analogues of cAMP (106) and of guanosine phosphate (107), hold much promise for studies directed at identifying receptors by photolabeling of membranes, whole cells, and nerve fibers.

HORMONE RECEPTORS   Hormone-receptor interactions are being investigated for membrane-bound and cytoplasmic receptors, in studies largely centered on steroid hormones (108, 109) and on peptide hormones, e.g. insulin, gonadotropin, and melanotropin (110, 111).

Steroid receptors   The use of photogenerated reagents in the study of estrogen receptors was introduced by Katzenellenbogen and co-workers (112–118). They prepared diazo and azido derivatives of estradiol, estrone, and hexestrol to try to photolabel the cytoplasmic receptor that, despite several different approaches by other workers, has so far proved too difficult to isolate. The binding affinities of these various derivatives were obtained by a competition assay; photolysis showed incorporation of radiolabel into the receptor to the extent of 5–20%. Studies with partially purified receptor however yielded better results, with decreased nonspecific labeling. A problem encountered in early experiments using crude cytoplasm was the hydrolytic lability of the diazoacyl group when present as the ester of the steroid molecule. This work on steroid receptors has been recently reviewed by Katzenellenbogen (119–121).

Edelman and co-workers have used photogenerated reagents to study corticosteroid receptors (122, 123). They used 21-diazo corticosteroids (α-diazoketones) which, on photolysis in methanol, yielded exclusively the product of addition of methanol to the ketene generated by Wolff rearrangement. As this model study shows, exclusive generation of ketene could be a test of the potential for nonspecific labeling by photogenerated ketene. The apparent K_d for 21-diazo-21-deoxy-[6,7-^{3}H]corticosterone was found to be 3.2×10^{-8} M, only 1.5 times greater than that of corticosterone itself. Photolysis led to incorporation of label into the corticosteroid-binding globulin. Polyacrylamide gel electrophoresis revealed label in three proteins, but photolysis in presence of competitive inhibitors showed that only one of the three had been labeled specifically. Furthermore, photolysis in the presence of tris buffer instead of phosphate buffer resulted in incorporation of label in the specifically labeled protein but very little in the others. Tris might be expected to scavenge ketene present in solution; the specifically labeled protein had apparently reacted with the ketene generated at the active site and not that equilibrated with such species in solution. Independent evidence for site-specific labeling was provided by fluorescence quenching experiments. This study suggests that when the binding is tight ($\sim 10^{-8}$ M) and when, presumably, reactive nucleophiles are present in the binding site, photoaffinity labeling with diazoketones via ketenes may prove to be specific enough to be useful. However, in the absence of product analysis, the results of labeling by way of a ketene should be regarded as preliminary. These investigations with steroids also demonstrate the utility of initial partial purification of receptors to reduce nonspecific labeling, and emphasize the need for reagents of high specific radioactivity to facilitate isolation of receptors found in low abundance.

Peptide hormones   Photolabile derivatives of peptide hormones have been synthesized, and labeling of specific receptors can be expected. Schwyzer and co-workers have synthesized p-azidophenylalanine, and incorporated the 3,5-ditritiated analogues into different peptides and peptide hormones (124, 128). In photolysis experiments using various ring substituted azido and nitro derivatives of phenylalanine, they observed irreversible incorporation of peptides containing the *p*-nitrophenyl moiety (126) into chymotrypsin. This unexpected result prompted a model study of the photochemistry of *p*-nitrophenylalanine and the corresponding N-acetyl ethyl ester (129). Photolysis in aqueous media led only to tar-like residues, and in aqueous ethanol, the exclusive identifiable product, isolated in only 4% yield, was *p,p*, '-azoxy-di(N-acetyl-phenylalanine ethyl ester), a coupling product not useful from the point of view of photoaffinity labeling. These results cast doubt upon the utility of the aromatic nitro moiety for photo-affinity labeling.

A diazomalonyl and a 2-nitro-5-azidobenzoyl derivative of the neurohypophyseal hormone, oxytocin, have been prepared and used to photolabel the receptor believed to mediate oxytocin-stimulated water transport in toad urinary bladder (130). In a separate study a tripeptide containing *p*-azidophenylalanine has been used recently to study the interaction of neurophysin II with oxytocin (131). Photolysis led to irreversible inactivation of the ligand-binding capacity of neurophysin II. These studies, although preliminary, hold promise for the elucidation of ligand receptor interaction at a molecular level.

Glucagon (132) and insulin (133) receptors have also been studied by using photolabile derivatives of these hormones. Both studies used an aromatic azido photolabile group, and appear to have led to specific labeling of the corresponding receptor. A 2-nitro-5-azidobenzoyl pentapeptide that mimics the action of the potent secretagogue cerulein in stimulating secretion of proteins from acinar cells of guinea pig pancreas in vitro, has been used to investigate the cerulein receptor by Galardy & Jamieson (134). Photolysis of the peptide in the presence of pancreatic lobules led to irreversible stimulation of protein discharge, although no protection against irreversible labeling was provided by cerulein. The absence of protection by cerulein and other peptide secretagogues raises questions as to the interpretation of these experiments.

Galardy and co-workers had earlier introduced the use of aryl ketone derivatives, and had obtained up to 50 mole% photolabeling of bovine serum albumin (known to bind carboxyl terminal tetrapeptide of gastrin) with arylazido and aryl ketone derivatives of pentagastrin (55). As Martyr & Benisek had suggested earlier, the triplet state of the ketone is relatively inert to reaction with water (53). The rate constant for hydrogen abstraction from water by benzophenone on photoactivation is $10^2 M^{-1} s^{-1}$, whereas that for abstraction from alcohol is 10^5–$10^7 M^{-1} s^{-1}$ (135). This, in principle, may be a major advantage since, as noted before, both carbenes and nitrenes are "wasted" to a considerable degree by reaction with water during photoaffinity labeling studies of biological systems. In model studies, Galardy and co-workers photolyzed acetophenone or benzophenone together with Nacetylglycine methyl ester in water but obtained C–H insertion products in only 6–8% yield after prolonged photolysis ($t_{1/2}$ = 55 hr for 0.03M acetophenone).

TRANSPORT PROTEINS   The identification and study of specific transport systems for inorganic ions, amino acids, and sugars is an active area of biochemical research (136–138). Like other specific receptors, these transport systems are found in low concentration and are usually imbedded in membranes; they are ideal targets for investigation by photoaffinity labeling. Photoaffinity labeling studies have been conducted on β-galactoside transport in *E. coli* (139, 140), anion transport in erythrocytes (141–144), glucose transport in erythrocytes (145) and adipocyte (146) plasma membranes, adenine nucleotide translocation (147–151), and peptide transport in *E. coli* (152). In initial studies, Kaback and co-workers showed inactivation of lactose transport on irradiation of *E. coli* membrane vesicles in the presence of 2-nitro-4-azidophenyl-1-thio-β-D-galactopyranoside and D-lactate (139). No inactivation was observed in the absence of D-lactate, which supports the hypothesis that the lac carrier system functions only when energized. The azidophenylgalactoside, although a competitive inhibitor of lactose transport (K_i = 75 μM), is itself accumulated in the vesicles; therefore labeling may have occurred from the inside surface. More recently, Kaback and co-workers (140) have repeated the study with 2'-N-(2-nitro-4-azidophenyl)-aminoethyl-1-thio-β-D-galactopyranoside. Although it is not transported, this compound is a competitive inhibitor of lactose transport (K_i = 30–40 μM). Photolysis leads again to inactivation of lac transport only in the presence of D-lactate or upon imposition of a membrane potential by valinomycin-induced potassium efflux, which supports the hypothesis concerning energized transport stated above.

Adenine nucleotide translocation in mitochondria has been investigated by using three different reagents: a photolabile derivative 8-azidoadenosine diphosphate (147), a 4-azido-2-nitrophenyl aminobutyrl derivative of the competitive inhibitor atractyloside (148), and a derivative of ADP that carries a photolabile group at the 2'-hydroxyl group (149). As the translocation system is readily damaged by ultraviolet light, the nitroarylazido derivative, which can be photoactivated by visible light, was utilized. The atractyloside derivative and the 2'-hydroxyl derivative of ADP appear to label the same protein, which supports the contention that the label was incorporated onto the specific translocation system.

Staros & Knowles have used glycyl-4-azido-2-nitro-L-phenylalanine to irreversibly inhibit the transport of glycylglycine by live *E. coli* W cells upon photolysis at 350 nm (152). The photolabile dipeptide is a reversible inhibitor of Gly-Gly transport in the dark and is itself transported. An analysis of the reversible inhibition suggests the presence of multiple transport systems; use of radiolabeled inhibitor is expected to lead to an identification of the dipeptide transport system of *E. coli.*

MISCELLANEOUS APPLICATIONS   Leonard and co-workers have synthesized 4-azido-2-chlorophenoxyacetic acid and shown that it has auxin activity (153). They hope to use the reagent to identify and isolate an auxin receptor. Recently, three different azido derivatives of adenine have been reported as possible photoaffinity labeling agents for cytokinin binding sites on plant cells (154, 155). The compounds have been shown to possess cytokinin-like activity.

In a fascinating new application of photoaffinity labeling, Menevse and co-workers have used aromatic azido compounds in an attempt to label frog olfactory receptors (156). Nakanishi and co-workers have synthesized the diazoacetyl analogue of (6E,11Z)-6,11-hexadecadienyl acetate, a sex pheromone for the moth *Antheraca polyphemus,* to study pheromone receptor interaction (157). By recording electrophysiological response from a single olfactory hair they have established that the photolabile analogue exhibits 10% of the activity of the natural pheromone and is specific in eliciting electrical response only from the acetate receptor cell dendrites and not from the aldehyde sensitive cells. These preliminary experiments are exciting in that they open a possible new area of application for photolabile reagents.

These studies on receptors and transport systems illustrate several important features of photogenerated reagents. For studies in vivo or with crude cytoplasm high specific radioactivity is necessary. The natural ligand, especially if it is small, should be perturbed as little as possible upon attachment of the photolabile group. Stringent controls are necessary to establish specific photoaffinity labeling; photolabile groups that generate reactive species of short lifetimes are particularly attractive. In systems where the dissociation constants are low, $\leqslant 10^{-8}$ M, and reactive nucleophiles are accessible in the binding site, longer-lived species may be acceptable, as seen in the labeling of the corticosteroid receptor.

Membrane Function and Structure

The structure, topographical distribution, and function of membrane-bound proteins is an area of current interest, as is the nature of the hydrophobic interaction of such proteins with the phospholipids of the bilayer (158–161). Photogenerated reagents of high indiscriminate reactivity are ideally suited to the study of the fluid mosaic of lipid and protein. Staros & Richards have used N-(4-azido-2-nitrophenyl)-2-aminoethyl sulfonate to label the surface proteins of human erythrocyte membrane (162). The permeability of the membrane to the reagent is temperature-dependent and in subsequent studies use was made of this fact to label the cytoplasmic surface of the membrane (163, 164). The results suggest that although some proteins are embedded either in the exterior or interior surface others may span the bilayer. Whole erythrocyte cells were incubated with the reagent at 37° (the membrane is permeable to the reagent at this temperature), then the cells were cooled to 0°, washed, and finally photolyzed. Electrophoresis of the photolyzed membranes revealed that oligomers ($n = 1$–4) of hemoglobin had been produced in significant yield. Polymerization is attributed to a "parallel side reaction accompanying the insertion process which is of principal interest for labeling." The authors suggest that radicals produced by the nitrene in the reaction with peptide chains could lead to polymerization by a radical recombination mechanism. The enhanced reactivity of the photogenerated species over conventional reagents was demonstrated by the labeling of proteins not previously tagged by other reagents.

Klip et al used 1-azidonaphthalene and 1-azido-4-iodobenzene in an attempt to photolabel membrane components from within the lipid core (165, 166). The idea in such studies and others subsequently published (167–171) is to diffuse into the lipid bilayer a hydrophobic photoaffinity labeling reagent that, on photolysis, will label protein components buried in the lipid core. Interpretation of such studies, however, may prove to be hazardous because such reagents are mobile in the bilayer and the lifetime of the nitrene or equivalent generated on photolysis will be an important variable.

Two careful studies by Bayley & Knowles highlight such concerns and cast doubt upon the usefulness of nitrenes in photolabeling hydrophobic regions of biological systems (172, 173). Phenylnitrene, generated by photolysis of phenylazide, was found to label fatty acid chains in phospholipid vesicles only in low yield (0.25–3.3%). In addition, the labeling was reduced to essentially zero when photolysis was conducted with glutathione present in the aqueous phase. Such scavenging of the photoactivated species in solution, even though the reagent may be generated in the bilayer, led the authors to conclude that "nitrenes are unsatisfactory reagents for the labeling not only of lipids but also of the hydrophobic amino acid chains of membrane proteins that are contiguous with lipid." Bayley & Knowles utilized 3-phenyl-3H-diazirine and spiro[adamantane-2,2'-diazirine] to generate carbenes in lipid bilayers and compared their utility as photolabeling reagents with that of phenylazide. These carbenes do undergo intramolecular rearrangement, but, nevertheless, label phospholipids in yields ranging from 3–10%; the yield, although significantly better than that obtained with nitrenes, is still quite low. Importantly, however, added glutathione had no effect on the yield. Carbenes, then, are clearly superior to nitrenes for photoaffinity labeling of hydrophobic regions of biological systems.

Khorana and co-workers synthesized fatty acids incorporating different photolabile groups (174) and used them to support the growth of auxotrophs of *E. coli* (175). Thus, viable biological membranes containing defined and characterized photolabile probes were obtained. Photolysis would lead to cross-linking with proteins in the immediate vicinity, thus providing a reliable picture of the membrane topography. This elegant approach has great potential, and these workers have outlined a comprehensive program directed at elucidating membrane structure, and lipid-lipid and lipid-protein interactions. Stoffel et al have also synthesized various fatty acids containing the azido group and demonstrated their incorporation into phospho- and spingholipids of eukaryotic cells by adding them to the growth medium in tissue culture (176). Preliminary results of experiments with high density apolipoprotein have been recently published (177).

A new α-diazo photolabile group, trifluorodiazopropionate, introduced by Chowdhry, Vaughan & Westheimer (40), has been used successfully to study membranes. Khorana and co-workers reported the synthesis of fatty acids of variable length, containing the trifluorodiazopropionyl and diazirinophenoxy groups; the photolabile fatty acids can be incorporated into mixed diacyl phospholipids, and into vesicles containing such phospholipids, either alone or together with ^{14}C-dipalmitoylphosphatidylcholine or ^{14}C-cholesterol (178). Photolysis of these vesicles led to insertion of the carbene into C–H bonds at the expected positions along the fatty acid chain. Further, fully reactivated Ca^{2+}/Mg^{2+} ATPase of sarcoplasmic reticulum and bacteriorhodopsin was obtained on treatment of delipidated proteins with the above-mentioned phospholipids and "photolysis of bacteriorhodopsin reconstituted with trifluorodiazopropionylphosphatidylcholine resulted in the expected level of phospholipid-protein crosslinking" (178). These results demonstrate the potential of appropriate photolabile groups to elucidate the lipid-lipid and phospholipid-protein interactions that are responsible for the stability, complexity, and function of biological membranes.

Erecinska and co-workers attached one to two 2,4-dinitrophenylazide moieties to cytochrome *c* (presumed to be at lysine residues on the protein surface) to investigate whether cytochrome *c* is active in the mitochondrial respiratory chain when bound to a mitochondrial site and, if so, to identify the binding site (179). The apparent dissociation constant of cytochrome *c* from the mitochondrial membrane is reported to be 5×10^{-8}M, and that of the derivatized cytochrome *c*, $\sim 10^{-7}$ M. Photolysis yielded cytochrome

c covalently bound to the mitochondria; subsequent fractionation in the presence of detergents and salts showed that cytochrome c had been covalently attached to cytochrome c oxidase, although in poor yield. Recently Erecinska has reported a higher yield of the covalent complex in this same system when a different arylazide derivative of cytochrome c was used (180). The cytochrome c:cytochrome oxidase complex was shown to be capable of mediating electron transfer between N,N,N',N'-tetramethyl-p-phenylenediamine/ascorbate and the oxidase. A similar independent study has been published recently by Bisson et al (181). In another approach to the study of protein complexes embedded in membranes Ji et al (182) have used flash photolysis of cleavable heterobifunctional reagents incorporating an arylazide as the photolabile group. The reagent is first attached covalently to membrane proteins by an imidoester function, and then subjected to flash photolysis of millisecond duration leading to cross-links in proximate proteins. As the specificity of such cross-linking depends on the diffusion rate of proteins in the membrane and the lifetime of nitrenes, neither of which is well documented, rigorous control experiments and cautious interpretation of results are necessary.

The studies discussed in this section illustrate the potential for the use of photogenerated reagents in the study of membrane topography, the structure of multienzyme complexes, and the topographical distribution of proteins in organelles. Photoaffinity labeling is likely to emerge as a major technique for elucidation of structure and function of biological membranes.

Ribosomes

The structure and function of ribosomes from *E. coli* have been intensively studied in recent years (184, 185). Bispink & Matthaei used ethyl-2-diazomalonyl Phe-tRNA in the first study of the *E. coli* ribosome by photogenerated reagents (186). Several groups have used both α-diazoacyl and arylazide derivatives of different ribosomal ligands to probe the structure of ribosomes (186–188). Despite the importance of this research, and the impressive literature on the subject, limitations of space do not permit a discussion of these studies; they have, however, been recently reviewed (189).

Nucleic Acids

Photoaffinity labeling has been used to study protein-nucleic acid interactions (62–64, 190, 191) and drug-nucleic acid interactions (192, 193). Studies directed at elucidating protein-nucleic acid interactions have been undertaken with DNA (62) and RNA (63), polymerase complexes with DNA, lac repressor-DNA complex (190, 191), and complexes of tRNA with aminoacyl tRNA synthetases (64, 194, 195). Usually these studies have utilized the photochemical lability of nucleic acids at short wavelength to bring about photochemical cross-linking of nucleic acid and protein. The mechanism of photochemical labeling in such studies is often not well understood. This raises doubts about how well the cross-linked complex reflects the geometry of the natural complex, especially because in many of these studies significant photoinduced damage accompanies cross-linking.

Yielding et al have photolyzed an azido derivative of ethidium bromide to covalently attach this intercalating drug to DNA, both in vivo and in vitro (197–199). Photolysis enhanced production of petite mutants in *Saccharomyces* and produced frameshift mutations in *Salmonella*. Production of these mutants by irreversible attachment of the intercalating drug, ethidium bromide, to DNA has been cited as evidence for the need to produce covalent attachment in mutagenesis. Such studies could prove useful in elucidating not only the mechanism of action of drugs that interact with DNA, but also the mechanism of mutagenesis induced by covalent attachment of small molecules to DNA.

Antibodies

The results of initial studies on photoaffinity labeling of antibodies are presented above. Several new studies have since been published (200–204). Knowles and co-workers have reported on the photoaffinity labeling of antibodies produced against the nitroazidophenyl haptenic group (200, 201). Antibodies exhibiting low dissociation constants ($\sim 10^{-7}$ M) were used and photolysis of the isolated antibody antigen complex led to labeling of the combining sites. These studies, together with those reported by Fisher & Press (202) show that when the ligand receptor complex is tight (dissociation constant of 10^{-6} M or less), photoaffinity labeling with the arylazide photolabile group does not appear to suffer from the problems of pseudophotoaffinity labeling discussed earlier. Applications of photogenerated reagents to the study of antibody combining sites have been recently reviewed (189c).

Enzymes

Enzymes catalyzing several different chemical reactions have been labeled with photogenerated reagents incorporating α-diazoacyl and arylazido groups. These applications have been listed in recent reviews (28, 29, 189c); only a few examples are presented here. Different azido derivatives of nicotinamide adenine dinucleotide have been prepared and their interactions with various dehydrogenases studied (205–207), although identification of the photochemically labeled amino acids has not as yet appeared. Several studies with photogenerated reagents have been directed at different adenosine triphosphatases; recent studies have utilized arylazido derivatives attached to the 3'-hydroxyl moiety of ATP (207–210). Such multiple investigations of specific enzymes by different reagents is expected to produce a more credible picture of the active sites. Bridges & Knowles photolyzed p-azido-^{14}C-cinnamoyl α-chymotrypsin to test the labeling characteristics of arylazides on a protein of known tertiary structure (211). Photolysis led to 60% incorporation of the radiolabel into the enzyme, and peptide analyses showed the radioactivity to be localized on the C chain in the tryptic fragment which forms the aromatic binding site of the enzyme. The high yield of label, localized in a hydrophobic pocket, further confirms the ability of photogenerated reagents to label biological receptor sites.

Henkin has recently introduced the diazoacyl mixed disulfide, VIII, to attach a photolabile reagent to thiol enzymes (212). This reagent was used successfully to label serine and threonine residues of creatine kinase, and should prove useful for the labeling of other sulfhydryl enzymes.

Hixson & Hixson had earlier introduced p-azidophenacyl bromide (IX) as a reagent suitable for photoaffinity labeling of sulfhydryl enzymes, and reported a preliminary study of its inactivation of glyceraldehyde 3-phosphate dehydrogenase (213). The extent of photoincorporation or the identity of labeled amino acid residues has not yet been reported. Barden and co-workers have prepared p-azidobenzoyl CoA and used it to photolabel acyl CoA : glycine N-acyltransferase (214). The enzyme has also been photolabeled by an 8-azidoadenine derivative of the coenzyme (215). Finally, transcarboxylase has been photolabeled by the radioactive analogue of p-azidobenzoyl CoA (216). The labeling was specific for the CoA ester sites on the carboxylase and revealed the presence of two binding sites per polypeptide in the 26S-transcarboxylase. This result is believed to support the theory of gene duplication and fusion leading to structural homology in the polypeptides of 12S$_\text{H}$ subunit.

New Photolabile Groups

The preceding discussion highlights the desirability of having several different photolabile groups of varying steric, electronic, and photochemical properties to facilitate a judicious choice, depending on the particular application being considered. Further, the reliability of results would be enhanced by studying the biological system of interest with different reagents and different photolabile groups, not only to ensure that the labeling patterns observed reflect true interactions but also because, in the absence of ideal reagents, negative results have little significance. The properties desirable in a photolabile group are chemical stability prior to photoactivation, rapid rate of photolysis at long wavelength, and very short half life for the photogenerated reactive species leading to labeling of the environment in which it is generated. The mechanism of labeling should not involve intramolecular rearrangement to a less reactive labeling species, such as ketene. None of the photolabile groups currently in use meet these requirements fully although some come closer than others. Arylazides are rapidly reduced to the corresponding amines by dithiothreitol at room temperature and physiological pH (105, 217). Such chemical instability is undesirable in a photoaffinity labeling reagent because dithiothreitol is commonly added to buffer solutions used in biochemical studies.

Smith & Knowles studied the photochemical behavior of aryl diazirines to evaluate their potential use in photoaffinity labeling studies (218, 219). Unlike the corresponding diazo compounds, these diazirines are stable for hours in 1 M acetic acid, and though of limited stability at room temperature in the pure state, are stable for several months as dilute ($<$0.1M) solutions in inert solvents at $-20°$. The diazirines show a characteristic absorption at 350–400 nm ($\epsilon \sim$ 200–300). Photolysis leads to some isomerization to the corresponding acid-labile diazo compound which is also however photolabile. Thus photolysis of phenyl diazirine in hexane/acetic acid led to a mixture of benzyl acetate and products of insertion of the benzyl carbene into the C–H bonds of hexane. In spite of these complications, the photolabile diazirine group holds much promise, as illustrated by a recent study on photolabeling of vesicles (172, 173).

Despite the inherent advantages in the use of photogenerated carbenes for photoaffinity labeling (26–29, 172, 173) the α-diazoesters most used so far suffer from three principal defects which have restricted their general utility. These defects are 1. instability to heat and acid, 2. the 30–60% Wolff rearrangement observed on photolysis of α-diazoesters (32, 220) and the 100% Wolff rearrangement on photolysis of α-diazothioesters (39, 221), and 3. the long time required for photolysis at 350 nm. Chemical instability, in addition to being a problem during synthesis and handling of the photolabile reagents, may lead to nonspecific labeling. The Wolff rearrangement decreases the amount of insertion into the macromolecule under study. The new photolabile groups, 2-diazo-3,3,3-trifluoropropionate, [X, (40)] and p-toluenesulfonyldiazoacetate, [XI, (222, 223)], have been recently introduced. They are essentially free of these defects, and hold much promise as precursors to carbenes for photoaffinity labeling of biological macro-molecules (178, 224).

$$CF_3-\overset{\overset{\displaystyle N_2}{\|}}{C}-\overset{\overset{\displaystyle O}{\|}}{C}-R \qquad\qquad CH_3-\langle\bigcirc\rangle-\overset{\overset{\displaystyle O}{\|}}{\underset{\underset{\displaystyle O}{\|}}{S}}-\overset{\overset{\displaystyle N_2}{\|}}{C}-\overset{\overset{\displaystyle O}{\|}}{C}-R$$

$$\mathbf{X} \qquad\qquad\qquad \mathbf{XI}$$

$$R = Cl, \quad -O-\langle\bigcirc\rangle-NO_2, \ OR', \ SR'$$

The compounds are stable in 1M hydrochloric acid! Photolysis of O-esters of trifluorodiazopropionic acid yields only 15% of the Wolff rearrangement product. In contrast to the photolysis of other α-diazothioesters (39, 221), photolysis of N-acetyl-O-methyl-cysteinyl-2-diazo-3,3,3-trifluoropropion-ate led to 40% insertion into the –OH bond of solvent methanol. α-Diazo-thioesters of biological thiols containing the photolabile group, X, may now be used as precursors of carbenes for photoaffinity labeling studies. The ^{19}F nucleus provides a sensitive NMR probe of the macromolecule under study (V. Chowdhry and R. A. Hudson, unpublished data). 2-Diazo-2-p-toluenesulfonyl diazoacetates are stable crystalline solids. Ethyl-2-diazo-2-p-toluenesulfonyl acetate yields 95% insertion into solvent on photolysis; no Wolff rearrangement product was detected. The thioester, thioethyl-2-diazo-2-p-toluenesulfonyl acetate, like the trifluorodiazopropionyl thio-ester, did not lead exclusively to the Wolff rearrangement product; 25% insertion into the –OH bond of solvent methanol was observed. p-Toluenesulfonyl diazoacetates, like other α-diazoesters, exhibit broad absorption maxima at long wavelength ($\sim$370 nm); the extinction coeffi-cients and rates of photolysis are however significantly greater than those of other diazoesters. This is a distinct advantage in photoaffinity labeling studies of macromolecules, particularly those that are especially sensitive to short wavelength UV radiation.

Recently, a series of photolabile α-diazophosphonate dianions has been synthesized (225, 226). Their chemical stability depends on the substituent attached to the diazo carbon. Breslow, Feiring & Herman have studied the photochemistry of phosphoryl azides (227a). Photolysis of the thermally stable alkoxy and phenoxy derivatives of these compounds in t-butanol produced no intramolecular rearrangement to the metaphosphoroimidate, and reasonable yields of the C–H insertion product on photolysis in hydro-carbon solvents were observed. The phosphoryl nitrenes also exhibited the lowest selectivity between primary, secondary, and tertiary carbon-hydro-gen bonds so far reported for nitrenes. The absence of intramolecular rear-rangement and indiscriminate reactivity suggest nitrenes derived from these compounds may be useful for photoaffinity labeling. Chládek and co-workers have synthesized 5'-phosphorylazide derivatives of guanosine and adenosine nucleotides (227b). Preliminary biochemical and photochemical studies suggest that these compounds may prove to be useful photoaffinity labeling reagents.

Nitrophenyl ethers undergo nucleophilic photosubstitution by aliphatic amines on photoactivation (228). Recently, new photoaffinity labeling reagents incorporating two nitrophenyl ethers, 4-nitro-methoxybenzene and 2-methoxy-4-nitro-methoxybenzene, have been used to cross-link proteins (229). Photoaffinity labeling reagents incorporating nitrophenyl ethers could prove useful in synthesizing covalent oligomers of proteins and studying topographical distribution of proteins in organelles.

CONCLUSION

Photoaffinity labeling has evolved into a widely used technique for the study of molecular interactions in complex biological systems. One of the more exciting areas of future application promises to be in vivo studies, including turning on specific receptors of specialized cells. Increased understanding of the mechanism of photoinactivation, through detailed studies on the photochemical behavior of reagents and photogenerated reactive species, should provide new capabilities, particularly for studying transient phenomena. Improvements in structural identification of small amounts of labeled products will greatly enhance the utility of photogenerated reagents. Their use in biochemical studies is now well established and is expected to grow both in volume and in level of sophistication.

ACKNOWLEDGMENTS

This review is drawn in part from the PhD thesis of V. Chowdhry (39); we thank the Institute of General Medical Sciences of the National Institutes of Health (grant 04712) and the donors of the Petroleum Research Fund, administered by the American Chemical Society, for support of the research in that thesis. We are grateful to Professors B. S. Cooperman, B. E. Haley, and J. R. Knowles for providing manuscripts reporting their work prior to publication, and to Dr. A. E. Feiring, Dr. T. Fukunaga, and Ms. S. Vladuchick for careful reading of the manuscript and helpful comments.

Literature Cited

1. Singer, S. J. 1967. *Adv. Protein Chem.* 22:1–54
2. Shaw, E. 1970. *The Enzymes* 1:91–146
3. Wold, F. 1977. *Methods Enzymol.* 46:3–14
4. Davies, D. R., Padlan, E. A., Segal, D. M. 1975. *Ann. Rev. Biochem.* 44: 639–67
5. Rossmann, M. G., Liljas, A., Branden, C., Banaszak, L. J. 1975. *The Enzymes* 11A:61–102
6. Kim, S. H., Suddath, F. L., Quigley, G. J., McPherson, A., Sussman, J. L., Wang, A. H. J., Seeman, N. C., Rich, A. 1974. *Science* 185:435–40
7. Robertus, J. D., Ladner, J. E., Finch, J. T., Rhodes, D., Brown, R. S., Clark, B. F. C., Klug, A. 1974. *Nature* 250: 546–51
8. Fink, A. L. 1977. *Acc. Chem. Res.* 10:233–39
9. Petsko, G. A. 1975. *J. Mol. Biol.* 96:381–92
10. Douzou, P., Hoa, G. H. B., Petsko, G. A. 1975. *J. Mol. Biol.* 96:367–80
11. Mildvan, A. S. 1977. *Acc. Chem. Res.* 10:246–52
12. Lilley, D. M. J., Pardon, J. F., Richards, B. M. 1977. *Biochemistry.* 16: 2853–60
13. Spiro, T. G., Gaber, B. P. 1977. *Ann. Rev. Biochem.* 46:553–72
14. Wu, C.-W., Yarbrough, L. R., Wu, F. Y.-H. 1976. *Biochemistry.* 15:2863–68
15. Brand, L., Gohlke, J. R. 1972. *Ann. Rev. Biochem.* 41:843–68
16. Dugas, H. 1977. *Acc. Chem. Res.* 10: 47–54
17. Butterfield, D. A. 1977. *Acc. Chem. Res.* 10:111–16
18. Engelman, D. M., Moore, P. B. 1976. *Sci. Am.* 235(4):44–54
19. Engelman, D. M., Moore, P. B. 1975. *Ann. Rev. Biophys. Bioeng.* 4:219–41
20. Helmkamp, G. M., Jr., Rando, R. R., Brock, D. J. H., Bloch, K. 1968. *J. Biol. Chem.* 243:3229–31
21. Abeles, R. H., Maycock, A. L. 1976. *Acc. Chem. Res.* 9:313–19
22. Rando, R. R. 1975. *Acc. Chem. Res.* 8:281–88
23. Walsh, C. T. 1977. In *Horizons in Biochemistry and Biophysics,* ed. E. Quagliariello, 3:36–81. Reading, Mass: Addison-Wesley. 340 pp.
24. Miesowicz, F. M., Bloch, K. E. 1975. *Biochem. Biophys. Res. Commun.* 65:331–35
25. Singh, A., Thornton, E. R., Westheimer, F. H. 1962. *J. Biol. Chem.* 237:PC3006–8

26. Knowles, J. R. 1972. *Acc. Chem. Res.* 5:155–60
27. Creed, D. 1974. *Photochem. Photobiol.* 19:459–62
28. Cooperman, B. S. 1976. In *Aging, Carcinogenesis and Radiation Biology,* ed. K. C. Smith, pp. 315–340. New York: Plenum 340 pp.
29. Bayley, H., Knowles, J. R. 1977. *Methods Enzymol.* 46:69–114
30. Balls, A. K., Aldrich, F. L. 1955. *Proc. Natl. Acad. Sci. USA* 41:190–96
31. Balls, A. K., Wood, H. N. 1956. *J. Biol. Chem.* 219:245–56
32. Shafer, J., Baronowsky, P., Laursen, R., Finn, F., Westheimer, F. H. 1966. *J. Biol. Chem.* 241:421–27
33. Hexter, C. S., Westheimer, F. H. 1971. *J. Biol. Chem.* 246:3928–33
34. Hexter, C. S. 1971. *Mapping of enzymic active sites with photochemically generated carbenes.* PhD thesis. Harvard Univ., Cambridge, Mass. 82 pp.
35. Hexter, C. S., Westheimer, F. H. 1971. *J. Biol. Chem.* 246:3934–38
36. Rajagopalan, T. G., Stein, W. H., Moore, S. 1966. *J. Biol. Chem.* 241:4295–97
37. Vaughan, R. J., Westheimer, F. H. 1969. *J. Am. Chem. Soc.* 21:217–18
38. Stefanovsky, Y., Westheimer, F. H. 1973. *Proc. Natl. Acad. Sci. USA* 70:1132–36
39. Chowdhry, V. 1977. *New reagents for photoaffinity labeling.* PhD thesis. Harvard Univ., Cambridge, Mass. 396 pp.
40. Chowdhry, V., Vaughan, R., Westheimer, F. H. 1976. *Proc. Natl. Acad. Sci. USA* 73:1406–8
41. Browne, D. T., Hixson, S. S., Westheimer, F. H. 1971. *J. Biol. Chem.* 246:4477–84
42. Hixson, S. S., Hixson, S. H. 1973. *Photochem. Photobiol.* 18:135–38
43. Cooperman, B. S., Brunswick, D. J. 1973. *Biochemistry* 12:4079–84
44. Fleet, G. W. J., Porter, R. R., Knowles, J. R. 1969. *Nature* 224:511–12
45. Converse, C. A., Richards, F. F. 1969. *Biochemistry* 8:4431–36
46. Ruoho, A. E., Kiefer, H., Roeder, P. E., Singer, S. J. 1973. *Proc. Natl. Acad. Sci. USA* 70:2567–71
47. Yoshioka, M., Lifter, J., Hew, C.-L., Converse, C. A., Armstrong, M. Y. K., Konigsberg, W. H., Richards, F. F. 1973. *Biochemistry* 12:4679–85
48. Hew, C.-L., Lifter, J., Yoshioka, M., Richards, F. F., Konigsberg, W. H. 1973. *Biochemistry* 12:4685–89

49. Lifter, J., Hew, C.-L., Yoshioka, M., Richards, F. F., Konigsberg, W. H. 1974. *Biochemistry* 13:3567–71
50. Richards, F. F., Lifter, J., Hew, C.-L., Yoshioka, M., Konigsberg, W. H. 1974. *Biochemistry* 13:3572–75
51. Amzel, L. M., Poljak, R. J., Varga, J. M., Richards, F. F. 1974. *Proc. Natl. Acad. Sci. USA* 71:1427–30
52. Hixson, S. H., Hixson, S. S. 1975. *Biochemistry* 14:4251–54
53. Martyr, R. J., Benisek, W. F. 1973. *Biochemistry* 12:2172–78
54. Ogez, J. R., Tivol, W. F., Benisek, W. F. 1977. *J. Biol. Chem.* 252:6151–55
55. Galardy, R. E., Craig, L. C., Jamieson, J. D., Printz, M. P. 1974. *J. Biol. Chem.* 249:3510–18
56. Guthrow, C. E., Rasmussen, H., Brunswick, D. J., Cooperman, B. S. 1973. *Proc. Natl. Acad. Sci. USA* 70:3344–46
57. Kallos, J. 1977. *Nature (London)* 265:705–10
58. Antonoff, R. S., Ferguson, J. J. Jr. 1974. *J. Biol. Chem.* 249:3319–21
59. Antonoff, R. S., Ferguson, J. J. Jr., Idelkope, G. 1976. *Photochem. Photobiol.* 23:327–29
60. Obrig, T. G., Antonoff, R. S., Kirwin, K. S., Ferguson, J. J. Jr. 1975. *Biochem. Biophys. Res. Commun.* 66:437–43
61. Smith, K. C. 1976. In *Photochemistry and Photobiology of Nucleic Acids,* ed. S. Y. Wang, Vols 1, 2. New York: Academic. 596 pp. 430 pp.
62. Markovitz, A. 1972. *Biochim. Biophys. Acta* 281:522–34
63. Strniste, G. F., Smith, D. A. 1974. *Biochemistry* 13:485–93
64. Schimmel, P. R., Budzik, G. P., Lam, S. S. M., Schoemaker, H. J. P. 1976. See Ref. 28, pp. 123–48
65. Singer, S. J. 1971. In *Structure and Function of Biological Membranes,* ed. L. I. Rothfield, pp. 145–222. New York: Academic. 486 pp.
66. Singer, S. J. Nicolson, G. L. 1972. *Science* 175:720–31
67. Lübke, K., Schillinger, E., Töpert, M. 1976. *Angew. Chem. Int. Ed. Engl.* 15:741–48
68. Karlin, A. 1974. *Life Sci.* 14:1385–1415
69. Cuatrecasas, P. 1974. *Ann. Rev. Biochem.* 43:169–214
70. Haber, E., Wrenn, S. 1976. *Physiol. Rev.* 56:317–38
71. Kahn, C. R. 1976. *J. Cell Biol.* 70:261–86
72. Frank, J., Schwyzer, R. 1970. *Experientia* 26:1207–9
73. Waser, P. G., Hofmann, A., Hopff, W. 1970. *Experientia* 26:1342–43
74. Kiefer, H., Lindstrom, J., Lennox, E. S., Singer, S. J. 1970. *Proc. Natl. Acad. Sci. USA* 67:1688–94
75. Hucho, F., Layer, P., Kiefer, H. R., Bandini, G. 1976. *Proc. Natl. Acad. Sci. USA* 73:2624–28
76. Witzemann, V., Raftery, M. A. 1977. *Biochemistry* 16:5862–68
77. Cohen, J. B., Changeux, J.-P. 1975. *Ann. Rev. Pharmacol.* 15:83–103
78. Hucho, F., Bergman, C., Dubois, J. M., Rojas, E., Kiefer, H. 1976. *Nature* 260:802–4
79. Hucho, F. 1977. *Nature* 267:719–20
80. Guillory, R. J., Rayner, M. D., D'Arrigo, J. S. 1977. *Science* 196:883–85
81. Reuben, J. P., Brandt, P. W., Girardier, L., Grundfest, H. 1967. *Science* 155:1263–66
82. Rayner, M. D. 1972. *Fed. Proc.* 31:1139–45
83. Robison, G. A., Butcher, R. W., Sutherland, E. W. 1968. *Ann. Rev. Biochem.* 37:149–74
84. Robison, G. A., Butcher, R. W., Sutherland, E. W. 1971. *Cyclic AMP,* New York: Academic. 531 pp.
85. Rubin, C. S., Rosen, O. M. 1975. *Ann. Rev. Biochem.* 44:831–87
86. Sheppard, J. R. 1971. *Proc. Natl. Acad. Sci. USA* 68:1316–20
87. Anderson, W. B., Russell, T. R., Carchman, R. A., Pastan, I. 1973. *Proc. Natl. Acad. Sci. USA* 70:3802–5
88. Daly, J. W. 1977. *Cyclic Nucleotides in the Nervous System,* New York: Plenum. 401 pp.
89. Nathanson, J. A., Greengard, P. 1977. *Sci. Am.* 237(2):108–19
90. Bourne, H. R., Lichtenstein, L. M., Melmon, K. L., Henney, C. S., Weinstein, Y., Shearer, G. M. 1974. *Science* 184:19–28
91. Brunswick, D. J., Cooperman, B. S. 1971. *Proc. Natl. Acad. Sci. USA* 68:1801–4
92. Brunswick, D. J., Cooperman, B. S. 1973. *Biochemistry* 12:4074–78
93. Haley, B. 1975. *Biochemistry* 14:3852–57
94. Haley, B. E., Hoffman, J. F. 1974. *Proc. Natl. Acad. Sci. USA* 71:3367–71
95. Rubin, C. S. 1975. *J. Biol. Chem.* 250:9044–52
96. Haley, B. E. 1977. *Methods Enzymol.* 46:339–46
97. Owens, J. R., Haley, B. E. 1976. *J. Supramol. Struct.* 5:91–102
98. Owens, J. R., Haley, B. E. 1978. *J. Supramol. Struct.* In press
99. Walkenbach, R. J., Forte, L. R. 1977. *Biochim. Biophys. Acta* 464:165–78

100. Walter, U., Uno, I., Liu, A. Y.-C., Greengard, P. 1977. *J. Biol. Chem.* 252:6494–500
101. Skare, K., Black, J. L., Pancoe, W. L., Haley, B. E. 1977. *Arch. Biochem. Biophys.* 180:409–15
102. Henion, W. F., Sutherland, E. W., Posternak, Th. 1967. *Biochim. Biophys. Acta* 148:106–13
103. Blecher, M., Ro'Ane, J. T., Flynn, P. D. 1970. *J. Biol. Chem.* 245:1867–77
104. Geahlen, R. L., Haley, B. E. 1977. *Proc. Natl. Acad. Sci. USA* 74:4375–77
105. Czarnecki, J., Geahlen, R., Haley, B. 1978. *Methods Enzymol.* In press
106. Keeler, E. K., Campbell, P. 1976. *Biochem. Biophys. Res. Commun.* 75:575–80
107. Wiegand, G., Kaleja, R. 1976. *Eur. J. Biochem.* 65:473–79
108. Gorski, J., Gannon, F. 1976. *Ann. Rev. Physiol.* 38:425–50
109. Yamamoto, K. R., Alberts, B. M. 1976. *Ann. Rev. Biochem.* 45:721–46
110. Gospodarowicz, D., Moran, J. S. 1976. *Ann. Rev. Biochem.* 45:531–58
111. Reichlin, S., Saperstein, R., Jackson, I. M. D., Boyd, A. E., III, Patel, Y. 1976. *Ann. Rev. Physiol.* 38:389–424
112. Katzenellenbogen, J. A., Myers, H. N., Johnson, H. J. Jr. 1973. *J. Org. Chem.* 38:3525–33
113. Katzenellenbogen, J. A., Johnson, H. J. Jr., Myers, H. N. 1973. *Biochemistry* 12:4085–92
114. Katzenellenbogen, J. A., Johnson, H. J. Jr., Carlson, K. E., Myers, H. N. 1974. *Biochemistry* 13:2986–94
115. Katzenellenbogen, J. A., Hsiung, H. M. 1975. *Biochemistry* 14:1736–41
116. Katzenellenbogen, J. A., Ruh, T. S., Carlson, K. E., Iwamoto, H. S., Gorski, J. 1975. *Biochemistry* 14:2310–16
117. Katzenellenbogen, J. A., Myers, H. N., Johnson, H. J. Jr., Kempton, R. J., Carlson, K. E. 1977. *Biochemistry* 16:1964–69
118. Katzenellenbogen, J. A., Carlson, K. E., Johnson, H. J. Jr., Myers, H. N. 1977. *Biochemistry* 16:1970–76
119. Katzenellenbogen, J. A., Carlson, K. E., Johnson, H. J. Jr., Myers, H. N. 1976. *J. Toxicol. Environ. Health Suppl.* 1:205–30
120. Katzenellenbogen, J. A. 1978. *Fed. Proc.* 37:174–78
121. Katzenellenbogen, J. A., Johnson, H. J. Jr., Myers, H. N., Carlson, K. E., Kempton, R. J. 1978. In *Bioorganic Chemistry,* ed. E. E. van Tamelan, 4:207–37
122. Wolff, M. E., Feldman, D., Catsoulacos, P., Funder, J. W., Hancock, C., Amano, Y., Edelman, I. S. 1975. *Biochemistry* 14:1750–59
123. Marva, D., Chiu, W.-H., Wolff, M. E., Edelman, I. S. 1976. *Proc. Natl. Acad. Sci. USA* 73:4462–66
124. Schwyzer, R. Caviezel, M. 1971. *Helv. Chim. Acta* 54:1395–1400
125. Escher, E., Jost, R., Zuber, H., Schwyzer, R. 1974. *Isr. J. Chem.* 12:129–38
126. Escher, E., Schwyzer, R. 1974. *FEBS Lett.* 46:347–50
127. Escher, E., Schwyzer, R. 1975. *Helv. Chim. Acta* 58:1465–71
128. Fischli, W., Caviezel, M., Eberle, A., Escher, E., Schwyzer, R. 1976. *Helv. Chim. Acta* 59:878–79
129. Escher, E. 1977. *Helv. Chim. Acta* 60:339–41
130. Stadel, J. M. 1977. *Photoaffinity labeling of the antidiuretic hormone receptor in the toad urinary bladder.* PhD thesis. Univ. Penn., Phila., Penn. 110 pp.
131. Klausner, Y. S., McCormick, W. M., Chaiken, I. M. 1978. *Int. J. Pept. Protein Res.* 11:82–90
132. Bregman, M. D., Levy, D. 1977. *Biochem. Biophys. Res. Commun.* 78:584–90
133. Yip, C. C., Yeung, C. W. T., Moule, M. L. 1978. *J. Biol. Chem.* 253:1743–45
134. Galardy, R. E., Jamieson, J. D. 1977. *Mol. Pharmacol.* 13:852–63
135. Helene, C. 1972. *Photochem. Photobiol.* 16:519–22
136. Oxender, D. L. 1972. *Ann. Rev. Biochem.* 41:777–814
137. Boos, W. 1974. *Ann. Rev. Biochem.* 43:123–46
138. Pressman, B. C. 1976. *Ann. Rev. Biochem.* 45:501–30
139. Rudnick, G., Kaback, H. R., Weil, R. 1975. *J. Biol. Chem.* 250:1371–75
140. Rudnick, G., Kaback, H. R., Weil, R. 1975. *J. Biol. Chem.* 250:6847–51
141. Cabantchik, Z. I., Knauf, P. A., Ostwald, T., Markus, H., Davidson, L., Breuer, W., Rothstein, A. 1976. *Biochim. Biophys. Acta* 455:526–32
142. Rothstein, A., Cabantchik, Z. I., Knauf, P. 1976. *Fed. Proc.* 35:3–10
143. Kaplan, J. H., Fasold, H. 1976. *Biochim. Biophys. Acta* 443:525–33
144. Knauf, P. A., Breuer, W., Davidson, L., Rothstein, A. 1976. *Biophys. J.* 16:107a
145. Farley, R. A., Collins, K. D., Konigsberg, W. H., 1976. *Biophys. J.* 16:169a
146. Trosper, T., Levy, D. 1977. *J. Biol. Chem.* 252:181–86

147. Schaefer, G., Schrader, E., Rowohl-Quisthoudt, G., Penades, S., Rimpler, M. 1976. *FEBS Lett.* 64:185–89
148. Lauquin, G., Brandolin, G., Vignais, P. 1976. *FEBS Lett.* 67:306–11
149. Lauquin, G. J. M., Brandolin, G., Lunardi, J., Vignais, P. V. 1978. *Biochim. Biophys. Acta* 501:10–19
150. Scala, A. M. 1977. *Modulation of the nucleoside transport system of mammalian cells by polyoma virus and photoaffinity probes.* PhD thesis. Univ. Rochester, Rochester, New York. 165 pp.
151. Rosenblit, P. D., Levy, D. 1977. *Biochem. Biophys. Res. Commun.* 77:95–103
152. Staros, J. V., Knowles, J. R. 1978. *Biochemistry* 17:3321–25
153. Leonard, N. J., Greenfield, J. C., Schmitz, R. Y., Skoog, F. 1975. *Plant Physiol.* 55:1057–61
154. Theiler, J. B., Leonard, N. J., Schmitz, R. Y., Skoog, F. 1976. *Plant Physiol.* 58:803–5
155. Sussman, M. R., Kende, H. 1977. *Planta* 137:91–96
156. Menevse, A., Dodd, G. H., Poynder, T. M., Squirrel, D. 1977. *Biochem. Soc. Trans.* 5:191–94
157. Ganjian, I., Pettei, M. J., Nakanishi, K., Kaissling, K.-E. 1978. *Nature (London)* 271:157–58
158. Singer, S. J., Nicolson, G. L. 1972. *Science* 175:720–31
159. Singer, S. J. 1974. *Ann. Rev. Biochem.* 43:805–33
160. DePierre, J. W., Ernster, L. 1977. *Ann. Rev. Biochem.* 46:201–62
161. Peters, K., Richards, F. M. 1977. *Ann. Rev. Biochem.* 46:523–51
162. Staros, J. V., Richards, F. M. 1974. *Biochemistry* 13:2720–26
163. Staros, J. V., Haley, B. E., Richards, F. M. 1974. *J. Biol. Chem.* 249:5004–7
164. Staros, J. V., Richards, F. M., Haley, B. E. 1975. *J. Biol. Chem.* 250:8174–78
165. Klip, A., Gitler, C. 1974. *Biochem. Biophys. Res. Commun.* 60:1155–62
166. Klip, A., Darszon, A., Montal, M. 1976. *Biochem. Biophys. Res. Commun.* 72:1350–58
167. Mikkelsen, R. B., Wallach, D. F. H. 1976. *J. Biol. Chem.* 251:7413–16
168. Mohinddin, G., Power, D. M., Thomas, E. M. 1976. *FEBS Lett.* 70:85–86
169. Nieva-Gomez, D., Gennis, R. B. 1977. *Proc. Natl. Acad. Sci. USA* 75:1811–15
170. Abu-Salah, K. M., Findlay, J. B. C. 1977. *Biochem. J.* 161:223–228
171. Bercovici, T., Gitler, C. 1978. *Biochemistry* 17:1484–89

172. Bayley, H., Knowles, J. R. 1978. *Biochemistry* 17:2414–19
173. Bayley, H., Knowles, J. R. 1978. *Biochemistry* 17:2420–23
174. Chakrabarti, P., Khorana, H. G., 1975. *Biochemistry* 14:5021–33
175. Greenberg, G. R., Chakrabarti, P., Khorana, H. G. 1976. *Proc. Natl. Acad. Sci. USA* 73:86–90
176. Stoffel, W., Salm, K., Körkemeir, U. 1976. *Hoppe-Seylers Z. Physiol. Chem.* 357:917–24
177. Stoffel, W., Därr, W., Salm, K.-P. 1977. *Hoppe-Seylers Z. Physiol. Chem.* 358:453–62
178. Gupta, C. M., Radhakrishnan, R., Gerber, G. E., Takagaki, Y., Khorana, H. G. 1977. *Natl. Meet. Am. Chem. Soc., 174th Chicago.* [Abstr. 179 (Biology)]
179. Erecinska, M., Vanderkooi, J. M., Wilson, D. F. 1975. *Arch. Biochem. Biophys.* 171:108–16
180. Erecinska, M. 1977. *Biochem. Biophys. Res. Commun.* 76:495–501
181. Bisson, R., Azzi, A., Gutweniger, H., Colonna, R., Montecucco, C., Zanotti, A. 1978. *J. Biol. Chem.* 253:1874–80
182. Ji, T. H. 1977. *J. Biol. Chem.* 252:1566–70
183. Kiehm, D. J., Ji, T. H. 1977. *J. Biol. Chem.* 252:8524–31
184. Nomura, M., Tissieres, A., Lengyel, P. 1974. *Ribosomes,* (Monograph Series) Cold Spring Harbor, NY: Cold Spring Harbor Lab. 930 pp.
185. Wittmann, H. G. 1976. *Eur. J. Biochem.* 61:1–13
186. Bispink, L., Matthaei, H. 1973. *FEBS Lett.* 37:291–94
187. Cooperman, B. S., Jaynes, E. N., Brunswick, D. J., Luddy, M. A. 1975. *Proc. Natl. Acad. Sci. USA* 72:2974–78
188a. Hsiung, N., Cantor, C. R. 1974. *Nucleic Acids. Res.* 1:1753–62
188b. Hsiung, N., Reines, S. A., Cantor, C. R. 1974. *J. Mol. Biol.* 88:841–55
188c. Sonenberg, N., Wilchek, M., Zamir, A. 1977. *Eur. J. Biochem.* 77:217–22
188d. Maassen, J. A., Möller, W. 1974. *Proc. Natl. Acad. Sci. USA* 71:1277–80
189a. Cooperman, B. S. 1978. In *Bioorganic Chemistry. A Treatise to Supplement Bioorganic Chemistry, an International Journal,* ed. E. van Tamelen, 4:81–115. New York: Academic. 478 pp.
189b. Cooperman, B. S., Grant, P. G., Goldman, R. A., Luddy, M. A., Minnella, A., Nicholson, A. W., Strycharz, W. A. 1979. *Methods Enzymol.* In press
189c. Jakoby, W. B., Wilchek, M. eds. 1977. *Methods Enzymol.* Vol. 46. 774 pp.

190. Lin, S.-Y., Riggs, A. D. 1974. *Proc. Natl. Acad. Sci. USA* 71:947–51
191. Anderson, E., Nakashima, Y., Konigsberg, W. 1975. *Nucleic Acids Res.* 2:361–71
192. Cantrell, C. W., Yielding, K. L. 1977. *Photochem. Photobiol.* 25:189–91
193. Bastos, R. N. 1975. *J. Biol. Chem.* 250:7739–46
194. Schimmel, P. R. 1977. *Acc. Chem. Res.* 10:411–18
195. Schimmel, P. R., Budzik, G. P. 1977. *Methods Enzymol.* 46:168–80
196. Yue, V. T., Schimmel, P. R. 1977. *Biochemistry* 16:4678–84
197. Hixon, S. C., White, W. E. Jr., Yielding, K. L. 1975. *J. Mol. Biol.* 92:319–29
198. Hixon, S. C., White, W. E. Jr., Yielding, K. L. 1975. *Biochem. Biophys. Res. Commun.* 66:31–35
199. Yielding, L. W., White, W. E. Jr., Yielding, K. L. 1976. *Mutat. Res.* 34:351–58
200. Fleet, G. W. J., Knowles, J. R., Porter, R. R. 1972. *Biochem. J.* 128:499–508
201. Smith, R. A. G., Knowles, J. R. 1974. *Biochem. J.* 141:51–56
202. Fisher, C. E., Press, E. M. 1974. *Biochem. J.* 139:135–49
203. Cannon, L. E., Woodard, D. K., Woehler, M. E., Lovins, R. E. 1974. *Immunology.* 26:1183–94
204. Lindeman, J. G., Woodard, D. K., Woehler, M. E., Chism, G. E., Lovins, R. E. 1975. *Immunochemistry.* 12:849–54
205. Koberstein, R. 1976. *Eur. J. Biochem.* 67:223–29
206. Chen, S., Guillory, R. J. 1977. *J. Biol. Chem.* 252:8990–9001
207. Guillory, R. J., Jeng, S. J. 1977. *Methods Enzymol.* 46:259–88
208. Jeng, S. J., Guillory, R. J. 1975. *J. Supramol. Struct.* 3:448–68
209. Russell, J., Jeng, S. J., Guillory, R. J. 1976. *Biochem. Biophys. Res. Commun.* 70:1225–34
210. Lunardi, J., Lauquin, G. J. M., Vignais, P. V. 1977. *FEBS Lett.* 80:317–23
211. Bridges, A. J., Knowles, J. R. 1974. *Biochem. J.* 143:663–68
212. Henkin, J. 1977. *J. Biol. Chem.* 252:4293–97
213. Hixson, S. H., Hixson, S. S. 1975. *Biochemistry* 14:4251–54
214. Lau, E. P., Haley, B. E., Barden, R. E. 1977. *Biochem.* 16:2581–85
215. Lau, E. P., Haley, B. E., Barden, R. E. 1977. *Biochem. Biophys. Res. Commun.* 76:843–49
216. Poto, E. M., Wood, H. G., Barden, R. E., Lau, E. P. 1978. *J. Biol. Chem.* 253:2979–83
217a. Staros, J. V., Bayley, H., Standring, D. N., Knowles, J. R. 1978. *Biochem. Biophys. Res. Commun.* 80:568–72
217b. Cartwright, I. L., Hutchinson, D. W., Armstrong, V. W. 1976. *Nucleic Acids Res.* 3:2331–39
218. Smith, R. A. G., Knowles, J. R. 1973. *J. Am. Chem. Soc.* 95:5072–73
219. Smith, R. A. G., Knowles, J. R. 1975. *J. Chem. Soc. Perkin Trans. 2* 686–94
220. Chaimovich, H., Vaughan, R. J., Westheimer, F. H. 1968. *J. Am. Chem. Soc.* 90:4088–93
221. Hixson, S. S., Hixson, S. H. 1972. *J. Org. Chem.* 37:1279–80
222. Chowdhry, V., Westheimer, F. H. 1978. *J. Am. Chem. Soc.* 100:309–10
223. Chowdhry, V., Westheimer, F. H. 1978. *Biorg. Chem.* 7:189–205
224. Westheimer, F. H. 1976. *21st Ann. Rep. Res. under Sponsorship of Pet. Res. Fund, Am. Chem. Soc.*, p. 2. (Research conducted by J. Stackhouse)
225. Goldstein, J. A., McKenna, C., Westheimer, F. H. 1976. *J. Am. Chem. Soc.* 98:7327–32
226. Bartlett, P. A., Long, K. P. 1977. *J. Am. Chem. Soc.* 99:1267–68
227a. Breslow, R., Feiring, A., Herman, F. 1974. *J. Am. Chem. Soc.* 96:5937–39
227b. Chládek, S., Quiggle, K., Chinali, G., Kohut, J. III., Ofengand, J. 1977. *Biochemistry* 16:4312–19
228a. Hajer, J. D., Shadid, O. B., Cornelisse, J., Havinga, E. 1977. *Tetrahedron* 33:779–86
228b. Cornelisse, J., Havinga, E. 1975. *Chem. Rev.* 75:353–88
229a. Jelenc, P. C. 1977. *High yield photoreagents for protein cross-linking and affinity labeling.* PhD thesis. Columbia Univ., New York. 188 pp.
229b. Jelenc, P. C., Cantor, C. R., Simon, S. R. 1978. *Proc. Natl. Acad. Sci. USA* 75:3564–68

Ann. Rev. Biophys. Bioeng. 1979. 8:165–93

CHEMICAL CROSS-LINKING
IN BIOLOGY ♦9131

Manjusri Das[1] and C. Fred Fox

Department of Microbiology and the Parvin Cancer Research Laboratories,
Molecular Biology Institute, University of California, Los Angeles,
California 90024

1 INTRODUCTION

The study of diverse biological phenomena by chemical cross-linking technology has greatly intensified during the past 5 years. A number of excellent, timely, and chemically oriented reviews of the cross-linking literature have appeared (4, 68, 87). Therefore, we have attempted to present a critical evaluation of the principles and strategies that govern the application of cross-linking technology to the solutions of biological problems.

The use of chemical cross-linking reagents as molecular rulers in the determination of quaternary structure in oligomeric protein complexes in solution and in membranes has enjoyed wide application. Another aspect of cross-linking technology is the exploitation of heterobifunctional reagents to identify ligand-binding components in complex biological systems. It is often difficult to determine how proteins function in multicomponent, complex systems. The classical biochemical approach of isolation and characterization of protein components does not always reveal transient interactions or migratory behavior of proteins, which occur in the natural environment of the cell. The covalent linkage of a ligand to a specific protein provides a strategy for visualizing this behavior.

2 PHOTOREACTIVE CROSS-LINKING REAGENTS

Arylazide reagents that can be employed for photochemical attachment of ligands to recognition sites on macromolecules are described in Table

---

[1] Present address: Department of Biochemistry and Biophysics, University of Pennsylvania School of Medicine, Philadelphia, Pa. 19104.

0084-6589/79/0615-0165$01.00
165

Table 1 Photoactivable, bifunctional cross-linking reagents

Cross-linker (Ref)	Cleavability of cross-link	Formula	Site specificity of the non-photoactivable group
4-Fluoro-3-nitrophenylazide (22)	—		amino
1,5-Diazidonaphthalene (62)	—		—
4,4′-Diazidobiphenyl (62)	—		—
4,4′-Dithiobisphenylazide (62)	+		—
N,N′-(4-azido-2-nitrophenyl-cystamine-dioxide (33)	+		sulfhydryl
p-Azidophenacyl bromide (31)	—		sulfhydryl
Methyl-4-azidobenzoimidate (36)	—		amino
Ethyl(4-azidophenyl)-1,4-dithiobutyrimidate (48)	+		amino

Compound		Structure	Reactive group
Methyl[3-(p-azidophenyl)dithio]propionimidate (15,17)	+		amino
N-succinimidyl-6-(4'-azido-2'-nitrophenylamino)hexanoate (50)	−		amino
N-5-azido-2-nitrobenzoyloxysuccinimide (48)	−		amino
N-(5-azido-2-nitrophenyl)ethylenediamine (14)	−		carboxyl
N-(4-azido-2-nitrophenyl)ethylenediamine (15)	−		carboxyl

1. In contrast to the more commonly used site-specific cross-linking reagents, many of which are highly water-soluble bisalkylimidates, the arylazides can react with components in a nonpolar, hydrophobic environment.
Arylazides are photolyzed at wavelengths (300–400 nm) that do not cause
direct photochemical damage to proteins or nucleic acids. Arylnitrenes
generated by photolysis of arylazides have lifetimes on the order of 10^{-4}
sec (71). Arylnitrene half-lives vary with substituents and increase by nearly
two orders of magnitude on going from p-acetyl (short lived) to p-N-
morpholine (long lived) substitution. The various reactions open to an
arylnitrene have been discussed by Knowles (47) and by Peters & Richards
(68). A nitrene can react with C-H bonds by abstraction and insertion
and therefore may create a cross-link in the absence of any particular
functional group on a protein or other reactant.

Knowles et al introduced the nitrophenylazide group as a nitrene precursor (22, 47) to label the recognition site on antibodies specific for the
4-azido-2-nitrophenyl haptenic group (22). Several authors (6, 45, 46)
synthesized the apolar radioactive azides [1–^{3}H]azidonaphthalene and
[5–^{125}I]iodonaphthylazide for radiolabeling portions of membrane proteins that are in contact with the lipid bilayer. Mikkelson & Wallach (62)
synthesized a series of bifunctional photoreactive reagents, i.e. 1,5-diazido-
naphthalene, 4,4'-diazidobiphenyl, and 4,4'-dithiobisphenylazide; cross-
links formed with the last of these can be reversed by reduction of the
disulfide bridge in the reagent. These lipophilic aromatic diazides were
used to cross-link proteins in erythrocyte membrane.

Heterobifunctional reagents, which attach initially by normal chemical
modification and secondarily by photolysis of an appropriate group, are
particularly useful in identifying ligand-binding components in complex
biological systems. One example, di-N-(2-nitro-4-azidophenyl)cystamine-
S,S-dioxide, was synthesized by Huang & Richards (33). It can undergo
sulfhydryl exchange with cysteine residues of proteins in the dark. The
azide group then can be photochemically activated to a nitrene, which
may react with another protein to complete the cross-link.

Hixson & Hixson (31) synthesized p-azidophenacylbromide to study
active sites of enzymes that contain sulfhydryl groups. α-Halo carbonyl
compounds react with nucleophilic amino acids, such as cysteine, allowing
study of the active sites of enzymes that possess a highly reactive cysteine
residue at the active site. When the reagent is irradiated after covalent
attachment to the active site, any portion of the protein chain labeled
by the resulting nitrene must be close to the residue to which the reagent
was initially attached.

Ji and co-workers (36, 44) synthesized two photosensitive heterobifunctional cross-linking reagents, methyl-4-azidobenzimidate and the reversible

reagent ethyl(4-azidophenyl)-1,4-dithiobutyrimidate. A similar reversible photosensitive reagent, methyl[3-(p-azidophenyl)dithio]propionimidate, was synthesized by Dos et al (15, 17). These arylazide reagents contain imidoesters selective for primary amino groups, and the principal reaction product is an amidine. The chemistry and reactivity of alkyl imidates have been studied by Hand & Jenkes (29) and Browne & Kent (10) and was reviewed recently by Peters & Richards (68). Imidoesters are rapidly inactivated by hydrolysis at pH ≤ 8.0. At higher pH (∼10), the rate of hydrolytic inactivation is much slower. The reactivity of imidates with amines is higher at pH 10.0 than at pH ≤ 8.0, and the yield of product amidine is also higher at pH 10.0. Since many proteins cannot tolerate even brief exposure to alkaline conditions, the utility of alkyl imidates in cross-linking and modification of protein ligands is somewhat limited.

The N-succinimidyl esters provide an alternative to the imidates. The synthesis and properties of the cleavable reagent [^{35}S]dithiobis(succinimidyl propionate) has been described by Lomant & Fairbanks (50). Amino groups are quantitatively acylated by this reagent at pH 7.0 within 2 min at 23°C. By contrast, the half-time for hydrolysis of the active ester terminus is 4–5 hr at pH 7.0, so that optimal reaction with protein can occur at low concentrations of reagent. These properties, high reactivity under mild conditions and long solution half-life, make the succinimidyl ester reagent particularly useful for cross-linking and modification of proteins in a variety of biological systems. Lomant also synthesized a photosensitive heterobifunctional cross-linker, N-succinimidyl-6-(4'-azido-2'-nitrophenylamino)hexanoate. A similar but somewhat shorter reagent, N-5-azido-2-nitrobenzoyloxysuccinimide, has been synthesized by Lewis et al (48).

Darfler & Marinetti (14) synthesized N-(5-azido-2-nitrophenyl)ethylenediamine, which condenses with carboxyl groups of proteins in the presence of a carbodiimide. A similar carboxyl-group-specific reagent, N-(4-azido-2-nitrophenyl)ethylenediamine, has been described (15).

3 PHOTOREACTIVE DERIVATIVES OF LIGANDS

3.1 Peptide Hormones

Heterobifunctional reagents containing a photolyzable group are extremely useful for preparing photoreactive derivatives of polypeptide ligands (9, 15, 17, 24, 33, 81, 93; Table 2). Primary amino, carboxyl, and sulfhydryl functional groups are most amenable for derivatization in polypeptides. Reagents suitable for reaction with these groups were described in Table 1. In polypeptide hormones, the groups most susceptible to selective modification may also be essential for biological activity. In certain instances,

Table 2 Photoreactive derivatives of peptide ligands and labeling of receptors

Ligand	Cross-linker used	Group derivatized	Ref
Concanavalin A	Methyl-4-azidobenzoimidate	8 amino groups per molecule of tetramer concanavalin A. Site of insertion not determined.	33
Murine EGF	Methyl[3-(p-azidophenyl)-dithio]propionimidate	α-Amino group at the NH_2-terminus.	15 16
Murine EGF	N-(4-azido-2-nitrophenyl)-ethylenediamine	Carboxyl groups. Sites of insertion not determined.	17 15a
Glucagon	N-Fluoro-3-nitrophenylazide	ϵ-Amino group of lysine-12.	9
Insulin	4-Azidobenzoyloxy-succinimide	Amino groups. Sites of insertion not determined.	93
Oxytocin	2-Nitro-5-azidobenzoyl-glycineoxysuccinimide	α-Amino group at the NH_2 terminus.	81

it may be necessary to protect these essential groups during derivatization to retain binding and biological activities in the photoreactive derivatives.

Ji (36) prepared a photoreactive derivative of concanavalin A by condensing methyl-4-azidobenzimidate to the amino groups. The extent of derivitization was measured spectrophotometrically. Simple arylazides absorb maximally at 268 nm. The covalent complex of concanavalin A and the reagent had an absorption maximum at 273 nm, probably produced by combination of the 268-nm maximum of the reagent and the 280-nm maximal absorbance of protein. Photolysis produced a gradual reduction of the 273-nm absorption peak, and the decrease ceased when photolysis neared completion. This property allowed estimation of the quantity of arylazide incorporated into concanavalin A. Maximum incorporation was achieved when 8 of the 40 available amino groups in tetrameric concanavalin A had reacted. This photoreactive derivative of concanavalin A retained its binding activity for glucosylated sepharose and also bound to erythrocyte ghost membranes. The quantitative aspects of carbohydrate binding

Binding affinity for receptors	Biological activity	Radiolabeling of receptor	Cross-linked complex formation as a linear function of specific binding of the derivatized ligand
Specific binding to carbohydrates, but binding kinetics not determined.	Not determined	Apparently labels the band 3 protein of erythrocyte membranes.	Not determined
No loss of binding activity.	No loss of biological activity.	Specific labeling of a single 3T3 cell surface protein (MW 190,000).	Established
No loss of binding activity.	Not determined	Specific labeling of a single 3T3 cell surface protein (MW 190,000).	Established
No loss of binding activity.	Total loss of adenyl cyclase stimulatory activity.	Labeling of a 25,000-dalton polypeptide and a high-MW (>500,000) polypeptide in hepatocyte membranes.	Not determined
Not determined	Not determined	High nonspecific labeling of adipocyte membrane proteins. A protein of MW 130,000 may be specifically labeled.	Not determined
Not determined	Partial loss of biological activity.	Not done	

with this derivative were not reported, nor were the biological properties of this derivative, e.g. initiation of mitogenesis in lymphocytes, studied. Irradiation of photoreactive concanavalin A bound to erythrocytes resulted in apparent cross-linking of concanavalin A to band 3 protein, the major glycoprotein in erythrocytes. The high-molecular-weight, cross-linked product remained at the top of the analytical gels, and the product was not analyzed or characterized further.

The ideal polypeptide ligand for photoaffinity labeling should be devoid of subunit structure and contain only a single derivatizable group. Murine epidermal growth factor (EGF), a single chain polypeptide of 6045 daltons, has no lysine residues, and the sole primary amino group is located at the N-terminus. A photoreactive derivative of this hormone was prepared by Das et al (16, 17) using methyl[3-(p-azidophenyl)dithio]propionimidate to selectively modify the N-terminal amino group. The maximal molar ratio achieved for reagent bound to EGF'was approximately 0.3, and this ratio was not increased by a second treatment with the reagent. This derivative and native unlabeled EGF had identical ability to bind to 3T3 cells, to down regulate EGF receptors, and to initiate DNA synthesis. The use of this derivative in the identification and characterization of EGF receptors in murine cells is described in a later section.

Glucagon, a single-chain polypeptide of MW 3500, has one internal lysine residue. The N-terminal α-amino group is apparently essential for retention of biological activity. Bregman & Levy (9) prepared an ϵ-amino arylazide derivative of glucagon using 4-fluoro-3-nitrophenylazide as the amino-group-specific reagent. Only the ϵ-amino group of lysine-12 was claimed to be modified with the arylazide moiety. This derivative and native glucagon had the same K_d for binding to hepatocyte plasma membranes, and the binding of the derivative was completely inhibited by the presence of high concentrations of unlabeled hormone. This derivative was biologically inactive since it did not stimulate adenyl cyclase activity. The derivative may prove to be extremely useful in studies where it is desirable to dissociate the binding phenomenon from the activation of adenyl cyclase.

Insulin contains two N-terminal α-amino groups and one internal lysine residue. The amino groups in insulin are apparently essential for its biological activity. Preparation of photolyzable derivatives of insulin with amino group site-specific reagents therefore has proved to be challenging. Yip et al (93) recently reported the synthesis of photoreactive insulin, although the product was not characterized thoroughly. The N-hydroxy-succinimidyl ester of 4-azidobenzoic acid was used for modification of the insulin amino groups. The product obtained was found to be a mixture of 30% unaltered insulin, 25% monoazidobenzoyl insulin, and 45% diazidobenzoylinsulin. The sites of insertion of arylazide into the molecule and its binding and biological characteristics were not reported.

A photoreactive analog of oxytocin, 2-nitro-5-azidobenzoylglycyl-oxytocin (NAB-Gly-oxytocin), has been synthesized and well characterized by Stadel et al (81). The N-hydroxysuccinimide ester of 2-nitro-5-azidobenzoylglycine was coupled to the N-terminal amino group of oxytocin, and NAB-Gly-oxytocin was purified from the reaction mixture by partition chromatography. NAB-Gly-oxytocin failed to form a fluorescent product with fluorescamine, confirming the pressure of the arylazide moiety at the amino terminus of oxytocin. A comparison of the electrophoretic mobilities of NAB-Gly-oxytocin and underivatized oxytocin at pH 10.5 and 5.0 also indicated single derivatization of oxytocin at the N-terminus. This photoreactive derivative of oxytocin stimulated osmotic water flow in the isolated toad bladder, but it was a weaker agonist than oxytocin. Although the K_m of NAB-Gly-oxytocin for optimal biological activity is increased, compared with oxytocin, NAB-Gly-oxytocin and oxytocin appear to bind to the same receptor. Repetitive photolysis of NAB-Gly-oxytocin incubating with toad bladder resulted in a permanent inhibition of oxytocin-stimulated urea permeability. The inhibition required photogeneration of the arylnitrene intermediate and was prevented by excess underivatized oxytocin during photolysis.

3.2   Nonpeptide Ligands

The germinal experiments in the field of photogenerated ligands were performed with carbene precursors. Highly reactive carbenes can be generated by photolysis of compounds, such as diazoalkanes and α-ketodiazo compounds, which produce carbenes on loss of nitrogen. Westheimer and his colleagues (76, 77, 88) synthesized the carbene precursor, p-nitrophenyldiazoacetate, and ethyl p-nitrophenyldiazomalonate to map the region around the active site of chymotrypsin and trypsin. Diazoketone derivatives of dinitrophenylglycine and dinitrophenylalanine were used by Converse & Richards (13) to study the combining sites of rabbit antidinitrophenyl antibodies. α-Diazoketones are stable and are photolyzed readily by irradiation above 350 nm. Unfortunately, the α-ketocarbene readily undergoes the intramolecular Wolff rearrangement to a ketene. The highly indiscriminate reactivity of the carbene is then lost, since ketenes are subject to attack principally by nucleophiles. A diazomalonyl derivative of cAMP, N^6-(ethyl-2-diazomalonyl)-cAMP, was synthesized by Brunswick & Cooperman (11) for photoaffinity labeling of cAMP binding proteins. Unfortunately, this derivative was subject to Dimroth rearrangement at pH ≥ 7.0. At pH ≥ 7.0, the diazo form isomerizes to the triazole form, and the failure of the triazole form to efficiently photolyze to yield a carbene poses a problem for practical use of this cAMP analog as a cAMP photoaffinity label at pH ≥ 7.0, where the triazole form predominates.

After the introduction of arylazides as stable, convenient photoaffinity labeling reagents, Haley (28) synthesized an azide photoaffinity analog of cAMP, 8-azido-cAMP. Unlike the diazomalonyl derivative, it did not undergo rearrangements at pH ≥ 7.0, allowing photolysis at physiological pH without noticeable formation of undesirable side products. A fluorescent azido analog of cAMP, 8-azido-1,N^6-ethenoadenosine-3'-5'-cyclic monophosphate, was synthesized by Dreyfuss et al (19). This compound combines the photoreactivity of the arylazide moiety with the fluorescence of a substituted 1,N^6-ethenoadenosine unit, yielding a highly specific photoaffinity label, which becomes an environment-sensitive fluorophore upon covalent attachment. This probe mimiced cAMP in its ability to stimulate the phosphotransferase activity of the protein kinase, and it strongly competed with cAMP for the binding site in all the preparations tested.

During the initial period of development of photoaffinity labeling techniques, Kiefer et al (43) synthesized two arylazide analogs of acetylcholine, 4-azido-2-nitrobenzyltrimethylammonium tetrafluoborate and 4-azido-2-nitrobenzyltriethylammonium tetrafluoborate. Both acetylcholine esterase activity and acetylcholine receptor activity were irreversibly inactivated by photoaffinity labeling with these two quaternary ammonium arylazides. The 4-azido-2-nitrobenayltriethylammonium tetrafluoborate derivative also irreversibly blocked potassium conductance in the node of Ranvier of frog sciatic nerve (34). A biologically active fluorescent photoaffinity analog of acetylcholine, bis-(3-azidopyridinium)-1,10-decane perchlorate, has been synthesized recently by Witzemann & Raftery (92).

Photoaffinity analogs of steroid hormones were introduced by Katzenellenbogen and his colleagues (40, 41). A number of photosensitive derivatives, 3-diazo-2-ketopropyl ether, and ortho azide derivatives of estradiol, estrone and hexestrol, were reasonably stable and could be purified easily. The binding affinity of these derivatives for the uterine receptor reflects the relative binding affinity of the parent ligands: hexestrol > estradiol > estrone. Of these derivatives, hexestrolazide had the highest binding affinity. In a subsequent article (42), Katzenellenbogen et al also described the radiochemical synthesis of [^{3}H]hexestrol azide and [^{3}H]hexestrol diazoketopropyl ether. These radioactive photoreactive derivatives were used to label the estrogen receptor in uterus.

A radiolabeled photoaffinity analog of corticosterone, 21-diazo-21-[6, 7-^{3}H]deoxycorticosterone, was synthesized by Marver et al (61) to label the high-affinity human corticosteroid binding globulin. Based on direct binding studies and cross-competition experiments, the diazo derivative exhibited the requisite affinity and site specificity to qualify as an affinity-labeling ligand.

Photoaffinity analogs of tRNA have been synthesized by a number of investigators. Most of these probes are positioned at the 3′ end of the aminoacyl-tRNA. These probes are useful for analyzing the P site, i.e. the peptidyl donor site, in ribosomes. An ultraviolet-reactive peptidyl-tRNA analog, N-(ethyl-2-diazomalonyl)[^{3}H]Phe-tRNA, was synthesized by Bispink & Matthaei (7). This photoderivative behaved like N-acetyl-Phe-tRNA in its kinetic properties and in the extent of poly(U)-stimulated complex formation with ribosomes. An arylazide analog of peptidyl-tRNA, 2-nitro-4-azidophenoxy-4′-phenylacetyl-[^{3}H]Phe-tRNA, was synthesized by Hsiung et al (32) and was as active as N-acetyl-Phe-tRNA in binding to ribosomes. Its binding to ribosomes was stimulated about fivefold by poly(U). Binding to the peptidyl site was indicated by the ability of puromycin to release the peptidyl moiety from nonphotolyzed samples. Synthesis of another biologically active arylazide peptidyl-tRNA analog, p-azido-N-tBOC-Phe-Phe-tRNA, has been described by Sonenberg et al (79).

The N-acyl-aminoacyl-tRNA analogs described above are useful for labeling the P site, but they cannot be used to analyze the ribosomal A site or the elongation factor Tu complexes. Ofengund et al (66) used a different approach for inserting photoaffinity probes into tRNA. The aryl-azide probes are attached to rare bases in tRNA. p-Azidophenacylbromide was used to modify the 4-thiouridine residue, and the N-hydroxysuccini-mide ester of N-(4-azido-2-nitrophenyl)glycine was used to derivatize the 3-(3-amino-3-carboxypropyl)uridine residue, which has a free α-NH$_2$ group. The derivatized tRNA was 90–100% as active as underivatized tRNA for aminoacylation, nonenzymatic binding to the ribosomal P site, and elongation factor Tu-dependent binding to the A site. These bases are located on opposite faces of the central region of the three-dimensional structure of tRNA. Thus, the covalent linking results should be approximately complementary and provide useful topographical information about tRNA binding sites.

Chakravarti & Khorana (12) synthesized a series of photosensitive aryla-zide derivatives of fatty acids to study interactions between phospholipids and proteins in membranes. The photosensitive fatty acids supported the growth of an auxotroph of *Escherichia coli* that requires unsaturated fatty acids (26). Analysis of phospholipids from cells grown with azido-substi-tuted fatty acids indicated incorporation at the 2 position of the glycerol moeity, i.e. the normal position for unsaturated fatty acids in phospholipids of *E. coli*. The incorporation of these fatty acid derivatives offers a new approach to the study of membrane structure, and in particular, phospho-lipid-protein interactions, by photolysis-induced cross-linking of the fatty acids to polypeptides and other components in the immediate vicinity.

4   SPECIFIC LABELING OF LIGAND BINDING RECEPTORS

4.1   General Principles

The field of receptor biochemistry has need for a method to selectively label receptors by using minute quantities of sample to permit study of the dynamic behavior of receptor-ligand complexes in cells or tissues. A complex can be formed by covalently cross-linking a photolyzable ligand to receptor before disruption or solubilization of cells or membranes (Figure 1; Table 2). The fate of the ligand-receptor complex may then be examined in situ. The availability of a variety of photoaffinity analogs of ligands should facilitate studies on receptor dynamics in a variety of systems.

Unlike ordinary affinity ligands, photoaffinity ligands create a covalent cross-link only on absorption of a photon and conversion to a reactive species, such as a nitrene or carbene. Therefore, the kinetics of reversible binding of the derivatized ligand to the receptor can be established in the dark, without the formation of irreversibly linked ligand-receptor complexes. Chemical inertness and metabolic stability of the arylazide moiety may create problems, especially if the ligand is susceptible to cellular degradation. The degradation products linked to the arylazide moiety may, on irradiation, give rise to covalent labeling of proteins that are not receptors for the undegraded ligand.

In photoaffinity labeling, the concentration of reagent is important. Labeling specificity at the expense of high extent of labeling is maximized by a high receptor concentration and a low ligand concentration. Repeated labeling or the use of reagent of very-high-specific radioactivity may be required to obtain interpretable results. After the first round of photochemical labeling, the noncovalently bound reaction products should be removed by dissociation before further photolysis in the presence of a second batch

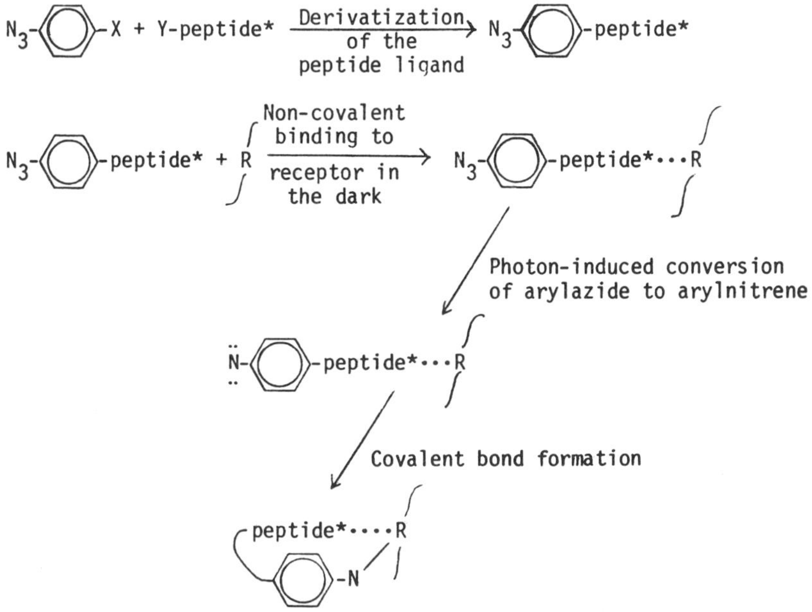

Figure 1   A schematic diagram for derivatization of peptide ligands with heterobifunctional arylazide cross-linking reagents, and covalent labeling of receptors using photoactivable peptide ligands. Extraction or solubilization of receptor-peptide complex using detergents such as SDS. Analysis of the radioactively labeled cross-linked complexes formed using SDS-polyacrylamide gel electrophoresis and autoradiography. X, Non-photoactivable functional group in the cross-linking reagent; Y, functional group ($-NH_2$, $-COOH$, or $-SH$) amenable for derivatization in the peptide; *, radioactive label in the peptide ligand; R, cell, tissue, or membrane containing a receptor for a peptide ligand.

of photoreactive ligand. However, these methods of repetitive labeling involve the exposure of samples to a large total radiation dose and light, which may have deleterious effects on both biological activity and ligand binding properties of the receptor.

One problem encountered in photoaffinity labeling is the nonspecific labeling of a variety of nonreceptor proteins discussed in detail by Ruoho et al (72) and Katzenellenbogen et al (39). Photoaffinity analogs of small ligands such as acetylcholine and steroid hormones often produce random labeling of proteins. This may be due to diffusion of the arylnitrenes from the binding site and reaction with remote groups. Generally, an increase in the reversible binding affinity of the photolyzable reagent for the active site of the receptor is likely to increase the likelihood of true photoaffinity labeling. Receptor binding affinity of the photolyzable derivative should be high, both in the photolyzed and unphotolyzed states, for it to qualify as a true photoaffinity reagent. Although a number of photoreactive hormone analogs have been synthesized recently, some have not been tested for binding affinity, and very few possess the high binding affinity required for true affinity labeling of receptors. Ideally, a photoreactive derivative of ligand should have the following characteristics: (a) a low K_d, unaltered from the underivatized form if possible; and (b) normal biological activity.

In attempts to identify ligand binding components in cells or unfractionated tissue extracts, the possibility of nonspecific associations must be excluded. The cross-linked ligand-receptor complex should meet the following two criteria: (a) The amount of cross-linked complex formed should decrease in accordance with kinetic predictions with increasing concentrations of unlabeled underivatized ligand; and (b) under a variety of conditions there should be a direct proportionality between photoreactive ligand binding activity and cross-linked complex formation. Immunoprecipitability of the cross-linked complex with antiligand antisera can provide additional evidence that the cross-linked complex contains the ligand in an undegraded form.

Nonspecific labeling can sometimes be minimized by performing photolabeling in the presence of scavengers. Scavengers are intended to destroy all photogenerated intermediates at places other than the ligand binding site. Molecules such as p-aminobenzoic acid, soluble proteins, and tris(hydroxymethyl)aminomethane have been proposed as scavengers (61, 72). Before use, however, scavengers should be tested to confirm that they do not bind to the receptor site or to the ligand.

Another major difficulty encountered in photochemical labeling studies is low extent of labeling. Bayley & Knowles (5) suggest that this may be due to the electrophilic nature of nitrenes, allowing preferential reaction with water or buffer components, thus reducing the chances of insertion into unactivated carbon-hydrogen bonds. Repetitive labeling experiments may sometimes be effective in overcoming this problem.

4.2 cAMP Receptor

8-Azido-cAMP, synthesized by Haley (28), proved to be a specific reagent for cAMP binding proteins in human erythrocytes. At low concentrations of $[^{32}P]$-8-N_3-cAMP, a single protein component (MW 55,000) was labeled, a result similar to the previous observations of Guthrow et al (27), with $[^3H]$-N^6-(ethyl-2-diazomalonyl)c-AMP. At high concentrations of $[^{32}P]$-8-N_3-cAMP, a second protein (MW 49,000) was also covalently labeled. Covalent incorporation into both these proteins was specific and was abolished in the presence of underivatized cAMP.

8-Azido-cAMP was also used for identification of cAMP receptor protein in cytosol fractions of various rat tissues (89). The $[^{32}P]$-8-N_3-cAMP was specifically incorporated into two protein bands (MW 47,000 and 54,000) in all tissues examined. These two proteins are the regulatory subunits of type 1 and type 2 cAMP-dependent protein kinases. The results suggested that most of the cAMP receptor proteins, at least in the mammalian tissues studies, represent regulatory subunits of cAMP-dependent protein kinases, a conclusion compatible with the idea that most effects of cAMP are mediated through these protein kinases.

4.3 Estrogen Receptor

Katzenellenbogen et al (38, 42) synthesized a series of photoreactive estrogen derivatives for covalent attachment to the uterine cytosol estrogen receptor. The two analogs used were $[^3H]$hexestroldiazoketopropylether and $[^3H]$hexestrolazide. No irreversible binding to receptor appeared to result from irradiation with $[^3H]$hexestroldiazoketopropylether. Irradiation with $[^3H]$hexestrol-N_3 does covalently label the estrogen site-specific receptor, but most of the $[^3H]$hexestrol-N_3 was bound to nonreceptor proteins. Both photoreactive derivatives were more lipophilic than estradiol, and this characteristic may be responsible for the nonspecific labeling of proteins other than receptor in the unfractionated cytosol preparations.

4.4 Acetylcholine Receptor

Witzemann & Raftery (92) used an arylazide analog of acetylcholine, bis-(3-azidopyridinium)-1,10-decane perchlorate, for covalent labeling of the acetylcholine receptor in membrane-bound and solublized states to learn more about functional and topographical aspects of the different receptor subunits. Photolysis of the ^3H-labeled bis-azido reagent in the presence of the solubilized and purified receptors resulted in covalent incorporation into two of the four subunits (MW 40,000 and 60,000). However, with the membrane-bound receptor, the subunits of MW 40,000 and 50,000 were labeled. The results favor the assumption that the specific ligand binding sites are located on the 40,000-MW subunit. Labeling of the other subunits appears to reflect their proximity to the ligand binding site, and alterations in subunit topography between membrane-bound and solubilized states.

4.5 EGF Receptor

Studies on the membrane receptor for EGF by Das et al (15–17) illustrate the range of applicability of photoaffinity labeling in cellular studies of biological phenomena. The EGF receptor in mouse 3T3 cells was identified using PAPDIP-EGF, a photoderivative of EGF containing an arylazide group at its N-terminus {PAPDIP, methyl[3-(p-azidophenyl)dithio] propionimidate}. Photolysis of ^{125}I-labeled PAPDIP-EGF bound to cells resulted in specific incorporation of EGF into a single species of MW 190,000. The amount of radioactivity incorporated into the 190,000-MW species was a linear function of the amount of radioactive EGF reversibly bound to receptors, indicating that the 190,000-MW band represents the covalently cross-linked EGF-receptor complex. This was confirmed by use of a nonresponsive and nonbinding variant of 3T3 cells. The cross-linked complex band was not observed with this variant cell line. The cross-linked complex can also be immunoprecipitated with anti-EGF antisera (P. Linsley, C. Blifeld, and C. F. Fox, unpublished data). Another photoreactive derivative of EGF, NAPEDE-^{125}I-labeled EGF, in which the arylazide groups were linked to the carboxyl groups in the EGF molecule [NAPEDE, N-(4-azido-2-nitrophenyl)ethylenediamine], was also specifically and irreversibly incorporated into the same 190,000-MW band (15). Treatment of the NAPEDE-EGF-receptor covalent complex with 2-mercaptoethanol did not lead to reduction of molecular weight.

Incubation of cells containing an in situ radiolabeled receptor at 37°C resulted in a time-dependent reduction of radioactivity from the receptor band at 37°C. The rate of loss of radioactivity was the same irrespective of whether the receptor had been radiolabeled using PAPDIP-EGF or NAPEDE-EGF. The loss of radioactivity from the receptor band was accompanied by appearance of low-molecular-weight bands of 60,000, 47,000, and 37,000. Approximately 90% of the radioactivity lost from the receptor-EGF complex was recovered in these low-molecular-weight species, suggesting a precursor-product relationship between these proteins. These low-molecular-weight proteins co-fractionated with the lysosomal enzyme markers during isopycnic banding of cellular organelles; all the 190,000-MW receptor banded with the plasmalemmal fraction. These results show that binding of EGF to its cell surface receptor leads to internalization of the EGF-receptor complex, possibly by endocytosis. This may be followed by fusion of the endocytic vesicles with lysosomes, leading finally to proteolytic processing of receptor by the lysosomal proteases. The kinetics of receptor processing induced by EGF were compatible with this process being responsible for the accumulation of an intracellular active substance responsible for the EGF-initiated synthesis of DNA (15). Specific radiolabeling of the EGF receptor, therefore, has provided an unusual opportunity for visualization of the metabolic fate of a receptor after binding to its hormone (Figure 2).

The photoaffinity labeling technique described above also revealed an interesting characteristic of the degradation products of the EGF receptor.

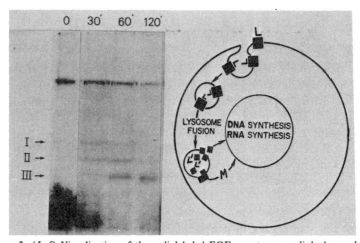

Figure 2 (*Left*) Visualization of the radiolabeled EGF-receptor cross-linked complex and its degradation products by autoradiography of 5–20% polyacrylamide gradient gels. Cells containing an in situ radiolabeled receptor (prepared using PAPDIP-^{125}I-labeled EGF) were incubated at 37° C for the indicated time periods. The band at the top (MW 190,000) represents the EGF-receptor cross-linked complex. The bands I, II, and III (MW 60,000, 47,000, and 37,000) are degradation products of the radiolabeled receptors. The diffuse band at the bottom represents free EGF. For experimental details, see (15). (*Right*) Sequential steps in receptor processing induced by EGF. Solid squares represent the cell surface receptors for EGF; L and L' represent the unprocessed and processed forms of the ligand (EGF), respectively. M denotes a catalytically derived second messenger. The triggering of both receptor processing and DNA synthesis by EGF is dependent upon the concentration of the ligand; in addition, both these processes achieve half maximal completion at the same concentration of ligand (15). These observations are consistent with the hypothe.' ' ' some event during the internalization and processing of receptor is limiting for the EGF-dependent activation of cellular DNA synthesis. This event could be the proteolytic activation of an internalized protein, possibly receptor, leading either to the catalytic production of a second messenger (M) or to the release of a polypeptide fragment that is itself the second messenger. See text and (15) for further details.

These retained EGF binding activity, since the low-molecular-weight receptor-derived products (principle products of MW 60,000, 47,000, and 37,000, and a minor product of MW 90,000) were covalently labeled with photoreactive ^{125}I-labeled EGF. Studies on the characterization of hormone receptors have been fraught with controversies regarding receptor molecular weights. Receptor processing by cellular proteases appears to be a likely explanation for the apparent discrepancies regarding molecular size of receptors.

Sahyoun et al (73) undertook the labeling of the EGF binding components in rat liver membranes by glutaraldehyde cross-linking followed by sodium borohydride reduction. In this type of reaction, the bifunctional reagent can cross-link not only ligand and receptor, but also receptor and many other macromolecules. Four labeled components with electrophoretic mobilities corresponding to species of 410,000, 200,000, 95,000, and 35,000 MW were observed. The higher-molecular-weight bands of 200,000 and 410,000 probably represent monomers and dimers of the EGF receptor, as they are in excellent accord with the value of MW 190,000 for the murine receptor. The low-molecular-weight bands (95,000 and 35,000) may represent degradation products of receptor that retain their binding activity.

4.6   Receptors for Glucagon and Insulin

Studies on hormone receptor identification by photoaffinity labeling have also been undertaken with glucagon and insulin. Bregman & Levy (9) used an arylazide derivative of glucagon (^{125}I-labeled N-4-azido-2-nitrophenylglucagon) to label a glucagon binding protein in hepatocyte plasma membranes. Photolysis of the derivative in the presence of membrane suspension resulted in the incorporation of radioactivity into a membrane component with a molecular weight range of 23,000-25,000 and another protein of MW $> 500,000$. Greater than 90% of the labeling was inhibited by unlabeled glucagon. Studies by Giorgio et al (25) on the lubrol-PX solubilized glucagon receptor from rat hepatocyte membranes indicated a binding component of MW 190,000 under nondissociating conditions.

Yip et al (93) used 4-azidobenzoyl-^{125}I-labeled insulin to label an insulin binding protein in adipocyte plasma membranes. A large number of proteins incorporated the label nonspecifically. Incorporation into one protein of MW 130,000 was reported to be inhibited in the presence of an excessively large concentration (8.3 μM) of unlabeled insulin (the ratio of labeled photoderivative to unlabeled insulin in this case was 1:100,000). The K_d for insulin binding is in the nanomolar range. Inhibition of covalent incorporation into the 130,000-MW protein in the presence of micromolar concentrations of unlabeled insulin therefore is not a rigorous proof for labeling of the true high-affinity receptor. Sahyoun et al (73) used the glutaraldehyde cross-linking technique for covalent linking of radiolabeled insulin to protein in rat liver membranes. Gel filtration analysis of detergent-solubilized, labeled extract demonstrated labeling of at least five components. The labeling of one of these, a component of Stokes radius, 72 Å, was markedly and preferentially inhibited by unlabeled insulin.

4.7 tRNA Binding Site in Escherichia coli Ribosomes

In photoaffinity labeling studies on ribosomes, different investigators using similar reagents have reported apparently contradictory results. Conclusive explanations have not been put forward to account for the divergencies. The photolyzable derivative, 2-nitro-4-azidophenoxy-4'-phenylacetyl-[^{3}H]Phe-tRNA, was used by Hsiung et al (32) for labeling the peptidyl site in ribosomes. The principal labeled products were two 50S ribosomal proteins, L11 and L18. There was no significant labeling of RNA of either 50S or 30S subunits. A totally different pattern of labeling was observed by Bispink & Matthaei (7) and Sonenberg et al (79) using the photoderivatives N-(ethyl-2-diazomalonyl)-[^{3}H]Phe-tRNA and p-azido-N-tBOC-Phe-[^{3}H]Phe-tRNA, respectively. After binding to 70S ribosomes in the presence of poly(U), both derivatives attached covalently to the 23S RNA of the 50S subunit upon irradiation. Both Bispink & Matthaei (7) and Sonenberg et al (79) used very high concentrations of tRNA photoderivatives (0.7–1.2 nmol/ml) for binding and cross-linking to ribosomes. In contrast, Hsiung et al (32) used a 10-fold lower concentration (15 pmol/ml) of derivatized tRNA. It is not clear if this difference in reaction condition determined the differences in labeling patterns. The peptidyl transferase center in ribosomes has also been investigated by Nicholson & Cooperman (65) using an arylazide analog of puromycin. The results are consistent with those observed by Hsiung et al (32), since the major puromycin site-specific protein labeled was L11.

S-(p-azidophenacyl)valyl-tRNA, an analog of aminoacyl tRNA that has a photoaffinity label attached to its 4-thiouridine residue, was used by Schwartz et al (74) to label the ribosomal A site. The analog was bound to ribosomes at 10 mM Mg^{2+}, and binding was stimulated 25-fold by the presence of elongation factor Tu. Covalent linking was dependent on the simultaneous presence of poly(U_2G) and elongation factor Tu-GTP. The covalently attached tRNA was distributed about equally between the 30S and 50S subunits. In the 30S subunit, 30% of the tRNA was bound to proteins, whereas 70% was linked to 16S RNA. In the 50S subunit, only the proteins were labeled. The proteins labeled in either the 30S or 50S subunits were not identified. Implications of the results have been discussed by Ofengund et al (66).

4.8   Other Systems

Arylazide photoaffinity analogs of cytochrome *c* have been used to label mitochondrial cytochrome *c* oxidase. A dinitroazidophenol analog of cytochrome *c*, containing one to two dinitroazidophenyl groups per cytochrome *c* molecule, was synthesized by Erecinska et al (21). Irradiation of cytochrome *c*-depleted rat liver mitochondrial membranes supplemented with an excess of photoaffinity labeled cytochrome *c* resulted in covalent binding of the derivative to cytochrome *c* oxidase. The labeled enzyme was not further analyzed for covalent incorporation into different subunits. Bisson et al (8) have attempted identification of the binding subunit of cytochrome *c* oxidase using cytochrome *c* derivatives labeled with a 3-nitrophenylazido group at the lysine 13 residue, or at both the lysine 13 and lysine 22 residues. The interactions of the cytochrome *c* derivatives with beef heart mitochondrial cytochrome *c* oxidase in the presence of ultraviolet light resulted in a loss of catalytic activity, accompanied by formation of a covalent complex between cytochrome *c* and subunit II of cytochrome *c* oxidase. Therefore, subunit II may be indicated as the binding site or may be close to the binding site of cytochrome *c* to cytochrome *c* oxidase in beef heart mitochondria.

Monovalent dimers of concanavalin A have been prepared by a combination of succinylation and photoaffinity labeling (23). Partial derivatization of native concanavalin A with the photoaffinity label, *p*-azidophenyl-α-D-mannopyranoside, followed by affinity chromatography, yielded a fraction consisting of dimers at pH 5.0 having a single saccharide binding site. These monovalent dimers formed divalent tetramers at pH 7. To achieve a monovalent dimer at this pH, the divalent tetramer was succinylated. The stable monovalent dimer thus obtained was used to study the effect of lectin valence on cell proliferation and cell-cell interactions.

Chemical cross-linking has been used to study the orientation of bacteriorhodopsin in purple membrane fragments (67). Short cross-linking reagents, such as glutaraldehyde (7.5 Å) and dimethyladipimidate (8.5 Å), inactivated the proton-pump activity of bacteriorhodopsin-liposomes, whereas the longer-chain-length cross-linker, dimethylsuberimidate (11.5 Å), did not. All three reagents conferred increased thermal stability. Implications of these results have been discussed by Packer et al (67). The shorter-chain-length molecules may permeate into the interior of the bacteriorhodopsin molecule and cause cross-linking of the group present in the interior of the molecule, but the longer-chain cross-linkers may cross-link outside of the molecule. Therefore the results indicate that the proton is transferred through a channel or pore present in the interior of the bacteriorhodopsin molecule rather than by a translocation mechanism.

Mast cells can bind monomeric immunoglobulin E (IgE), but binding per se does not lead to release of histamine, serotonin, or other active components enclosed within the basophilic granules. Secretion is stimulated by multivalent reagents capable of reacting with the Fab portion of IgE, thereby causing aggregation of bound IgE on the cell surface. To determine the minimal extent of aggregation or cross-linking of IgE required, Segal et al (75) treated IgE with dimethylsuberimidate and fractionated the cross-linked IgE into monomers, dimers, trimers, and higher oligomers. The monomer did not stimulate release of histamine or serotonin from mast cells, but the dimers and higher polymers gave excellent and approximately equivalent responses on a weight basis. The results suggest that the bridging of two molecules of IgE is sufficient to generate a unit signal; the summation of such signals leads to degranulation of mast cells.

5   NEAREST NEIGHBOR INTERACTIONS BETWEEN PROTEINS IN SUPRAMOLECULAR BIOLOGICAL STRUCTURES

5.1 Techniques and General Principles

The applications of cross-linking to the study of nearest neighbor interactions between proteins in erythrocyte membranes and ribosomes were reviewed recently by Peters & Richards (68). This section focuses on the more recent developments in these and related areas. Synthesis of cleavable cross-linking reagents by Wang & Richards (90), Sommer & Traut (78), and Lutter et al (54) and the development of two-dimensional diagonal gel electrophoresis have yielded technology for determining the composition of cross-linked products. The cross-linked oligomers resolved in the first dimension are cleaved during an initial phase of separation in the second dimension. Cross-linked complexes can be recognized by the position of the off-diagonal elements in the final, two-dimensional pattern. The pattern of cross-linking depends to a large extent on the specificity and length of the cross-linking reagent, its concentration, and the availability of the suitable functional groups in proper geometry in the neighboring proteins. Although the formation of an oligomer is usually evidence for contact between components, the failure to demonstrate an oligomer cannot be used with confidence to indicate the lack of this contact.

Ordinary polyacrylamide gels are often not suitable for clear resolution of complex mixtures of cross-linked oligomers. A polyacrylamide gel with a gradient of decreasing pore size from top to bottom may be a better substitute. The low exclusion limit of sodium dodecyl sulfate (SDS) polyacrylamide gels is another problem in resolution of cross-linked oligomers. In most cross-linking studies of membranes, an intense band of cross-linked product can be detected on top of the gels. Kiehm & Ji (44) have developed an agarose-polyacrylamide gel electrophoresis technique, which may permit analysis of these cross-linked complexes up to MW 5×10^6, without sacrificing the resolution of monomeric polypeptide bands seen in polyacrylamide gels.

Because of the difficulty of specifying composition solely on the basis of gel electrophoresis, Sun et al (83), Lutter & Kurland (53), and Takemoto et al (84) used immunologic procedures for identification of components of cross-linked oligomers. Specific immunoadsorption of a cross-linked complex serves two purposes: (a) It clearly identifies the primary component; and (b) it separates this component from a heterogenous mixture of proteins, increasing the resolution of the system. With this immunologic technique, several pairs of ribosomal proteins have been unequivocally identified (53), and single cross-linked oligomers have been resolved from complex membrane systems (84).

5.2   Erythrocyte Membranes

The erythrocyte membrane is the most common model system used for testing the efficacy of cross-linkers of varying size and specificity. Until recently, the reagents most commonly used were the highly water-soluble bisalkylimidates, such as DTBP (90). When applied to membranes, these reagents may react primarily with groups that are accessible to the aqueous environment. This could stem from a lack of amino groups on those amino acids that lie within the membrane hydrocarbon core (55). Therefore, several investigators have explored the application of aromatic diazides as cross-linkers than can react in an apolar milieu. Mikkelson & Wallach (62) used a series of symmetrical bisazides, 1,5-diazidonaphthalene, 4,4'-diazidobiphenyl, and the reversible 4,4'-dithiobisphenylazide. However, a symmetrical reagent with two photolyzable groups may have a low probability for forming cross-links, since many reactions are open to the reactive groups. A successful insertion reaction would be required to occur twice in the same reagent molecule. With an unsymmetrical reagent, however, the two dissimilar cross-linking reactions can be controlled individually, and such reagents can be expected to induce a greater degree of cross-linking. One such compound, di-N-(2-nitro-4-azidophenyl)cystamine-S-S-dioxide, was synthesized by Huang & Richards (33). When applied to erythrocyte membranes, a series of cross-linked complexes were produced by this reagent, which were similar to, but not identical with, those produced by the water-soluble imidates, or Cu-P catalyzed air oxidation of intrinsic −SH groups (90). Membrane permeability of cross-linking reagents is an additional problem encountered with membrane systems. Miyakawa et al (64) have recently studied this property for a series of diazide tartrate derivatives. One of these, tartryl-di(glycylazide), was not permeable to erythrocyte membranes, but lower- and higher-chain-length members of the series readily permeated erythrocyte membranes.

One of the problems in cross-linking studies is the discrimination of naturally occurring cross-linked oligomers from those formed during accidental collisions between independent molecules in fluid membranes. Kiehm & Ji (44) approached this problem by using flash photolysis with a xenon flash lamp to cross-link proteins in erythrocyte ghosts. The flash discharged within a millisecond, and the time period for cross-linking was estimated to be of the same order. The same cross-linked products were observed with photolysis at 4° or 23°C, indicating the presence of naturally occurring complexes.

Other means for cross-linking membrane proteins have been reported by several investigators. Ca^{++}-mediated cross-linking of human erythrocyte proteins was observed by Lorand et al (51), who demonstrated cross-linking due to Ca^{++}-activated transglutaminase activity, which yielded protein-protein cross-linking by formation of γ-glutamyl-ϵ-lysine bridges. Spontaneous cross-linking of proteins in human erythrocyte membranes at low pH (pH 4.0–5.0) has been reported by Liu et al (49).

5.3   Fibroblast and Lympocyte Cell Surface Membrane

Identification and resolution of cross-linked species on the basis of their molecular weights in SDS-polyacrylimide gel electrophoresis is difficult in complex systems, e.g. fibroblasts and lymphocytes, where many proteins may have similar mobilities. Analysis of fibroblast (LM cell) surface membranes by Takemoto et al (85a) revealed numerous native disulfide-linked oligomers, but only a few species that formed oligomers when cells were exposed to DTBP. Among the native oligomers was a glycoprotein of MW 70,000 linked to a polypeptide of MW 15,000. Of all resolvable cell surface components, only this MW 85,000 complex was cross-linked, forming apparent homodimers and homotrimers. An extension of this work showed that the MW 85,000 complex is the major envelope glycoprotein of the murine C-type viruses (84). These viral proteins (gp70 and gp15) are commonly expressed as surface components of murine cells. The identity of this surface displayed protein complex of MW 85,000 and its cross-linked oligomers was assessed using formaldehyde-fixed *Staphylococcus aureus* and goat antiserum monospecific for gp70. A coat protein on *S. aureus* has high affinity for the Fab fragment of immunoglobulin. This characteristic facilitates rapid immune precipitation of the antibody-antigen complex while introducing only trivial quantities of additional protein solubilized when the immune precipitate is exposed to SDS solution. A similar approach was also used to study the organization of murine histocompatibility antigen H-2 in murine lymphosarcoma (EL-4) cells. After cross-linking with DTBP and solubilization with nonionic detergent, addition of anti-H2 or anti-β_2 microglobulin antisera followed by formaldehyde-fixed S. aureus resulted in immune precipitation of a complex of H-2 and anti-β_2 microglobulin, which accounted for up to 40% of the total H-2 protein solubilized (35,85). Springer et al (80a) have shown human histocompatibility antigen (HLA) formed a 1:1 dimer with β_2-microglobulin when a highly purified HLA preparation was treated with dithiobis-(succinimidyl propionate) (Lomant's reagent). These studies with membrane systems (35, 84) and the immunoprecipitation studies on cross-linked oligomers formed by cross-linking of ribosomes (53, 83) indicate that immune precipitation may enjoy general applicability in facilitating the identification of the individual protein components of cross-linked oligomers from complex systems.

5.4   Viruses

Chemical cross-linking in conjunction with diagonal gel electrophoresis has been used for studying supramolecular organization of proteins in animal viruses (20, 56, 63, 70, 91). The virions of the *Paramyxoviridae* and *Rhabdovirus* family are composed of an outer lipoprotein envelope and a nucleoprotein core. A glycoprotein (G or HN) of MW $\sim$ 70,000 is present on the outer surface of the membrane envelope. The nonglycosylated membrane protein M (MW $\sim$ 30,000) is associated with the inner, matrix side of viral membranes and is relatively inaccessible to labeling by surface-specific radioiodination. The major structural protein of nucleocapsid is N or NP (MW $\sim$ 55,000). An elaborate analysis of vesicular stomatitis virus proteins was performed by Dudovi & Wagner (20) with three different reversible heterobifunctional cross-linkers: methyl-4-mercaptobutyrimidate, dithiobissuccinimidyl propionate, and tartryldiazide, which generated qualitatively similar viral protein complexes. They observed covalently linked homooligomers of M, N, and G and two heterodimers, M-N and G-M. The existence of N-M and G-M heterodimers is consistent with the hypothesis that the matrix M protein may bridge between the outer envelope glycoprotein G and the nucleocapsid protein N in assembly of this virion.

An analysis of Newcastle disease virus using the reversible cross-linker DTBP was reported by Miyakawa et al (63). They observed homooligomers of M, NP, and HN, and in addition a heterooligomer of MW 140,000, which appeared to be a 1 : 1 dimer of HN and NP. No HN-M or M-NP heterodimers were observed. They concluded, therefore, that a stable transmembrane association occurs between the major nucleocapsid protein NP and an externally displayed intrinsic viral glycoprotein HN. A reexamination of this work was performed by Markwell & Fox (56, 57) using an improved gradient gel system for analysis of the cross-linked products. Cross-linking with either dimethyl-3,3'-dithiobispropionimidate or with methyl[3-(p-azidophenyl)dithio]propionimidate produced homodimers of NP, HN, and M, and a heterodimer of NP and M. Markwell & Fox (56, 57) observed that NP-M heterodimer formation was more predominant in early than in late harvest virus preparations and in freshly harvested preparation than in those frozen for several months. The failure to observe this specific heterodimer by Miyakawa et al could be due to loss of viral integrity during long storage. Markwell & Fox (56, 57) also presented evidence that the MW 140,000 oligomer of MN and NP reported by Miyakawa et al is in fact a mixture of homodimers (MW 154,000 and 127,000) of HN and NP, which did not separate in the lower resolution gel system used by Miyakawa et al (63).

5.5   Chromatin

Cross-linking studies of histones in chromatin by Thomas & Kornberg (86) revealed that the basic histone unit in nucleosomes is an octamer (MW 110,000) with the composition $(H_2A, H_2B, H_3, H_4)_2$. The cross-linking reagent dimethylsuberimidate revealed a histone octamer in chromatin. The interactions between different histones in this complex have been studied by Martinson et al (58–60) using tetranitromethane and ultraviolet light (280 nm) to form cross-links. Both tetranitromethane and ultraviolet light are effective "zero length" cross-linkers and presumably act on tyrosine residues to produce tyrosine-free radicals, which insert directly onto appropriately situated neighbors. Since tyrosine is predominantly localized in the hydrophobic regions of the histones, the cross-linking events probably occur within a tight hydrophobic binding site (58-60). Treatment of chromatin or intact cells growing in culture with tetranitromethane resulted in a cross-linked product identified as the H_2B-H_4 dimer (58); irradiation of either whole cells or chromatin at 280 nm resulted in a covalent linkage of H_2A and H_2B (60). Characterization of the cyanogen bromide peptide fragment of H_2B-H_4 and H_2B-H_2A cross-linked dimers showed that the C-terminal half of H_2B contains the link to H_4, whereas the N-terminal half contains the link to H_2A (59). These data suggest that H_2A-H_2B-H_4 association may be an important underlying structural feature of chromatin.

The details of condensations of DNA by the octameric histone complex in nucleosomes are of considerable interest. Stein et al (82) prepared a chemically cross-linked histone octamer complex by treating purified core particles with dimethylsuberimidate and used the cross-linked core as a model for studying histone-DNA interactions. DNA could be separated from the cross-linked octamer under nondenaturing conditions, and the nucleosome structure reconstituted from isolated DNA and the cross-linked protein core. If the histones in the cross-linked core particles are rather tightly held together by a sufficient number of cross-links, the DNA extractability by increased ionic strength, and the occurrence of reconstitution under nondenaturing conditions makes it unlikely that any portion of DNA is buried inside the protein core of the nucleosome. The results support the accepted model in which DNA is wound about the outside of a protein core.

5.6 Enzyme Crystals

Crystallographic studies have been useful in determining the static position of purported catalytically essential residues in enzymes. To deduce possible mechanisms of action from detailed structural information, models of substrates have been superimposed onto three-dimensional structural models. Most mechanistic conclusions are based on the kinetic and chemical properties of enzyme solutions, and it is assumed that these properties are conserved in crystals. This assumption is clearly critical when assigning a functional significance to specific residues discerned from X-ray analysis of crystals. Therefore, studies on the catalytic characteristics of enzyme crystals are necessary and indispensable for the design of mechanisms based on enzyme structure and function. One of the difficulties in measuring catalytic activity of enzyme crystals is their fragility. They also dissolve if the composition of the immersion medium is much changed from that in which they were grown. Quiocho & Richards (69) showed that cross-linking of enzyme crystals with gluteraldehyde markedly increased their mechanical stability and completely suppressed their solubilization under enzyme assay conditions. Moreover, the quality of the X-ray diffraction pattern was changed only slightly by cross-linking. Vallee and his co-workers (1, 80) studied the catalytic properties of cross-linked crystals of carboxypeptidases A and B. Crystallization reduced K_{cat} dramatically, 20- to 1,000-fold, but it had little effect on the K_m. A similar result was also obtained by Kasvinsky & Madsen (37) with gluteraldehyde cross-linked crystals of muscle phophorylase a and b. The kinetic parameters, K_{cat} and K_m, were determined under conditions that obviate artifacts due to diffusion limitation of substrates or products. Since the K_m generally is not altered by crystallization, the substrate binding sites in the cross-linked crystals and soluble enzyme are likely to be similar. Loss of catalytic efficiency, however, clearly points to differences in the active site of the enzymes caused by crystallization. This may not be a static difference, but rather the crystal lattice may restrain a conformational change that is an essential part of the catalytic cycle, requiring more energy to achieve the enzyme structure required for the transition state. Also, an enzyme in solution may be an equilibrium mixture of a number of different conformations, and the process of crystallization may lock the enzyme into one of these. These results indicate that X-ray crystallographic analysis alone may be unable to detect certain dynamic aspects of the mechanism of action, since the technique itself precludes such studies.

5.7   Other Systems

Davis & Stark (18) showed that SDS gel analysis of cross-linked samples could reveal quaternary structures in soluble oligomeric enzymes. With the introduction of cleavable cross-linking reagents and diagonal gel electrophoresis, the technique has been further improved and refined. Oligomeric multicomponent complex enzymes that have been studied by using this approach include *Escherichia coli* RNA polymerase holoenzyme (30), spinach chloroplast coupling factor I (2), and beef mitochondrial coupling factor I (3). Chemical cross-linking has also been used to study the composition of tubulin dimer (52). Two forms of 55,000-dalton monomers of α and β are found in all microtubule preparations. Thus the dimers could be either heterodimers ($\alpha\beta$) or homodimers ($\alpha\alpha$ and $\beta\beta$). A bifunctional reagent, dimethyl-3-3'-(tetramethylenedioxy)dipropionimidate, was able to produce tubulin dimers. Electrophoretic analysis showed that 60–90% of the cross-linked dimers formed were $\alpha\beta$, indicating that soluble tubulin dimers are largely heterodimers.

6   CONCLUDING REMARKS

Photoaffinity labeling has two major advantages over ordinary chemical affinity labeling. First, the vast majority of chemical affinity labels are electrophilic species and a nucleophile at the binding site is required for labeling. In photoaffinity labeling, the reactive group (nitrene or carbene) is generated at the ligand binding site and may react relatively indiscriminately with any of the chemical groups present at that site. Second, some biological problems require reagents in which the reactivity remains quiescent until the experimenter chooses to activate it. With photoaffinity reagents, the transient interactions of the photoactivable ligand with various cellular components can be monitored directly. It is possible to develop strategies that allow the generation of a reactive reagent only at the ligand binding site of interest. Studies of dynamic behavior of ligands and their receptors in living cells may then be possible. The use of photoactivable heterobifunctional cross-linking reagents in studies of complex biological phenomena is obviously a conceptually attractive approach that has not yet achieved its full potential.

Photosensitive heterobifunctional cross-linkers have also been used to some extent in structural studies, but here they suffer many of the problems encountered upon cross-linking with bis-site-specific cross-linking reagents. The site specific end of the heterobifunctional reagent is limited in its range of reactivity with available sites on oligomeric structures. Thus, heterobifunctional reagents share the experimental deficiency wherein a failure to demonstrate cross-linking between any two given species cannot provide evidence for failure of these components to exist as an oligomeric structure.

Literature Cited

1. Alter, G. M., Leussing, D. L., Neurath, H., Vallee, B. L. 1977. *Biochemistry* 16:3663–68
2. Baird, B. A., Hammes, G. G. 1976. *J. Biol. Chem.* 251:6953–62
3. Baird, B. A., Hammes, G. G. 1977. *J. Biol. Chem.* 252:4743–48
4. Bayley, H., Knowles, J. R. 1977. *Methods Enzymol.* 46:69–114
5. Bayley, H., Knowles, J. R. 1978. *Biochemistry* 7:2414–19
6. Bercovici, T., Gilter, C. 1978. *Biochemistry* 7:1484–89
7. Bispink, L., Matthaei, H. 1973. *FEBS Lett.* 37:291–94
8. Bisson, R., Azzi, A., Gutweniger, H., Colonna, R., Montecucco, C., Zanotti, A. 1978. *J. Biol. Chem.* 253:1874–80
9. Bregman, M. D., Levy, D. 1977. *Biochem. Biophys. Res. Commun.* 78:584–90
10. Browne, D. T., Kent, B. H. 1975. *Biochem. Biophys. Res. Commun.* 67:126–32
11. Brunswick, D. J., Cooperman, B. S. 1971. *Proc. Natl. Acad. Sci. USA* 68:1801–4
12. Chakrabarti, P., Khorana, H. G. 1975. *Biochemistry* 14:5021–33
13. Converse, C. A., Richards, F. F. 1969. *Biochemistry* 8:4431–36
14. Darfler, F. J., Marinetti, G. V. 1977. *Biochem. Biophys. Res. Commun.* 79:1–7
15. Das, M., Fox, C. F. 1978. *Proc. Natl. Acad. Sci. USA* 75:2644–48
15a. Das, M., Fox, C. F. 1978. In *Transmembrane Signalling*, ed. M. Bitensky, R. J. Collier, D. F. Steiner, C. F. Fox. New York: Liss. In press
16. Das, M., Miyakawa, T., Fox, C. F. 1978. In *Cell Surface Carbohydrates and Biological Recognition*, ed. V. T. Marcheri, V. Ginsburg, D. C. Robbins, C. F. Fox, pp. 647–56. New York: Liss
17. Das, M., Miyakawa, T., Fox, C. F., Pruss, R. M., Aharonov, A., Herschman, H. R. 1977. *Proc. Natl. Acad. Sci. USA* 74:2790–94
18. Davis, G. E., Stark, G. R. 1970. *Proc. Natl. Acad. Sci. USA* 66:651–56
19. Dreyfuss, G., Schwartz, K., Blant, E. R., Barrio, J. R., Liu, F. T., Leonard, N. J. 1978. *Proc. Natl. Acad. Sci. USA* 75:1199–203
20. Dudovi, E. J., Wagner, R. R. 1977. *J. Virol.* 22:500–9
21. Erecinska, M., Vanderkooi, J. M., Wilson, D. F. 1975. *Arch. Biochem. Biophys.* 171:108–16
22. Fleet, G. W. J., Knowles, J. R., Porter, R. R. 1972. *Biochem. J.* 128:499–508
23. Fraser, A. R., Hemperly, J. J., Wang, J. L., Edelman, G. M. 1976. *Proc. Natl. Acad. Sci. USA* 73:790–94
24. Galardy, R. E., Craig, L. C., Jamieson, J. D., Printz, M. P. 1974. *J. Biol. Chem* 249:3510–18
25. Giorgio, N. A., Johnson, C. B., Blecher, M. 1974. *J. Biol. Chem.* 249:428–37
26. Greenberg, G. R., Chakrabarti, P., Khorana, H. G. 1976. *Proc. Natl. Acad. Sci. USA* 73:790–94
27. Guthrow, C. E., Rasmussen, H., Brunswick, D. J., Cooperman, B. S. 1973. *Proc. Natl. Acad. Sci. USA* 70:3344–46
28. Haley, B. E. 1975. *Biochemistry* 14:3852–57
29. Hand, E. S., Jencks, W. P. 1962. *J. Am. Chem. Soc.* 84:3050–514
30. Hillel, Z., Wu, C. W. 1977. *Biochemistry* 16:3334–42
31. Hixson, S. H., Hixson, S. S. 1975. *Biochemistry* 14:4251–54
32. Hsiung, N., Reines, S. A., Cantor, C. R. 1974. *J. Mol. Biol.* 88:841–55

192   DAS & FOX

33. Huang, C. K., Richards, F. M. 1977. *J. Biol. Chem.* 252:5514–21
4. Hucho, F., Bergman, C., Dubois, J. M., Rojas, E., Kiefer, H. 1976. *Nature* 260:802–4
35. Huggins, J. W., Fox, C. F. 1978. *J. Supramol. Struct.* 2:282 (Abstr.)
36. Ji, T. H. 1977. *J. Biol. Chem.* 252:1566–70
37. Kasvinsky, P. J., Madsen, N. B. 1976. *J. Biol. Chem.* 251:6852–59
38. Katzenellenbogen, J. A., Johnson, H. J., Carlson, K. E., Myers, H. N. 1974. *Biochemistry* 16:1970–76
39. Katzenellenbogen, J. A., Johnson, H. J., Carlson, K. E., Myers, H. N. 1974. *Biochemistry* 13:2986–94
40. Katzenellenbogen, J. A., Johnson, H. J., Myers, H. N. 1973. *Biochemistry* 12:4085–91
41. Katzenellenbogen, J. A., Myers, H. N., Johnson, H. J. 1973. *J. Org. Chem.* 38:3525–33
42. Katzenellenbogen, J. A., Myers, H. N., Johnson, H. J., Kempton, R. J., Carlson, K. E. 1977. *Biochemistry* 16:1964–70
43. Kiefer, H., Lindstrom, J., Lennox, E. S., Singer, S. J. 1970. *Proc. Natl. Acad. Sci. USA* 67:1688–94
44. Kiehm, D. J., Ji, T. H. 1977. *J. Biol. Chem.* 252:8524–31
45. Klip, A., Gitler, C. 1974. *Biochem. Biophys. Res. Commun.* 60:1155–62
46. Klip, A., Darszon, A., Montal, M. 1977. *Biochem. Biophys. Res. Commun.* 72:1350–58
47. Knowles, J. R. 1972. *Acc. Chem. Res.* 5:155–60
48. Lewis, R. V., Roberts, M. F., Dennis, E. A., Allison, W. S. 1977. *Biochemistry* 16:5650–54
49. Liu, S. C., Fairbanks, G., Paleu, J. 1977. *Biochemistry* 16:4066–74
50. Lomant, A. J., Fairbanks, G. 1976. *J. Mol. Biol.* 104:243–61
51. Lorand, L., Weissmann, L. B., Epel, D. L., Bruner-Lonard, J. 1976. *Proc. Natl. Acad. Sci. USA* 73:4479–81
52. Luduena, R. F., Shooter, E. M., Wilson, L. 1977. *J. Biol. Chem.* 252:7006–14
53. Lutter, L. C., Kurland, C. G. 1974. *Mol. Gen. Genet.* 129:167–76
54. Lutter, L. C., Kurland, C. G., Stoffler, G. 1975. *FEBS Lett.* 54:144–50
55. Marchesi, V. T., Furthmayr, H., Tomita, M. 1976. *Ann. Rev. Biochem.* 45:667–98
56. Markwell, M. A. K. 1978. *Fed Proc.* 37:2757 (Abstr.)
57. Markwell, M. A. K., Fox, C. F. Manuscript in preparation
58. Martinson, H. G., McCarthy, B. J. 1975. *Biochemistry* 14:1073–78
59. Martinson, H. G., McCarthy, B. J. 1976. *Biochemistry* 15:4126–31
60. Martinson, H. G., Shotler, M. D., McCarthy, B. J. 1976. *Biochemistry* 15:2002–7
61. Marver, D., Chiu, W. H., Wolff, H. E., Edelman, I. S. 1976. *Proc. Natl. Acad. Sci. USA* 73:4462–66
62. Mikkelson, R. B., Wallach, D. F. H. 1976. *J. Biol. Chem.* 251:7413–16
63. Miyakawa, T., Takemoto, L. J., Fox, C. F. 1976. In *Animal Virology*, ed. D. Baltimore, A. S. Huang, C. F. Fox, pp. 485–97. New York: Academic
64. Miyakawa, T., Takemoto, L. J., Fox, C. F. 1978. *J. Supramol. Struct.* 8:301–8
65. Nicholson, A. W., Cooperman, B. S. 1978. *FEBS. Lett.* 90:203–8
66. Ofengund, J., Schwartz, I., Chinelli, G., Hixson, S. S., Hixson, S. H. 1977. *Methods Enzymol.* 46:683–702
67. Packer, L., Konishi, T., Shich, P. 1977. *Fed. Proc.* 36:1819–23
68. Peters, K., Richards, F. M. 1977. *Ann. Rev. Biochem.* 46:523–51
69. Quiocho, F. A., Richards, F. M. 1964. *Proc. Natl. Acad. Sci. USA* 52:833–39
70. Raghow, R., Kingsbury, D. W. 1976. In *Animal Virology*, ed. D. Baltimore, A. S. Huang, C. F. Fox, pp. 471–84. New York: Academic
71. Reiser, A., Willets, F. W., Terry, G. C., Williams, V., Marley, R. 1968. *Trans. Faraday Soc.* 64:3265–75
72. Ruoho, A. E., Kiefer, H., Roeder, P. E., Singer, S. J. 1973. *Proc. Natl. Acad. Sci. USA* 70:2567–71
73. Sahyoun, N., Hoch, R. A., Hollenberg, M. D. 1978. *Proc. Natl. Acad. Sci. USA* 75:1675–79
74. Schwartz, I., Gordon, E., Ofengund, J. 1975. *Biochemistry* 14:2907–14
75. Segal, D. M., Taurog, J. D., Metzger, H. 1977. *Proc. Natl. Acad. Sci. USA* 74:2993–97
76. Shafer, J., Baronowsky, P., Laursen, R., Finn, F., Westheimer, F. H. 1966. *J. Biol. Chem.* 241:421–27
77. Singh, A., Thornton, E. R., Westheimer, F. H. 1962. *J. Biol. Chem.* 237:3006–8
78. Sommer, A., Traut, R. R. 1974. *Proc. Natl. Acad. Sci. USA* 71:3946–50
79. Sonenberg, N., Wilchek, M., Zamir, A. 1975. *Proc. Natl. Acad. Sci. USA* 72:4332–36
80. Spilburg, C. A., Bethune, J. L., Vallee, B. L. 1977. *Biochemistry* 16:1142–50
80a. Springer, T. A., Robb, R. J., Terhorst, C., Strominger, J. L. 1977. *J. Biol. Chem.* 252:4694–700
81. Stadel, J. M., Goodman, D. B. P., Ga-

lardy, R. E., Rasmussen, H. 1978. *Biochemistry* 17:1403–8

82. Stein, A., Bina-Stein, M., Simpson, R. T. 1977. *Proc. Natl. Acad. Sci. USA* 74:2780–84

83. Sun, T. T., Traut, R. R., Kahan, L. 1974. *J. Mol. Biol.* 87:509–22

84. Takemoto, L. J., Fox, C. F., Jensen, F. C., Elder, J. H., Lerner, R. A. 1978. *Proc. Natl. Acad. Sci. USA* 75:3644–48

85. Takemoto, L. J., Huggins, J. W., Fox, C. F. Unpublished observations

85a. Takemoto, L. J., Miyakawa, T., Fox, C. F. 1977. In *Cell Shape and Surface Architecture,* ed. J. P. Revel, U. Henning, C. F. Fox, pp. 605–14. New York: Liss

86. Thomas, J. D., Kornberg, R. D. 1975. *Proc. Natl. Acad. Sci. USA* 72:2626–30

87. Uy, R., Wold, F. 1977. In *Protein Crosslinking,* Part A, ed. M. Friedman, pp. 169–86. New York: Plenum

88. Vaughan, R. J., Westheimer, F. H., 1968. *J. Am. Chem. Soc.* 91:217–18

89. Walter, U., Uno, I., Liu, A. Y. C., Greengard, P. 1977. *J. Biol. Chem.* 252:6494–500

90. Wang, K., Richards, F. M. 1974. *J. Biol. Chem.* 249:8005–18

91. Wiley, D. C., Skehal, J. J., Waterfield, M. 1977. *Virology* 79:446–48

92. Witzemann, V., Raftery, M. A. 1977. *Biochemistry* 16:5862–68

93. Yip, C. C., Yeung, C. W. T., Moule, M. L. 1978. *J. Biol. Chem.* 253:1743–45

Ann. Rev. Microbiol. 1978. 32:19–39
Copyright © 1978 by Annual Reviews Inc. All rights reserved

PHAGOCYTOSIS AS A SURFACE PHENOMENON

♦1720

C. J. van Oss

Department of Microbiology, State University of New York at Buffalo, Buffalo, New York 14214

CONTENTS

0066-4227/78/1001-0019$01.00

19

INTRODUCTION

Phagocytosis is the ingestion (and subsequent digestion) of particles by single cells. Phagocytosis by circulating granulocytes and monocytes and by fixed macrophages is an organism's most important means of defense against invading matter, after the defense provided by the skin and mucous membranes. In the presence or absence of opsonins most bacterial species become readily ingested by circulating granulocytes [or polymorphonuclear leukocytes (PMNs)] and therefore are generally nonpathogenic. Bacteria that are easily ingested but that owe their pathogenicity to resistance to phagocytic digestion are not discussed here. Bacteria of only a relatively small number of species resist phagocytic ingestion by means of capsular or other surface components (75) and therefore can be potential pathogens. Specific antibodies, assisted by complement, can "opsonize" such bacteria for subsequent phagocytosis, which helps the animal host to resist or overcome overt infections by pathogens (17, 43, 90).

One of the major questions in phagocytosis centers around the mechanism by which phagocytes (*a*) recognize all the nonpathogenic bacteria they readily ingest, and (*b*) recognize phagocytosis-resisting bacteria only after they are opsonized. An attractive, albeit speculative, answer to (*b*) postulates the existence of immunoglobulin and complement receptors on the phagocyte surfaces for the purpose of binding the particles that should be ingested, e.g. see Murphy (57). However, with respect to (*a*) it is not conceivable that phagocytic cells are endowed with the infinite number of receptors with the many specificities required not only for the different determinants of innumerable nonpathogenic bacterial species, but even for surface determinants of various synthetic plastic beads, e.g. polystyrene latex particles (74). It could still be supposed that immunoglobulins might adsorb nonspecifically to the surfaces of bacteria and latex particles, and so provide the recognition factor (110). However, encapsulated microorganisms readily absorb nonspecific immunoglobulins as well as specific antibodies, but only specific anticapsular antibodies induce phagocytosis (78). It is known that the reactivity of specific anticapsular antibody at the outer periphery of the capsule strongly accentuates the visibility of the "Quellung" reaction (59). The peculiarity of the phagocytosis-inducing property of certain immunoglobulins therefore would appear to be situated at the outermost surface of the particle that is to become phagocytized. The physicochemical surface properties of the outermost interface of bacteria and other particles, as well as of phagocytic cells, can essentially be of only two kinds: (a) electrical surface potential, and (b) interfacial tension.

(a) The strength of the electrical surface (ζ) potential of particles does not appear to be directly linked to the facility with which these particles become phagocytosed. For instance, rough strains of various bacteria generally have a much higher negative ζ-potential than smooth strains (37, 52), in apparent contradiction to their propensity to become readily phagocytized by leukocytes that are equally negatively charged (71). The connection between phagocytosis and ζ-potential (if any) thus appears far from simple, and its measurement does not promise to be fruitful in yielding a direct and obvious correlation between the two phenomena. As discussed below, the pleomorphic and irregular shape of phagocytic cells plays a much more important role in surmounting electrostatic repulsion forces than do the absolute values of the electrokinetic potentials.

(b) Presumably, interfacial tension is then the major physicochemical cell surface property likely to play a crucial role in the decision a phagocyte makes between ingestion and noningestion. It has long been conjectured that interfacial tensions play an important role in the engulfment of bacteria and other particles by leukocytes (21, 53–55), or sea-urchin eggs (15). The semiquantitative determination of the hydrophobicity of various bacteria by penetrability measurements with two-phase systems (53–55) showed a correlation between the degree of hydrophobicity and proneness to phagocytic engulfment. Sorting out and other morphogenetic rearrangements of embryonic cells have also been attributed to the tendency of interacting cells toward a minimal interfacial free energy; Phillips & Steinberg have devised a method for estimating intercellular adhesiveness through equilibrium centrifugation of such embryonic cell aggregates (66).

The solid-liquid interfacial tension of solids can best be studied by contact angle measurements at gas-liquid-solid interface, using a technique for investigating the nature of solid surfaces first proposed in 1805 by Thomas Young (115). This method has been applied to the study of the interfacial properties of monolayers of phagocytic cells and of various bacteria since 1970, and the first results were published in 1972 (94).

THE SINGLE LIQUID CONTACT ANGLE METHOD

In the last 20 years, Young's technique (115), which involves the measurement of the contact angle made between a sessile drop of liquid and a layer of solid material in air, has been developed to some degree of sophistication

(116–118). For osmotic and biochemical reasons, one labors under the current impossibility or impracticability of measuring contact angles with a wide variety of organic liquids of known surface tensions. Although Baier and his collaborators (7) have attempted to extend Zisman's method (116–118) in their measurement of critical surface tensions of materials coated with substances of biological origin, only saline water can reasonably be contemplated as the liquid to be used for measuring contact angles on monolayers of living cells (94, 102).

A contact angle (θ) is the angle between a solid surface and a liquid drop. The contact angle made with a saline drop of a standard size (10 μl), sessile on a flat layer of a variety of microorganisms, phagocytes, or other cells, is measured (through the drop) as the angle between the tangent to the drop and the cell surface at the three-phase solid/liquid/air meeting point (94, 102) (see Figure 1). The measurements are best done with the aid of a telescope with cross-hairs, attached to a goniometer (Gaertner Scientific Corp., Chicago, Ill.) (94, 102). The angles of at least 10 sessile drops of physiological saline should be measured and the averages taken; the results then are quite reproducible and the contact angles, with care, can be estimated within $\pm 1°$ SE for layers of bacteria and within $\pm 0.5°$ SE for phagocytes and other mammalian cells (94, 102).

Prior to measuring contact angles on monolayers of bacteria as well as of phagocytes, air drying is required to eliminate a surface layer of water that otherwise would give rise to a contact angle of 0°. The length of time of air drying required prior to contact angle measurement is easily judged by the disappearance of surface glossiness and the appearance of a matted-looking surface. On agar layers, once the matted aspect appears, contact angles on bacterial cell layers remain constant for several hours (102).

Monolayers of human PMNs are obtained on glass coverslips from a few drops of fingerprick blood as the first step of the in vitro phagocytosis

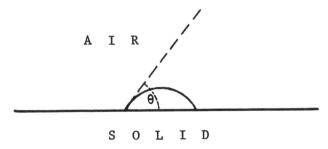

Figure 1   Measurement of the contact angle of a sessile liquid drop on a flat, solid surface. The contact angle θ is the angle of the tangent to the drop with the solid surface (which can be a flat layer of microorganisms, as well as a monolayer of phagocytes or other cells) at the solid/liquid/air meeting point. The angle is measured through the profile of the drop.

method described by Newsome (64) (see also 94, 102, 110). After 25 min in a moist chamber at 37°C, the phagocytic cells adhere firmly to the coverslip and the erythrocytes and the other nonphagocytic cells can be washed away with saline. This procedure yields monolayers of 200–400/mm^2 of phagocytes (mainly neutrophils) (94, 102). In this case one must also wait until the glossy wetness has subsided (which takes approximately 1 hr at room temperature); a plateau of constant contact angles then prevails during at least the entire second hour (102). With phagocytic cells, layers thicker than monolayers should be avoided (102). The contact angle thus obtained for normal human PMNs, which varies between 17.3 and 18.7°, is independent of the contact angle with waterdrops on the glass on which the cells repose (102).

For practical purposes all contact angles, on phagocytes as well as on bacteria, are most conveniently determined at room temperature. When contact angles on PMNs and on bacteria were measured at 20° and 37°C, no significant differences were detected (102)

Monolayers of other cells can be obtained in a variety of ways. Macrophage monolayers form easily when these cells are deposited on glass coverslips. Nonphagocytic blood cells can also be deposited by centrifugation on glass, or on cellulose acetate membranes (92). Monolayers of cells grown in tissue culture can be used directly for contact angle measurement, after an appropriate drying period. Here also, the reproducibility of the contact angles generally is within ±1° (102).

Contact angles can also be measured on layers of dissolved protein. To that effect the protein solution should be ultrafiltered (without stirring) through a cellulose acetate membrane of sufficiently low porosity to preclude the passage of the protein under study (92). Contact angles can then be measured on the protein-clogged ultrafilter membrane after the usual air drying. Alternatively, and more expediently, small amounts of a protein solution can be deposited on such an ultrafiltration membrane and allowed to dry; after a relatively short time the contact angle can then be measured. The latter method requires less protein although the initial protein concentration should be at least 1%. The ultrafiltration method can be used to concentrate the protein. Desiccation of the protein should be avoided since this might cause denaturation, which tends to give rise to inordinately increased contact angles (102).

OTHER METHODS FOR MEASURING SURFACE TENSILE PROPERTIES OF CELLS

Multi-Liquid Contact Angle Method

Although the multi-liquid contact angle method, developed by Zisman (116–118), has the considerable drawback of exposing cell surfaces to a variety of non-physiological liquids that can interact chemically and physically with them in numerous ways, the one advantage of the method is that by extrapolation to cos $\theta = 1$, a Zisman plot will directly yield a critical surface tension for the surface. Instead of organic solvents, various concentrations of $NaNO_3$ in water have been used, and values analogous to those found with the single liquid (saline) contact angle method were obtained with bacteria, as well as with lymphocytes (102). Baier & Zisman (8) studied the wetting properties of collagen and gelatin surfaces with the help of 12 different liquids, and Baier and co-workers (7) studied the surfaces of blood vessel walls as well as of thromboresistant synthetic materials with 8 and 12 different liquids, respectively.

Cell Adhesiveness

van den Tempel (88) obtained information about the surface properties of particles by centrifugally detaching them after adsorption onto well-defined surfaces (see also 50). Earlier, Weiss measured adhesion by subjecting cells to shearing forces in a rotating device (112). McKeever measured the degree of macrophage adherence to flat surfaces by determining the force it takes to detach these cells with calibrated glass needles (49), and van Oss and associates compared McKeever's results with those obtained with contact angle measurements (104). The proportion of phagocytic cells that adhere to glass (89, 102) or plastic surfaces (19), or to nylon (30) or glass fibers (13), has also been utilized as a measure of cell adhesiveness.

Immiscible Liquids

Mudd & Mudd (53–55) used immiscible liquids (generally water and oil) and obtained a semiquantitative estimate of the interfacial tension of cells according to the phase in which they preferentially congregated (see also 47). Immiscible aqueous systems, developed by Albertsson (2) and used in partition (countercurrent distribution) methods, can also be used to obtain at least qualitative information about cellular interfacial properties (76). These methods have more recently been compared with the contact angle method, and the correlation between bacterial hydrophobicity, colony "roughness," and phagocytability of different strains of salmonellae has been confirmed (16).

Finally, an elegant method was developed by Gingell & Todd (27). They used a toroid ring with cells adsorbed to the surface. After immersion of the ring at water-oil interface, a completely flat meniscus can be obtained at one given level at the interface; the angle of this meniscal interface with the surface of the torus is a measure of the cellular interfacial tension (27).

PHAGOCYTOSIS AND CONTACT ANGLES
OF NONOPSONIZED BACTERIA

When the contact angles of about 20 different species or strains of bacteria are compared with the degree to which they become phagocytosed by human PMNs, a strong correlation emerges, and the bacteria clearly fall into two different classes (94, 102). (*a*) The ones with contact angles >18° readily become phagocytosed. These are, in the order of increasing Θ, *Shigella flexneri* (18.1°), *Haemophilus influenzae* (rough) (18.6°), *Staphylococcus aureus* (18.7°), *Arizona arizonae* (19.0°), *Streptococcus faecium* (20.0°), *Salmonella typhimurium* (rough) (20.0°), *Streptococcus pyogenes* (21.3°), *Enterobacter aerogenes* (21.5°), *Escherichia coli* (group 07) (23.0°), *Staphylococcus epidermidis* (24.5°), *Listeria monocytogenes* (rough) (26.5°), *Neisseria gonorrhoeae* (26.7°), *Brucella abortus* (27.0°), and *Mycobacterium butyricum* (70.0°) (94, 102). (*b*) The ones with θ < 18°, which resist phagocytosis, are in order of decreasing θ: *H. influenzae* (group B) (17.6°), *Streptococcus pneumoniae* (type unknown) (17.3°), *E. coli* (group 0111) (17.2°), *S. pneumoniae* (type 1) (17.0°), *Klebsiella pneumoniae* (17.0°), *S. typhimurium* (smooth) (17.0°), and *S. aureus* (Smith strain) (16.5) (94, 102).

The most important aspect of the contact angles of bacteria (in connection with the degree to which they become phagocytized) is not the absolute value of θ, but its value as compared to the θ of phagocytic cells: bacteria more hydrophobic than the phagocytes easily become phagocytized; bacteria more hydrophilic than the phagocytic cells resist phagocytosis (94, 102). This was demonstrated by comparing θ's and the consequence of phagocytosis, i.e. the number of bacteria ingested per phagocyte. Accordingly, a number of bacterial species (θ, 18.1–24.5°) were assessed with human PMNs ($\theta = 18.0$°), and with guinea pig macrophages ($\theta = 21.3$°). Human PMNs easily ingested all the bacteria in the series, whereas guinea pig macrophages ingested only those with $\theta > 21.3$° (102). (It should be kept in mind that a higher θ, measured with drops of saline water, corresponds to a greater surface hydrophobicity.)

Apart from the definite correlation between the contact angle and degree of phagocytosis, a more general picture also emerged from this study, namely the fact that those bacteria that have a significantly higher contact angle than PMNs can generally be considered either to have rather low virulence, or to have special mechanisms of pathogenicity independent of the ease with which they become phagocytized (e.g. *L. monocytogenes, N. gonorrhoeae,* and *M. butyricum*) (92, 102). On the other hand, bacteria that have a significantly lower contact angle than PMNs are virulent. In the last class particularly are encapsulated microorganisms. A striking example is

S. aureus (Smith strain), which has a pronounced capsule, is thus quite hydrophilic ($\theta = 16.5°$), and strongly resists phagocytosis, whereas after decapsulation (78) it acquires a high contact angle (26.0°) and becomes easily phagocytized (94, 102). The results of these investigations are in accord with the concept that most nonvirulent bacteria are so because their surfaces are more hydrophobic than the peripheral phagocytes of their mammalian hosts. As a result, these microorganisms become speedily ingested (94, 102).

OPSONIZATION BY IMMUNOGLOBULINS AND COMPLEMENT COMPONENTS

General

Virulent, encapsulated, smooth, or otherwise hydrophilic bacteria that resist phagocytosis are phagocytized after exposure to heat-stable opsonins [specific antibodies (17, 43)] and heat-labile opsonins [complement (25, 38)]. Virulent, smooth, or encapsulated bacteria [*S. pneumoniae* (type 1), *K. pneumonie* (type 2), *E. coli* (group 055), *S. typhimurium* (type C5S and 395 MS smooth strain), and *S. aureus* (Smith strain)] become more hydrophobic (θ increased from $\simeq 17$ to $\simeq 21°$) and are more readily phagocytized after treatment with specific antisera. Further treatment with complement (guinea pig serum) renders the sensitized bacteria even more hydrophobic ($\theta = 25°$) and enhances their phagocytosis. Heat-inactivated complement has no influence on either hydrophobicity or phagocytosis of the sensitized bacteria, and whole complement alone has no measurable influence on unsensitized bacteria (16, 95, 97, 102).

These results appear to clarify the immunological mechanism of defense against smooth and encapsulated bacteria. After antibodies are formed to a hydrophilic strain of bacteria, these antibodies render the bacteria more hydrophobic (which is further enhanced by the action of complement), and phagocytosis then readily ensues (97). It is pertinent to note that specific antibodies also enhance the ingestion of bacteria by amoebae (24).

Although current information strongly supports the opsonizing role of antibodies (17, 43) and complement in phagocytosis (25, 38), it is acknowledged that there may well be other as yet undefined physiological mechanisms that play an additional role in mediating or enhancing opsonization. With a microorganism such as *listeria,* antibody and complement cannot further increase its high contact angle ($\theta = 25°$); however, specific antiserum does cause an increase in its phagocytosis that is not enhanced by complement (102). It is possible that *tuftsin,* a tetrapeptide "hormone" that stimulates phagocytosis by aspecifically binding to γ-globulin (58), plays a role here.

Immunoglobulins

The antibody-linked opsonizing effect is mainly a function of immunoglobulin (Ig) G and, in human IgG, of the subclasses IgG_1 and IgG_3 (77, 91). The part of the IgG molecule with opsonic properties is the Fc portion (111), which is also the portion responsible for increasing the hydrophobicity of bacteria (102). Of course IgG_2 by binding complement can indirectly cause opsonization (91). Cell wall proteins (protein A) of *S. aureus* have been reported to bind IgG by attaching to its Fc portion (22); this causes the hydrophilic Fab fraction to stick out (102) and thwarts the opsonic power of IgG-class antibodies.

IgM alone, in the absence of complement, does not appear to opsonize (110); its contact angle is 18° (102). However, via complement activation IgM does play an important role in opsonization (110).

IgA, because of its low contact angle ($\theta = 15.6°$) (102), actually depresses phagocytosis (110); this property may help to explain why antibodies of this class appear to act as antiviral rather than antibacterial antibodies, in particular in the upper respiratory and the lower digestive tracts (97).

Complement Components

By using the purified guinea pig complement (C) components C1 through C9, the precise C components responsible for the opsonization and the hydrophobization of sensitized *E. coli* have been determined (96, 102). In agreement with the reported function of C1423 as a heat-labile opsonin (25), it was found that C1423 was the one combination that strongly increased the hydrophobicity and the phagocytability of sensitized *E. coli*. Addition of C5 or any other C component(s) had no further effect on either phagocytosis or contact angle (96, 97, 102). The reported need for C5 in opsonization (65) is difficult to assess. It contradicts earlier work by Johnston and associates (38), and it does not agree with the results of Gigli & Nelson (25) and of van Oss & Gillman (96). In both of the latter studies guinea pig C components were used. C3 and C5 are much more unequivocably separable in guinea pig than in human complement. Therefore, it seems reasonable to accept that the opsonic function of C resides solely in C3, and not in C5. The C3 fraction responsible for opsonization and enhancement of hydrophobicity must be C3b, as that is the only fraction of C3 that remains attached to the cells (48).

Thus, the increase in hydrophobicity caused by specific tagging by antibodies can be further enhanced by the interaction of the antigen-antibody complex with complement and the sequence C1423 is required for the attainment of maximum hydrophobicity as well as for maximum opsonization. The effector molecule appears to be C3b. In all likelihood C3 can play the same role when activated through the alternate pathway (4, 102).

OPSONIZING ROLE OF OTHER PLASMA COMPONENTS

Albumin

Albumin has a relatively low contact angle ($\theta = 15°$) (102), but in low concentrations (e.g. 0.1%, in which it is frequently used in Hanks' balanced salt solution) it does not appear to influence the contact angles of either phagocytes or bacteria to any significant degree. In whole serum or plasma, in which albumin normally occurs in concentrations of 3.5–4.3%, its influence may be quite important. Indeed, as discussed below, in certain cases increasing the ambient serum albumin concentration by $\simeq 10\%$ in vitro (26, 107) and even in vivo (107) can have a profound influence on the contact angle, as well as on the phagocytic activity of the PMNs of certain individuals.

Altered Albumin

The influence of serum albumin that has been either physically or chemically altered can differ greatly from that of native serum albumin. Heat-aggregated albumin is cleared much more rapidly by the reticuloendothelial system than unaltered albumin (36). Chemically modified albumin is much more readily phagocytized in vivo (82), and methylated albumin enhances phagocytosis of microorganisms in vitro (23, 102). Methylated albumin raises the contact angle of E. coli from 17.0 to 23.5° (102).

Glycoproteins

The influence of a few isolated serum glycoproteins on cellular contact angles and on in vitro phagocytosis has been tested. α-2 HS glycoprotein raises the contact angle and opsonizes bacteria (99). α-1 acid glycoprotein, on the other hand, lowers the contact angle of bacteria and diminishes the degree to which they become phagocytized (98). It is interesting to note that patients suffering trauma tend to have increased levels of α-1 acid glycoprotein and decreased levels of α-2 HS glycoprotein (93), which may contribute to their decreased resistance to bacterial infections. It would not appear that a relationship exists between the phagocytosis-promoting α-globulin described by Tullis & Surgenor (86) and/or Saba's aspecific opsonins (72) and α-2 HS glycoprotein (T. M. Saba, private communication).

Hageman Factor

Hageman factor, or clotting factor XII, enhances the adhesiveness of PMNs (3). Isolated Hageman factor causes a decrease in the contact angle of PMNs to 14.3 and strongly enhances their phagocytic activity towards S. typhimurium, E. coli (group 055), S. aureus (Smith strain), and Candida albicans (102).

Fibrinogen and Fibrin

The contact angles of fibrinogen and fibrin are 24.4 and 31.0°, respectively (102). The hydrophobicity of insoluble fibrin most likely plays a considerable role in phagocytic ingestion as well as in cellular adhesiveness, e.g. in its interaction with platelets.

ROLE OF LYMPHOKINES

One of the most important lymphokines is the macrophage migration inhibition factor (MIF) (67), which appears in part to be responsible for the activation of macrophages [one of the most important manifestations of cell-mediated immunity (33, 51)] and affects macrophage spreading, adherence, motility, and phagocytosis. Thrasher and her collaborators (83) demonstrated a direct correlation between the inhibition of macrophage migration through glass capillaries, the increase in macrophage hydrophilicity (as judged by the lowering of the contact angle from 21.3 to 17.6°), and macrophage activation (as judged from the doubling of the phagocytic index) upon treatment with MIF-rich supernatants (see also 102). It is interesting to note that contrary to the considerable time needed for the standard MIF assay (44), the contact angle test requires only a 1-hr incubation of a macrophage monolayer with MIF prior to the contact angle measurement (83, 102). It seems likely that increased macrophage adhesiveness (19, 113), decreased macrophage contact angle (83), macrophage migration inhibition, and macrophage activation are all consequences of the same underlying mechanism, i.e. a strong increase in the surface hydrophilicity (102).

EFFECT OF ANTIBIOTICS

Munoz & Geister (56) may have been the first to announce that an antibiotic (aureomycin) could inhibit phagocytosis. Louria (41), in a study on the influence of antibiotics on superinfectability, uncovered the untoward effect in bacterial pneumonia of high doses of oral phenethicillin and injectable penicillin; the rate of superinfection was increased >20%. On the other hand, an enhancement of phagocytosis of *Listeria monocytogenes* by human macrophages was noted in the presence of subinhibitory doses of ampicillin, tetracycline, and chloramphenicol (1).

The action of a number of antibiotics on the contact angles of grampositive and gram-negative bacteria, as well as of phagocytic cells, together with in vitro phagocytosis has been studied (102). Ampicillin makes phagocytes somewhat more hydrophilic, but it makes bacteria much more hydrophilic, which results in an overall depression of phagocytosis. Penicillin, chloromycetin, polymyxin, and bacitracin have no influence on the surface of phagocytes; however, these agents make bacteria more hydrophilic and, as expected, phagocytosis is depressed. Only gentamycin was found to make phagocytes more hydrophilic and bacteria more hydrophobic, thereby resulting in much enhanced phagocytosis (102).

EFFECT OF OTHER ADDITIVES

Heparin

Heparin has been reported to enhance the in vitro phagocytic activity of Kupffer cells (39). Moreover, incubation of guinea pig macrophages with 0.3 mg of heparin per 100 ml results in a strong decrease of their contact angle (from 21.8 to 18.8°) and a concomittant increase in their phagocytic activity for *S. aureus*. Heparin does not influence the contact angle of *S. aureus* (102).

Lectins

Phytohemagglutinin has an immunosuppressive effect in animals (35), and it is known that macrophages are among the cells that play a role in the immune response (28). Concanavalin A also interacts with macrophages (73). Both phytohemagglutinin and concanavalin A render macrophages considerably more hydrophobic and, as a result, depress their phagocytic activity (102). Therefore, the immunosuppressive effect of these lectins may well be due, in part, to their interaction with macrophages, as well as with lymphocytes (28).

Levamisole

Levamisole [the 1-isomer of 2, 3, 5, 6-tetrahydro-6-phenylimidazo (2, 1-*b*) thiazole hydrochloride] has been shown to have immunostimulating (68, 69) as well as tumor-inhibiting properties (69). One of its principal actions appears to be aspecific stimulation of macrophages (70, 80). Levamisole activates guinea pig macrophages in vitro (it causes their contact angle to decrease from 21.4 to 17.6°) and strongly enhances their phagocytic capacity for *S. aureus* (102).

Surfactants

If a detergent (such as Tween, or sodium desoxycholate) is added to PMNs before incubation with bacteria, an enhancement of phagocytosis ensues as a consequence of lowering the contact angle of the PMNs, without altering that of the bacteria. But if a detergent is added at the same time as, or immediately after, the introduction of bacteria, the result generally is inhibition of phagocytosis, or even exocytosis (expulsion of already ingested bacteria). In these cases the contact angle of the bacteria as well as that of the PMNs is reduced to the same low value of $\simeq 13°$ (102). Thus surfactants, which induce the same contact angle in all cell types, decrease the adhesion between bacteria and PMNs and make exocytosis almost as likely as phagocytosis.

Hydrophobic Particles and Droplets

The ingestion of very hydrophobic particles, such as polystyrene latex particles or *Mycobacterium butyricum,* with contact angles of 66 and 70° (but not of particles of a much smaller contact angle, such as staphylococci), strongly decreases the contact angle of PMNs and of macrophages and results in an increased phagocytic activity for staphylococci over and above the already ingested hydrophobic particles (108). These findings may serve to explain the crucial influence of the presence of *Mycobacteria* sp. (or their cell-wall lipids) in adjuvants of the Freund type. They may also explain the efficacy of polystyrene particles as a replacement for *Mycobacteria* sp. in Freund's adjuvant, in the induction of antibodies to human IgG in rabbits (109). This phenomenon can be interpreted as follows: when particles become phagocytized, part of the phagocyte's cell membrane disappears into the cell's interior. This stretches the components that make up the cell membrane and dilutes them with water, which renders the membrane more hydrophilic. After the exceptionally strong phagocytosis elicited by very hydrophobic particles, the increase in membrane hydrophilicity caused by pronounced stretching is measurable (102).

Lipid droplets (e.g. glycerol trioleate, methyl stearate) have the same effect as the earlier-mentioned hydrophobic latex and mycobacterial particles (102) (see also 79).

INFLUENCE OF CELL CHARGE AND SHAPE

Under physiological conditions all human blood cells have an electrokinetic (ζ) potential >10 mV (103); ζ for platelets, PMNs, lymphocytes, and erythrocytes is 11, 12, 16, and 18 mV, respectively (102, 103). Therefore, through simple electrostatic repulsion these cells (provided they are reasonably spherical or discoid shaped) cannot approach one another more closely than to a separation of $\simeq 50$–80 Å (29, 103), which is too far to allow cellular interaction (102, 103). However, cellular protrusions with radii of curvature <500Å will enable cells to overcome this electrostatic repulsion, pierce the diffuse electrical double layer, and establish molecular contact (9, 29, 100, 102, 103).

Granulocytes have a medium-low ζ potential as well as a strong tendency to extrude pseudopods of a small radius of curvature; of all cells they are the most suited to make molecular contact with other cells or particles and engulf them (at least if these other cells or particles are more hydrophobic than the PMNs, i.e. have a contact angle $\theta > 18°$) (100, 102, 103). Platelets also have a propensity to stick to other cells and surfaces, but only after they have become "sticky" under the influence of, e.g. ADP. ADP does not change the contact angle of platelets ($\theta = 16.3–17.0°$) (100, 102), but it causes spiculation with multiple microvilli with small radii of curvature (100, 102, 114).

Pili on gonococci (75) as well as the thin appendages that protrude from a variety of viruses (e.g. adenoviruses) (100) also are likely to be instrumental in the attachment of these microorganisms to cell membranes by the same mechanism (100, 102).

Hyperglycemic concentrations of glucose diminish the phagocytic activity and the adhesiveness of PMNs in vitro (and probably in vivo as well) (89), without causing a change in contact angle or in ζ potential. The reason for this decreased adhesiveness and diminished phagocytic activity appears to be in the tendency of glucose to render phagocytic cells more spherical and to decrease their power to extrude pseudopods (100, 102). As long as phagocytes remain spherical under the influence of glucose, their surface potential appears sufficient to prevent contact with other cells or with other negatively charged surfaces, so that hydrophobic-hydrophilic interactions simply cannot take place. Not only does uninterrupted exposure of phagocytic cells to hyperglycemic glucose levels cause a decrease in phagocytic activity, but intermittent contact with glucose (e.g. during 5 or 10 sec every 2 min for a few hours) has the same effect (C. J. van Oss, manuscript in preparation). This fact may have some bearing on the increased susceptibility to bacterial infections among patients with trauma and following surgery (3, 5) who undergo frequent and sustained glucose infusions. Other intravenous infusion liquids, such as amino acid mixtures, have no detrimental effect on phagocytosis (C. J. van Oss, manuscript in preparation), nor does ethanol (89, 102), however see MacGregor et al (42).

THERMODYNAMICS OF ENGULFMENT

Independent of the shape of a bacterium B originally embedded in saline water W, an overall free energy change ΔF_{net} exists for the process of engulfing a bacterium of unit surface area by a phagocyte P, so that

$$\Delta F_{net} = \gamma_{PB} - \gamma_{BW}, \qquad 1.$$

where γ_{BW} = bacterium/water interfacial tension, and γ_{PB} = phagocyte/bacterium interfacial tension. Complete engulfment of the bacterium by the phagocyte can only ensue when $\Delta F_{net} < 0$ (60, 62, 63, 84, 85, 102). Via the approach of Neumann and collaborators (61), contact angles obtained with a single liquid (in this case saline water) suffice for the derivation of γ_{PB} and γ_{BW}, as well as of γ_{PW} (=phagocyte/water interfacial tension).

The experimental value for the contact angle of human PMNs with respect to water is 18°, whereas the contact angles for bacteria (with respect to water) generally vary between 15 and 27° (94, 102). By using the derivation of Neumann and collaborators (61), this yields $\gamma_{PW} = 0.20$ ergs/cm². For this value of γ_{PW}, γ_{PB} can be derived for all applicable angles. The following three different situations can occur: θ bacterium $>$ θ phagocyte; θ bacterium $=$ θ phagocyte; and θ bacterium $<$ θ phagocyte.

In the first case ΔF_{net} is more negative than $- 0.20$ ergs/cm², a situation that favors engulfment. In the second case $\Delta F_{net} \simeq -0.20$ ergs/cm², a situation that may still give rise to rare episodes of engulfment, or to simple phagocyte/bacterium attachment. In the third case ΔF_{net} is less negative than -0.20 ergs/cm², in which situation engulfment is no longer favored (60, 62, 63, 102).

INFLUENCE OF PARTICLE SIZE

Minimum Size of Particles Liable to be Engulfed

All single molecules and particles regardless of their size have (at a given temperature) the same translational kinetic (Brownian or thermal) energy, $3/2\ kT$ (20) (where $K =$ Boltzmann's constant $= 1.38 \times 10^{-16}$ ergs/degree, and $T =$ the absolute temperature in degrees kelvin). Therefore, a critical particle size must exist below which that kinetic energy ($3/2\ kT = 642 \times 10^{-16}$ ergs, at 37°C) per unit of surface area is larger than the interfacial energy required for particle attachment and ingestion by PMNs. Because of their high kinetic energy per unit of surface area, particles smaller than this critical size will resist attachment, escape engulfment, and remain freely dispersed or dissolved in the suspending medium or solvent. Hydrophilic particles or molecules oponized or complexed with three IgG-class antibodies have a thermal energy of $\simeq 0.19$ ergs/cm² of contacting surface area (40, 87) of three Fc tail extremities, which is insufficient to overcome the interfacial free energy of -0.20 ergs/cm² required for engulfment. Therefore, single complexes that contain three or more IgG molecules with the Fc extremities sticking out have a kinetic energy per contactable surface area that is too low to avoid phagocytosis. On the other hand, because of their high kinetic energy per contactable surface area, solitary IgG molecules, or immune complexes with only two IgG molecules, will escape phagocytic ingestion (97, 101, 102). Similarly, in the presence of complement, two IgG molecules, or one IgM molecule, will suffice to make phagocytic ingestion possible (101, 102). These calculations are in close agreement with the experimental findings of Mannik et al (6, 45, 46) on the correlation between the size and composition of antigen-antibody complexes and the time span during which these remain in circulation.

Therefore, it seems superfluous to postulate the existence of Fc receptors on PMNs because for purely thermodynamic reasons PMN surfaces should (and do) attach to immune complexes that expose three or more Fc extremities. Also, receptor hypotheses cannot account for the failure of solitary IgG molecules to attach to PMNs to any significant extent. On the other hand, macrophages may indeed have Fc receptors, as their surfaces can, under certain conditions, bind to single molecules of guinea pig γ_2-type antibodies (10).

Effect of Agglutination

From the preceding considerations it is clear that microbial agglutination is not a mechanism that through increasing particle size makes phagocytosis possible where it was not possible before. That seems to be more the function of immune complex formation (see the preceding section). However, as phagocytes are capable of ingesting rather large particles, the clamping of microorganisms by means of immune agglutination can nevertheless be of some advantage; if a clump of microbes is as easily ingested as one single microbe, more agglutinated microbes can be engulfed per ingestion than would be possible with monodispersed particles (105).

ERYTHROPHAGOCYTOSIS

Mammalian erythrocytes are quite hydrophilic (102, 103). They are also somewhat more negatively charged than other blood cells (71, 102, 103), as well as (normally) quite smooth (106). These combined properties tend to make them highly resistant to phagocytosis by PMNs, as long as these properties remain unaltered.

Aged erythrocytes are removed by phagocytes (12), probably because of an increase in surface hydrophobicity with age, which accounts for the increased susceptibility of effete erythrocytes to phagocytosis. Erythrocytes incubated in physiological saline for 24 hr at 37°C become more susceptible to phagocytosis in vitro (32). After such a treatment their contact angle increases from 15 to 23°, which correlates well with their enhanced phagocytability, and also with the observations of Greenwalt & Steane (31), who studied the connection between in vivo aging of erythrocytes and the decreasing sialic acid content of their surfaces. Erythrocytes subjected to various adverse conditions, e.g. an acid pH (which is known to cause sickling in vitro) (81), also become more hydrophobic and thus more susceptible to phagocytosis (102). However, the contact angle of erythrocytes of a patient homozygous for hemoglobin S shows no significant difference from that of normal human erythrocytes (102). Therefore, the increased erythrophagocytosis among patients with hemoglobin S disease can only be ascribed to the multiple spicules and other processes with small radii of curvature that are characteristic of sickle cells (12).

Erythrocytes coated with specific antibodies of the IgG class to antigenic determinants on the cell surface (e.g. blood group D antigens) become more hydrophobic than phagocytes and thus are engulfed by them (102). Considerably diluted anti-D antisera can still cause a significant increase in the contact angle of D-positive cells (102). The contact angle method thus appears quite sensitive for the determination of the presence of antibodies on erythrocytes. The increase in hydrophobicity also tends to explain the enhanced phagocytosis of antibody-coated erythrocytes, and the occurrence of erythrophagocytosis in autoimmune anemias (12). In addition, certain types of antibodies (e.g. anti-A, anti-B) induce spiculation in erythrocytes (106), which further enhances their susceptibility to phagocytosis.

ACTION OF ANTILYMPHOCYTE ANTISERA

Human lymphocytes show an increase in contact angle similar to that of erythrocytes when treated with specific antibodies of the IgG class (102). This allows the prediction that the in vivo administration of antilymphocyte antiserum, as it enhances the phagocytosis of lymphocytes, should cause a decrease in lymphocyte count. This is indeed the case (18, 34).

DYSFUNCTION OF PHAGOCYTES RELATED TO THEIR SURFACE PROPERTIES

In 1976 a number of cases were reported of children with chronic upper respiratory infections, with a significant increase in contact angle (1.5 to 3° above normal) of their PMNs and a decreased phagocytic activity (26). In one case studied in depth, a defect in chemotaxis was also noted (11). Since then several more cases have been studied, and it has emerged that the surface defect of the patients' PMNs is induced by a factor (or by deprivation of a factor) in the patients' own sera. After incubation in normal serum, the patients' PMNs function normally in vitro. After incubation of normal PMNs in the patients' sera, the phagocytic activity of the normal PMNs often is somewhat depressed, and the contact angle is increased (107). Not only incubation in normal serum but also in the patients' sera supplemented with an extra 0.5% human serum albumin causes the patients' PMNs phagocytic activity as well as contact angle to revert to normal values (107). Intravenous administration of serum albumin to one of these patients also caused the PMNs to revert to normal, accompanied by a striking clinical improvement during the first 2 weeks post-administration (J. M. Bernstein & C. J. van Oss, unpublished results). Very similar findings were recently noted in a number of young people affected with localized idiopathic juvenile periodontosis (14).

CONCLUSION

An expedient and precise method of studying the solid-liquid interfacial tensions of cells is by measuring the contact angles of sessile drops of fluid on flat layers of phagocytes or microorganisms. There is a significant correlation between differences in interfacial free energy and the capacity of phagocytes to engulf microorganisms, other cells, or inert particles. Bacteria more hydrophobic than phagocytes readily become phagocytized; bacteria more hydrophilic than phagocytes resist phagocytosis. Of clinical relevance is the knowledge that virulent, encapsulated, and smooth strains of bacteria comprise the latter class. Bacteria are made more hydrophobic by specific antibodies to their hydrophilic surface components; complement ($\overline{C1423}$) further enhances this hydrophobicity, thus helping to elucidate the mechanism of the opsonic action of antibodies (IgG in particular), and complement.

Because the main influence of the electrokinetic (ζ) potential of cells is repulsive, it tends to prevent cell-cell contact. This electrostatic repulsion can be overcome when at least one of the interacting cell types has pseudopods or other processes with small radii of curvature, as is the case with all phagocytic cells. After cell contact is made, the difference in interfacial tension becomes the major factor in the decision between engulfment and nonengulfment. Glucose (in concentrations $>0.2\%$) has been shown to promote a spherical shape in phagocytes. This causes an effective increase in electrostatic repulsion and a concomitant decrease in cell contact, which results in diminished phagocytic adhesion and ingestive activity. These findings significantly relate to the mode of development of infection and inflammation among, e.g. diabetics. Also important to our understanding of pathogenesis is the knowledge that many other substances (e.g. acute-phase proteins, various other plasma proteins, heparin, antibiotics) influence the interfacial tension of phagocytes and/or bacteria and subsequent phagocytosis.

A number of other phenomena have been elucidated by contact angle measurement, e.g. macrophage activation by MIF, by levamisole, and by mycobacteria and other hydrophobic particles and droplets; erythrophagocytosis; action of antilymphocyte antisera. The clinical implications of these findings are supported by the observation of a concurrent and inordinate hydrophobicity of peripheral granulocytes in a number of children with chronic bacterial infections.

There is little doubt that much more can be done with this simple and powerful technique, e.g. determining, in clinical samples, which of several microorganisms isolated is the most hydrophilic and therefore likely to be the most pathogenic or etiologic; ascertaining in neoplastic, metastatic, or "transformed" cells whether or not differences in cellular interfacial tension exist between these and normal cells; continuing studies of interfacial tensions of cells before and after infection by viruses; correlating cellular interfacial tensions with the degree of "arming" or activation of macrophages, granulocytes, and/or various types of lymphocytes; and pursuing investigations into the action of plasma proteins, antibiotics, hormones, vitamins, and other pharmaceutical products on phagocytic ingestion. A number of these studies currently are in progress.

ACKNOWLEDGMENTS

I am much indebted to my colleagues, R. K. Cunningham and E. A. Gorzynski, for fruitful discussions.

Literature Cited

1. Adam, D., Schaffert, W., Marget, W. 1974. *Infect. Immun.* 9:811–14
2. Albertsson, P.-Å. 1971. *Partition of Cell Particles and Macromolecules.* New York: Wiley-Interscience
3. Alexander, J. W., Good, R. A. 1970. *Immunobiology for Surgeons,* p. 10, Philadelphia: Saunders
4. Alper, C. A. 1975. *Int. Convoc. Immunol.* 4:479–88
5. Altemeier, W. A. 1972. *Bull. Am. Coll. Surg.* 7:7–16
6. Arend, W. P., Mannik, M. 1971. *J. Immunol.* 107:63–75
7. Baier, R. E., Dutton, R. C., Gott, V. L. 1970. *Surface Chemistry of Biological Systems,* ed. M. Blank, pp. 235–60. New York: Plenum
8. Baier, R. E., Zisman, W. A. 1975. *Adv. Chem. Ser.* 145:155–74
9. Bangham, A. D. 1964. *Ann. NY Acad. Sci.* 116:945–49
10. Berken, A., Benacerraf, B. 1966. *J. Exp. Med.* 123:119–44
11. Bernstein, J. M., Gillman, C. F. 1976. *Trans. Am. Acad. Ophthalmol. Otol.* 82:509–17
12. Bessis, M. 1973. *Living Blood Cells and Their Ultrastructure.* New York: Springer
13. Broxmeyer, H. E., van Zant, G., Schultz, E. F., Koltun, L. A., LoBue, J.,

Gordon, A. S. 1975. *J. Reticuloendoth. Soc.* 18:118–24
14. Cianciola, L. J., Genco, R. J., Patters, M. R., McKenna, J., van Oss, C. J. 1977. *Nature* 265:445–47
15. Chambers, R., Kopac, M. J. 1937. *J. Cell Physiol.* 9:331–61
16. Cunningham, R. K., Söderström, T. O., Gillman, C. F., van Oss, C. J. 1975. *Immunol. Commun.* 4:429–42
17. Davis, B. D., Dulbecco, R., Eisen, H. N., Ginsberg, H. S., Wood, W. B. 1973. *Microbiology,* pp. 633–34. New York: Harper/Hoeber
18. Denman, A. M., Frenkel, E. P. 1968. *Immunology* 14:115–26
19. Dy, M., Dimitriu, A., Thomson, N., Hamburger, J. 1974. *Ann. Immunol. Inst. Pasteur* 125(C):451–59
20. Einstein, A. 1956. *Investigation on the Theory of the Brownian Movement,* p. 64. New York: Dover
21. Fenn, W. O. 1922. *J. Gen. Physiol.* 4:373–85
22. Forsgren, A., Sjöquist, J. 1967. *J. Immunol.* 99:19–24
23. Gambrill, M. R., Wisseman, C. L. 1973. *Infect. Immun.* 8:631–40
24. Gerisch, G., Lüderitz, O., Ruschmann, E. 1967. *Z. Naturforsch. Teil B* 22:109
25. Gigli, I., Nelson, R. A. 1968. *Exp. Cell Res.* 51:45–67

38   VAN OSS

26. Gillman, C. F., Bernstein, J. M., van Oss, C. J. 1976. *Fed. Proc.* 35:227
27. Gingell, D., Todd, I. 1975. *J. Cell Sci.* 18:227–39
28. Golub, E. S. 1977. *The Cellular Basis of the Immune Response.* Sunderland, Mass.: Sinauer
29. Good, R. J. 1972. *J. Theoret. Biol.* 37:413–34
30. Greenwalt, T. J., Gajewski, M., McKenna, J. L. 1962. *Transfusion* 2: 221–29
31. Greenwalt, T. J., Steane, E. A. 1973. *Br. J. Haematol.* 25:217–26
32. Habeshaw, J., Stuart, A. E. 1971. *J. Reticuloendoth. Soc.* 9:528–43
33. Hibbs, J. B. 1974. *Science* 184:468–71
34. James, K., Jubb, V. S. 1967. *Nature* 215:367–71
35. Jennings, J. F., Oates, C. M. 1967. *Clin. Exp. Immunol.* 2:334–53
36. Jeunet, F. J., Good, R. A. 1969. *J. Reticuloendoth. Soc.* 6:96–107
37. Joffe, E. W., Mudd, S. 1935. *J. Gen. Physiol.* 18:599–613
38. Johnston, R. B., Klemperer, M. R., Alper, C. A., Rosen, F. S. 1969. *J. Exp. Med.* 129:1275–90
39. Kitchen, A. G., Megirian, R. 1971. *J. Riticuloendoth. Soc.* 9:13–22
40. Labaw, L. W., Davies, D. R. 1971. *J. Biol. Chem.* 246:3760–62
41. Louria, D. B. 1974. *Opportunistic Pathogens,* ed. J. E. Prier, H. Friedman, pp. 1–18. Baltimore: University Park Press
42. MacGregor, R. R., Spagnulo, P. J., Lentnek, A. L. 1974. *N. Engl. J. Med.* 291:642–46
43. MacLeod, C. M. 1958. *Bacterial and Mycotic Infections of Man,* ed. R. J. Dubos, pp. 230–47. Philadelphia: Lippincott
44. Maini, R. N., Roffe, L. M., Magrath, I. T., Dumonde, D. C. 1973. *Int. Arch. Allergy* 45:308–21
45. Mannik, M., Arend, W. P. 1971. *J. Exp. Med.* 134:19s–31s
46. Mannik, M., Arend, W. P., Hall, A. P., Gilliland, B. C. 1971. *J. Exp. Med.* 133: 713–39
47. Marshall, K. C. 1976. *Interfaces in Microbiology,* pp. 12–21. Cambridge, Mass.: Harvard University Press
48. Mayer, M. M. 1978. *Principles of Immunology,* ed. N. R. Rose, F. Milgrom, C. J. van Oss. New York: Macmillan
49. McKeever, P. E. 1974. *J. Reticuloendoth. Soc.* 16:313–17
50. McKeever, P. E., Gee, J. B. L. 1975. *J. Reticuloendoth. Soc.* 18:221–29

51. Mooney, J. J., Waksman, B. H. 1970. *J. Immunol.* 105:1138–45
52. Moyer, L. S. 1936. *J. Bacteriol.* 32: 433–64
53. Mudd, E. B. H., Mudd, S. 1933. *J. Gen. Physiol.* 16:625–36
54. Mudd, S., Mudd, E. B. H. 1924. *J. Exp. Med.* 40:633–60
55. Mudd, S., Mudd, E. B. H. 1930–1931. *J. Gen. Physiol.* 14:733–51
56. Munoz, J., Geister, R. 1950. *Proc. Soc. Exp. Biol. Med.* 75:367–70
57. Murphy, P. 1976. *The Neutrophil,* pp. 139–43. New York: Plenum
58. Najjar, V. A., Constantopoulos, A. 1972. *J. Reticuloendoth. Soc.* 12:197–215
59. Neufeld, F. 1902. *Z. Hyg.* 40:54–72
60. Neumann, A. W., Gillman, C. F., van Oss, C. J. 1974. *J. Electroanal. Chem.* 49:393–400
61. Neumann, A. W., Good, R. J., Hope, C. J., Sejpal, M. 1974. *J. Colloid Interface. Sci.* 49:291–304
62. Neumann, A. W., van Oss, C. J., Szekely, J. 1973. *Kolloid Z. Z. Polym.* 251:415–23
63. Neumann, A. W., van Oss, C. J., Zingg, W. 1975. *Klin. Wochenschr.* 53: 1021–27
64. Newsome, J. 1967. *Nature* 214:1092–94
65. Nilsson, U. R., Miller, M. E., Wyman, S. 1974. *J. Immunol.* 112:1164–76
66. Phillips, H. M., Steinberg, M. S. 1969. *Proc. Natl. Acad. Sci. USA* 64:121–27
67. Remold, H. G., David, J. R. 1974. *Mechanisms of Cell-Mediated Immunity,* ed. R. T. McCluskey, S. Cohen, pp. 25–42. New York: Wiley
68. Renoux, G., Renoux, M. 1971. *CR Acad. Sci.* 272(D):349–50
69. Renoux, G., Renoux, M. 1972. *Nature New Biol.* 240:217–18
70. Renoux, G., Renoux, M., Aycardi, D. 1976. *Fed. Proc.* 35:366
71. Ruhenstroth-Bauer, G. 1965. *Cell Electrophoresis,* ed. E. J. Ambrose, pp. 66–84. Boston: Little, Brown
72. Saba, T. M. 1975. *Int. Convoc. Immunol.* 4:489–504
73. Sethi, K. K., Pelster, B. 1974. *Activation of Macrophages,* ed. W. H. Wagner, H. Hahn, pp. 269–79. New York: Elsevier
74. Singer, J. M., Adlersberg, L., Hoenig, E. M., Ende, E., Tchorsch, Y. 1969. *J. Reticuloendoth. Soc.* 6:561–89
75. Smith, H. 1977. *Bacteriol. Rev.* 41:475–500
76. Stendahl, O., Magnusson, K. E., Tagesson, C., Cunningham, R. K., Edebo, L. B. 1973. *Infect. Immun.* 7:573–77

77. Steward, M. W. 1974. *Immunochemistry*, p. 56. New York: Wiley
78. Stinson, M. W., van Oss, C. J. 1971. *J. Reticuloendoth. Soc.* 9:503–12
79. Stuart, A. E., Cooper, G. N. 1963. *Exp. Mol. Pathol.* 2:215–18
80. Symoens, J. 1977. *Control of Neoplasia by Modulation of the Immune System*, ed. M. A. Chirigos, pp. 1–24. New York: Raven Press
81. Tavassoli, M., Weiss, L. 1970. *Formation and Destruction of Red Cells*, ed. T. J. Greenwalt, G. A. Jamieson, pp. 108–24. Philadelphia: Lippincott
82. Thorbecke, G. J., Maurer, P. H., Benacerraf, B. 1960. *Brit. J. Exp. Pathol.* 41:190–97
83. Thrasher, S. G., Yoshida, T., van Oss, C. J., Cohen, S., Rose, N. R. 1973. *J. Immunol.* 110:321–26
84. Torza, S., Mason, S. G. 1969. *Science* 162:813–14
85. Torza, S., Mason, S. G. 1970. *J. Colloid Interface Sci.* 33:67–83
86. Tullis, J. L., Surgenor, D. M. 1956. *Ann. NY Acad. Sci.* 66:386–90
87. Valentine, R. V., Green, N. M. 1967. *J. Mol. Biol.* 27:615–17
88. van den Tempel, M. 1972. *Adv. Colloid Interface Sci.* 3:137–59
89. van Oss, C. J. 1971. *Infect. Immun.* 4:54–59
90. van Oss, C. J. 1973. *Principles of Immunology*, ed. N. R. Rose, F. Milgrom, C. J. van Oss, pp. 93–102. New York: Macmillan
91. van Oss, C. J. 1978. *Principles of Immunology*, ed. N. R. Rose, F. Milgrom, C. J. van Oss. New York: Macmillan
92. van Oss, C. J., Bronson, P. M. 1970. *Sep. Sci.* 5:63–75
93. van Oss, C. J., Bronson, P. M., Border, J. R. 1975. *J. Trauma* 15:451–55
94. van Oss, C. J., Gillman, C. F. 1972. *J. Reticuloendoth. Soc.* 12:283–92
95. van Oss, C. J., Gillman, C. F. 1972. *J. Reticuloendoth. Soc.* 12:497–502
96. van Oss, C. J., Gillman, C. F. 1973. *Immunol. Commun.* 2:415–19
97. van Oss, C. J., Gillman, C. F. 1975. *Int. Convoc. Immunol.* 4:505–11
98. van Oss, C. J., Gillman, C. F., Bronson, P. M., Border, J. R. 1974. *Immunol. Commun.* 4:321–28
99. van Oss, C. J., Gillman, C. F., Bronson, P. M., Border, J. R. 1974. *Immunol. Commun.* 3:329–35
100. van Oss, C. J., Gillman, C. F., Good, R. J. 1972. *Immunol. Commun.* 1:627–36
101. van Oss, C. J., Gillman, C. F., Neumann, A. W. 1974. *Immunol. Commun.* 3:77–84
102. van Oss, C. J., Gillman, C. F., Neumann, A. W. 1975. *Phagocytic Engulfment and Cell Adhesiveness*. New York: Marcel Dekker
103. van Oss, C. J., Good, C. F., Neumann, A. W. 1972. *J. Electroanal. Chem.* 37:387–91
104. van Oss, C. J., Good, R. J., Neumann, A. W., Wieser, J. D., Rosenberg, A. L. 1977. *J. Colloid Interface Sci.* 59:505–15
105. van Oss, C. J., Grossberg, A. L. 1978. *Principles of Immunology*, ed. N. R. Rose, F. Milgrom, C. J. van Oss. New York: Macmillan
106. van Oss, C. J., Mohn, J. F. 1970. *Vox Sang.* 19:432–43
107. van Oss, C. J., Park, B. H., Bernstein, J. M., Gillman, C. F. 1977. *Proc. 51st Colloid Surf. Sci. Symp.*, pp. 100–1
108. van Oss, C. J., Rose, N. R., Cohen, S., Thrasher, S. G., Gillman, C. F. 1972. *Abstr. Ann. Meet. Am. Soc. Microbiol.*, p. 896
109. van Oss, C. J., Singer, J. M., Gillman, C. F. 1976. *Immunol. Commun.* 5:181–88
110. van Oss, C. J., Stinson, M. W. 1970. *J. Reticuloendoth. Soc.* 8:397–406
111. van Oss, C. J., Woeppel, M. S., Marquart, S. E. 1973. *J. Reticuloendoth. Soc.* 13:221–30
112. Weiss, L. 1961. *Exp. Cell Res.* 8: Suppl., 141–53
113. Weiss, L., Glaves, D. 1975. *J. Immunol.* 115:1362–65
114. White, J. G. 1968. *Blood* 31:604–22
115. Young, T. 1805. *Phil. Trans. R. Soc. London* 95:65–87
116. Zisman, W. A. 1962. *Adhesion and Cohesion*, ed. P. Weiss, pp. 176–208. New York: Elsevier
117. Zisman, W. A. 1963. *Ind. Eng. Chem.* 55:18–38
118. Zisman, W. A. 1964. *Adv. Chem. Ser.* 43:1–51

Ann. Rev. Genet. 1977. 11:127–60

IMMUNOGENETICS OF CELL ◆3118
SURFACE ANTIGENS
OF MOUSE LEUKEMIA

Lloyd J. Old and Elisabeth Stockert
Memorial Sloan-Kettering Cancer Center, New York, New York 10021

CONTENTS

8243-2502/80/0310-0177$01.00
127

INTRODUCTION

This review deals with a description of the various categories of cell surface antigens that have now been defined on mouse leukemia. Because of the range of inbred mouse strains with known susceptibility to spontaneous or induced tumor development, analysis of cell surface antigens is most advanced with tumors of this species. Much of this work has been motivated by the search for antigens that are distinctive for malignant cells. Although initial evidence for such antigens came from experiments involving transplant rejection, serological techniques have proved far more powerful in sorting out the array of gene products that are expressed on the surface of tumor cells. As with so many areas of cancer research, the study of cancer illuminates much about normal cells, and this has certainly been true for the serological study of surface antigens of leukemia cells (1). A few examples suffice to illustrate this point. The surface markers that have come to be known as differentiation antigens, because their appearance relates to particular pathways of cellular differentiation, were initially recognized during an analysis of antisera to leukemia cells. The realization that other surface components of normal mouse cells were products of integrated viral genes came from the study of leukemias induced by murine leukemia virus (MuLV). The TL (thymus-leukemia) antigen, another surface marker of normal cells that was discovered during a study of mouse leukemia, is a product of a structural gene universally present in the mouse, but normally expressed in only certain strains. The surprising appearance of TL in the leukemias of strains that ordinarily do not express the antigen revealed the presence of the normally silent TL gene and represents the clearest example of genetic derepression or activation in malignant cells. Analysis of the TL system also gave rise to the recognition that surface markers of mammalian cells can undergo rapid and reversible changes following exposure to antibody comparable in some ways to those originally observed with protozoa, and antigenic modulation—as the phenomenon of TL antibody–induced suppression of TL came to be called—can now be viewed in relation to the fluidity of the surface membrane and the mobility of many of its constituents.

Our emphasis in this review is on surface antigens defined serologically. Because leukemia cells can be easily obtained in free cell suspension and are highly sensitive to cytotoxic antibody, they have been a favorite object of serological study. Mouse leukemias frequently arise in the thymus, and this permits comparative serological study of leukemia cells and normal thymocytes, two cell populations of similar derivation. Of the various surface antigens that have been recognized on mouse leukemia, those related to the MuLV-Gross and TL systems are among the most important with regard to natural leukemogenesis, and for this reason their discovery and analysis are the main topics of this review.

TECHNIQUES FOR THE IN VITRO ANALYSIS OF SURFACE ANTIGENS OF LEUKEMIA CELLS

Antibody Detection Systems

A variety of serological techniques have been devised to detect antibody to cell surface antigens. Nearly all depend on two properties of the attached antibody: (*a*) reaction with anti-immunoglobulin reagents labeled with visual (fluorescein, red blood cells, ferritin), radioactive (^{125}I, etc), or enzymatic (horseradish peroxidase) markers, or (*b*) ability to fix complement. Although fixation of complement can be detected by immune adherence, anticomplement reactions, or complement consumption assays, the consequence of complement fixation that has been most useful for analyzing surface antigens is cell lysis. This ability of antibody directed to components of the cell surface to kill target cells in the presence of complement is the basis for the cytotoxic test originally devised by Gorer & O'Gorman to demonstrate H-2 antigens on nucleated cells (2). Since its description, the cytotoxic test has been subject to considerable modification and improvement and has evolved into a powerful technique with exquisite sensitivity and reliability for the demonstration and quantitation of cell surface antigens. In fact, almost without exception, the surface antigens that have now been defined on nucleated cells of the mouse were initially discovered through application of this fundamentally very simple test.

Preparation of Antisera

The antisera that recognize the systems of surface antigens on thymocytes and leukemia cells of the mouse were raised by a variety of immunization procedures. Table 1 illustrates ten general categories of immune sera that have been useful in defining non-H-2 specificities on nucleated cells. Because antibody to products of the H-2 complex are usually the dominant ones formed during alloimmunization, the search for surface antigens determined by other loci has depended on the use of antisera that lack H-2 antibody or on serological test systems that make it irrelevant whether H-2 antibody is present or not. The recognition of TL and GCSA antigens was based on this latter procedure (Category 1, Table 1). In both cases, C57BL/6 (C57BL) mice were immunized with H-2 incompatible leukemia cells, resulting in antisera with high H-2 titers and, as subsequent analysis showed, anti-TL and anti-GCSA antibodies as well. Although absorption procedures, either in vivo or in vitro, could have been used to remove anti-H-2, this turned out to be unnecessary. Selected C57BL leukemias were found that expressed TL or GCSA and, by using these target cells in cytotoxic tests with the C57BL antisera, reactions due to H-2 antibodies were eliminated and the GCSA and TL specificities could be defined without interference by irrelevant alloantibodies. Of course, this method of antiserum analysis is possible only under conditions where the same antigen is expressed on the allogeneic cells used for immunization and on the syngeneic cells used for serological testing. The initial detection of the surface antigens related to Friend, Moloney, or Rauscher murine leukemia viruses (FMR complex) also came about through the application of this procedure of H-2 incompatible immunization (5). However, because these viruses induce leukemias with uniquely strong immunogenicity (6, 7), it was possible to produce cytotoxic antiserum by immunizing

Table 1 General description of immunization procedures for the production of cyto-toxic antibody to cell surface antigens of the mouse

| Category | Examples | | | |
	Antiserum preparation	Test cell	Cell surface antigen detected	Reference
1 H-2 incompatible immunization	C57BL anti-A strain spontaneous leukemia	C57BL X-ray leukemia	TL	3
	C57BL anti-AKR spontaneous leukemia	C57BL MuLV-Gross leukemia	GCSA	4
2 Syngeneic immunization	C57BL anti-MuLV-Rauscher leukemia	C57BL MuLV-Rauscher leukemia	FMR	6
3 Syngeneic immunization (rat)	(W/Fu × BN) F_1 anti-W/Fu MuLV leukemia absorbed in vitro	129 thymocyte	G_{IX}	8, 9
4 Congenic immunization	C57BL-TL$^+$ anti-C57BL X-ray leukemia	C57BL X-ray leukemia	TL.4	10
5 F_1 hybrid immunization	(BALB/c × C57BL) F_1 anti-BALB/c X-ray leukemia	BALB/c X-ray leukemia	X.1	11
6 H-2 compatible immunization	C3H anti-AKR thymocytes	AKR thymocyte	Thy-1 (formerly θ)	12
	DBA/2 anti-BALB/c myeloma	BALB/c myeloma	PC.1	13
7 H-2 incompatible immunization: in vivo absorption	C57BL anti-AKR spontaneous leukemia absorbed in vivo in AKR	I strain thymocyte	Lyt-1 (formerly Ly-A, Ly-1)	14
8 Heteroimmunization with mouse cells	Rabbit anti-mouse thymocytes ab-sorbed in vivo in donor strain	thymocyte	MSLA	16
9 Heteroimmunization with MuLV structural components	Goat or rabbit anti-MuLV gp70, p30, p15	thymocyte or leukemia cell	gp70, p30, p15	20–23
10 Natural antibody to MuLV-related antigens	(C57BL-G_{IX}^+ × 129) F_1 normal serum	129 thymocyte	G_{IX}	27
	Swiss mouse normal serum	A strain X-ray leukemia	$G_{(RADA1)}$	Obata, Y., unpublished

mice with syngeneic FMR leukemias (Category 2). These FMR reagents proved of considerable value, not only because of high titer but also because they lack alloan-tibodies. For similar reasons, antisera prepared in inbred rats against syngeneic leukemias induced by MuLV-Gross have been widely used, and analysis of these rat antisera has resulted in the recognition of the G_{IX} antigenic system (Category 3).

Syngeneic immunization would appear to be the method of choice for producing antibody with specificity for leukemia cells. However, with the notable exception of FMR leukemias in the mouse, it has generally not been possible to detect specific antibody after syngeneic immunization with spontaneous, radiation-, or chemically induced mouse leukemias. Why this should be so is not known, but it may have to do with the inability of certain surface determinants to trigger a humoral immune response in the absence of additional, perhaps stronger, antigenic differences or be related to the absence of *Ir* genes necessary for antigen recognition. Experience with mice that are congenic for surface alloantigens, such as Thy-1 or Ly, may help to clarify this matter. We had expected that as the number of unrelated alloantigenic differences between donor and recipient were reduced, the immune response to a single surface determinant would be correspondingly increased. Although this proved to be true in several instances, immunization of congenic pairs exhibiting Thy-1 or single Ly differences results in little or no antibody. If, however, the congenic recipient is crossed to an unrelated mouse, the hybrid produces a good immune response to the determinant, and this result has been ascribed to heterozygosity at *Ir* loci. In this regard, one specificity of the TL system, TL.4, was recognized by immune sera produced in TL congenic mice (Category 4), but this cannot be considered a strictly congenic immunization, because C57BL and its congenic partner C57BL-TL$^+$ differ at more than the *Tla* locus. The most striking example of an immune response to a leukemia-associated antigen being determined by *Ir* genes relates to the X.1 system of BALB/c leukemias (Category 5). Syngeneic mice are incapable of forming anti-X.1, whereas hybrids with C57BL can produce the antibody. Genetic analysis shows that *H-2* linked *Ir* genes contributed by the C57BL partner are essential for X.1 recognition.

The definition of surface alloantigens characteristic of lymphocytes of T or B lineage and their malignant derivatives resulted from other methods of antisera preparation and analysis. Thy-1 and PC.1 alloantigens were detected and originally defined with antisera prepared in H-2–compatible mice (Category 6). The Ly series of T-cell alloantigens were recognized during analysis of antisera against leukemia cells prepared in H-2–incompatible mice. To remove H-2 antibody, these antisera were absorbed in vivo in normal mice of the strain in which the leukemia arose (Category 7). The absorbed sera retained antibody that reacted strongly with thymocytes and, in lower titers, with peripheral lymphocytes. Later tests proved that these antisera defined antigens that were restricted to T lymphocytes, and the two systems they identified were called Ly-A and Ly-B. Once the strain distribution of these systems was known, antisera could be prepared in H-2–compatible combinations that did not require in vivo absorption (15). These antisera, as well as others that have been defined subsequently, are proving of considerable value in distinguishing the various functionally distinct populations of T cells.

Heteroimmune sera prepared against mouse cells have been of only limited value in the analysis of cell surface antigens (Category 8). Properly absorbed, they can be useful markers for different cell populations in the mouse; absorbed heteroantisera with specificity for T lymphocytes (MSLA), B lymphocytes (MBLA), or plasma cells (MSPCA) have been described (16–19). As species antigens, they are not amenable to conventional genetic analysis, but for the study of interspecies hybrids in somatic cell genetics, they may find considerable use. In addition, a range of heteroantisera to individual structural proteins of MuLV are available and are now being used to study the expression of viral antigens on the cell surface (Category 9).

Since the original detection of antibody to MuLV-related antigens in normal mouse serum (24), naturally occurring antibody to MuLV structural antigens and to MuLV cell surface antigens has been found in a number of mouse strains, particularly those with low incidence of spontaneous leukemia (25, 26) (Category 10). Two such natural antibodies of the mouse are of particular interest. One is directed to the G_{IX} antigen which was originally defined by rat antiserum. Anti-G_{IX} had not previously been detected in inbred mice, and attempts at deliberate immunization of G_{IX}^- mice with G_{IX}^+ cells failed to induce antibody. However, certain $G_{IX}^+ \times G_{IX}^-$ or G_{IX}^+ hybrids form G_{IX} antibody, and this finding has also been explained on the basis of Ir genes necessary for G_{IX} recognition. The other naturally occurring antibody which defines a new system of MuLV-related antigens, $G_{(RADA1)}$, is found in the sera of random-bred Swiss mice (Category 10).

Qualitative and Quantitative Absorption Analysis In Vitro

Once an antiserum with sufficiently high titer for a target cell has been selected, the specificity of the cytotoxic antibody can be analyzed by absorption tests. With this technique, cells, cellular membranes, tissue homogenates, or isolated viral or cellular antigens can be tested for the presence of the relevant antigen by determining whether specific antibody for the target cell is removed or not from the antiserum. Absorption tests are invaluable for defining antigenic systems, particularly because of greater sensitivity of antigen detection than direct tests and because solid tissues such as liver, brain, and lung (where it would be impossible to obtain suitable target cells for direct tests) can be examined by absorption. Absorption tests to detect presence or absence of antigen are called qualitative absorptions. Absorption techniques can also be performed to quantitate the amount of surface antigen in a cell population. These quantitative absorption procedures have been useful in analyzing genotypic and phenotypic aspects involving cell surface antigens and in developing a method for mapping their spatial relations on the cell surface.

Standard Test Cells

Several lines of transplanted tumors have become prototype cells for the definition of certain cell surface antigens, and, for this reason, their surface antigenic structure is well characterized. The surface phenotype for some of these cells is given in Table 2. Even though many of these lines have been transplanted for a decade or so, their surface phenotype is remarkably stable. In a sense, these transplanted tumors represent the modern counterpart of the genetically undefined Ehrlich tumor and S-180 sarcoma so widely used by a former generation of cancer investigators. Although growing emphasis is being placed on using tumors of more recent origin in studies of cancer immunology, cells with well-characterized antigenic structure greatly facilitate the analysis of immune reactions to specific antigens and the definition of new antigenic systems. In fact, a good case could be made for the collective use of a limited number of these prototype cells by laboratories addressing various aspects of cell surface antigens, so that a comprehensive picture of the surface structure of a neoplastic mammalian cell could be constructed.

Table 2 Surface phenotype of standard transplantable tumor cell lines of the mouse

Designation	Strain of origin	Tumor induction	H-2	TI 1 2 3 4	Thy-1	Lyt 1 2 3 4	PC.1	G_{IX}	GCSA	$G_{(RADA1)}$	MuLV gp70	MuLV p30	MuLV p15
ERLD	C57BL/6	X-ray leukemia	b	1 2 - 4	2	1 2 3 4	-	-	-	-	+	-	-
EδG2	C57BL/6	MuLV Gross leukemia	b	- - - -	2	1 - - 4	-	+	+	+	+	+	+
EL4	C57BL	DMBA leukemia	b	- - - -	2	1 2 3 4	-	-	-	-	+	-	-
K36	AKR	Spontaneous leukemia	k	- - - -	-	- - - -	-	+	+	+	+	+	+
RLδ1	BALB/c	X-ray leukemia	d	1 2 - -	2	1 2 3 4	-	+	+	-	+	-	+
Meth A	BALB/c	Methylcholanthrene sarcoma	d	- - - -	-	- - - -	-	-	-	-	-	-	-
MOPC-70A	BALB/c	Mineral oil myeloma	d	- - - -	-	- - - -	1	-	+	-	-	-	+
ASL1	A	Spontaneous leukemia	a	1 2 3 -	2	1 2 3 4	-	-	-	-	+	-	-
RADA1	A	X-ray leukemia	a	1 2 3 -	2	- - - 4	-	+	-	+	+	-	-

Other Techniques for Analyzing Cell Surface Antigens

After a new surface antigen has been serologically identified and distinguished from known systems by its strain and tissue distribution, the procedure for its further analysis is becoming rather straightforward. *Biochemical characterization* is possible by techniques that were originally developed to analyze the product of the *H-2* locus. *Relation to MuLV* can be assessed by absorption tests with known MuLV$^+$ and MuLV$^-$ cells and with structural components of MuLV, as well as by determining whether the antigen can be induced in cells by MuLV infection. *Chromosomal mapping* of genes determining surface antigens is facilitated by the extensive range of biochemical markers that distinguish inbred strains and the availability of recombinant inbred lines of mice. The techniques of somatic cell genetics will undoubtedly become increasingly useful for mapping genes specifying cell surface antigens, particularly those that are not amenable to conventional genetic analysis (e.g. species antigens and tumor-specific antigens). *Construction of congenic mice* on defined genetic background is now a standard approach to the immunogenetic analyses of serologically defined cell surface alloantigens, and congenic stocks for TL, G_{IX}, the Ly series, Thy-1 and PC.1, in addition to those related to the H-2 complex, are available.

Several years ago, there was considerable hope that the topographical relationship of cell surface antigens could be visualized by immunoelectronmicroscopy (1, 28). The introduction of a double labeling technique with two visually distinguishable markers made it possible to think about visual maps of antigens on the cell surface. However, the realization that the antibody probes themselves caused aggregation and rearrangement of the surface antigens led to the discontinuation of such studies and to the current search for methods that will give a picture of the antigenic mosaic as it exists in the unperturbed state. A method that may be of considerable value in determining the spacial relationship of cell surface antigens is the antibody-blocking technique, and the current status of these studies is discussed below.

CELL SURFACE ANTIGENS RELATED TO NATURALLY OCCURRING MURINE LEUKEMIA VIRUSES

Background

Murine leukemia viruses (MuLV) belong to a family of structurally related RNA viruses that are known to infect an extraordinary range of animals, from snakes and birds to higher apes. Although overt disease is a rare manifestation of infection by these viruses, they can under appropriate circumstances induce cancer, and it is this feature that has led to their being called *oncornaviruses*. In the mouse, three types of cancers (leukemia, sarcoma, and mammary adenocarcinoma) are closely associated with oncornaviruses, and there are indications that they may also play a role in autoimmune diseases as well. The presence of a DNA intermediary in the life cycle of oncornaviruses provides opportunity for close interaction with the genome of the host cell, and there is considerable evidence that genetic information related to these viruses resides in an integrated state in most, if not all, mice (29). The degree to which viral genes are expressed is determined by other factors, some clearly under the control of host genes. The picture that is emerging from the analysis of MuLV is one of extensive polymorphism of endogenous viruses, with several distinct classes of MuLV having been identified on the basis of host range, interference patterns, antigenicity, nucleic acid hybridization, and peptide mapping.

Serological study of MuLV-related antigens began after L. Gross demonstrated that leukemogenic virus could be isolated from mice of the high leukemic AKR strain (30). Subsequently, Friend, Moloney, Rauscher and others isolated MuLV variants with properties that distinguished them from Gross's original isolate (31). In these early studies, rabbit antisera to viral filtrates resulted in antibody of low titer, undoubtedly a consequence of little viral antigen in the immunizing inocula. Because of the difficulties in obtaining potent heteroantibody to MuLV, attention turned to the immune response of mice to surface antigens of MuLV-induced leukemias. It soon became evident that cytotoxic antisera could be easily raised to leukemias induced by Friend, Moloney, and Rauscher (FMR) viruses, whereas it proved more difficult to produce high titered antibody to leukemias induced by Gross virus. These early serological studies indicated that mouse leukemias could be placed into two groups on the basis of their surface antigens: (a) leukemias induced by FMR viruses sharing the FMR complex of antigens and (b) leukemias induced by Gross virus or occurring spontaneously in high leukemia incidence strains sharing G(Gross) antigen (4, 6, 32). As FMR antigens were restricted to leukemias induced by FMR viruses and could not be found in any other normal or neoplastic cell, it was concluded that these viruses played no role in the development of naturally occurring leukemia. The occurrence of G antigen in spontaneous and induced leukemias and in sarcomas of low leukemia incidence strains indicated widespread infection of mouse populations with MuLV and provided an explanation for the poor immunological reactivity of mice to MuLV-Gross-related antigens.

An important step in MuLV serology was taken when it was found that rat antisera to syngeneic MuLV-induced leukemias detected a far broader range of MuLV antigens than did mouse antisera (8). Rats, which lack endogenous MuLV, are highly susceptible to leukemia induction by MuLV. The transplantation behavior of these induced rat leukemias suggested strong immunogenicity; in order to maintain transplanted lines of certain rat leukemias, it was necessary to serially pass them in immunologically immature recipients. If, however, sufficiently large numbers of leukemia cells were transplanted to adult animals, progressively growing tumors resulted and the sera of these rats contained high levels of cytotoxic, neutralizing, and precipitating MuLV antibodies. Analyses of these rat antisera gave rise to the recognition of the G_{IX} antigenic system (9), the major group-specific core antigen of MuLV (8, 20), and the interspecies antigen shared by mammalian leukemia-sarcoma viruses (33). With the development of methods to concentrate and purify MuLV, heteroimmune sera prepared in rabbits and goats to intact virus and to isolated structural components have become valuable reagents to identify and quantitate virion antigens (22, 34).

GCSA: Recognition and Initial Analysis

The first attempts to detect cell surface antigens related to MuLV-Gross were carried out with antisera prepared in C3H mice by repeated sublethal inocula of syngeneic virus-induced leukemia cells (35). These antisera showed weak and variable reactivity, most likely a reflection of the high susceptibility of this strain to Gross virus leukemogenesis. For this reason, C57BL mice were chosen as a source of antibody, since it was known from the work of Gross that mice of this strain were exceptionally resistant to MuLV. From a large series of C57BL mice injected as newborns with Gross virus, a small number of leukemias were induced and, from one of the leukemic mice, a transplanted leukemia line designated E♂G2 was established. The C57BL antiserum showing highest titer against E♂G2 was prepared against a transplanted AKR spontaneous leukemia, K36 (Table 2 and 3). Absorption analysis of this antiserum showed that all leukemias induced by MuLV-Gross and all spontaneous leukemias occurring in mice of high leukemia incidence strains absorbed cytotoxic activity. In tests of normal young mice from different inbred strains, occurrence of antigen in spleen and other lymphoid tissues correlated closely with the incidence of spontaneous leukemia (Table 4). All high incidence strains, AKR, C58, PL, C3H/Figge, and F, were antigen positive, whereas low incidence strains, e.g. C57BL, A, and BALB/c, lacked antigen. In view of its obvious relationship to the leukemia virus originally described by Gross, the antigen was named G (Gross) cell surface antigen (GCSA) (4). It soon became clear that GCSA was not restricted to high incidence strains, but could also be found in normal and malignant tissues of low incidence strains. In fact, typing for GCSA provided some of the earliest evidence for the widespread infection of mouse population with MuLV. Spontaneous and X-ray–induced leukemias and chemically induced sarcomas of GCSA$^-$ strains were occasionally GCSA$^+$. Cell cultures derived from GCSA$^-$ mice frequently became GCSA$^+$ after in vitro passage. Age was also found to play a role in determining GCSA expression in certain GCSA$^-$ strains of mice. C3Hf/Bi, which are GCSA$^-$ at 2 months of age, became GCSA$^+$ later in life (36) and strains showing this age-related GCSA$^-$ → GCSA$^+$ change are referred to as *conversion strains* (Table 4). Electronmicroscopy revealed a good correlation between GCSA and occurrence of MuLV particles in both normal and tumor tissue, and much subsequent study has substantiated the early impression that GCSA is an almost invariable marker for MuLV replication in the mouse.

Table 3 Cell surface antigens related to MuLV-Gross defined by cytotoxic tests with antisera from mice or rats

Designation	Antiserum	Standard test cell	Relation to MuLV structural component	Reference
GCSA	C57BL anti-AKR spontaneous leukemia K36	E♂G2 leukemia	p15, p30	4, 46, 47
G$_{IX}$	1 (W/Fu × BN)F$_1$ anti-W/Fu MuLV induced leukemia (C58NT)D^a	129 or C57BL-G$_{IX}^+$ thymocyte	gp70	9, 39, 45
	2 (C57BL-G$_{IX}^+$ × 129)F$_1$ normal mouse serum			27
X.1	(BALB/c × C57BL)F$_1$ anti-RL♂1	RL♂1 leukemia	?	11, 53
G$_{(RADA1)}$	Swiss mouse normal serum^b	RADA1 leukemia	gp70	Obata, Y., unpublished
G$_{(ERLD)}$	(C57BL × 129)F$_1$ normal serum	ERLD leukemia	?	

^{a}Absorbed in vitro with G$_{IX}^-$ thymocytes.
^{b}Absorbed in vitro with G$_{IX}^+$ thymocytes

Table 4 Strain distribution of cell surface antigens related to MuLV-Gross

	Inbred strains	GCSA	G_{IX}	X.1	$G_{(RADA1)}$	$G_{(ERLD)}$
High leukemia incidence strains	AKR, C58, C3H/Figge	+	+	+	+	+
Low leukemia incidence strains	A	−	+	−	−	+
	BALB/c	−	−	−	−	−
G_{IX} congenic strains	129	−	+	+	−	+
	129-G_{IX}^-	−	−	+	−	−
	C57BL	−	−	−	−	+
	C57BL-G_{IX}^+	−	+	−	−	+
Conversion strains	C3Hf/Bi young	−	−	−	−	+
	old	+	+		+	+
	NZB young	−	+			
	old	+	+	+	−	

Expression of GCSA in GCSA⁺ × GCSA⁻ Crosses

In contrast to the codominant expression of other cell surface antigens, F_1 hybrids derived from GCSA⁺ × GCSA⁻ crosses show either a GCSA⁻ or GCSA⁺ phenotype (Table 5). Certain GCSA⁻ strains, such as C57BL, suppress GCSA in AKR or C58 hybrids, whereas other GCSA⁻ strains do not (4). This effect of GCSA⁻ strains on GCSA expression can now be ascribed to the *Fv-1* locus and its control over MuLV replication (37). The two alleles at *Fv-1*, *Fv-1ⁿ* and *Fv-1ᵇ*, determine the susceptibility of mouse cells to infection by N-tropic or B-tropic MuLV. AKR and other high leukemia strains share the *Fv-1ⁿ* allele and leukemogenic virus from these strains have N-tropic properties. Low incidence strains have either the *Fv-1ⁿ* or *Fv-1ᵇ* allele and both N- and B-tropic MuLV have been isolated from these strains, although it is unclear whether these viruses have leukemogenic activity. AKR or C58 hybrids with Fv-1ⁿ low incidence strains are GCSA⁺, whereas hybrids with Fv-1ᵇ low incidence strains are GCSA⁻. An important exception to this rule has been found. The CBA strain is Fv-1ⁿ, but crosses with AKR are GCSA⁻. This absence of GCSA is surprising and deserves further study, especially since (AKR × CBA)F_1 mice are reported to have a low incidence of leukemia but a high level of MuLV (38).

Table 5 GCSA phenotype* of AKR or C58 crosses with GCSA⁻ strains

GCSA⁺ hybrids	GCSA⁻ hybrids
129 × AKR†	A × AKR†
C3Hf/Bi × AKR†	BALB/c × AKR†
AKR × DBA/2	C57BL × AKR†
AKR × GR	C57BL-G_{IX}^+ × AKR
C57L × AKR	C57BL-H–2ᵏ × AKR
129-G_{IX}^- × AKR	CBA × AKR†
129 × C58†	C57BL × C58
C58 × C3Hf/Bi	A × C58

*Based on absorption tests with spleen.
†Reciprocal crosses tested.

The G_{IX} Antigenic System

The G_{IX} antigen was recognized during the analysis of the polyvalent MuLV anti-sera produced in (W/Fu X BN)F_1 rats immunized with a W/Fu leukemia originally induced by MuLV (9) (Table 3). Initial tests with this antiserum gave rise to the impression that its specificity was similar to anti-GCSA, i.e. cytotoxic for GCSA$^+$ leukemias but not for GCSA$^-$ leukemias. Further analysis, however, indicated that its pattern of reactivity was distinct, and this was most evident in cytotoxic tests with normal thymocytes from different inbred mouse strains. Although thymocytes from the high leukemia incidence GCSA$^+$ strains were positive, thymocytes from some GCSA$^-$ strains (e.g. 129, A) were equally and, in some instances, more reactive. Because 129 thymocytes showed maximal sensitivity, they were selected as the prototype cell for defining the specificity of the rat antiserum in absorption tests, and this choice of target cells gave rise to the original designation of $G_{(129)}$ for this antigenic system. The later decision to rename it G_{IX} came from evidence that one of the two genes responsible for antigen expression resided in linkage group IX of the mouse. However, now that this genetic assignment must be questioned, the $G_{(129)}$ designation might be more appropriate. Nevertheless, to avoid unnecessary confusion, the designation G_{IX} will be preserved until a more definitive nomenclature can be devised.

Based on absorption tests with normal thymocytes, inbred mouse strains can be classified as G_{IX}^+ or G_{IX}^- (Table 4). Quantitative absorption analysis provided an explanation for the variable reactivity of thymocytes from different G_{IX}^+ strains detected in direct cytotoxic tests. G_{IX}^+ mouse strains are found to differ in the amount of G_{IX} expressed on thymocytes, and because absorption capacity follows a ratio of $3:2:1$ these strains are designated G_{IX}^3, G_{IX}^2, or G_{IX}^1 (Table 6). As all cytotoxic activity for G_{IX}^3 cells can be removed by G_{IX}^1 or G_{IX}^2 thymocytes, and vice versa, the G_{IX} test system apparently detects a single determinant with variable expression. The thymocytes of F_1 hybrids from G_{IX}^+ X G_{IX}^- matings express 50% of the amount found in the G_{IX}^+ partner and crosses between G_{IX}^3 X G_{IX}^2 or G_{IX}^1 strains also express 50% of the parental G_{IX} levels. In the GCSA$^+$ strains (AKR, C58), G_{IX} is found in spleen and other lymphatic tissue as well as thymus, and levels in the spleen are, in fact, higher than in the thymus. In GCSA$^-$ strains, the thymus is the only lymphoid tissue that expresses G_{IX}. Recent evidence indicates that antigen with G_{IX} specificity is found also in serum, on sperm, and in seminal vesicle fluid of G_{IX}^+ mice (27, 39).

Genetics of G_{IX}

The G_{IX} trait has been the subject of considerable genetic analysis (9, 40–43). The prototype G_{IX}^+ strain 129 has been the object of most study because the G_{IX}^3 thymocyte phenotype facilitates typing and because productive MuLV infection, which itself can cause G_{IX} appearance, does not occur in 129 mice. In backcross and F_2 populations with C57BL (the prototype G_{IX}^- strain), segregation ratios indicate that G_{IX} is specified by two unlinked genes, designated $Gv-1$ and $Gv-2$ (Gv = Gross virus related). Both $Gv-1$ and $Gv-2$ are required for G_{IX} expression, but $Gv-1$

Table 6 Strain distribution of the $G_{IX}{}^3$, $G_{IX}{}^2$, $G_{IX}{}^1$, and $G_{IX}{}^-$ phenotype of mouse thymocytes

$G_{IX}{}^+$			$G_{IX}{}^-$	
$G_{IX}{}^3$	$G_{IX}{}^2$	$G_{IX}{}^1$		
129	AKR (and AKR.K, AKR-H-2^b)	SJL/J	C57BL (and C57BL-TL$^+$, C57BL-H-2^k, C57BL-Ly-1.1,	
C57BL-$G_{IX}{}^+$	AKR. T1ALD	DBA/2	C57BL-Ly-2.2, C57BL-Ly-2.1, Ly-3.1)	
CE	C58	C3H/An	C57BL/10	
	C3H/Figge	101	C57BL/Ka	GR
	C3H/He		C57BR	MA
	A (and A-TL$^-$, A-Thy-1.1)		C57L	Swiss/NIH
	NZB*		129-$G_{IX}{}^-$	SWR
	C57BR-$G_{IX}{}^{+M*}$		BALB/c (and BALB/c-T)	HSFS
	C57BL-$G_{IX}{}^{+M*}$		RF	B10BR
			CBA (and CBA-T6)	HTG
			DBA/1	HTH
				HTI
				C3Hf/Bi young[†]

*In quantitative absorption tests, these strains fall between $G_{IX}{}^3$ and $G_{IX}{}^2$ phenotype.
†Conversion strain.

behaves as a semidominant gene (50% G_{IX} expression in heterozygotes) and *Gv-2* as a dominant gene (full G_{IX} expression in heterozygotes). Comparable crosses with BALB/c ($G_{IX}{}^-$) mice give a one-gene ratio for G_{IX} and genetic analysis shows that this strain possesses the *Gv-2* allele. Thus, $G_{IX}{}^-$ strains are either *Gv-1$^-$/Gv-2$^-$* (C57BL and CBA) or *Gv-1$^-$/Gv-2$^+$* (BALB/c, C57L, and the 129-$G_{IX}{}^-$ congenic strain). An extensive search for the *Gv-1$^+$/Gv-2$^-$* genotype has not been productive, even in crosses that should have revealed them, and it has been suggested that this genetic constellation is lethal. The original linkage studies indicated that *Gv-1* was located on chromosome 17 (linkage group IX), 37 units from *H-2* (gene order centromere:*H-2:Gv-1*) and that *Gv-2* was located on chromosome 7, 34 units from *Hbb* (gene order *Gpi-1:Hbb:Gv-2*). However, when the G_{IX} trait of AKR mice ($G_{IA}{}^2$ strain) was studied, crosses with C57BL or BALB/c showed no linkage of *Gv-1* to *H-2* but indicated a chromosome 4 locus for *Gv-1*, approximately 19 units from the *Fv-1/Gpd-1* region. Two possibilities were considered to explain this discrepancy. Either *Gv-1* occupies different chromosomal sites in AKR and 129 mice or the assignment of *Gv-1* to chromosome 17 in 129 mice was incorrect. Because the *Fv-1* allele of C57BL and BALB/c (*Fv-1^b*) has a marked suppressive effect on MuLV production in crosses involving AKR (*Fv-1^n*) and this might influence the expression of G_{IX} in segregating populations, backcrosses of AKR to C57L (a $G_{IX}{}^-$:*Gv-1$^-$/Gv-2$^+$/Fv-1^n* strain) were analyzed. In this *Fv-1^n* homozygous cross, no linkage of *Gv-1* with chromosome 4 (marker Gpd-1) or with chromosome 17 (marker H-2) was noted. Similar findings have resulted from the further analysis of the *Gv-1/H-2* association of 129 mice. Linkage of *Gv-1* to *H-2* is noted when heterozygosity at the *H-2* locus is involved, but disappears when the crosses are homozygous for *H-2* (marker TL; < 2 map units from *H-2*). These results on the association of *Gv-1* with *Fv-1* and *H-2* must therefore be viewed as examples of pseudo- or quasi-linkage, in which certain combinations of unlinked genes appear to be inherited together. In light of this newer information, the initial assignment of *Gv-2* to chromosome 7 must also be reexamined.

Relation of GCSA and G_{IX} to MuLV Structural Components

The finding that G_{IX} and GCSA could be induced in rats by MuLV infection made it likely that MuLV genes directly code for these antigens (8, 9). Although the possibility was considered that G_{IX} and GCSA represented structural components of the virus incorporated into the cell surface during virus maturation, evidence at the time suggested that they were nonstructural products of MuLV. Immunoelectronmicroscopy with GCSA antibody showed labeling of the cell surface but no labeling of the envelope of budding or more mature viral particles (44). In contrast, both viral envelope and cell surface were labeled with broadly reactive anti-MuLV sera. In the case of G_{IX}, the antigen was classified as a nonvirion component because electronmicroscopy and infectivity studies revealed no evidence for MuLV in 129 thymocytes, the prototype G_{IX}^+ cell. With advances in the biochemical analysis of MuLV and new methods to define cell surface molecules, it has now been shown that both G_{IX} and GCSA are in fact viral structural components incorporated into the cell surface. G_{IX} is a type-specific antigen of the major envelope glycoprotein of MuLV, gp70 (39, 45). GCSA is related to the internal core proteins of MuLV, p30, and p15, which occur as glycosolated polyproteins on the surface of infected cells (46, 47). The failure of anti-GCSA to label intact virus can now be understood in relation to the internal location of the antigenically related structural components in the virion. Although GCSA has never been found in the absence of replicating MuLV, viral genes coding for G_{IX} can be expressed independently of other MuLV genes.

GCSA and G_{IX} Phenotype of Mouse Leukemia

Table 7 summarizes our accumulated evidence on expression of GCSA and G_{IX} in leukemias of various inbred and hybrid strains. Leukemias arising in the GCSA$^+$/G_{IX}^+ high leukemia incidence strains invariably express both antigens. In G_{IX}^3, G_{IX}^2, or G_{IX}^1 strains, where G_{IX} appears as a differentiation alloantigen of normal thymocytes, the leukemias are commonly G_{IX}^+, an expected finding in view of the T-cell origin of these leukemias. GCSA and G_{IX} may also occur in leukemias arising in strains that ordinarily do not express these antigens during normal life, revealing the presence of viral structural genes in these mice that are activated as a consequence of leukemogenesis. In some low leukemia strains (BALB/c), GCSA, and G_{IX} activation is common, whereas in others (C57BL), these antigens are only rarely found. In the 129 strain, GCSA activation has never been observed in a leukemia, and this correlates with the fact that MuLV has not been isolated from mice of this strain. (C57BL × AKR)F$_1$ mice resemble C57BL in the GCSA phenotype of their leukemias, indicating marked suppression of MuLV replication. (C57BL × A)F$_1$ resemble A mice in showing GCSA activation in a proportion of leukemias. The exceptional leukemia phenotype GCSA$^+$/G_{IX}^- may reflect activation of an MuLV that does not induce G_{IX}.

GCSA and G_{IX} Induction by MuLV

GCSA and G_{IX} can be induced in mouse fibroblasts by MuLV, and this consequence of viral infection has been useful in distinguishing various isolates of MuLV

Table 7 GCSA and G_{IX} phenotype of mouse leukemia

Strains	Thymocyte phenotype GCSA/G_{IX}	Leukemia induction	Leukemia cell phenotype			
			$GCSA^+/G_{IX}^+$	$GCSA^+/G_{IX}^-$	$GCSA^-/G_{IX}^+$	$GCSA^-/G_{IX}^-$
High leukemia incidence strains			Number of leukemias tested			
AKR, C58, PL, C3H/Figge	+/+	Spontaneous and urethan	>100			
Low leukemia incidence strains						
BALB/c, RF, DBA/1	−/−	Spontaneous and X-ray	3		2	2
A,A.BY, DBA/2	−/+	Spontaneous and X-ray	5	2	5	2
G_{IX} congenic strains						
129 (G_{IX}^+)	−/+	X-ray			9	
129-G_{IX}^-	−/−	X-ray			2	10
C57BL (G_{IX}^-)	−/−	X-ray	2	1		21
		Spontaneous				2
C57BL-G_{IX}^+	−/+	X-ray			26	
F_1 hybrids						
C57BL × A	−/− × −/+	X-ray	2	1	2	6
C57BL × AKR	−/− × +/+	X-ray			3	7

(48). Two G_{IX} phenotypes (G_{IX}^-, G_{IX}^+) and three GCSA phenotypes (GCSA$^-$, GCSA$^+$, GCSA^{2+}) can be scored in MuLV-infected fibroblasts by absorption of cytotoxic antibody, and five of the six possible G_{IX}/GCSA phenotypes have been found. (The missing phenotype is G_{IX}^+/GCSA$^-$.) With virus isolated from normal mouse tissues, N-tropic MuLV usually induces the G_{IX}^+/GCSA^{2+} phenotype, and B-tropic MuLV the G_{IX}^-/GCSA^{2+} phenotype, although N- and B-tropic MuLV isolates have been identified that do not follow this rule. G_{IX} and GCSA typing of fibroblasts infected with FMR viruses give results that parallel the phenotype of leukemias induced by these viruses—G_{IX}^-/GCSA$^+$. Xenotropic MuLV, a class of MuLV that cannot infect mouse cells but replicates well in certain heterologous cells, does not induce G_{IX}, and this is also true for the recently recognized amphotropic class of MuLV derived from wild mice (49). However, these viruses can be distinguished on the basis of GCSA typing and, in the case of xenotropic MuLV, this appears to correlate with their classification by nucleic acid hybridization and type-specific heteroantisera. Quantitative differences in GCSA levels induced by various MuLV undoubtedly reflect type-specific differences in the core protein of various MuLV, with all N- and B-tropic MuLV being most closely related (GCSA^{2+}), FMR viruses and MuLV isolated from wild mice and certain xenotropic MuLV more distantly related (GCSA$^+$), and AT124 and Caroli xenotropic MuLV being unrelated (GCSA$^-$). Presumably these latter viruses induce type-specific core protein of distinct antigenicity on the cell surface. Cell surface typing for G_{IX} and GCSA, as well as for other type-specific antigens specified by MuLV, may be of considerable value for analyzing MuLV recombinants. In this regard, the new MCF class of MuLV, originally recognized in preleukemic AKR mouse thymus, appears to represent a stable recombinant between a xenotropic and an N-tropic MuLV, having the properties of both classes by neutralization tests, host range, and interference patterns (50). MCF MuLV can induce G_{IX} antigen in infected cells, behaving therefore like an ecotropic virus and not a xenotropic MuLV in this respect.

Preleukemic Changes in Surface Alloantigens and MuLV-Related Antigens on AKR Thymocytes

The study of AKR mice during the preleukemic period (4–6 months) has revealed characteristic changes in the pattern of surface antigens expressed by thymocytes (51, 52). In contrast to the low H-2/high Thy-1 phenotype of normal thymocytes of young AKR mice, thymocytes from 6-month-old AKR show high H-2/low Thy-1 levels. In addition, expression of G_{IX}, GCSA, and other MuLV-related antigens on the surface of thymocytes is greatly amplified in preleukemic AKR mice. As a result of these changes, the surface phenotype of the preleukemic thymocyte comes to resemble the surface characteristics of AKR leukemia cells. Assays for MuLV reveal that the level of N-tropic MuLV remains constant during the 2- to 6-month period. However, virus with xenotropic properties appears in the thymus of 6-month-old animals, and the level of this virus correlates well with amplified MuLV-antigen expression (52). Further characterization of virus isolated from the preleukemic thymus led to the recognition of the MCF class of MuLV (discussed above).

X.1 System

This system was detected during the study of the transplantation behavior of X-ray-induced BALB/c leukemias (11). Although no evidence for resistance to transplants could be elicited in BALB/c mice, (BALB/c × C57BL)F$_1$ hybrids were found to reject large numbers of BALB/c leukemia cells. Considerable evidence points to the conclusion that this hybrid resistance to leukemic transplants is controlled by the H-2-linked Ir locus contributed by the C57BL partner. Serum from hybrids that had rejected repeated inocula of BALB/c leukemia RL♂1 defined an antigen, designated X.1, that was present on BALB/c, A, and AKR leukemias (Table 3). X.1 is unrelated to the GCSA or G_{IX} system as the standard $G_{IX}{}^+$/GCSA$^+$ leukemia E♂G2 types X.1$^-$. X.1 is present in normal tissues of high leukemia strains, but unlike GCSA and G_{IX}, in very low levels. For this reason, mouse strains were typed for X.1 by the method of in vivo absorption (Table 4). All high leukemia strains are GCSA$^+$/$G_{IX}{}^+$/X.1$^+$, whereas low incidence GCSA$^-$ strains may be $G_{IX}{}^+$/X.1$^+$ (129 mice), $G_{IX}{}^+$/X.1$^-$ (A mice), $G_{IX}{}^-$/X.1$^+$ (129-$G_{IX}{}^-$ mice), or $G_{IX}{}^-$/X.1$^-$ (BALB/c mice). X.1 antisera also detects a gp70 molecule (designated X-gp70) on the surface of leukemia cells that is distinguishable from G_{IX}-gp70 (53). However, as leukemia cells that type X-gp70$^+$/X.1$^-$ have been found, it appears likely that X-gp70 and X.1 represent distinct antigenic systems. Although the presence of X.1 in the normal tissues of high leukemia incidence strains and its appearance in leukemias of X.1$^-$ strains suggest an association with MuLV, more direct evidence that X.1 is an MuLV-related antigen (i.e. induction in MuLV-infected fibroblasts) is lacking.

$G_{(RADA1)}$ and $G_{(ERLD)}$

The serum of normal mice, particularly F_1 hybrids and random-bred Swiss mice, is proving to be an exceptional source of antibody capable of distinguishing new cell surface antigens related to MuLV. As discussed before, this may have to do with heterozygosity at Ir loci, permitting a broader range of immune reactions to antigens of endogenous and exogenous origin. We know that $(C57BL\text{-}G_{IX}{}^+ \times 129)F_1$ mice produce G_{IX} antibody, and there is indication that X.1 antibody is found in normal $(BALB/c \times C57BL)F_1$ mice. Antibody with GCSA specificity has not as yet been detected in normal mouse serum, but we expect that it too will be found in the appropriate hybrid. Several new systems of MuLV-related cell surface antigens have now been detected and two of these are sufficiently well analyzed to be briefly described. They are designated $G_{(RADA1)}$ and $G_{(ERLD)}$ to indicate their relation to MuLV-Gross and to the prototype leukemia cell lines that were used in their definition (Table 3). Random-bred Swiss mice are the source of $G_{(RADA1)}$ antibody, and $(C57BL \times 129)F_1$ mice are the source of $G_{(ERLD)}$ antibody. Both $G_{(RADA1)}$ and $G_{(ERLD)}$ are found in normal and leukemic lymphoid tissues of strains with a high incidence of leukemia, and both of these can be induced in fibroblasts by infection with MuLV. The distinct pattern of occurrence of these two antigens in the normal tissues of low incidence strains clearly distinguishes them from one another as well as distinguishing them from G_{IX}, GCSA, and X.1 (Table 4). Past studies with heteroantibody to MuLV-gp70 have indicated that all inbred mouse strains tested, with the exception of $129\text{-}G_{IX}{}^-$ and BALB/c, expressed gp70-like molecules (54). $G_{(ERLD)}$ has an equally widespread strain distribution and is similarly absent from $129\text{-}G_{IX}{}^-$ and BALB/c. We had originally assumed that $G_{(ERLD)}$ might be related to the 0-gp70 species defined by heteroantibody to gp70 on C57BL and other thymocytes (55), but as 129 thymocytes are $G_{(ERLD)}{}^+/0\text{-}gp70^-$, the two systems are serologically distinguishable. Present evidence indicates that the $G_{(RADA1)}$ antigen is related to a gp70 molecule on the surface of RADA1 cells that is not expressed by normal A strain cells. The relation of this gp70 to $G_{IX}\text{-}gp70$, X-gp70, and 0-gp70 remains to be determined.

PC.1 Antigen: Relation to MuLV?

The need to discuss this differentiation alloantigen arises from the suggestion that PC.1 is related to a class of MuLV that is widespread in mice. The PC.1 antigen was originally identified during a study of the surface antigens of myeloma cells (13). Antisera prepared against the BALB/c myeloma MOPC-70A in H-2–compatible DBA/2 mice were cytotoxic for BALB/c myeloma cells but not for normal thymocytes or thymic leukemias. Absorption tests showed that the antigen was present in normal BALB/c mice and that it had a distinctive tissue distribution in comparison with other known surface antigens. Because normal plasma cells as well as malignant plasma cells (myelomas) were marked by this antigen, it was called PC.1. Typing of mouse strains by absorption tests with normal spleen or liver distinguished PC.1$^+$ and PC.1$^-$ strains, and genetic studies indicated conventional single-gene specification (as yet not mapped) of the PC.1 system. After the PC.1 system was defined, it was observed that the serum of BALB/c mice, the prototype PC.1$^+$ strain, had cytotoxic antibody to BALB/c myelomas and that this BALB/c antibody appeared to be detecting an antigen with a strain and tissue distribution that was identical with PC.1 (56). Antibody of similar specificity was found in a number of other mouse strains, both PC.1$^+$ and PC.1$^-$. The suggestion was made that viral induction of PC.1 may be responsible for the widespread distribution of naturally occurring antibody to PC.1$^+$ myelomas and that the MuLV frequently found in myelomas is the likely candidate. If a PC.1 inducing virus does in fact exist, PC.1 might be expected to occur in myelomas arising in PC.1$^-$ strains, and one such instance was reported (56). However, we have tested 7 myelomas from PC.1$^-$ strains in the standard PC.1 typing system and they have all been PC.1$^-$. In addition, we have been unable to detect PC.1 antibody in normal BALB/c serum under the conditions of our cytotoxic test. If PC.1 is indeed virus-induced rather than the product of a conventional Mendelian gene, one might not expect to find an allelic product in PC.1$^-$ strains. Thus the definition of such an allele may be important in distinguishing these two alternatives.

CELL SURFACE ANTIGENS OF THE TL SYSTEM

Background

Recognition of the TL system of cell surface antigens came about during a study of radiation-induced leukemias of C57BL mice (3). Because resistance to transplants of these leukemias could not be induced in C57BL, it seemed unlikely that syngeneic immunization would give rise to antibody with specificity for the leukemia cells. For this reason, C57BL mice were immunized with radiation leukemia cells of (C57BL × A)F$_1$ origin, with the idea that radiation leukemias of the mouse share a common antigen. During rejection of the histoincompatible leukemia cells, antibody would be produced to alloantigenic differences and, if present, to leukemia-specific antigens as well. Reactions due to conventional alloantibodies could be eliminated by testing the resulting immune sera on syngeneic leukemia cells. In initial tests with these antisera prepared against F$_1$ leukemia cells, cytotoxic reactions were observed with several transplanted C57BL radiation leukemias, most notably ERLD, but not with any normal C57BL lymphoid cell. In examining the reactions of other C57BL antisera, highest titer for ERLD was found with an antiserum prepared against ASL1, a transplanted A strain spontaneous leukemia, and absorption tests with this antiserum and ERLD target cells formed the basis for the original analysis of the TL system. In C57BL mice, the antigen was strictly leukemia-specific; no normal tissue absorbed cytotoxic antibody. In A strain mice, absorption tests revealed the surprising fact that the antigen was found on normal thymocytes as well as on leukemia cells. Normal cells other than thymocytes lacked the antigen. Restriction of antigen to thymocytes and leukemia cells suggested the name thymus-leukemia or TL for this antigenic system.

We then showed that inbred mouse strains could be typed TL$^-$ (like C57BL) or TL$^+$ (like A strain) on the basis of absorption tests with normal thymocytes and that TL$^+$ leukemias can occur in TL$^-$ strains other than C57BL (57). In normal mice,

TL is inherited as a Mendelian dominant trait, and linkage studies have placed the TL locus, designated *Tla,* on chromosome 17 < 2 units from the D end of the *H-2* complex (58). The generally accepted explanation for the anomalous appearance of TL$^+$ leukemias in mice of TL$^-$ strains is that all mice possess the structural gene for TL, but that in TL$^-$ strains, the gene is not normally expressed. As a consequence of leukemogenesis, the *Tla* locus is derepressed or activated, resulting in the appearance of the TL product on the surface of leukemia cells. According to this view, a regulatory gene controls expression of the TL structural gene, and allelism for the trait in normal mice is based on *expression* versus *nonexpression* alleles at the regulatory locus (1, 28). The possibility has been raised that the *Tla* locus on chromosome 17 represents the TL regulatory gene and that the TL structural gene, since it is present in all mice, could be elsewhere in the genome (59). Although this has not been formally excluded, current understanding of the TL system makes it most unlikely (60).

Antigens Specified by the Tla Locus

Initial serological study of TL indicated detection of a single antigenic determinant. However, subsequent tests have shown that the *Tla* locus specifies at least four serologically distinguishable determinants, TL.1, TL.2, TL.3, and TL.4 (Table 8). Antibodies detecting TL.2 and TL.3 were found in C57BL anti-ASL1 serum during analysis of this antiserum by the technique of in vivo absorption. Absorption in normal A mice eliminated all H-2 antibody but did not remove cytotoxic activity for TL$^+$ cells, such as ERLD. In direct tests with the absorbed antiserum, thymocytes from BALB/c mice, formerly classified TL$^-$, showed weak reactivity. Using this as a basis for absorption tests, it was found that thymocytes from all TL$^+$ strains expressed the new specificity and that several other strains, also previously typed TL$^-$, were positive. Formal demonstration that the new determinant, called *TL.2,* belonged to the TL system came from co-typing segregating populations from TL$^-$

Table 8 Antisera defining the four antigens of the TL system

Antiserum	Standard test cell	TL specificity detected
1 (C57BL × A-TL$^-$)F$_1$ anti-ASL1 (A strain spontaneous leukemia)	Strain A thymocyte	TL.1,2,3
	ERLD (C57BL X-ray leukemia)	TL.1
	BALB/c thymocyte	TL.2
2 (BALB/c × C3H/An)F$_1$ anti-ASL1 absorbed in vivo in (C57BL × A)F$_1$ mice bearing advanced transplants of ERLD	Strain A thymocyte	TL.3
3 (C57BL × A-TL$^-$)F$_1$ anti-ASL1 absorbed in vitro with ERLD	Strain A thymocyte	TL.3
4 C57BL-TL$^+$ anti-ERLD	ERLD	TL.4

X TL$^+$ crosses. Recognition of TL.3 resulted from the analysis of (BALB/c X C3H/An)F$_1$ anti-ASL1 serum absorbed in vivo in (C57BL X A)F$_1$ mice growing ERLD leukemia. It was expected that all TL antibody would be eliminated from this antiserum when absorbed in this way, and, in fact, cytotoxic activity for ERLD was removed. However, strong cytotoxicity for thymocytes of A strain mice remained. Genetic tests similar to those performed with TL.2 showed that TL.3, as the antigen came to be called, was also specified by the *Tla* locus. With the recognition of TL.2 and TL.3, it became clear that the original typing system for TL (C57BL anti-ASL1 versus ERLD) was detecting a distinct specificity, TL.1, because ERLD cells lacked TL.3 and, for purposes of typing, TL.2. Thus, three phenotypes can now be distinguished in normal mice on the basis of thymocyte typing, TL$^-$, TL.2, TL.1,2,3 and the corresponding genotypes have been designated *Tla^b*, *Tla^c*, and *Tla^a*.

The strain distribution of the three TL phenotypes based on TL typing in our laboratory is given in Table 9. The TL congenic stocks (C57BL-TL$^+$ and A-TL$^-$), which were derived from *H-2D/Tla* crossovers occurring in C57BL X A crosses, are proving valuable in mapping the region between *Tla* and *H-2D*. New specificities coded for by this region have been defined by skin graft rejection (61, 62) and by cytotoxic tests (63, 64). However, the occurrence of these antigens in tissues other than thymus clearly sets them apart from products of the *Tla* locus. TL.4, the most recently recognized TL specificity, has not been found on normal thymocytes of TL$^+$ or TL$^-$ strains, and in this regard, is the only antigen of the TL series that is restricted to leukemia cells. It is strongly represented on ERLD and other C57BL leukemia cells but has not been found on leukemias of A strain mice, and this accounts for the absence of anti-TL.4 in anti-ASL1 serum. The antiserum that detects TL.4 was produced in the TL congenic strain, C57BL-TL$^+$, by immunization with ERLD. Because TL.4 does not occur on normal thymocytes, formal genetic proof that it is specified by the *Tla* locus has not been possible to obtain. However, evidence from analyses of H-2/TL-loss variants, modulation of TL.4 by TL antibody, and assignment of TL.4 to the TL.1/H-2D region of the cell surface by antibody blocking tests indicates that TL.4 clearly belongs to the TL system.

Table 9 Strain distribution of the TL.1,2,3, TL.2, and TL$^-$ phenotype of mouse thymocytes

TL.1,2,3 (*Tla^a*)	TL.2 (*Tla^c*)	TL$^-$ (*Tla^b*)	
A (and A-Thy-1.1)	129 (and 129-G$_{IX}$$^-$)	C57BL (and C57BL-G$_{IX}$$^+$, C57BL-G$_{IX}$$^+$M,	
C57BL-TL$^+$	BALB/c (and BALB/c-T)	C57BL-H-2^k, C57BL-Ly-1.1, C57BL-Ly-2.1,	
C57BR (and C57BR-G$_{IX}$$^+$M)	DBA/2	C57BL-Ly-2.1,Ly-3.1)	
C58	C57L	C57BL/Ka	ASW
SJL/J	A.BY	A-TL$^-$	HTH
HSFS	GR	BALB/H-2^b	HTG
PL	C × BD	C3H/An	101
NZB	C × BE	C3Hf/Bi	CE
HTI	C × BH	C3H/Figge	C × BG
AKR.K		CBA (and CBA-T6)	C × BI
		AKR (and AKR H-2^b)	C × BJ
		I	C × BK
		RF	

Influence of Tla Haplotype on Expression of TL and H-2 Antigens by Thymocytes

Quantitative absorption analysis has provided the means to study the expression of TL and H-2 on normal thymocytes from mice of various *Tla* haplotypes (65). Different *Tla^a^* strains do not vary in the quantity of TL.1,2, or 3 found on thymocytes. *Tla^c^* strains also do not show interstrain variation in TL.2, although the amount of TL.2 expressed by *Tla^c^* thymocytes is lower than by *Tla^a^* thymocytes. *Tla^b^* X *Tla^a^* or *Tla^c^* heterozygotes express one half the quantity of individual TL specificities detected on thymocytes of *Tla^a^* or *Tla^c^* homozygotes. These findings are what one would expect from conventional gene dose effects, with no positive or negative interaction between *Tla* alleles. A different result occurs in *Tla^a^* X *Tla^c^* heterozygotes, where intermediate levels of TL.2, heterozygous levels of TL.3, but homozygous levels of TL.1 were found. The reason for a homozygous TL.1 phenotype in a mouse with a heterozygous genotype is unknown but could reflect interactions at the level of genetic regulation, antigen synthesis, or antigen insertion. The *Tla* haplotype also influences the expression of H-2D antigen on the thymocyte. The amount of H-2D antigen on TL⁻ *(Tla^b^)* thymocytes is significantly greater than on TL.1,2,3 or TL.2 (*Tla^a^* or *Tla^c^* thymocytes). In contrast, the level of H-2K and Thy-1 antigens is constant and unrelated to TL genotype. This inverse association between TL and H-2D may relate to the close spatial relation of these two molecules on the cell surface (see below). Absence of TL might relieve a steric hindrance to attachment of the H-2D antibody used to measure the amounts of H-2D by quantitative absorption tests. This idea receives support from the finding that TL⁺ cells undergoing phenotypic suppression of TL by TL antibody (antigenic modulation) show a corresponding increase in the level of H-2D antigen (66).

Antigenic Modulation

This name was given to a phenomenon originally thought unique for TL antigens, but now considered likely to be of a more general significance. It refers to reversible changes in the sensitivity of cells to the cytotoxic action of TL antibody and complement brought about by prior exposure to TL antibody. Antigenic modulation was recognized while investigating the reason TL-immunized mice with high levels of TL antibody showed no resistance to transplants of syngeneic TL⁺ leukemia cells (67). An explanation for this paradox became apparent when the leukemia cells were recovered from the immunized mice and found to be totally resistant to TL antibody and complement. As long as the cells were passed in animals with TL antibody, they remained TL⁻, but when passed back to nonimmune mice, they reverted to TL⁺ and high sensitivity to TL antibody. Passive transfer of TL antibody can also induce antigenic modulation, and, in this way, it was shown that normal thymocytes and leukemia cells of TL⁺ mice (which are incapable of forming TL antibody) undergo modulation (68).

Antibody-mediated change in TL phenotype can also be brought about in vitro, and much that we know about antigenic modulation comes from such studies (66, 69). Loss of sensitivity to complement-mediated cytotoxicity occurs rapidly, in certain cases within 30 min after exposure to TL antibody. When TL antibody is removed, TL sensitivity returns after one to two cell divisions. The process is temperature-dependent and can be inhibited by certain metabolic antagonists, particularly actinomycin. Antibody to an individual specificity of the TL complex causes modulation of other TL antigens, and this is consistent with the current thinking that all TL specificities reside on a single molecule. Different TL$^+$ cell types modulate at different rates; leukemia cells undergo modulation more rapidly than normal thymocytes, a reflection most likely of the greater metabolic activity of leukemia cells.

A number of explanations have been proposed to account for antigenic modulation. With the recognition that antibody to certain cell surface antigens causes rearrangement of these molecules into patches and caps, there has been speculation that TL modulation represents a similar process. However, as monovalent Fab fragments of TL antibody can modulate TL but fail to cause patching and capping, antigenic modulation appears to represent a more subtle consequence of antibody attachment to surface molecules. Although there is some indication that the amount of TL remaining after modulation is reduced, considerable TL antigen can still be accounted for on the surface of modulated cells (70). Rather than antigen loss, current evidence points to antibody-induced conformational changes in TL sites that reduce the efficiency with which lytic complement components can be engaged. However, whatever the mechanism of antigenic modulation, it provides a remarkably effective mechanism for TL$^+$ leukemia cells to escape the consequence of their antigenicity.

TL Phenotype of Mouse Leukemia

Table 10 summarizes our accumulated information on the TL phenotypes of leukemias occurring in various mouse strains. The key feature of the TL system in regard to malignancy is the anomalous occurrence of TL$^+$ leukemias in strains with

Table 10 TL phenotype of mouse leukemia

	Tla haplotype	Thymocyte phenotype	Leukemia induction	Leukemia cell Phenotype				
				1,2,3,4	1,2,3	1,2,4	1,2	–
TL congenic strains				Number of leukemias tested				
A (TL$^+$)	a	TL.1,2,3	Spontaneous		4			1
			X-ray		3			
A-TL$^-$	b	TL$^-$	X-ray			3		4
C57BL (TL$^-$)	b	TL$^-$	Spontaneous			1		3
			X-ray			45		8
C57BL-TL$^+$	a	TL.1,2,3	X-ray		4			
TL.2 strains								
129, BALB/c, DBA/2	c	TL.2	Spontaneous			2	2	1
			X-ray			9	13	6
			DMBA					6
TL$^-$ high leukemia incidence strain								
AKR	b	TL$^-$	Spontaneous			10		78
			Urethan			10		2
F$_1$ hybrids								
C57BL × A	b × a	TL$^-$ × TL.1,2,3	X-ray	7	6			1
C57BL × AKR	b × b	TL$^-$ × TL$^-$	X-ray			9		4

the TL⁻ phenotype. The frequency of TL^+ leukemias varies among inbred strains. For example, X-ray-induced leukemias of C57BL mice are frequently TL^+, whereas most spontaneous leukemias of AKR mice are TL⁻. Urethan-induced AKR leukemias, however, are commonly TL^+. This relation of TL appearance to different modes of leukemia induction requires more direct study.

Each of the TL specificities can be distinguished on the basis of appearance on normal thymocytes and on leukemia cells (Table 11). In normal mice, TL.1 is an antigen of normal differentiation, appearing on thymocytes of Tla^a (phenotype TL.1,2,3) strains. TL.2 is also an antigen of normal differentiation, appearing on normal thymocytes of Tla^a and Tla^c (phenotype TL.2) strains and is the only TL specificity that occurs alone on normal thymocytes. TL.1 and 2 are also antigens of leukemic differentiation, because they may occur anomalously on leukemias of Tla^b (phenotype TL⁻) strains and, in the case of TL.1, on the leukemias of Tla^c mice. It is this evidence that has led to the supposition that structural information for TL.1 and 2 is present in all mice. TL.3 is an antigen of normal differentiation only, its occurrence on leukemia cells being restricted to Tla^a strains where the antigen is a marker of normal thymocytes. Structural genes for TL.3 may not be universal, because TL.3 leukemias have never been found in mice of Tla^b or Tla^c haplotypes. An alternative explanation is that TL.3 structural genes may not be subject to derepression or activation during leukemogenesis. TL.4 is an antigen of leukemic differentiation only, having never been found on normal thymocytes of any strain. Its occurrence is restricted to leukemic mice of Tla^b and Tla^c haplotypes, suggesting that the structural gene for TL.4, like that for TL.3, is not present universally in mice.

The anomalous appearance of TL antigens on leukemias and the clearly distinctive behavior of individual TL components allow certain questions to be asked in regard to the relation of the Tla locus to leukemogenesis. The occurrence of TL⁻ leukemias of thymic derivation in both TL^+ and TL⁻ strains indicates that TL activation is not an invariable consequence of T-cell leukemogenesis in the mouse.

Table 11 Conclusions derived from a comparison of the TL phenotypes of normal thymocytes and leukemia cells

Tla haplotype	Prototype strain	Normal thymocyte	TL^+ leukemia	Conclusions
Tla^a	A, C57BL-TL⁺	TL.1,2,3	TL.1,2,3	Phenotype of TL^+ leukemia resembles normal thymocyte. No evidence for appearance of anomalous TL components.
Tla^b	C57BL, A-TL⁻	TL⁻	TL.1,2,4	Invariable appearance of anomalous TL.1, TL.2, and TL.4 on TL^+ leukemias.
Tla^c	BALB/c	TL.2	TL.1,2, or TL.1,2,4	No leukemia found with a TL.2 phenotype only, indicating that anomalous TL.1 appearance (but not TL.4) is an invariable consequence of leukemogenesis of the type involving TL activation in mice with the Tla^c haplotype.
$Tla^b \times Tla^a$	(C57BL × A)F₁	TL.1,2,3	TL.1,2,3, or TL.1,2,3,4	The TL phenotype TL.1,2,3,4 is found only in leukemias of (Tla^b or $^c \times Tla^a$) heterozygotes.
$Tla^b \times Tla^b$	(C57BL × AKR)F₁	TL⁻	TL.1,2,4	Otherwise the TL phenotype of F₁ leukemias is similar to those arising in Tla homozygotes.

With regard to the transformation pathway that leads to TL$^+$ leukemias, one can ask whether anomalous TL antigens are invariably expressed. TL$^+$ leukemias arising in mice of Tla^a strains are not revealing, because no anomalous TL products have been recognized in these mice. In Tla^c strains, however, where thymocytes are marked by TL.2, all TL$^+$ leukemias are both TL.1 and TL.2 and never TL.2 alone, indicating that the structural gene for TL.1 is invariably activated during leukemogenesis involving this class of T cell. Given that there are two TL structural genes in a diploid cell, are both Tla loci activated in a TL$^+$ leukemia arising in a TL$^-$ mouse? Although quantitative absorption tests should be able to distinguish homozygous from heterozygous amounts of TL in such leukemias, studies of this sort have not given clear results. An indication that both loci need not be activated, however, comes from the analysis of leukemias occurring in Tla^a X Tla^b mice, where TL.4 can be used as the marker for activation of the Tla^b haplotype (Tables 10 and 11). Leukemias of both TL.1,2,3 and TL.1,2,3,4 phenotypes are found, indicating that the Tla^b locus need not be involved.

Another question relates to whether the product of the Tla locus is essential for the continued malignant behavior of TL$^+$ leukemia cells. TL expression per se is apparently not critical, since the TL phenotype of TL$^+$ leukemias can be suppressed by TL antibody (antigenic modulation) without the cell losing malignant characteristics. The isolation of a TL$^-$ variant from an originally TL$^+$ leukemia by in vitro immunoselection does not help in this regard because the leukemia came from a mouse of Tla^a genotype where Tla activation is not known to occur (71). TL variants can also be isolated by immunoselection in vivo (72) and Table 12 shows the results of our analysis of 3 TL$^+$ leukemias of (C57BL X A)F$_1$ origin and the 6 H-2/TL-loss variants derived from them. The selection method, which has been extensively used to analyze H-2 variants (73), involved the passage of the F$_1$ leukemias into mice that are homozygous for the H-2^b (C57BL) haplotype or for the H-2^a (A strain) haplotype. In this way, stable variants that do not express one or the other H-2 haplotype escape immunological destruction and can be recovered from the original population of leukemia cells. A variety of explanations have been

Table 12 TL and H-2 phenotypes of three (C57BL X A)F$_1$ X-ray induced leukemias and the TL/H-2-loss variants derived from them by immunoselection in vivo

	TL.1	TL.3	TL.4	H-2^b	H-2^a
(C57BL X A)F$_1$ leukemia A	1	3	4	b	a
H-2^a-loss variant	1	–	4	b	–
H-2^b-loss variant	1	3	–	–	a
(C57BL X A)F$_1$ leukemia B	1	3	4	b	a
H-2^a-loss variant	1	–	4	b	–
H-2^b-loss variant	1	3	–	–	a
(C57BL X A)F$_1$ leukemia C	1	3	–	b	a
H-2^a-loss variant	–	–	–	b	–
H-2^b-loss variant	1	3	–	–	a

put forward to account for these antigenic loss variants, but at the moment their origin is unclear (74). Nonetheless, they have proved to be valuable in the study of TL for, as Table 12 shows, the process leading to the loss or inactivation of the *H-2* locus also leads to the loss of the closely linked *Tla* locus. Thus, H-2ᵃ-loss variants lack products of the *Tlaᵃ* locus (marker TL.3) and H-2ᵇ-loss variants lack products of the *Tlaᵇ* locus (marker TL.4). Parental variants of reciprocal type were obtained with all three leukemias, indicating that the presence of both *Tla* loci is not required to maintain the malignant phenotype. The H-2ᵇ-loss variants of leukemia A and B show that the activated *Tlaᵇ* locus is also unnecessary. With leukemia C, a TL⁻ variant could be isolated from an originally TL⁺ leukemia (H-2ᵃ-loss variant), suggesting that TL is irrelevant as far as the malignant behavior of this leukemia is concerned. However, as there is no evidence for anomalous TL activation in this leukemia, it will be critical to show whether TL⁻ variants can be isolated from TL⁺ leukemias arising in *Tlaᵇ* X *Tlaᵇ* heterozygotes, such as (C57BL X AKR)F₁ mice.

Mapping of TL Antigens on the Surface of Thymocytes and Leukemia Cells

In 1968, our group proposed a map designating the relative positions of various alloantigens on the surface of mouse thymocytes (75). The method we used to develop this map was based on the idea that antibody to one antigenic site would inhibit or block the subsequent attachment of antibody to a second unrelated site if the two sites were sufficiently close to one another on the cell surface. The test (which has come to be called the *antibody blocking test*) is performed by exposing thymocytes to saturating levels of antibody directed to a particular surface alloantigen. After the cells are washed, they are tested for the amount of an unrelated surface antigen by quantitative absorption assays with antibody to the second specificity. Cells that are not exposed to antibody serve as the standard to measure the degree of blocking induced by attachment of antibody to the first specificity. Study of different antigenic systems by such pair-by-pair blocking tests gave rise to instances of no blocking, reciprocal blocking, or nonreciprocal blocking. The pattern that emerged from this analysis and forms the basis for the map is shown in Figure 1.

Based on ten distinct alloantigenic specificities, four regions of the map can be distinguished. Antigens defining region I, III, and IV are not within blocking range of one another. Thy-1 alloantigens appear to be proximal to antigens in region I and III, but the nonreciprocal nature of blocking suggests that its surface representation may be far greater than other alloantigens. This interpretation is consistent with the finding that the ratio of Thy-1 to H-2 antigenic sites on thymocytes, as estimated by the uptake of tritiated labeled alloantibody, is approximately 5 to 1 (76). At the time the map was constructed, it came as somewhat of a surprise that H-2D and H-2K were in separate blocking regions, but subsequent genetic, biochemical, and other studies have shown that these antigens do in fact reside on separate molecules. Two examples of surface association related to genetic linkage are found in region I. The *Tla* and *H-2D* loci are within 2 map units from one another, and this is reflected in the close proximity of their products on the cell surface. Lyt-2 and Lyt-3,

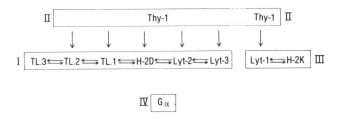

Figure 1   Spatial relation of alloantigens on the surface of mouse thymocytes as determined by antibody-blocking tests. *Arrow* indicates direction of antibody blocking (for example, antibody to the specificity at the arrow tail blocks attachment of antibody to the specificity at the arrowhead). *Arrows in both directions* (⇆) indicate reciprocal blocking. A *single arrow* (→) indicates nonreciprocal blocking. No blocking was found between alloantigens comprising region I and those in region III and IV.

determined by closely linked genes that have not as yet been resolved by crossing-over, are also closely linked on the cell surface. However, genetic linkage is not necessarily associated with surface linkage (e.g. H-2D/H-2K) and conversely, surface linkage does not necessarily reflect genetic linkage (e.g. H-2D/Lyt-2 and Lyt-1/H-2K). If current evidence indicating that the 3 TL specificities on normal thymocytes reside on a single molecule is correct, then their relative positions on the TL molecule is also resolved by the blocking test.

Blocking tests also permit questions to be asked about changes in the alloantigenic map following appearance of new tumor antigens on the cell surface. The TL system provides a unique opportunity to compare the surface site of TL on a leukemia cell that arose in a TL⁻ mouse with its known site on a TL⁺ thymocyte. For this purpose, the TL.1/H-2D surface association was explored with five TL⁺ leukemias (Table 13). In TL⁺ leukemias of TL⁻ mice, anomalous TL.1 mapped adjacent to H-2D. However, blocking is not reciprocal; H-2D antibody blocks TL sites, but TL antibody does not block H-2D sites. This can be interpreted to indicate that TL occupies the correct site (so that every TL molecule has an adjacent H-2D molecule), but not every H-2D site has an adjacent TL molecule, as if only one *Tla* locus had been activated during leukemogenesis. In TL⁺ leukemias of TL⁺ mice, nonreciprocal blocking was also observed, but, in the opposite direction; TL antibody blocked H-2D sites, whereas H-2D antibody did not block TL sites. The appearance of unrecognized anomalous TL components could explain this result, although other possibilities can be envisioned. Thus, the blocking technique may prove useful in mapping other tumor antigens, including viral antigens, that appear as a consequence of malignancy.

With the recognition that many of the protein constituents of the plasma membrane are highly mobile and that their distribution can be selectively altered by the attachment of antibody, doubt has been cast on the significance of the associations revealed by the blocking test. However, we now know that the temperature at which the test is performed (0°C) minimizes antibody-induced surface changes and that

Table 13 Spatial relation of TL.1 and H-2D antigens on the surface of normal thymocytes and TL⁺ leukemia cells

Strain of origin (*Tla* haplotype)	Leukemia induction	Results of TL.1/H-2D blocking tests[a]	
		Normal thymocytes	Leukemia cells
C57BL (*Tla*^{b})	X-ray (ERLD)	−	TL.1 ⟵ H-2D
C57BL (*Tla*^{b})	X-ray	−	TL.1 ⟵ H-2D
AKR (*Tla*^{b})	Spontaneous	−	TL.1 ⟵ H-2D
A (*Tla*^{a})	Spontaneous (ASL1)	TL.1 ⟷ H-2D	TL.1 ⟶ H-2D
C57BL-TL⁺ (*Tla*^{a})	X-ray	TL.1 ⟷ H-2D	TL.1 ⟶ H-2D

[a] See Figure 1.

alloantigens, such as H-2 and Thy-1, in contrast to Ig and TL, undergo little surface rearrangement as a consequence of attached mouse antibody alone (77). Most important, a consistent pattern emerges from these blocking studies that indicates a preferential association of certain surface alloantigens which cannot be easily explained as an artifact of the technique. Clearly what is needed are other methods that can more directly assess the supramolecular organization of surface constituents on normal and malignant cells.

Preleukemic Expression of TL Antigens

Ever since the recognition of the TL system, it has been assumed that the anomalous appearance of TL antigen coincided with the transformation event and signaled the emergence of leukemia cells. However, the striking preleukemic changes in alloantigens and MuLV-related antigens in AKR thymus (51, 52) prompted us to examine this point directly in relation to X-ray leukemogenesis. In a study of C57BL mice that received fractionated whole body irradiation according to a schedule resulting in a high incidence of leukemia, TL⁺ cells were found in the thymus long before the development of overt leukemia (78). Thus TL should be considered a marker for preleukemic changes occurring in a population of cells at high risk for leukemia transformation.

TL and MuLV: Two Mechanisms of Leukemogenesis?

A comparison of the GCSA/G_{IX} phenotype and the TL phenotype of the leukemias that have now been studied (Table 7 and 10) distinguishes two major classes of mouse leukemia. One is exemplified by spontaneous leukemias of high incidence strains, such as AKR, which are primarily GCSA⁺/G_{IX}⁺/TL⁻ and the other by X-ray-induced leukemias of low incidence TL⁻ strains, such as C57BL, which are GCSA⁻/G_{IX}⁻/TL⁺. An important question for future investigation is whether this difference reflects two distinct pathways of T-cell leukemogenesis, one a direct or indirect consequence of MuLV and the other not involving MuLV. There has been speculation that the *Tla* locus may represent the integration site of a defective

MuLV genome (28), but this appears unlikely in view of the similar biochemical characteristics of the TL products and the products of the closely linked *H-2* genes (79). Another possibility is that the *Tla* locus is activitated by a special class of MuLV involved in X-ray leukemogenesis. The fact that most C57BL leukemias lack GCSA, G_{IX}, and other MuLV structural antigens as well as infectious MuLV speaks against this idea (78). However, there is growing evidence that MuLV appears transiently during the preleukemic phase of X-ray leukemogenesis, and it could be at this time that *Tla* activation by MuLV might occur. If a TL-inducing MuLV can be identified, the relation between the TL-class and the MuLV-class of mouse leukemias would be clarified. In this regard, the frequent occurrence of trisomy 15 in spontaneous AKR leukemias (80) and X-ray-induced C57BL leukemias (81) suggests a common genetic basis for these leukemias.

ML SURFACE ANTIGEN OF MOUSE LEUKEMIA

Recognition of the ML system came about during the study of spontaneous leukemias of DBA/2 mice (82). Antisera were prepared in histoincompatible mice and were absorbed in vivo to remove alloantibody. The absorbed antisera retained cytotoxic activity for the immunizing leukemia and other DBA/2 leukemias. Absorption tests revealed that the antigen could not be detected in spontaneous or induced leukemias of any other mouse strain but was found in normal mammary tissue and spontaneous mammary tumors of mice infected with the mammary tumor virus (MTV). This restriction of antigen to leukemias of DBA/2 mice and MTV-infected cells prompted the designation ML for mammary-leukemia. The classical mode of MTV transmission is through the milk of infected mothers, and this permitted a more direct approach to the relation of MTV to ML antigen (32). When newborn mice of MTV⁻ strains were foster nursed on MTV⁺ females, infection with MTV was accompanied by expression of ML in mammary tissue. Furthermore, in reciprocal crosses between MTV⁺ and MTV⁻ strains, the mammary tissue of (MTV⁺ X MTV⁻)F₁ mice was ML⁺/MTV⁺ and the mammary tissue of (MTV⁻ X MTV⁺)F₁ mice was ML⁻/MTV⁻, showing that maternal transmission of MTV led to ML antigen expression as well. Although there is little doubt that the ML antigen is coded directly or indirectly by MTV, the reason for ML appearance in DBA/2 leukemias is not clear. There are indications from molecular hybridization studies that genetic information related to MTV is present in all mouse strains (83), but that expression is restricted to certain strains (MTV⁺ strains) and in these strains to certain tissues. Occurrence of ML antigen in leukemia cells could represent derepression of MTV genetic information in malignant lymphoid cells, although this leaves unanswered why this should occur only in DBA/2 mice and, as recently reported, in GR mice (84). Another possibility is that these mice carry a variant leukemogenic virus that arose through genetic interaction with MTV. Biochemical definition of the ML antigen, its relation to MTV structural components, and analysis of oncornaviruses from ML⁺ leukemias should resolve some of these questions.

GENERAL COMMENTS

Several categories of surface antigens can now be recognized on mouse leukemia (Table 14). As leukemia has been the subject of the most intense scrutiny, we have a more comprehensive picture of the surface antigens of the leukemia cell and its normal counterpart, the thymocyte, than of any other cell type in the mouse. Serological study of nonlymphoid tumors of the mouse is at a very early stage and even rudimentary questions, such as expression of known alloantigens, have not been asked in relation to many classes of experimental cancer. Through the application of the serological techniques and approaches that have given us our present, albeit limited, view of surface antigens on leukemia cells, analysis of other tumor cell populations will undoubtedly uncover a large series of new differentiation alloantigens, as well as additional classes of tumor antigens that may have more immediate relevance to malignancy.

A diverse array of MuLV-related cell surface antigens has now been identified in mouse leukemia and there is every indication that the list will continue to grow. This complexity parallels comparable diversity of MuLV envelope antigens (85) and reflects the extensive MuLV polymorphism that has been recognized to exist in the mouse. None of the MuLV-related surface antigens can be considered to be transformation-specific, because they are also found on MuLV-infected cells that are not malignant. As it appears increasingly likely that cells transformed by avian and feline oncornaviruses express transformation-specific surface antigens that are unrelated to viral structural antigens (86, 87), search for this category of antigen on mouse leukemia needs to continue.

Knowledge of the TL and MuLV systems of antigens and the recognition that these antigens occur in leukemias and solid tumors of mice whose normal tissues do not express them have added considerable sophistication to our discussion of tumor-specific antigens and their genetic origin. They provide a secure basis for searching for other examples of distinctive tumor products that are determined by

Table 14   Categories of serologically demonstrable surface antigens on mouse leukemia

Conventional alloantigens	H-2D, H-2K
Differentiation alloantigens	Lyt-1,2,3,4, Thy-1, TL.1,2,3
MuLV-structural antigens	MuLV-gp70, p30, p15
MuLV-related antigens	GCSA, G_{IX}, X.1, $G_{(RADA1)}$, $G_{(ERLD)}$
Transformation-specific MuLV antigens	None defined
MTV-related antigens	ML
Derepression antigens	TL.1,2,4 (in TL$^-$ strains)
	GCSA, G_{IX}, $G_{(RADA1)}$, X.1 (in strains not expressing MuLV-related antigens in normal tissue)
Individually unique antigens	None defined
Species antigens	MSLA
Embryonic and fetal antigens	None defined

genes that are never expressed in normal life or expressed for only a limited period during some developmental phase. Much speculation has centered on the possibility that tumor-specific antigens may arise from derepressed fetal genes, but the evidence from transplantation and serological studies that has been presented to support this idea does not exclude other interpretations. For example, MuLV antigens, which are found so widely in mouse tumors, might be expressed during restricted periods of fetal development and so would mimic a fetal gene product. A serological definition of the surface antigens of embryonic and fetal cells will clarify such questions and permit us to know whether unique embryonic- or fetal-specific surface antigens not expressed by adult cells do in fact exist and, if so, whether these reappear on malignant cells. The analysis of mouse teratocarcinoma cells and preimplantation embryos shows much promise as a way to approach these important issues (88, 89).

Genes determining histocompatibility antigens, particularly those of the H-2 complex, have been considered another source of genetic information for tumor-specific antigens. Given the TL model, it is not difficult to imagine that structural genes for certain H-2 components are present in all mice but expressed in only some strains, and that anomalous appearance of H-2 antigens may occur as a consequence of malignancy. Suggestive evidence for this possibility comes from the study of chemically induced tumors, where immunization with normal tissues from an H-2 incompatible strain led to transplantation resistance against syngeneic tumor (90, 91). With the highly developed state of H-2 serology and biochemistry, identification of anomalous H-2 antigens on the tumor cell surface should be straightforward, and by analyzing a number of similarly but independently derived tumors, one could determine how frequently this phenotypic change occurs and whether a particular region of the H-2 complex is invariably involved.

The tumor antigens that have not as yet been defined serologically are the individually unique antigens that represent the classic tumor-specific transplantation antigens of cancer immunology (92). Since the discovery of these antigens in sarcomas induced by polycyclic hydrocarbons, individually distinct transplantation antigens have been detected in spontaneous mammary tumors (93, 94) and spontaneous reticulum cell sarcomas (95). The remarkable feature of these antigens is their polymorphism, even two tumors arising in the same inbred mouse being antigenically distinguishable. Their serological analysis is complicated by the frequent and unpredictable presence of MuLV and its antigens in these tumors, and past studies that did not take this fact into account are impossible to interpret. The genetic origin of these unique antigens in mouse tumors has been the subject of much discussion, and the commonly held view is that they represent the products of derepressed or mutated genes. Another possibility not involving genetic change relates their origin to a self-perpetuating phenotypic error in membrane synthesis or assembly (96). The view that they represent preexisting antigenic diversity in the normal cell population seems to have been excluded by the demonstration that transformed cell populations derived from the same clone have noncrossreacting antigenicity (97). Although antigens of this class have not been detected on leukemia cells, their presence may have been obscured by other systems of antigens, particularly those related to MuLV, and planned immunizations can now be devised to detect their existence.

Literature Cited

1. Old, L. J., Boyse, E. A. 1973. Current enigmas in cancer research. *Harvey Lect.* 67:273–315
2. Gorer, P. A., O'Gorman, P. 1956. The cytotoxic activity of isoantibodies in mice. *Transplant. Bull.* 3:142–43
3. Old, L. J., Boyse, E. A., Stockert, E. 1963. Antigenic properties of experimental leukemias. I. Serological studies *in vitro* with spontaneous and radiation-induced leukemias. *J. Natl. Cancer Inst.* 31:977–86
4. Old, L. J., Boyse, E. A., Stockert, E. 1965. The G (Gross) leukemia antigen. *Cancer Res.* 25:813–19
5. Old, L. J., Boyse, E. A., Lilly, F. 1963. Formation of cytotoxic antibody against leukemias induced by Friend virus. *Cancer Res.* 23:1063–68
6. Old, L. J., Boyse, E. A., Stockert, E. 1964. Typing of mouse leukemias by serological methods. *Nature* 201:777–79
7. Klein, E., Klein, G. 1964. Antigenic properties of lymphomas induced by the Moloney agent. *J. Natl. Cancer Inst.* 32:547–68
8. Geering, G., Old, L. J., Boyse, E. A. 1966. Antigens of leukemias induced by naturally occurring murine leukemia virus: Their relation to the antigens of Gross virus and other murine leukemia viruses. *J. Exp. Med.* 124:753–72
9. Stockert, E., Old, L. J., Boyse, E. A. 1971. The G$_{IX}$ System. A cell surface alloantigen associated with murine leukemia virus; implications regarding chromosomal integration of the viral genome. *J. Exp. Med.* 133:1334–55
10. Boyse, E. A., Stockert, E., Old, L. J. 1969. Properties of four antigens specified by the *Tla* locus: Similarities and differences. In *International Convocation on Immunology*, Buffalo, New York, ed. N.R. Rose, F. Milgrom, pp. 353–57. Basel & New York: Karger
11. Sato, H., Boyse, E. A., Aoki, T., Iritani, C., Old, L. J. 1973. Leukemia-associated transplantation antigens related to murine leukemia virus. *J. Exp. Med.* 138:593–606
12. Reif, A. E., Allen, J. M. V. 1964. The AKR thymic antigen and its distribution in leukemias and nervous tissues. *J. Exp. Med.* 120:413–33
13. Takahashi, T., Old, L. J., Boyse, E. A. 1970. Surface alloantigens of plasma cells. *J. Exp. Med.* 131:1325–41

14. Boyse, E. A., Miyazawa, M., Aoki, T., Old, L. J. 1968. Ly-A and Ly-B: Two systems of lymphocyte isoantigens in the mouse. *Proc. R. Soc. London Ser. B.* 170:175–93
15. Shen, F.-W., Boyse, E. A., Cantor, H. 1975. Preparation and use of Ly antisera. *Immunogenetics* 2:591–95
16. Shigeno, N., Arpels, C., Hämmerling, U., Boyse, E. A., Old, L. J. 1968. Preparation of lymphocyte-specific antibody from antilymphocyte serum. *Lancet* 2:320–23
17. Raff, M. C., Nase, S., Mitchison, N. A. 1971. Mouse-specific bone marrow-derived lymphocyte antigen as a marker for thymus-independent lymphocytes. *Nature* 230:50–51
18. Takahashi, T., Old, L. J., Hsu, C.-J., Boyse, E. A. 1971. A new differentiation antigen on plasma cells. *Eur. J. Immunol.* 1:478–82
19. Watanabe, T., Yagi, Y., Pressman, D. 1971. Antibody against neoplastic plasma cells. I. Specific surface antigens on mouse myeloma cells. *J. Immunol.* 106:1213–21
20. Gregoriades, A., Old, L. J. 1969. Isolation and some characteristics of a group-specific antigen of murine leukemia viruses. *Virology* 37:189–202
21. Strand, M., August, J. T. 1973. Structural proteins of oncogenic ribonucleic acid viruses. Interspec II, a new interspecies antigen. *J. Biol. Chem.* 248:5627–33
22. Fleissner, E., Ikeda, H., Tung, J.-S., Vitetta, E. S., Tress, E., Hardy, W. D. Jr., Stockert, E., Boyse, E. A., Pincus, T., O'Donnell, P. 1975. Characterization of murine leukemia virus-specific proteins. *Cold Spring Harbor Symp. Quant. Biol.* 39:1057–66
23. Hunsmann, G., Claviez, M., Moennig, V., Schwarz, H., Schäfer, W. 1976. Properties of mouse leukemia viruses. X. Occurrence of viral structural antigens on the cell surface as revealed by a cytotoxicity test. *Virology* 69:157–68
24. Aoki, T., Boyse, E. A., Old, L. J. 1966. Occurrence of natural antibody to the G (Gross) leukemia antigen in mice. *Cancer Res.* 26:1415–19
25. Hanna, M. G. Jr., Ihle, J. N., Batzing, B. L., Tennant, R. W., Schenley, C. K. 1975. Assessment of reactivities of natural antibodies to endogenous RNA tumor virus envelope antigens and virus-

induced cell surface antigens. *Cancer Res.* 35:164–71
26. Nowinski, R. C., Klein, P. A. 1975. Anomalous reactions of mouse alloantisera with cultured tumor cells. II. Cytotoxicity is caused by antibodies to leukemia viruses. *J. Immunol.* 115: 1261–68
27. Obata, Y., Stockert, E., Boyse, E. A., Tung, J.-S., Litman, G. W. 1976. Spontaneous autoimmunization to G_{IX} cell surface antigen in hybrid mice. *J. Exp. Med.* 144:533–42
28. Boyse, E. A., Old, L. J. 1969. Some aspects of normal and abnormal cell surface genetics. *Ann. Rev. Genet.* 3: 269–90
29. Rowe, W. P. 1977. Leukemia virus genomes in the chromosomal DNA of the mouse. *Harvey Lect.* 71: In press
30. Gross, L. 1951. "Spontaneous" leukemia developing in C3H mice following inoculation in infancy with AK leukemic extracts or AK embryos. *Proc. Soc. Exp. Biol. Med.* 76:27–32
31. Gross, L. 1970. In *Oncogenic Viruses.* Oxford, New York: Pergamon. 2nd ed
32. Old, L. J., Boyse, E. A. 1965. Antigens of tumors and leukemias induced by viruses. *Fed. Proc.* 24:1009–17
33. Geering, G., Aoki, T., Old, L. J. 1970. Shared viral antigen of mammalian leukemia viruses. *Nature* 226:265–66
34. Bolognesi, D. P. 1974. Structural components of RNA tumor viruses. *Adv. Virus Res.* 19:315–59
35. Slettenmark-Wahren, B., Klein, E. 1962. Cytotoxic and neutralization tests with serum and lymph node cells of isologous mice with induced resistance against Gross lymphomas. *Cancer Res.* 22:947–54
36. Nowinski, R. C., Old, L. J., Boyse, E. A., de Harven, E., Geering, G. 1968. Group-specific viral antigens in the milk and tissues of mice naturally infected with mammary tumor virus or Gross leukemia virus. *Virology* 34:617–29
37. Lilly, F., Pincus, T. 1973. Genetic control of murine viral leukemogenesis. *Adv. Cancer Res.* 17:231–77
38. Barnes, R. D., Tuffrey, M. A., Crewe, P., Dawson, L., Brown, K., Joyner, J. 1976. Levels of C-type viral p30 antigens in lymphoma-resistant mice. *Cancer Res.* 36:3622–24
39. Obata, Y., Ikeda, H., Stockert, E., Boyse, E. A. 1975. Relation of G_{IX} antigen of thymocytes to envelope glycoprotein of murine leukemia virus. *J. Exp. Med.* 141:188–97

40. Stockert, E., Sato, H., Itakura, K., Boyse, E. A., Old, L. J., Hutton, J. J. 1972. Location of the second gene required for expression of the leukemia-associated mouse antigen G_{IX}. *Science* 178:862–63
41. Ikeda, H., Stockert, E., Rowe, W. P., Boyse, E. A., Lilly, F., Sato, H., Jacobs, S., Old, L. J. 1973. Relation of chromosome 4 (linkage group VIII) to murine leukemia virus-associated antigens of AKR mice. *J. Exp. Med.* 137:1103–7
42. Ikeda, H., Rowe, W. P., Boyse, E. A., Stockert, E., Sato, H., Jacobs, S. 1976. Relationship of infectious murine leukemia virus and virus-related antigens in genetic crosses between AKR and the Fv-1 compatible strain C57L. *J. Exp. Med.* 143:32–46
43. Stockert, E., Boyse, E. A., Sato, H., Itakura, K. 1976. Heredity of the G_{IX} thymocyte antigen associated with murine leukemia virus: Segregation data simulating genetic linkage. *Proc. Natl. Acad. Sci. USA* 73:2077–81
44. Aoki, T., Boyse, E. A., Old, L. J., de Harven, E., Hämmerling, U., Wood, H. A. 1970. G (Gross) and H-2 cell surface antigens: Location on Gross leukemia cells by electron microscopy with visually labeled antibody. *Proc. Natl. Acad. Sci. USA* 65:569–76
45. Tung, J.-S., Vitetta, E. S., Fleissner, E., Boyse, E. A. 1975. Biochemical evidence linking the G_{IX} thymocyte surface antigen to the gp69/71 envelope glycoprotein of murine leukemia virus. *J. Exp. Med.* 141:198–205
46. Tung, J.-S., Yoshiki, T., Fleissner, E. 1976. A core polyprotein of murine leukemia virus on the surface of mouse leukemia cells. *Cell* 9:573–78
47. Snyder, H. W. Jr., Stockert, E., Fleissner, E. 1977. Characterization of molecular species carrying Gross cell surface antigen (GCSA). *J. Virol.* 23: 302–14
48. O'Donnell, P. V., Stockert, E. 1976. Induction of G_{IX} antigen and Gross cell surface antigen after infection by ecotropic and xenotropic murine leukemia viruses *in vitro. J. Virol.* 20:545–54
49. Hartley, J. W., Rowe, W. P. 1976. Naturally occurring murine leukemia viruses in wild mice: Characterization of a new "amphotropic" class. *J. Virol.* 19:19–25
50. Hartley, J. W., Wolford, N. K., Old, L. J., Rowe, W. P. 1977. A new class of murine leukemia virus associated with development of spontaneous lym-

phomas. *Proc. Natl. Acad. Sci. USA* 74:789–92

51. Kawashima, K., Ikeda, H., Stockert, E., Takahashi, T., Old, L. J. 1976. Age-related changes in cell surface antigens of preleukemic AKR thymocytes. *J. Exp. Med.* 144:193–208

52. Kawashima, K., Ikeda, H., Hartley, J. W., Stockert, E., Rowe, W. P., Old, L. J. 1976. Changes in expression of murine leukemia virus antigens and production of xenotropic virus in the late preleukemic period in AKR mice. *Proc. Natl. Acad. Sci. USA* 73:4680–84

53. Tung, J.-S., Shen, F.-W., Fleissner, E., Boyse, E. A. 1976. X-gp70: A third molecular species of the envelope protein gp70 of murine leukemia virus, expressed on mouse lymphoid cells. *J. Exp. Med.* 143:969–74

54. Strand, M., Lilly, F., August, J. T. 1974. Host control of endogenous murine leukemia virus gene expression: Concentrations of viral proteins in high and low leukemia mouse strains. *Proc. Natl. Acad. Sci. USA* 71:3682–86

55. Tung, J.-S., Fleissner, E., Vitetta, E. S., Boyse, E. A. 1975. Expression of murine leukemia virus envelope glycoprotein gp69/71 on mouse thymocytes: Evidence for two structural variants distinguished by presence versus absence of G_{IX} antigen. *J. Exp. Med.* 142:518–23

56. Herberman, R. B., Aoki, T. 1972. Immune and natural antibodies to syngeneic murine plasma cell tumors. *J. Exp. Med.* 136:94–111

57. Boyse, E. A., Old, L. J., Stockert, E. 1965. The TL (thymus leukemia) antigen: A review. In *Immunopathology, IV Int. Symp.*, ed. P. Grabar, P. A. Miescher, pp. 23–40. Basel: Schwabe

58. Boyse, E. A., Old, L. J., Luell, S. 1964. Genetic determination of the TL (thymus-leukemia) antigen in the mouse. *Nature* 201:779

59. Schlesinger, M. 1970. How cells acquire antigens. *Prog. Exp. Tumor Res.* 13:28–83

60. Boyse, E. A., Old, L. J. 1971. A comment on the genetic data relating to expression of TL antigens. *Transplantation* 11:561–62

61. Boyse, E. A., Flaherty, L., Stockert, E., Old, L. J. 1972. Histo-incompatibility attributable to genes near *H-2* that are not revealed by hemagglutination or cytotoxicity tests. *Transplantation* 13:431–32

62. Flaherty, L., Wachtel, S. S. 1975. *H(Tla)* System: Identification of two new loci *H-31* and *H-32,* and alleles. *Immunogenetics* 2:81–85

63. Stanton, T. H., Boyse, E. A. 1976. A new serologically defined locus, *Qa-1,* in the *Tla*-region of the mouse. *Immunogenetics* 3:525–31

64. Flaherty, L. 1976. The *Tla* region of the mouse: Identification of a new serologically defined locus, *Qa-2. Immunogenetics* 3:533–39

65. Boyse, E. A., Stockert, E., Old, L. J. 1968. Isoantigens of the *H-2* and *Tla* loci of the mouse. Interactions affecting their representation on thymocytes. *J. Exp. Med.* 128:85–95

66. Old, L. J., Stockert, E., Boyse, E. A., Kim, J. H. 1968. Antigenic modulation: Loss of TL antigen from cells exposed to TL antibody. Study of the phenomenon *in vitro. J. Exp. Med.* 127:523–39

67. Boyse, E. A., Old, L. J., Luell, S. 1963. Antigenic properties of experimental leukemias. II. Immunological studies *in vivo* with C57BL/6 radiation-induced leukemias. *J. Natl. Cancer Inst.* 31:987–95

68. Boyse, E. A., Stockert, E., Old, L. J. 1967. Modification of the antigenic structure of the cell membrane by thymus-leukemia (TL) antibody. *Proc. Natl. Acaa. Sci. USA* 58:954–57

69. Lamm, M. E., Boyse, E. A., Old, L. J., Lisowska-Bernstein, B., Stockert, E. 1968. Modulation of TL (thymus-leukemia) antigens by Fab-fragments of TL antibody. *J. Immunol.* 101:99–103

70. Stackpole, C. W., Jacobson, J. B. 1977. Antigenic modulation. In *Handbook of Cancer and Immunology,* ed. H. Waters, Vol. 1. New York: Garland. In press

71. Hyman, R., Stallings, V. 1976. Characterization of a TL⁻ variant of a homozygous TL⁺ mouse lymphoma. *Immunogenetics* 3:75–84

72. Boyse, E. A., Stockert, E., Iritani, C. A., Old, L. J. 1970. Implications of TL phenotype changes in an H-2-loss variant of a transplanted H-2ᵇ/H-2ᵃ leukemia. *Proc. Natl. Acad. Sci. USA* 65:933–38

73. Bjaring, B., Klein, G. 1968. Antigenic characterization of heterozygous mouse lymphomas after immunoselection *in vivo. J. Natl. Cancer Inst.* 41:1411–29

74. Hauschka, T. S., Hitt, S. A., Zumpft, M., Shows, T. B., Boyse, E. A. 1975. Immunoselective loss of parental H antigens by somatic reduction in an

H-2ᵃ/H-2ᵇ hybrid mouse leukemia. *Transplant Proc.* 7:165–71

75. Boyse, E. A., Old, L. J., Stockert, E. 1968. An approach to the mapping of antigens on the cell surface. *Proc. Natl. Acad. Sci. USA* 60:886–93

76. Hämmerling, U., Eggers, H. J. 1970. Quantitative measurement of uptake of alloantibody on mouse lymphocytes. *Eur. J. Biochem.* 17:95–99

77. Stackpole, C. W. 1977. Topographical differentiation of the cell surface. *Prog. Surf. Membr. Sci.* 12: In press

78. Stockert, E., Old, L. J. 1977. Preleukemic expression of TL antigens in X-irradiated C57BL/6 mice. *J. Exp. Med.* 146:271–76

79. Snell, G. D., Dausset, J., Nathenson, S. 1976. Biochemical and structural properties of the cell membrane located alloantigens of the major histocompatibility complex. In *Histocompatibility,* pp. 275–321. New York: Academic

80. Dofuku, R., Biedler, J. L., Spengler, B. A., Old, L. J. 1975. Trisomy of chromosome 15 in spontaneous leukemia of AKR mice. *Proc. Natl. Acad. Sci. USA* 72:1515–17

81. Chang, T. D., Biedler, J. L., Stockert, E., Old, L. J. 1977. Trisomy of chromosome 15 in X-ray-induced mouse leukemia. *Proc. Am. Assoc. Cancer Res.* 18: 225

82. Stück, B., Boyse, E. A., Old, L. J., Carswell, E. A. 1964. ML—A new antigen found in leukaemias and mammary tumours of the mouse. *Nature* 203: 1033–34

83. Varmus, H. E., Quintrell, N., Medeiros, E., Bishop, J. M., Nowinski, R. C., Sarkar, N. H. 1973. Transcription of mouse mammary tumor virus genes in tissues from high and low tumor incidence mouse strains. *J. Mol. Biol.* 79:663–79

84. Hilgers, J., Haverman, J., Nusse, R., van Blitterswijk, W. J., Cleton, F. J., Hageman, P. C., van Nie, R., Calafat, J. 1975. Immunologic, virologic and genetic aspects of mammary tumor-virus-induced cell surface antigens: Presence of these antigens and the Thy-1.2 antigen on murine mammary gland and tumor cells. *J. Natl. Cancer Inst.* 54: 1323–33

85. Aoki, T., Huebner, R. J., Chang, K. S. S., Sturm, M. M., Liu, M. 1974. Diversity of envelope antigens on murine type-C RNA viruses. *J. Natl. Cancer Inst.* 52:1189–97

86. Stephenson, J. R., Essex, M., Hino, S., Hardy, W. D. Jr., Aaronson, S. A. 1977. Feline oncornavirus-associated cell membrane antigen (FOCMA). VII. Distinction between FOCMA and the major virion glycoprotein. *Proc. Natl. Acad. Sci. USA* 74:1219–23

87. Rohrschneider, L. R., Kurth, R., Bauer, H. 1975. Biochemical characterization of tumor-specific cell surface antigens on avian oncornavirus transformed cells. *Virology* 66:481–91

88. Artzt, K., Bennett, D., Jacob, F. 1974. Primitive teratocarcinoma cells express a differentiation antigen specified by a gene at the T-locus in the mouse. *Proc. Natl. Acad. Sci. USA* 71:811–14

89. Jacob, F. 1977. Mouse teratocarcinoma and embryonic antigens. *Immunol. Rev.* 33:3–32

90. Martin, W. J., Gipson, T. G., Rice, J. M. 1977. H-2ᵃ-associated alloantigen expressed by several transplacentally-induced lung tumours of C3Hf mice. *Nature* 265:738–39

91. Parmiani, G., Invernizzi, G. 1975. Alien histocompatibility determinants on the cell surface of sarcomas induced by methylcholanthrene. I. *In vivo* studies. *Int. J. Cancer* 16:756–67

92. Old, L. J., Boyse, E. A. 1964. Immunology of experimental tumors. *Ann. Rev. Med.* 15:167–86

93. Vaage, J. 1968. Nonvirus-associated antigens in virus-induced mouse mammary tumors. *Cancer Res.* 28:2477–83

94. Morton, D. L., Miller, G. F., Wood, D. A. 1969. Demonstration of tumor-specific immunity against antigens unrelated to the mammary tumor virus in spontaneous mammary adenocarcinomas. *J. Natl. Cancer Inst.* 42:289–302

95. Carswell, E. A., Wanebo, H. J., Old, L. J., Boyse, E. A. 1970. Immunogenic properties of reticulum cell sarcomas of SJL/J mice. *J. Natl. Cancer Inst.* 44: 1281–88

96. Boyse, E. A., Old, L. J. 1970. The invitation to surveillance. In *Immune Surveillance,* ed. R. T. Smith, M. Landy, pp. 5–30. New York: Academic

97. Basombrio, M. A., Prehn, R. T. 1972. Antigenic diversity of tumors chemically induced within the progeny of a single cell. *Int. J. Cancer* 10:1–8

Ann. Rev. Med. 1979. 30:269–77

CONTROL OF THE IMMUNE SYSTEM BY INHIBITOR AND INDUCER T LYMPHOCYTES

♦7322

H. Cantor, M.D.

Department of Medicine, Harvard Medical School,
Boston, Massachusetts 02115

The field of immunology has its historical roots in clinical medicine. It grew directly out of modern medicine's greatest success: diagnosis and prevention of bacterial diseases, which began at the turn of the century. Since then the field has expanded enormously. Analysis of the immunologic system is now recognized as a distinct field of biology. Studies of the biochemical regulation of immunologic cells promise to be the key approach to understanding how genes work in mammalian cells. Nonetheless, the historical connection between immunology and clinical medicine has been maintained as well, perhaps more vigorously than in any other field of biology. There is a constant interchange among scientists doing "basic" immunologic research and those engaged in "applied" research who study the disease processes that ensue when the immune system malfunctions. Over the past ten years, an explosion of information from basic experimental studies has resulted in a entirely new view of the immune system that promises to have an important impact upon applied or clinical immunology. The following is a summary of some of these developments.

The important cells in the immune system are lymphocytes and macrophages. Macrophages line the tissues of the body, ingest foreign material, and present it to lymphocytes. Lymphocytes circulate freely through the blood and lymphatic vessels of the body and bear clonally distributed receptors for antigen. Lymphocytes are directly responsible for all specific immune responses. They are divisible into two sorts: (a) the T lymphocytes

0066-4219/79/0401-0269$01.00   269

(or T cells), so-called because their maturation requires processing in the thymus; and (*b*) the B lymphocytes (or B cells), which in mammals are probably generated mainly in bone marrow.

It should be emphasized that although the field of immunology began at the turn of the century, identification of the lymphocyte as the immunological cell was clearly established only 15–20 years ago. This means that cellular immunology is an extraordinarily young discipline, and a coherent view of the cellular basis of the immune response is only just beginning to emerge. Until recently, immunologists generally held that the immune system was comprised of clones of lymphocytes that, when activated by antigen, produced antibody or initiated a cell-mediated response (such as an inflammatory response). According to this view, the duration and strength of a response depended only on the number of lymphocyte clones in the host that carried receptors for a particular antigen, and the absence of immunity to "self" reflected deletion at birth of all lymphocytes bearing receptors for self-antigens.

Over the past decade, evidence refuting this view of the immune system has increased. More accurately described, the immune system is composed of many sets of regulatory lymphocytes that respond mainly to signals generated from within the system itself, and for the most part these interactions inhibit both antibody and cellular immune responses; these interactions also serve to prevent B lymphocytes from producing antibody against host antigens. In other words, the absence of autoimmune reactions may be, in part, due to continuous and active suppression rather than the absence of self-reactive cells within the system.

One approach supporting this view of the immune system involves the dissection and definition of T cells and the various immune functions they perform. Despite their uniform morphology, T cells are by no means a homogeneous population; they comprise subclasses or sets of lymphocytes with different and even seemingly opposing functions. Thus, one property of T cells, called helper function, is to assist B cells to make antibody. A second function of T cells was also suspected from investigations of immunologic tolerance or unresponsiveness. These studies indicated that the adoptive transfer of T lymphocytes from an animal unresponsive to a given antigen to a normal animal could render the recipient specifically unresponsive. This property of T cells, termed "suppressor" function, has been subsequently observed in a large number of immunologic experiments. It is likely that suppressor function is a necessary homeostatic control mechanism that keeps the immune system "in trim" and prevents untoward autoimmune reactions. Another property of T cells is the generation of cells capable of damaging or destroying those cells recognized as antigenically foreign after, for example, infection by a virus. This is associated with the cytotoxic or killer function of T cells. Yet another function of T cells involves inducement or activation of other cells to participate in inflammatory responses.

A crucial point arises: Are all these functions invested in a single set of T cells differentiated in the thymus, and are these diverse responses governed entirely by extraneous conditions such as a mode or type of antigen stimulation? Alternatively, are these immunologic functions invested in distinct sets of T cells programmed to respond in different ways during their differentiative history? According to this latter idea, thymus-dependent differentiation may give rise to a number of separate sublines of mature T cells, each genetically programmed to mediate one or another T-cell response.

In the mouse, this question has resolved itself into the practical problem of finding out whether it is possible to subdivide the T-cell population into different sets that, when confronted with antigens, are able to make only one or another of the possible T-cell responses. Presently, the most effective technique for identifying and separating subpopulations of peripheral T cells comes from studies of the cell surface components, which are expressed on cells undergoing thymus-dependent differentiation. This classification is based upon the use of alloantisera to define cell surface differentiation components expressed on T cells. Since these components have not been detected on cells of other tissues such as brain, kidney, liver, or epidermal cells, they are evidently specified by genes expressed exclusively during T-cell differentiation. These are called the Ly systems. The Ly1 component is coded for by a gene on chromosome 19, and the Ly2,3 components are both coded for by genes on chromosome 6. These last two are tentatively treated together because the two genes are tightly linked, and these two systems have not yet exhibited any differences other than the fact that they are genetically coded for by distinguishable loci.

In general, the approach involves a cytotoxicity assay similar to the complement-dependent hemolytic test used to identify markers on red cells. As with hemolysis by antierythrocyte antibody and complement, lymphocytes exposed to, say, anti-Ly1 sera in the presence of complement are lysed. This lysis can be monitored by the use of trypan blue, which stains lysed but not living cells, or by the release of a radioactive label from the lysed cells. More recently, these antisera to Ly1 or Ly2 components have been used to "positively" select cells bearing these components: Columns containing beads coated with anti-Ly1 or anti-Ly2 selectively retain lymphocytes expressing the relevant Ly surface component.

Analysis of this sort revealed that the peripheral T-cell pool contains at least three separate T-cell sets. We refer to them as the Ly123 set, the Ly1 set, and the Ly23 set. They compose respectively 50%, 30%, and approximately 10% of the peripheral T-cell pool. Thus, according to the criterion of selective expression of gene products on the cell surface, the T-cell pool is divisible into three groups of cells, each following a different set of genetic instructions. The question then becomes whether these individual differentiative programs include information that decides what the function of each T-cell set should be. Evidence to date indicates that cells of the Ly1 set are genetically programmed to help or amplify activity of other cells after stimulation by antigen. Ly1 cells are most aptly called "inducer" cells since they will induce or activate other cell sets to fulfill their respective genetic programs: Ly1 cells induce B cells to secrete antibody; they induce macrophages and monocytes to participate in delayed-type-hypersensitivity responses; they can, under appropriate circumstances, induce precursors of killer cells to differentiate to killer-effector cells; most recently, and perhaps most importantly, Ly1 cells were also found to induce a set of resting, nonimmune T cells to generate potent "feedback" suppressive activity. Analysis of isolated Ly1 inducer cells from nonimmune donors indicates that these cells are already programmed for helper/inducer function *before* overt immunization with antigen.

By contrast, cells of the Ly23 set are specially equipped both to develop alloreactive cytotoxic activity and to suppress humoral and cell-mediated immune responses. Whether cytotoxicity and suppression are two manifestations of one genetic program or whether they represent the phenotype of two separate genetic programs is not yet established.

It is of particular interest that both sets of T cells see antigen in the context of the host's own major histocompatibility (MHC) gene products. In other words, these T cells screen the host for "foreignness" as judged by alterations of their own MHC antigens as, for example, when these MHC products have been "modified" by association with a virus. Ly1 cells are selectively activated and bind to the so-called I-region products of the MHC, which correspond to HLA-D products in man. I-region products may be recognized as foreign because of either polymorphic variation (alloantigens) or modification by foreign antigens such as viruses. By contrast, Ly23 cells bind to and react against H2/KD gene products of the MHC which roughly correspond to HLA-A and B antigens in man.

Proof that these two cell sets, which are marked by different surface Ly phenotypes and different functional potentials, in fact represent two branches of thymus-directed differentiation comes from experiments in which isolated Ly1 cells and Ly23 cells are used to repopulate the lymphoid tissues of mice depleted of their T-cell system. These recipients lack detectable numbers of T cells and are called B mice. Recipients of Ly1 cells are called B-Ly1 mice and recipients of Ly23 cells are called B-Ly23 mice. For as long as we have observed them, B-Ly1 mice have been equipped for helper function but not killer function, and B-Ly23 mice have been equipped for primary killer function but not for helper function. These findings show that Ly1 and Ly23 cells have already exercised differentiative options that prevent them from giving rise to one another. In other words, these two T-cell sets belong to different lines of differentiation and are not sequential stages of a single progression.

Until recently cells of the Ly123 set have been the least well defined of the various T-cell sets. Most likely at least some Ly123 cells represent a store of receptor-positive intermediary cells that regulate the supply and function of more mature Ly1 and Ly23 cells. This is supported in part by experiments showing that (*a*) after stimulation with virus-infected syngenic cells, some Ly123 cells give rise to Ly23 progeny; and (*b*) purified populations of Ly123 cells can give rise to Ly1 cells after polyclonal activation by concanavalin A. That at least a portion of Ly123 cells represent a precursor pool is also consistent with earlier observations that cells of the Ly123 subclass are detectable in the spleens of mice within the first week of life, while neither Ly1 nor Ly23 cells reach maximal numbers until adult life (8–12 weeks of age).

More recently, it has been demonstrated that antigen-stimulated Ly1 cells, or supernatants of activated Ly1 cells, in addition to inducing B cells to secrete antibody, can induce or activate resting Ly123 T cells to develop profound feedback-suppressive activity. The term "feedback suppression" is appropriate here since the degree of suppressive activity exerted by a fixed number of nonimmune Ly123 cells increases in direct proportion to the numbers of antigen-activated Ly1 cells in the system. This Ly1:Ly123 interaction has also been shown to influence the immune response in vivo in mice and may well represent the central cell interaction that governs the duration and intensity of immune reactions. After stimulation of the immune system by foreign materials, activated antigen-specific Ly1 cells induce B cells to form antibody and also induce resting Ly123 cells to inhibit T-helper cell activity. Reduction in T-helper activity is accompanied by decreased induction of B cells as well as progressively decreasing induction of resting Ly123 cells; the net result is progressive decrease in both antibody formation and suppressor cell induction. These findings also indicate that, like the formation of antibody, the generation of immunologic suppression after stimulation by antigen is not an autonomous function; both require induction by Ly1 cells.

These negative feedback circuits suggest also that the response to any given antigen may reflect in part the amount of feedback inhibition generated after exposure to that antigen. The response to many antigens is regulated by MHC-linked genes: Each inbred strain of mouse will not respond to a certain proscribed list of antigens. In some cases, this lack of response reflects exaggerated induction of feedback-inhibitory cells that mask delivery of the T-helper signal to the B cell.

The ability of Ly1 inducer cells to activate various effector cell systems on the one hand, and suppressive systems on the other, is essential to the regulation of both the intensity and type of the immune response. It therefore has become critically important to know whether Ly1 cells that induce suppressive activity represent a specialized fraction of Ly1 cells. A direct approach to this question comes from the finding that some Ly1 cells also express a newly defined antigen called Qa1. This antigen, or antigen system, is coded for by genes that are closely linked to MHC genes of the mouse. Studies of $Ly1:Qa1^+$ cells show that these cells are responsible for induction of feedback inhibition and that $Ly1:Qa1^-$ cells are not. In addition, these studies show that signals from both $Ly1:Qa1^+$ and $Ly1:Qa1^-$ cells are required for optimal formation of antibody by B cells. Thus, the ability of antigenic determinants to induce a detectable antibody response may depend largely on the ratio of $Ly1:Qa1^+$ and $Ly1:Qa1^-$ T-cell clones that bear receptors for that antigen. Recent work also suggests that the ability of $Ly1:Qa1^+$ inducer cells to elicit strong suppressive responses is likely to be particularly important in governing the duration and intensity of inflammatory reactions such as delayed-type hypersensitivity and IgE-mediated hypersensitivity. Analysis of the cell-free products of homogeneous populations of $Ly1:Qa1^+$ cells is currently of intense interest since these materials may well prove useful in strategies designed to selectively suppress hypersensitivity or antibody responses to defined antigens.

This analysis indicates that perturbation of the immune system by antigen results in stimulation of two distinct inducer T-cell sets; both deliver signals that activate B cells to produce antibody, but only one activates the T-suppressive system, and it is the strength of this latter interaction that ultimately sets the level and the duration of an immune response.

In sum, these experiments established that (*a*) the genetic program for a single differentiated set of cells, in this case immunologic cells, combines information coding for a surface antigenic profile associated with particular physiologic functions; (*b*) the majority of T cells are not effector cells poised to respond to foreign antigen, but regulatory cells that respond mainly to signals or messages generated from within the T-cell system itself; and (*c*) detectable immune responses reflect perturbations of these signals after the Ly1 inducer system is stimulated by "antigen." The net effect of these T-T interactions after perturbation by antigen is to restore the homeostatic balance of the system, usually at a new level reflecting differentiation of antigen-specific T- and B-cell clones belonging to the sets described above.

We have just begun to delineate the circuits involved in the regulatory system summarized above. The picture beginning to emerge is that Ly1 cells act as sentinel cells that screen the surfaces of other cells, particularly macrophages, for foreign material associated with MHC molecules (Figure 1). When activated, these sentinel cells can induce a variety of effector cells

T CELL
REGULATORY NETWORK

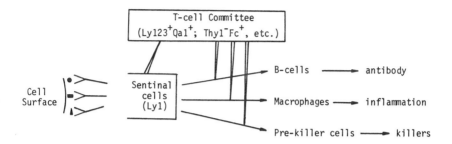

Figure 1   T-cell regulatory network.

(e.g. B cells that make antibody, or macrophages and monocytes that participate in inflammatory responses) to produce a specific immune response. In addition, they activate a "committee" of resting T cells that are probably relatively immature.[1] This committee of cells emits inhibitory signals. The intensity of inhibition depends mainly on the genetic background of the host, the nature of the antigenic stimulus, and the intensity of the inducing signal emitted by the sentinel cells. The observed immune response depends upon the relative potency and timing of feedback-suppressive inhibitory signals.

What happens when this system goes wrong? There are, so far, two examples of disorders of this immunoregulatory circuit. NZB mice spontaneously develop an autoimmune disorder characterized by the production of a variety of autoantibodies and a clinical syndrome resembling human systemic lupus erythematosus. The major T-cell deficit of NZB mice is the absence or malfunction of an Ly123 T-cell set responsible for feedback inhibition.

A second example comes from experiments in which Ly123 regulatory cells were deliberately eliminated from the host: Mice depleted of all T cells were repopulated with either Ly1 inducer cells or all T-cell sets (including Ly123 regulatory cells). Within the first two weeks after repopulation, sera from the former but not from the latter mice contained autoantibodies against erythrocytes and thymocytes. Thus, elimination of the regulatory T cells that participate in feedback inhibition results directly in the formation of autoantibodies.

[1]The term "committee" is used here because it is virtually certain that Ly123 cells are themselves a heterogeneous set, and perhaps not the sole members of this system. Moreover, the response of a committee is generally suppressive.

It should be emphasized that a number of critical questions remain to be answered. Are feedback-inhibitory interactions among T-cell sets responsible, in part, for self-tolerance beginning at birth? What is the molecular basis underlying communication among these T-cell sets? And, finally, how can we use this information to improve our understanding and treatment of autoimmune disorders in man?

Recent studies using antisera specific for subsets of human T lymphocytes revealed that human T cells are separable into sets of functionally distinct populations that so far appear analogous to those identified in mice. One set exerts suppressive activity, as judged by the ability of these cells to inhibit the in vitro production of immunoglobulin by human B cells. A second set of cells helps human B cells to secrete immunoglobulin. Recently, it was demonstrated that sera from children suffering from rheumatoid arthritis contain antibodies that selectively react with suppressor T cells found in normal individuals. Moreover, patients with active disease, but not those in remission, have high titers of antisuppressive cell antibody and lack T cells that suppress the in vitro production of immunoglobulin by B cells. Whether removal of suppressor T cells by this autoantibody plays a key role in the pathogenesis of this disease remains to be established. Selective dysfunction of T-suppressor activity was also reported in studies of patients with systemic lupus erythematosus, and there is reason to suspect that other major diseases such as multiple sclerosis, certain types of diabetes mellitus, and perhaps a subset of essential hypertension may reflect, in part, disorders of the immunoregulatory system.

No one can say with certainty whether these new insights into the workings of the immune system will have an important impact upon treatment of autoimmune disorders in man. Dissection of regulatory T-cell circuits is currently the subject of intense experimentation and debate. And perhaps this is the most hopeful and encouraging aspect of this new phase of immunobiology.

Selected References

Alter, B. J., Bach, F. H. 1974. Role of H-2 lymphocyte defined and serologically defined components in the generation of cytotoxic lymphocytes. *J. Exp. Med.* 140:1410

Bach, F. H., Bach, M. L., Sondel, P. M. 1976. Differential function of major histocompatibility complex antigens and T lymphocyte activation. *Nature* 259:273

Boyse, E. A., Old, L. J. 1969. Some aspects of normal and abnormal cell surface genetics. *Ann. Rev. Genet.* 3:269

Broder, S., Humphrey, R., Durm, M., Blackman, M., Meade, B., Goldman, C.,

Strober, W., Waldmann, T. A. 1975. Impaired synthesis of polyclonal immunoglobulins by circulating lymphocytes from patients with multiple myeloma. *N. Engl. J. Med.* 293:887

Chess, L., Schlossman, S. F. 1977. *Adv. Immunol.*, pp. 125–213

Cantor, H., Boyse, E. A. 1977. Regulation of cellular and humoral immunity by T-cell subclasses. In *Proc. 41st Cold Spring Harbor Symp. Origin of Lymphocyte Diversity,* Vol. XLI, p. 23. Cold Spring Harbor Lab., NY

Cantor, H., McVay-Boudreau, L., Hugenberger, J., Naidorf, K., Shen, F. W., Gershon, R. K. 1978. Immunoregulatory circuits among T-cell sets. II. Physiologic role of feedback inhibition in vivo: Absence in NZB mice. J. Exp. Med. 147:1116

Cantor, H., Weissman, I. 1976. Development and function of subpopulations of thymocytes and T cells. Prog. Allergy 20:1

Eardley, D. D., Hugenberger, J., McVay-Boudreau, L., Shen, F. W., Gershon, R. K., Cantor, H. 1978. Immunoregulatory circuits among T-cell sets. I. T-helper cells induce other T-cell sets to exert feedback inhibition. J. Exp. Med. 147:1106

Engleman, E. G., McMichael, A. J., Batey, M. E., McDevitt, H. O. 1978. A suppressor T cell of the mixed lymphocyte reaction in man specific for the stimulating alloantigen. J. Exp. Med. 147:137

Evans, R. L., Breard, J. M., Lazarus, H., Schlossman, S. F., Chess, L. 1977. Detection, isolation and functional characterization of two human T cell subclasses bearing unique differentiation antigens. J. Exp. Med. 145:2221

Evans, R. L., Lazarus, H., Penta, A. C., Schlossman, S. F. 1978. Two functionally distinct subpopulations of human T cells that collaborate in the generation of cytotoxic cells responsible for cell-mediated lympholysis. J. Immunol. 120:1423

Good, R. A. 1973. Immunodeficiency in developmental perspective. The Harvey Lecture Series 67, p. 1. New York: Academic

Gershon, R. K. 1974. T cell suppression. Contemp. Top. Immunobiol. 3:1

Möller, G., ed. 1977. Immunology and Differentiation. Immunologic Reviews #33. Copenhagen: Munksgaard. 145 pp.

Moretta, L., Ferrarini, M., Mingari, M. C., Moretta, A., Webb, S. R. 1976. Subpopulations of human T cells identified by receptors for immunoglobulins and mitogen responsiveness. J. Immunol. 117:2171

Paul, W. E., Benacerraf, B. 1977. Functional specificity of thymus dependent lymphocytes. Science 195:1293

Shou, L. S., Schwartz, A., Good, R. A. 1976. Suppressor cell activity after concanavalin A treatment of lymphoctyes from normal donors. J. Exp. Med. 143:1100

Shreffler, D., David, C. S. 1975. The H-2 major histocompatibility complex in the immune region. Adv. Immunol. 20:125

Stanton, T. H., Boyse, E. A. 1977. A new serologically defined locus, Qa1, in the TL-A region of the mouse. Immunogenetics 3:525

Strelkauskas, A. J., Schauf, V., Wilson, B. S., Chess, L., Schlossman, S. F. 1978. Isolation and characterization of naturally occurring subclasses of human peripheral blood T cells with regulatory functions. J. Immunol. 120:1278

Ann. Rev. Microbiol. 1979. 33:439–57

PERSPECTIVES ON THE ❖1762
IN VIVO LOCATION
OF CELLULAR INTERACTIONS
IN THE HUMORAL
IMMUNE RESPONSE

Judith Rae Lumb[1]

Department of Biology, Atlanta University, Atlanta, Georgia 30314

CONTENTS

[1]Recipient, Research Career Development Award, National Cancer Institute.

439

INTRODUCTION

The purpose of this review is to consider the available data on the structure and function of the lymphoid system to learn where cellular interactions in the humoral immune response occur in vivo. The questions currently receiving the most attention from immunologists are those that deal with the functions of lymphocyte subpopulations in the immune response. For example, thymus cells appear to have two opposing functions in the humoral response, either as helper cells or as suppressor cells. Most of this work involves in vitro experiments. It seems appropriate at this time to return to the whole animal and, using the knowledge gained by these in vitro experiments, to consider the location and mechanism of cellular interactions in vivo. To do this, the structure of the lymphoid tissue is described with regard to the location and pathways of migration of (a) antigen, (b) antibody, (c) antibody-forming cells, (d) memory cells, (e) suppressor cells, and (f) helper cells.

HISTOLOGICAL DESCRIPTION

Cells of the Lymphoid System

The following is a brief description of the cells found in lymphoid tissues (90, 124). For a more complete description, the reader is referred to the excellent volume by Weiss (156).

RETICULAR CELLS   The reticular meshwork of lymphoid tissues consists of reticular cells and the collagen-like fibers they produce. These cells are variable in shape, often showing long cytoplasmic processes. The meshwork is continuous with the trabeculae and the capsule, which form the border of the lobules and the entire lymphoid organ. Reticular cells are seldom phagocytic, although the dendritic reticular cells of the germinal centers and secondary follicles retain antigen on their surfaces (24). Veldman (149) described a reticular cell type with interdigitating processes that was found in the thymus-dependent area of the lymph nodes. The same pattern has been observed on the periarteriolar lymphatic sheath (PALS) of the spleen. In addition to the collagen-like fibers, elastic fibers are found throughout the reticular mesh. These fibers are thought to have some function in the maintenance of flow of lymph through the nodes and spleen.

MACROPHAGES   Phagocytic cells in the lymphoid tissues are either macrophages, if mobile, or histiocytes, if sessile. The relationship between reticular cells, macrophages, histiocytes, and blood monocytes is unclear. Occasionally the dendritic reticular cells of the follicles are referred to as dendritic histiocytes, because of their retention of antigen. Evidence indicates that the interdigitating cells in the thymus-dependent areas of the spleen and nodes are derived from mononuclear phagocytic cells (145). The distinctive features of all phagocytic cells are the presence of lysosomes and phagocytic vacuoles. The confusion concerning classification of these cells comes from their ability to transform from resting cells with few organelles to activated phagocytic cells with many organelles. The macrophages of the marginal zone and marginal sinus are distinguishable from the other macrophages by their ability to take up uncharged polysaccharides in contrast to acidic polysaccharides (59).

ENDOTHELIAL CELLS   Endothelial cells form the lymphatic and blood vessels. They bound a variety of vessels from the very thin lymphatics to the thick high endothelium postcapillary venules of the lymph nodes, across which cells migrate between the blood and lymph (3, 76, 109).

LYMPHOCYTES   Lymphocytes are cells with a large, round nucleus and little cytoplasm. They are known to carry specific immunologic information. Lymphocytes are divided into two lines according to their pattern of migration. T-lymphocytes migrate from the bone marrow through the thymus before populating the thymus-dependent areas of the lymphoid tissues. B-lymphocytes are cells that migrate through the Bursa of Fabricius in birds and are the precursors of the antibody-forming plasma cells. In mammals no bursal equivalent has been specifically identified, although several tissues associated with the digestive system have been suggested. These two populations of lymphocytes are distinguished by different surface markers. T-cells show θ antigen, whereas B-cells possess surface immunoglobulin. Morphological differences between these cells have been described (147); B-lymphocytes are said to be generally smaller, are more likely to show microvilli, and are more likely to have sphaeridia (nuclear bodies containing both DNA and RNA) than are the T-lymphocytes. Early scanning electron micrographs of human peripheral blood indicated that B-lymphocytes were covered with microvilli whereas T-lymphocytes had a smooth surface (106). However, it has become clear that the presence of microvilli relates instead to the activated state of the cell. Quiescent lymphocytes tend to have smooth surfaces (136). Lymphocytes also appear to withdraw their microvilli while passing through the endothelium of the postcapillary venules of lymphoid tissues (4, 10). Recent scanning electron micrographs reveal polyhedral-shaped cortical thymus lymphocytes and more rounded lymphocytes in the medulla of the thymus (10), and detailed surface morphology of bone marrow and spleen small lymphocytes (65).

LYMPHOBLASTS Lymphocytes, when stimulated with antigen or a mitogen, transform into blast cells that are larger than mature lymphocytes and stain with methyl green pyronin. These pyroninophilic cells are capable of rapid proliferation with a doubling time as low as 6 hr. These blasts may then differentiate into mature small lymphocytes, if they were derived from T-lymphocytes, or mature plasma cells or memory cells, if they were derived from B-lymphocytes.

PLASMA CELLS Plasma cells are the major antibody-producing cells. Therefore they are well equipped with a considerable amount of rough endoplasmic reticulum and a Golgi apparatus. Since plasma cells are derived from B-lymphocytes, which have very little cytoplasm, transitional cells appear that have varying amounts of cytoplasm that contain endoplasmic reticulum.

Spleen

The circulation of blood through the spleen has been known in detail for over 50 years (31, 67, 113–115, 121, 122). Blood is introduced into the spleen through the coeliac axis to the splenic artery, the trabecular arteries, the central arteries, and the pencillary arterioles. At this point it empties into capillaries that are somewhat porous and provide the border between the PALS and the marginal zone. The porosity of these capillaries allows some of the blood elements to be distributed through the marginal zone to the red pulp. The remaining blood is emptied into the red pulp at the end of the capillaries, which are associated with ellipsoids in some species (16). The blood then enters the venous sinusoids in the red pulp and proceeds through the pulp veins, the trabecular veins, the splenic vein and into the portal vein. Detailed descriptions of the ultrastructure of the vascular pathways have been provided by Weiss (152–156) and Kellner (66). Only the circulation pattern is relevant to the purpose of this review.

The entire pulp of the spleen is interlaced with reticular cells and the fibers produced by them. The fibrous tissue appears to be composed of fibrils similar to collagen fibrils (44, 88, 112, 153). Although the fibrous material appears to provide only an inert support matrix, the surface of reticular cells may be important in the immune response.

In addition to the reticular and vascular tissue, the red pulp contains all the cellular elements of the blood, including polymorphonuclear cells, macrophages, monocytes, plasma cells, lymphocytes, and large numbers of red blood cells. One of the main functions of the spleen appears to be the destruction and metabolism of defective red blood cells (89, 154). This function seems unrelated to the immune response and is not considered in this review. In addition, the red pulp contains a large number of macrophages and antibody-producing plasma cells. Since the red pulp is the area where the bulk of the blood enters the spleen, it is a logical place for a large concentration of antibody-producing and phagocytosing cells.

The white pulp of the spleen contains the majority of the lymphocytes and is highly organized. The PALS appears to be almost exclusively composed of T-cells, whereas the follicles are mostly composed of B-cells. Germinal centers are formed in the follicles during an immune response. Later sections review the evidence that germinal centers are the source of memory cells, and the evidence for the specific localization of T- and B-lymphocytes. The structure of the spleen is most dramatically shown in scanning electron micrographs (157).

Lymph Nodes

The following generalized description of lymph nodes disregards some differences between nodes such as the quantitative relationships between areas of cortex and medulla and sizes of the septa and sinuses (80). Lymph nodes basically function as filters in the line of lymph flow (34). As in the spleen, the supporting matrix is composed of reticular cells and reticular fibers (27, 33, 42, 86, 87, 124). Again, the surfaces of reticular cells appear to be important in the retention of antigen in the immune response. The lymph flows into the node from efferent vessels into the subcapsular sinuses. Early evidence indicates that the subcapsular sinuses are the only porous ones (35). Thus cells are able to migrate between the endothelial cells that form the subcapsular sinus wall to enter the cortex of the node. The lymph proceeds through the node into the medulla and exits via the medullary sinuses and the afferent lymphatic vessel. Blood is also circulated through lymph nodes. The blood flow is in the opposite direction to that of the lymph and it appears to be a completely closed circulation. However, there is evidence that fluid and cells are exchanged across the high endothelium of the postcapillary veins (3, 76, 109).

The parenchyma of lymph nodes is divided into cortex and medulla (87). In addition to the reticular tissue, the cortex contains mainly closely packed lymphocytes. Some are organized into follicles that are surrounded by a thin reticular cell process. Some of these follicles, especially during an immune response, contain areas of cellular proliferation called germinal centers. The evidence that the follicular cells are B-cells and the cortical cells outside organized follicles (parafollicular) are T-cells is presented later. In addition, macrophages are commonly found throughout the cortex.

In addition to the reticular elements, the medulla of the lymph node contains most of the plasma cells. These are often found in clusters associated with macrophages (124, 128).

Gut- and Bronchial-Associated Lymphoid Tissues

Throughout the epithelial tissue of the gastrointestinal tract, lymphocytes and plasma cells are found associated with the epithelium. Lymphocytes may constitute as much as 23% of the cells in the epithelium in the rabbit, or as little as 5% in rats (39). In addition, structures such as Peyer's Patches, the appendix, and the palatine tonsils contain lymphoid follicles and germinal centers similar to those in the spleen and lymph nodes. These structures also appear to be analogous to spleen and nodes in terms of the distribution of B-cells in follicles and T-cells in parafollicular areas (50, 63, 74, 93).

Similar lymphoid structures have been described in the bronchial epithelium (13, 14). As in the gut-associated lymphoid tissue, the bronchial epithelium includes follicular structures and parafollicular lymphocytes (110). It is supposed that the B- and T-cell localization is analogous to that in the other lymphoid tissue, although specific localization studies have not been done (12).

LYMPHOCYTE SUBPOPULATIONS

Distribution in Tissues

The parafollicular area of the lymph nodes and the PALS have been termed thymus dependent since it was first shown that these areas were depleted of lymphocytes in thymectomized animals (81, 103). This conclusion was supported by experiments in which the thymus cells were labeled in vivo and then detected later in lymphoid tissues (102, 158).

Specific cell surface markers such as θ antigen on T-cells have been used to localize these subpopulations in the lymphoid tissue by immunofluorescent techniques (47, 49). Although most of the earlier conclusions were supported by the immunofluorescent studies, two surprising observations were made. In addition to the localization of T-cells in the paracortical and medullary areas of the lymph nodes and PALS of the spleen, Gutman & Weissman (49) found a few cells in the central area of the germinal centers and occasionally in the primary follicles that stained with their anti-T serum. Gutman & Weissman (49) found very bright staining with anti-immunoglobulin in the germinal centers; in contrast, Goldschneider &

McGregor (47) found the germinal center lymphocytes did not stain with fluorescein-conjugated anti-immunoglobulin, but they did find staining of dendritic reticular cells. They attributed this to receptors for cytophilic antibodies on these cells rather than to specific staining. However, the staining pattern shown by Gutman & Weissman (49) appears circular, as if outlining lymphocytes, rather than reticular as one would expect if the dendritic reticular cells were nonspecifically absorbing the fluorescent antibody. An alternative explanation would be that the round cells staining were lymphocytes with Fc receptors. The inconsistencies between these two reports might be explained by differences in the specificity of the antiserum used. Further evidence for the localization of a few T-cells in the center of germinal centers is provided by the adherence of sheep red blood cells to a few cells in this location (64).

More recently, Veerman & van Ewijk (147) distinguished between the central portion of the PALS, which contains only very fine interdigitating reticular cells, and the peripheral portion, which contains reticular cells arranged in cylindrical shells. They concluded, on a morphological basis, that the central area contains T-lymphocytes only and the peripheral area contains T- and B-lymphocytes. They suggest that the distinctive reticular tissue in the central PALS and in the follicles plays a part in the specific homing of T- and B-cells to these areas.

In addition to the traditional categorization of lymphocytes as thymus-derived and bone marrow derived, these cells are also subdivided by functional markers. Dukor et al (36) have determined the localization of cells with complement (C'3) receptors by treating tissue sections with erythrocytes coated with antibody and complement under conditions where little hemolysis occurred. They found localization of sensitized erythrocytes only in the marginal zone and in the follicular areas, especially in active follicles. No binding of the sensitized erythrocytes occurred in the thymus-dependent areas of the spleen, nodes, or Peyer's Patches or in the thymus itself.

More recently, Christensen et al (26) have distinguished between cells that absorb unsensitized sheep erythrocytes (E), E coated with rabbit immunoglobulin (EA), E coated with immunoglobulin and complement 3d (EAC3d), and E coated with immunoglobulin and complement 3b (EAC3b). The cells that absorb E have the same distribution as T-cells. The cells that adsorb EA are presumed to have Fc receptors; these are evenly distributed throughout the splenic red and white pulp. The cells that adsorb EAC3d are exclusively lymphocytes outside the T-dependent area but near arterioles. EAC3b is adsorbed to these cells, and also to cells throughout the red pulp.

It is suggested that the cells with C'3 receptors are B-cells; they make up 20–40% of the lymphocytes in the spleen and 5–20% of the lymphocytes in the nodes (11). These percentages are similar to those found in the spleen and nodes on staining with anti-immunoglobulin serum (11, 47). Ultrastructural studies of the cells with C'3 receptors have revealed nuclear bodies, called sphaeridia, which contain both DNA and RNA (37, 129). These sphaeridia increase in number after immunization. In NZB mice in the presence of an autoimmune reaction, the number of cells with C'3 receptors decreases (6).

Migration Patterns

The route of migration of thoracic duct cells was studied by draining the thoracic duct cells, labeling them in vitro, and returning them to the thoracic duct (46). The results show that thymus cells migrate into the marginal sinus in the spleen, through the marginal zone, and into the PALS. T-cells appear to stay in the central PALS for at least 36 hr (91). B-cells also enter the spleen through the marginal sinus, the marginal zone, and the periphery of the PALS. Within 1–6 hr, the B-cells have moved to the lymphocyte corona in the follicular area. They are then distributed into the follicles (91). One can distinguish in both the B- and T-cell populations between long-lived, recirculating cells and short-lived, non-recirculating cells. It appears that in both populations the recirculating cells are the primed cells and the short-lived cells are the virgin cells (108, 111, 127). Evidence indicates that the cells of the germinal centers do not originate from the recirculating population, but are follicular cells (68). It seems that the follicles are storage points for memory cells produced in the germinal centers.

In an analysis of data from Ford (41), Hammond (53) calculated that 80% of the cells that entered the spleen migrated through within 5 min. The remaining lymphocytes were divided, approximately in half, between those that traversed the red pulp in 2.3 hr and those that crossed the marginal zone in 50 min and then spent an average of 4.6 hr in the white pulp. Presumably the cells entering the white pulp would be divided between those thymus-derived cells that migrate through to the central portion of the PALS and those that migrate through the follicles. These data include the total population of lymphocytes in the spleen. Sainte-Marie (120) has recently studied the differential traffic of B- and T-cells through a rat lymph node and found that T-cells traversed the node much more rapidly than did B-cells. Lymphocyte traffic is also radically altered by the presence of antigen. Antigen-specific memory cells (107) and bone marrow cells (17) accumulate in the draining lymph node (131). One can remove the regional node and get a significantly reduced antibody response (40). This specific trapping may be inhibited by pretreatment of the cells with concanavalin A, but no correlation occurs between the binding of concanavalin A by particular cells and the trapping of those cells (118). Inflammation of the peritoneal cavity causes a tremendous change in the lymphocyte traffic (23). For more detailed considerations of lymphocyte movement, the reader is referred to reviews by Ford (41) and Bell (9).

LOCALIZATION OF THE HUMORAL IMMUNE RESPONSE

Lymphoid Tissue Change

Dramatic changes occur in the spleen and lymph nodes during a humoral immune response. In the first 24 hr after administration of antigen, the existing germinal centers become disorganized, reticular cells in those areas proliferate, numerous mitotic figures appear throughout the white pulp, the number of large lymphocytes increases, capillaries and postcapillary venules enlarge, the number of tingible bodies in macrophages (phagocytosed cells being degraded) increases, and the cells in the marginal zone appear swollen (29, 58, 88, 105, 106). After the initial disorganization, the number and size of organized germinal centers progressively increase until at about 9 days the volume of germinal center area reaches a peak of approximately four times that of the unstimulated control (55). Cellular proliferation in the lymph nodes and spleen continues for about 10 days, after which it declines (88). The histological change that correlates best with the peak of detectable serum antibody is the proliferation of plasma cell blasts in the red pulp and marginal zone of the spleen and the medulla and the corticomedullary border of the nodes (29, 71, 133).

Formation of Germinal Centers

It has been clear for some time that germinal centers develop in the spleen and lymph nodes in relation to antigen deposits (83). Hanna (55) studied the role of germinal centers in the immune response in detail. He found that the germinal center can be considered to have two sections: In one, cells divide with a generation time of 5 to 7 hr; in the other, cells divide at a rate similar to the rest of the lymphocytic population in the spleen (every 9 to 10 hr). He suggested that the cells in the rapidly dividing section are precursor cells that migrate through the other section to the rest of the spleen.

Immediately following antigen injection, an increase in volume and number of germinal centers occurred. This was followed by a dissociation of the centers in the first 24 hr, and by subsequent recovery of germinal center number and volume, exceeding the control values, by 4 days following injection.

Several studies have been performed to determine the role of germinal centers in the immune response. Hanna et al (56) showed that early germinal centers are specific for the localization of one antigen. Several workers have suggested that the cells being produced in the germinal center are memory B-cells and that the center therefore is required for the secondary response (56, 61, 150, 151). Buerki et al (21) have shown specifically that the cells produced in the germinal center are not likely to be directly involved in antibody production, because no correlation occurs between the production of cells in the germinal center and the serum levels of antibody. Alternatively, they suggest that the proliferation of cells in the marginal zone and red pulp correlates in time with the levels of antibody in the circulation. This supports the suggestion that the cells produced in the germinal center are memory cells, derived from B-lymphocytes, which then migrate into the circulation to be stimulated on a second encounter with the same antigen. These conclusions are supported by the work of Nieuwenhuis & Keuning (92), who have followed the migration and capabilities of cells leaving germinal centers. They found that these cells migrate through the mantle, which was referred to as the thinly populated area by Hanna (55), into the marginal zone and then join the recirculating population of B-cells. These cells are destined to become plasmablasts following antigenic stimulation with the same antigen.

Germinal center cells do not appear to comprise a single clone, because in the same center exist cells that make different classes of immunoglobulins with different classes of light chains (25, 104). In contrast, Burton & Buffe (22) have shown only one L chain and one H chain type in each germinal center.

Although the cells in germinal centers are probably B-cells, the formation of the centers depends on thymus function. Thus, they are rare in neonatally thymectomized, irradiated, bone marrow-reconstituted mice (159). In addition, germinal centers occur in immunized or unimmunized nude mice only when they have been reconstituted with thymus cells (60, 85, 125). In a study designed to determine the precursor cell of the germinal center, it was shown that bone marrow cells would initiate a center, but only if T-cells were available (45). Since thymus function is required for immunoglobulin (Ig)G synthesis (48), it is understandable that in breaking tolerance, germinal center formation is correlated with the recovery of IgG synthesis and not with IgM synthesis (135). It has also been shown that germinal center formation requires histocompatibility between the cells involved (134). Hence, it has been concluded that germinal centers result from the interaction between histocompatible thymus-derived cells or their soluble products and memory B-cells, and that the proliferating cell in the germinal center is the activated memory B-cell.

Antigen

The initial localization of antigen depends upon the route of injection (28). For example, following a subcutaneous injection, the amount of antigen in the draining lymph node is 10 times that in the aortic lymph node and 100 times that in the spleen (1). The antigen is first found in the medulla and subcapsular sinus histiocytes of the draining node (1, 2, 8).

In a primary exposure to antigen it generally stays in the medulla for about 7 days until antigen-antibody complexes are found in the circulation (30, 77, 78, 95, 97). Then the antigen becomes localized in the follicles (8, 30, 96). During a secondary response, the localization of antigen in the follicles occurs by 4–6 hr (2, 8, 57). The antigen appears first on the outer edge of the follicle and moves to the center. It is ultimately localized on the surface of dendritic histiocytes in the center of the follicles where it remains for a long time (84, 98, 161). During this period the antigen remains functionally antigenic if transferred to another system (132). These follicles often become germinal centers that show a high level of cellular proliferation at their centers.

When antigen is injected intravenously, it localizes mainly in the spleen. The pattern of localization in this organ is similar to that in lymph nodes. The antigen is first found in the red pulp and marginal zone (99, 117). In the primary response the antigen becomes localized in the cap of the germinal center by 7 days (99), but during a secondary response antigen has been observed in germinal centers as early as 6 hr after injection (8). Rodak (116) found antigen localization in follicles at 2 hr after a secondary immunization.

Additional evidence that lymphocytes are involved in antigen trapping comes from experiments in which isotopically labeled antigen-antibody complexes were injected intravenously (144). The complexes were found in the marginal zone in heavily labeled cells within 30 min following injection. These cells progressively lost their label, but they remained in the marginal zone over the next hour and a half while heavily labeled cells appeared in periphery of the follicles. Electron microscopy showed the labeled antigen to be associated with lymphocytes at this stage (148). During the next week a migration of the label from the periphery to the center of the follicle was observed. It was suggested that this migration within the follicle occurs on the surface of dendritic reticular cells, and that new dendritic cells appear at the periphery to replace those that migrated with antigen-antibody complexes to the center of the follicle (144).

Salmonella endotoxin, a thymus-independent antigen, causes the B-cells to migrate from the marginal zone into the follicles (146). When the same antigen is injected prior to the administration of labeled antigen-antibody complex, the follicular trapping is inhibited (143). This inhibition cannot be reversed by increasing the amount of labeled complex administered (142).

The localization of antigen in the center of germinal centers is correlated with the immune response. Non-immunogenic substances are cleared completely from the lymph nodes and spleen without any evidence of follicular localization (2, 83). The only exception is the fact that homologous immunoglobulin shows follicular localization. The reason for this is probably related to its role as antibody rather than to antigen localization.

Results are contradictory concerning whether or not antigen becomes localized in germinal centers in the tolerized animal. Early work (1) indicated some localization of flagellin in germinal centers when tolerance had been previously induced. However, White et al (162) found that repeated injections of human serum albumin, which induced tolerance, was not followed by germinal center localization of the antigen. More recently, Vainio, Viljanen & Toivanen (135) showed a complete correlation between tolerance to bovine serum albumin and the absence of germinal centers. As tolerance was broken, the germinal centers reappeared.

Antigen localization in germinal centers depends on the presence of (*a*) specific antibody (8, 138, 162), (*b*) complement (C'3) (43), and (*c*) cells with receptors for either the Fc portion of the antibody or for the C'3 (19, 139). van Rooijen (141) concluded that another cell beside the dendritic histiocyte was responsible for the migration of antigen into the follicle, because his experiments showed exactly the same localization of the same antigen labeled with two different isotopes and given at 2-week intervals. He suggested that this additional cell is a lymphocyte on the basis of an autoradiographic and ultrastructural study. This revealed lymphocytes containing labeled antigen; the arrangement of the uropods of these cells suggested that the direction of migration was toward the follicle (148). B-lymphocytes are probably the cells concerned, since the phenomenon is not interfered with by neonatal thymectomy, antilymphocyte serum treatment, or irradiation combined with bone marrow reconstitution (62). These cells must have receptors for either the antibody-antigen complex or the antigen-antibody-complement complex. However, it was noted that specific antibody was not localized in the same cell with the antigen (77). It has also been observed that one cell may bind more than one antigen (32, 140).

Jesus et al (62) and Brown et al (18) have used heat-aggregated human gamma-globulin to study antigen trapping. They concluded that the cells involved are cells with receptors for the Fc portion of antibody which has undergone a conformational change by combining with antigen or by heat aggregation. However, the immunologic significance of cells with Fc receptors has been questioned (119). Other workers have suggested that the cells become involved through their C'3 receptor (43, 101). Both techniques may be measuring the same phenomenon, that of uptake of an antigen-antibody-complement complex.

Antibody and Antibody-Secreting Cells

Antibody synthesis is first found in the lymph node draining the site of antigen administration (126). Antibody has been noted in the germinal centers of lymph nodes and the spleen since the advent of fluorescent antibody techniques (73, 100, 160). However, it is now clear that the immunoglobulin localized on the dendritic cells in the germinal centers is not synthesized there. Intracellular antibody is first seen in isolated cisternae of the endoplasmic reticulum of a few plasma cells located in the red pulp of the spleen and the medulla of lymph nodes (30, 69, 160). As long as 10 months after a single antigen injection, mature plasma cells with specific antibody still persist in the lymph nodes (70).

The possibility that these cells might be multipurpose plasma cells that provide early antibody with low avidity for a number of different antigens appears to have been missed in interpretation of the immune response in vivo. A related phenomenon is the increase in synthesis of immunoglobulin that has no specific antibody activity during the primary response (5). This synthesis of nonspecific immunoglobulin occurs only in the primary immune response, is unrelated to the adjuvant used, and is produced in proportion to the amount of primary antigen administered. There is no interaction of that immunoglobulin with the antigen.

Antibody is next seen in the perinuclear space in plasmablasts located in the germinal centers and marginal zone (117). As these cells mature, antibody is found in all the cisternae of the endoplasmic reticulum (69, 123). The peak of antibody in the circulation is coincident with the peak of plasma cell proliferation in the marginal zone (21, 72, 117, 133). Langevoort (71) observed plasmablasts also in the PALS within 24 hr after the administration of antigen. Later these cells were observed in the periphery of the PALS. Since Veerman & van Ewijk (147) identified the periphery of the PALS as having both T- and B-lymphocytes, it is suggested that this area is one where T-B cellular interactions may take place.

To determine the tissue specificity of synthesis of different immunoglobulin classes, Brown & Bourne (20) have localized cells containing IgG, IgA, and IgM in the alimentary tract, spleen, and mesenteric lymph node of the pig. All three classes of immunoglobulin were found in mature plasma cells throughout the lamina propria of the alimentary tract in large numbers. IgM- and IgA-containing plasma cells usually outnumbered IgG-containing plasma cells. All three classes of immunoglobulin were found in the red pulp and peripheral white pulp areas of the spleen, but these cells were usually lymphoblasts or transitional cells rather than mature plasma cells. Immature cells were also stained in the mesenteric lymph nodes. There were approximately equal numbers of cells staining with each of the antisera. These cells often occurred as clusters in the subtrabecular sinuses and also at the periphery of germinal centers.

Evidence for Cellular Interactions

Aronson (7) showed evidence of cellular interactions during an immune response when he demonstrated the transfer of bacille Calmette-Guérin between histiocytes in vitro. This transfer appeared to take place in long cytoplasmic bridges that contained label when the bacteria had previously been treated with [^{3}H]uridine. Cell clusters have also been observed during in vitro immune responses. Hanitin & Cline (54) observed clusters containing macrophages and lymphocytes in the presence of purified protein derivative of the turbercle bacillus. Blastogenesis appeared to be occurring among lymphocytes associated with macrophages and antigen in these clusters. Similarly, McIntyre et al (79) observed blast cells in clusters with macrophages and either small lymphocytes or plasma cells in an in vitro humoral response against sheep red blood cells. Clusters that included plasma cells, lymphoblasts, and macrophages were hemolytic against the antigen whereas clusters that contained small lymphocytes instead of plasma cells were nonhemolytic. The number of hemolytic clusters increased with time during the immune response, while the numbers of nonhemolytic clusters decreased. Electron micrographs of these clusters show junctional formations such as desmosomes between the cells of the clusters.

As early as 1960, cellular interactions were observed during in vivo immune responses. In an ultrastructural study, Sorenson (124) noted that macrophages in the medulla of the responding rabbit popliteal lymph node were surrounded by plasma cells. He suggested that a transfer of material occurs between the macrophage and plasma cell. Later it was found that in immunized animals macrophages that had taken up antigen were in the center of clusters of plasma cells that were producing specific antibody (69, 82). Farr & de Bruyn (38) compared the clusters formed in vivo with those found in vitro. They showed that macrophages attached to the trabeculae in the lumen of lymphatic sinuses form clusters with lymphocytes. This provides considerably more cell contact in vivo than is seen in clusters formed in vitro.

In thymus-dependent areas, cellular interactions have also been shown. In the paracortex of rabbit lymph nodes, mononuclear phagocytic cells with long, narrow processes have been demonstrated (149). These "interdigitating cells" seem to be in contact with lymphoblasts. Small finger-like projections extend from the lymphoblast, making indentations in the membrane of the interdigitating cells (137). Also in tuberculous lesions, lymphoblastic cells in mitosis were those surrounding epithelial cells (75). Thus, microscopy has shown not only that cellular interactions exist in vivo, but that these interactions are associated with immunologic functions such as blastogenesis or antibody synthesis.

CONCLUSIONS

Table 1 summarizes the basic events of the humoral immune response and their proposed in vivo locations. As antigen circulates, it first encounters the immune system in the blood or the lymph. The antigen in the blood is filtered through the spleen where it enters the red pulp. The antigen in the lymph enters the medulla of the lymp node. In the medulla of the node or the red pulp of the spleen, the antigen encounters any specific antibody that is already being synthesized. Complexes are then formed between the antigen, specific antibody, and complement. The pathway of migration of the antigen and lymphocytes through the organs takes them through the cortico-medullary border of the lymph nodes and the marginal zone of the

Table 1   Location of humoral immune functions in lymphoid tissues

Function	Compartment	
	Lymph node	Spleen
Primary immune response		
Macrophage processing	medulla	
T-cell/B-cell/macrophage	cortico-medullary	marginal zone,
interactions	border	periphery of PALS
Plasmablast proliferation	cortico-medullary	marginal zone,
	border	periphery of PALS
Antibody synthesis	medulla	red pulp
B-memory cell differentiation	mantle layer	mantle layer
Secondary immune response		
B-cell storage	primary follicle	primary follicle
T-cell storage	paracortical	PALS
Activated B-cell proliferation	germinal center	germinal center
Activated T-cell proliferation	paracortical	PALS
T-cell/B-cell/macrophage	cortico-medullary	marginal zone,
interaction	border	periphery of PALS
Antibody synthesis	medulla	red pulp

spleen where interactions probably take place. The antigen is then trapped on the dendritic cells of the follicles, and presumably, T-cells migrate to the PALS of the spleen and the parafollicular area of the lymph nodes. B-memory cells migrate to and proliferate in the germinal centers, and plasmablasts proliferate and migrate to the red pulp of the spleen and medulla of the lymph node, where they mature into plasma cells. Thus, antibody is produced in the red pulp and medulla where the antigen is first introduced into the spleen and lymph nodes.

This is merely a best-guess general description of the location of the humoral immune process. The separate locations of helper and suppressor T-cells have not yet been determined, the details of T-cell/B-cell/macrophage interactions are not at all clear, and the details of the processing of antigens have not yet been determined. As these aspects of the immune response are revealed, this generalized description should become more specific.

ACKNOWLEDGMENT

I wish to acknowledge the help of George Bell, Alan Perelson, and Byron Goldstein in the preparation of this review.

Literature Cited

1. Ada, G. L., Nossal, G. J. V., Pye, J. 1964. *Aust. J. Exp. Biol. Med. Sci.* 42:295–310
2. Ada, G. L., Nossal, G. J. V., Pye, J. 1964. *Aust. J. Exp. Biol. Med. Sci.* 42:267–82
3. Anderson, A. O., Anderson, N. D. 1975. *Am. J. Pathol.* 80:387–418
4. Anderson, A. O., Anderson, N. D. 1976. *Immunology* 31:731–48
5. Antoine, J. C., Avrameas, S. 1976. *Immunology* 30:537–47
6. Arnaiz-Villena, A., Sheldon, P. 1975. *Immunology* 29:1103–10
7. Aronson, M. 1963. *J. Exp. Med.* 118:1083–88
8. Balfour, B. M., Humphrey, J. H. 1967. In *Germinal Centers in Immune Responses,* ed. H. Cottier, R. Schindler, C. C. Congdon, pp. 80–85. New York: Springer-Verlag
9. Bell, G. I. 1977. In *Theoretical Immunology,* ed G. I. Bell, A. Perlson. New York: Marcel Dekker
10. Bhalla, D. K., Karnovsky, M. J. 1978. *Anat. Rec.* 191:203–20
11. Bianco, C., Patrick, R., Nussenzweig, V. 1970. *J. Exp. Med.* 132:702–20
12. Bienenstock, J., Clancy, F. L., Percy, D. Y. E. 1976. In *Immunological and In-fectious Reactions in the Lung,* ed. C. H. Kirkpatrick, H. Y. Reynolds. New York: Marcel Dekker
13. Bienenstock, J., Johnston, N., Percy, D. Y. E. 1973. *Lab. Invest.* 28:686
14. Bienenstock, J., Johnston, N., Percy, D. Y. E. 1973. *Lab. Invest.* 28:693
15. Deleted in proof
16. Blaustein, A. 1963. *The Spleen.* New York: McGraw-Hill
17. Brahim, F., Osmond, D. G. 1976. *Clin. Exp. Immunol.* 24:515–26
18. Brown, J. C., de Jesus, D. G., Holborow, E. J., Harris, G. 1970. *Nature* 228:367–69
19. Brown, J. C., Harris, G., Papamichail, M., Sljivic, V. S., Holborow, E. J. 1973. *Immunology* 24:955–68
20. Brown, P. J., Bourne, F. J. 1976. *Am. J. Vet. Res.* 37:9–13
21. Buerki, H., Cottier, H., Hess, M. W., Laissue, J., Stoner, R. D. 1974. *J. Immonol.* 112:1961–70
22. Burtin, P., Buffe, D. 1967. In *Germinal Centers in Immune Responses,* ed. H. Cottier, R. Schindler, C. C. Congdon, pp. 10–25. New York: Springer-Verlag
23. Catanzaro, P. J., Agniel, L. D., Hogrefe, W. R., Phillips, S. M. 1978. *J. Reticuloendothel. Soc.* 23:459–68

24. Chen, L. L., Adams, J. C., Steinman, R. M. 1978. *J. Cell Biol.* 77:148–64
25. Chiappino, G., Pernis, B. 1964. *Pathol. Microbiol.* 27:8–15
26. Christensen, B. E., Jonsson, V., Matre, R., Tonder, O. 1978. *Scand. J. Haematol.* 20:246–57
27. Clark, S. L. 1962. *Am. J. Anat.* 110:217–57
28. Cohen, S., Vassalli, P., McCluskey, R. T., Benacerraf, B. 1966. *Lab. Invest.* 15:1143–55
29. Congdon, C. C., Makinodan, T. 1961. *Am. J. Pathol.* 39:697–709
30. Coons, A. H., McCluskey, R. T. 1971. *Prog. Immunol. 1st Int. Cong. Immunol.,* ed. B. Amos, pp. 1523–25
31. Dameshek, W., Estren, S. 1947. *The Spleen and Hypersplenism.* New York: Grune & Stratton
32. DeLuca, D., Miller, A., Sercarz, E. 1975. *Cell. Immunol.* 18:255–73
33. Downey, H. 1922. *Haematology* 3: 431–68
34. Drinker, C. K., Field, M. E., Ward, H. K. 1934. *J. Exp. Med.* 59:393–405
35. Drinker, C. K., Wislocki, G. B., Field, M. E. 1933. *Anat. Rec.* 56:261–74
36. Dukor, P., Bianco, C., Nussenzweig, V. 1970. *Proc. Natl. Acad. Sci. USA* 67:991–97
37. Dukor, P., Dietrich, F. M., Suter, E., Probst, H. 1973. In *Advances in Experimental Biology and Medicine,* ed. B. D. Jancovic, K. Isakovic. New York: Plenum
38. Farr, A. G., de Bruyn, P. P. H. 1975. *Am. J. Anat.* 144:209–32
39. Eichlelius, K. E., Finstad, J., Good, R. A. 1969. *Int. Arch. Allergy Appl. Immunol.* 35:119–33
40. Fontalin, L. N. 1962. *B. Eksp. Biol. Med.* 54:81–84
41. Ford, W. L. 1975. *Prog. Allergy* 19:1–59
42. Fresen, O., Wellensiek, H. J. 1959. *Verh. Duetsch. Ges. Pathol.* 42:353–63
43. Gajl-Peczalsko, K. J., Fish, A. J., Meuwissen, H. J., Frommel, D., Good, R. A. 1969. *J. Exp. Med.* 130:1367–93
44. Galindo, B., Freeman, J. A. 1963. *Anat. Rec.* 147:25–41
45. Gastkemper, N. A., Wubbena, A. S., Nieuwenhuis, P. 1978. *Z. Immunitaetsforsch. Allerg. Klin. Immunol.* 154: 314–15
46. Goldschneider, I., McGregor, D. D. 1968. *J. Exp. Med.* 127:155–68
47. Goldschneider, I., McGregor, D. D. 1973. *J. Exp. Med.* 138:1443–65
48. Grumet, F. C., Mitchell, G. F., McDevitt, H. O. 1971. *Ann. NY Acad. Sci.* 190:170–77
49. Gutman, G. A., Weissman, I. L. 1972. *Immunology* 23:465–79
50. Guy-Grand, D., Gricelli, C., Vassalli, P. 1974. *Eur. J. Immunol.* 4:435–43
51. Deleted in proof
52. Deleted in proof
53. Hammond, B. J. 1975. *Cell Tissue Kinet.* 8:153–69
54. Hanifin, J. M., Cline, M. J. 1970. *J. Exp. Med.* 135:200–19
55. Hanna, M. G. 1964. *ORNL-3595.* Oak Ridge, Tenn: Oak Ridge Natl. Lab.
56. Hanna, M. G., Francis, M. W., Peters, L. C. 1968. *Immunology* 15:75–91
57. Hanna, M. G., Szakal, A. K. 1968. *J. Immunol.* 101:949–62
58. Herman, P. G., Yamamoto, I., Mellins, H. Z. 1972. *J. Exp. Med.* 136:697–714
59. Humphrey, J. H. 1978. *Z. Immunitaetsforsch. Allerg. Klin. Immunol.* 154: 323–24
60. Jacobson, E. B., Caporale, L. H., Thorbecke, G. J. 1974. *Cell Immunol.* 13:416–30
61. Jacobson, E. B., Thorbecke, G. J. 1968. *Lab. Invest.* 19:635–42
62. Jesus, D. G. de, Holborow, E. J., Brown, J. C. 1972. *Clin. Exp. Immunol.* 11:507–22
63. Joel, D. D., Hess, M. W., Cottier, H. 1971. *Nature* 231:24
64. Jonsson, V., Christensen, B. E. 1978. *J. Haematol.* 20:5–12
65. Kammerer, W. A., Osmond, D. G. 1978. *Anat. Rec.* 192:423–34
66. Kellner, G. 1963. *Wien Klin. Wochenschr.* 75:616–20
67. Knisely, M. H. 1934. *Proc. Soc. Exp. Biol. Med.* 32:212
68. Koburg, E. 1967. In *Germinal Centers in Immune Responses,* ed. H. Cottier, R. Schindler, C. C. Congdon, pp. 176–82. New York: Springer-Verlag
69. Kuhlmann, W. D., Avrameas, S. 1972. *Cell. Immunol.* 4:425–41
70. Kuhlmann, W. D., Avrameas, S. 1975. *Cell Tissue Res.* 156:391–402
71. Langevoort, H. L. 1963. *Lab Invest.* 12:106–18
72. Langevoort, H. L., Asofsky, R. M., Jacobson, E. B., de Vries, T., Thorbecke, G. J. 1963. *J. Immunol.* 90:60–71
73. Leduc, E. H., Coons, A. H., Connolly, J. M. 1955. *J. Exp. Med.* 102:64–72
74. Leene, W. 1971. *Z. Zellforsch Mikrosk. Anat.* 116:502–22
75. Levaditi, J. C., Destombes, P., Balouet, G. 1973. *Bull. Inst. Pasteur Paris* 71:5–20
76. Marchesi, V. T., Gowans, J. L. 1964. *Proc. R. Soc. London Ser. B* 159:283–90

77. McDevitt, H. O., Askonas, B. A., Humphrey, J. H., Schechter, I., Sela, M. 1966. *Immunology* 11:337–51
78. McDevitt, H. O., Sela, M. 1965. *J. Exp. Med.* 122:517–31
79. McIntyre, J. A., La Via, M. F., Prater, T. F., Niblack, G. D. 1973. *Lab. Invest.* 29:703–13
80. Meneghelli, V. 1961. *Acta Anat.* 47:164–82
81. Metcalf, D. 1960. *Br. J. Haemotol.* 6:324–33
82. Miller, H. R. P., Avrameas, S. 1971. *Nature New Biol.* 229:184–85
83. Miller, J. J. III, Nossal, G. J. V. 1964. *J. Exp. Med.* 120:1075–86
84. Mitchell, J., Abbot, A. 1965. *Nature* 208:500–2
85. Mitchell, J., Pye, J., Holmes, M. C., Nossal, G. J. V. 1972. *Aust J. Exp. Biol. Med. Sci.* 50:637–50
86. Moe, R. E. 1963. *Am. J. Anat.* 112:311–35
87. Moe, R. E. 1964. *Am. J. Anat.* 114:341–69
88. Moore, R. D., Lamm, M. E., Lockman, L. A., Schoenberg, M. D. 1963. *Br. J. Exp. Pathol.* 44:300–11
89. Moore, R. D., Mumaw, V. R., Schoenberg, M. D. 1964. *Exp. Mol. Pathol.* 3:31–50
90. Movat, H. Z., Fernando, N. V. P. 1964. *Exp. Mol. Pathol.* 3:546–68
91. Nieuwenhuis, P., Ford, W. L. 1976. *Cell. Immunol.* 23:254–67
92. Nieuwenhuis, P., Keuning, F. J. 1974. *Immunology* 26:509–19
93. Nieuwenhuis, P., van Nouhuijs, C. E., Eggens, J. H., Keuning, F. J. 1974. *Immunology* 26:497–519
94. Deleted in proof
95. Nossal, G. J. V., Abbot, A., Mitchell, J. 1968. *J. Exp. Med.* 127:263–76
96. Nossal, G. J. V., Abbot, A., Mitchell, J., Lummus, Z. 1968. *J. Exp. Med.* 127:277–90
97. Nossal, G. J. V., Ada, G. L., Austin, C. M. 1964. *Aust. J. Exp. Biol. Med. Sci.* 42:283–94
98. Nossal, G. J. V., Ada, G. L., Austin, C. M. 1964. *Aust. J. Exp. Biol. Med. Sci.* 42:311–30
99. Nossal, G. J. V., Austin, C. M., Pye, J., Mitchell, J. 1966. *Int. Arch. Allergy* 29:368–83
100. Ortega, L. G., Mellors, R. C. 1957. *J. Exp. Med.* 106:627–39
101. Papamichail, M., Gutierrez, C., Embling, P., Johnson, P. M., Holborow, E. J., Pepys, M. B. 1975. *Scand. J. Immunol.* 4:343–47
102. Parrott, D. M. V. 1967. In *Germinal Centers in Immune Responses,* ed H. Cottier, R. Schindler, C. C. Congdon, pp. 168–75. New York: Springer-Verlag
103. Parrott, D. M. V., de Sousa, M. A. B., East, J. 1966. *J. Exp. Med.* 123:191–204
104. Pernis, B., Chiappino, G. 1964. *Immunology* 7:500–6
105. Policard, A., Collet, A., Martin, J. C. 1962. *Nouv. Rev. Fr. Hematol.* 2:159–71
106. Polliack, A., Fu, S. M., Douglas, S. D., Bentwich, Z., Lampen, N., de Harven, E. 1974. *J. Exp. Med.* 140:146–58
107. Ponzio, N. M., Chapman-Alexander, J. M., Thorbecke, G. J. 1977. *Cell. Immunol.* 34:79–92
108. Press, O. W., Rosse, C., Clagett, J. 1977. *Cell. Immunol.* 33:114–24
109. Pressman, J. J., Simon, M. B., Hand, K., Miller, J. 1962. *Surg. Gyn. Obstet.* 115:207–14
110. Racz, P., Tenner-Racz, K., Myrvik, Q. N., Fainter, L. K. 1977. *J. Reticuloendothel. Soc.* 22:59–83
111. Raff, M. C. 1970. *Immunology* 19:637–50
112. Roberts, D. K., Latta, J. S. 1964. *Anat. Rec.* 148:81–101
113. Robinson, W. 1926. *Am. J. Pathol.* 2:341–55
114. Robinson, W. 1928. *Am. J. Pathol.* 4:309–19
115. Robinson, W. 1930. *Am. J. Pathol.* 6:19–25
116. Rodak, L. 1976. *Z. Immunitaetsforsch. Allerg. Klin. Immunol.* 151:46–60
117. Rodak, L. 1975. *J. Immunol. Methods* 8:307–17
118. Rodriguez, B. A., Rich, R. R. 1977. *Clin. Immunol. Immunopathol.* 8:300–10
119. Rubin, B., Hertel-Wulff, B. 1975. *Scand. J. Immunol.* 4(5-6):451–62
120. Sainte-Marie, G. 1978. *Z. Immunitaetsforsch. Allerg. Klin. Immunol.* 154:359
121. Snook, T. 1944. *Anat. Rec.* 89:413–27
122. Snook, T. 1950. *Am. J. Anat.* 87:31–78
123. Sordat, B., Sordat, M., Hess, M. W., Stoner, R. D., Cottier, H. J. 1970. *J. Exp. Med.* 131:77
124. Sorenson, G. D. 1960. *Am. J. Anat.* 107:73–96
125. Sousa, M. A. B. de, Parrott, D. M. V., Pantelouris, E. M. 1969. *Clin. Exp. Immunol.* 4:637–44
126. Stavitsky, A. B., Folds, J. D. 1972. *J. Immunol.* 108:152–60
127. Strober, S. 1975. *Transplant. Rev.* 24:84–112
128. Sundberg, R. O. 1960. In *Lymphocytes and Lymphocytic Tissue,* ed. J. W. Rebuck. New York: Hoebner

129. Suter, E. R., Probst, H., Dukor, P. 1972. *Eur. J. Immunol.* 2:189–90
130. Deleted in proof
131. Taub, R. N., Gershon, R. K. 1972. *J. Immunol.* 108:377–86
132. Tew, J. G., Mandel, T., Burgess, A., Hicks, J. D. 1978. *Z. Immunitaetsforsch. Allerg. Klin. Immunol.* 154:371–72
133. Thorbecke, G. J., Asofsky, R. M., Hochwald, G. M., Siskind, G. W. 1962. *J. Exp. Med.* 116:295–310
134. Toivanen, A., Toivanen, P. 1977. *J. Immunol.* 118:431–36.
135. Vainio, O., Viljanen, M. K., Toivanen, A. 1978. *Z. Immunitaetsforsch. Allerg. Klin. Immunol.* 154:374–75
136. van Ewijk, W., Brons, N. H. C., Rozing, J. 1975. *Cell. Immunol.* 19:245–61
137. van Ewijk, W., Verzijden, J. H. M., van der Kwast, T. H., Luijcs-Meijer, S. W. M. 1974. *Cell Tissue Res.* 149:43–60
138. van Rooijen, N. 1972. *Immunology* 22:757–65
139. van Rooijen, N. 1973. *Immunology* 25:847–52
140. van Rooijen, N. 1973. *Immunology* 25:853–67
141. van Rooijen, N. 1974. *Immunology* 27:617–22
142. van Rooijen, N. 1975. *Int. Arch. Allergy Appl. Immunol.* 49:754–62
143. van Rooijen, N. 1975. *Immunology* 28:1155–63
144. van Rooijen, N. 1977. *J. Reticuloendothel. Soc.* 21:143 51
145. Veerman, A. J. P. 1974. *Cell Tissue Res.* 148:247–57
146. Veerman, A. J. P., de Vries, H. 1976.

147. Veerman, A. J. P., van Ewijk, W. 1975. *Cell Tissue Res.* 156:417–41
148. Veerman, A. J. P., van Rooijen, N. 1975. *Cell Tissue Res.* 161:211–17
149. Veldman, J. F. 1970. Histophysiology and electron microscopy of the immune response. PhD thesis. Univ. Groningen, Groningen, Netherlands
150. Wakefield, J. D., Thorbecke, G. J. 1968. *J. Exp. Med.* 128:153–69
151. Wakefield, J. D., Thorbecke, G. J. 1968. *J. Exp. Med.* 128:171–87
152. Weiss, L. 1957. *J. Biophys. Biochem. Cytol.* 3:599–610
153. Weiss, L. 1959. *J. Anat.* 93:465–77
154. Weiss, L. 1962. *Am. J. Anat.* 111:131–79
155. Weiss, L. 1963. *Am. J. Anat.* 113:51–59
156. Weiss, L. 1972. *The Cells and Tissues of the Immune System: Structure, Functions and Interactions.* Englewood Cliffs, NJ: Prentice-Hall
157. Weiss, L. 1974. *Blood* 43:665–91
158. Weissman, I. 1967. *J. Exp. Med.* 126:291–304
159. Weissman, I. 1970. In *Developmental Aspects of Antibody Formation and Structure,* ed. J. Sterzl, I. Riha, p. 55. Prague: Czechoslovak Acad. Sci.
160. White, R. G. 1960. In *Mechanisms of Ab Antibody Formation,* ed. M. Holub, L. Jaroskova, pp. 25–29. Prague: Czechoslovak Acad. Sci.
161. White, R. G. 1963. In *The Immunologically Competent Cell: Its Nature and Origin,* ed. Wolstenholme Knight. CIBA Symposium, Vol. 16
162. White, R. G., French, V., Stark, J. M. 1970. *J. Med. Micro.* 3:65–83

Z. *Immunitaetsforsch. Allerg. Klin. Immunol.* 151:202–18

Ann. Rev. Microbiol. 1979. 33:201–13

ASSOCIATIONS BETWEEN   ❖1752
MAJOR HISTOCOMPATIBILITY
ANTIGENS AND SUSCEPTIBILITY
TO DISEASE

R. M. Zinkernagel

Department of Immunopathology, Scripps Clinic and Research Foundation,
La Jolla, California 92037

CONTENTS

INTRODUCTION

The incidence of certain diseases is somehow linked with major transplantation antigens coded by the major histocompatibility gene complex (MHC)
(reviewed in 15, 40, 47, 55, 63, 73). Why the two phenomena are associated
and how T-cell immunity, which also seems closely related, fits into the
picture are still unclear and subject to many speculations (1, 2, 7, 12, 15,

0066-4227/79/1001-0201$01.00   201

20, 29, 40, 64, 67–69). The explanatory hypotheses span several possibilities: Infectious agents mimic MHC products, so disease is a consequence of tolerance (61, 61a); MHC products act as virus-receptors and so determine susceptibility to infection (25, 61, 61a); and MHC-linked immune response (*Ir*) genes—including immune surveillance against altered self—reflect both the polymorphism of MHC and the restriction specificity and MHC-regulated responsiveness of T-cells (2, 3, 20, 32a, 40, 61a, 68, 69). These models have all been described in detail and have been reviewed extensively.

This review emphasizes work with acute infectious viral diseases in which immunoprotective as well as immunodestructive mechanisms function. The experimental diseases described here are mediated principally by T-cells, subject to control by MHC-linked (*Ir*) genes. The discussion and explanations are obviously biased and are based on the following assumptions. (*a*) The association between MHC and susceptibility to disease is relatively direct; thus we largely disregard the possibility that such susceptibility must be a multifactorial phenomenon in which the MHC is only one decisive factor among many [e.g. macrophages, immunoglobulin (Ig) allotypes, concurrent infection, etc] (*b*) The association between MHC and disease reflects an MHC dependence of the host's immunologic responsiveness. To simplify the present argument, I assume that the association in question is caused by defects affecting only one class of immune responses, in this case, responses mediated by cytotoxic thymus-derived (T) lymphocytes. I do not deal principally with non lytic cellular responses here, but the argument can be readily extended to all T-cell responses and combinations thereof. (*c*) Viral or other intracellular infections are often the instigators of diseases for which susceptibility is linked to the MHC.

The empirical clinical findings, some experimental analytical models, and arguments on the role of polymorphic MHC products in cellular immunity are reviewed briefly. Thereby the stage is set for the proposal: Many diseases preferentially associated with certain MHC haplotypes are of autoaggressive[1] character, and increased or decreased susceptibility may directly reflect MHC restriction of T-cells.

EMPIRICAL CLINICAL FINDINGS

As summarized in recent reviews (15, 47, 55, 63), susceptibility to many diseases characterizes individuals of particular MHC haplotypes (HLA

---

[1]I use the term autoaggressive here to describe the fact that T-cells attack host cells when the latter express foreign antigenic determinants; the term autoimmune is avoided because of its implied meaning of immune reactivity against normal cells or self-structures. I think that autoimmunity in the strict sense may exist only very rarely and that most of the autoimmune pathology is in fact of autoaggressive character as defined here.

type in man). The association and incidence of specific diseases with certain HLA antigens have been compiled in a report from the *HLA and Disease Registry of Copenhagen* and in a summary thereof (55, 63). The most significant (relative risk, >5) degrees of susceptibility or resistance linked to certain HLA antigens have been found for the following diseases: ankylosing spondylitis; Reiter's disease; *Yersinia* arthritis; *Salmonella* arthritis; psoriatic arthritis; acute anterior uveitis; psoriasis vulgaris; and dermatitis herpetiformis.

Other less pointed linkages (relative risk between 2 and 5) have been described for systemic lupus erythematosus, thyrotoxicosis, juvenile insulin-dependent diabetes, ulcerative colitis, psoriasis vulgaris, myasthenia gravis, and multiple sclerosis.

Even though this list is incomplete, each disease presents salient features regarded as characteristically autoimmune or autoaggressive.

MHC, ITS ROLE IN T-CELL-MEDIATED IMMUNITY, AND AN EXPLANATION FOR MHC POLYMORPHISM

The murine MHC (H-2) is a gene region located on chromosome 17 (the human HLA counterpart is on chromosome 6) and is of a size approximating the genome of *Escherichia coli*. More than 10 loci are known in H-2 coded in some 10 subregions, *H-2K, I-A, I-B, I-J, I-E, I-C, S, G*, and *D*, but other subregions (e.g. Tl, Q, etc) that code for similar products are included in the MHC (reviewed in 23, 30, 32, 59, 62). The murine *K,D*, regions (corresponding to *HLA-A,B* in man) code for the serologically defined classical major transplantation antigens that are expressed on all cells and serve as targets for lytic T-cells. The murine I region (corresponding to the *HLA-D,DWR* regions in man) codes for serologically defined determinants expressed only by lymphohemopoietic cells (Ia-antigens), for antigens involved in proliferative and other nonlytic T-cell responses, and for genes that regulate several other nonlytic T-cell responses. The I region also codes for *Ir* genes that regulate immune responsiveness of nonlytic T-cells.

MHC products were originally detected in their role as the cell surface antigens most responsible for rejection of foreign cell and tissue grafts, therefore their name, major histocompatibility or transplantation antigens. However, during the last 10 to 15 years, it has become increasingly clear that the prime biological function of MHC products is not to frustrate transplantation surgery, but rather to function in all immune responses mediated by T-lymphocytes (reviewed in 18, 20, 29, 35, 44, 45, 48, 52, 53, 58, 60, 65, 68).

All research on T-cell function reaffirms that T-cells are specific not only for a foreign antigen but also for a self-MHC product (self-H). This phenomenon is perhaps best illustrated by the following example: During acute virus infections in mice, virus-specific T-cells are generated that can destroy (lyse) virus-infected target cells in vitro (reviewed in 4, 50). Interestingly, virus-specific cytotoxic T-cells from an inbred $H-2^k$ mouse lyse only infected $H-2^k$ target cells, not target cells infected with the same virus but originating from different inbred strains of mice (72). Thus, T-cells express two specificities, one for self-H and one for a foreign antigenic determinant, X. It is not clear whether this dual specificity lies in two separate receptor sites, one for self-H and one for the foreign antigenic determinant X, or is combined into a single receptor site specific for a neoantigenic determinant of the complex between self-H and X (18, 57, 58, 72). Whether or not any of these receptors are products of genes that code variable regions of Ig heavy chains is equally unclear. However, several facts have emerged. (a) Different classes of effector T-cells are specific for different self-H antigens; lytic T-cells are specific for H-2K,D products in mice (or HLA-A,B in man), whereas nonlytic (proliferative, cooperative, etc) T-cells are specific for self-H-2I (HLA-D,DWR). Thus, the effector function of T-cells is determined by their restriction specificity. (b) In general, the responsiveness of T-cells against particular antigens is regulated by genes coded in the MHC (3, 36, 40–43, 53, 68). These Ir genes and the genes coding for the restricting self-H seem to map to the same MHC region and therefore may be identical (3, 32a, 68, 71). (c) The capacities to recognize self-H and the Ir-phenotype are not determined by the genotype of the stem cells from which T-cells derive, but rather by the MHC of the thymus (9, 28, 68). Thus, recognition of self-H is selected ontogenetically in the thymus and is independent of antigen recognition.

These findings have been explained with the two theories of T-cell recognition mentioned. Unfortunately, since the molecular nature of T-cell receptors is still unknown, these interpretations have not been too revealing. However, these findings and speculations have led to a rationale as to how to explain MHC polymorphism, i.e. the fact that in a population multiple allelic forms of MHC gene products exist. One hypothesis proposes that MHC products influence antigen presentation. Self-H binds to foreign antigens (or fragments thereof) to form or expose the immunogenic determinant(s); low responder MHC alleles fail to complex immunogeneically and therefore do not induce a proper response. In this model polymorphism and gene duplication optimally guarantee the formation of immunogenic antigen presentation in association with self-H. This idea was applied first to an altered-self model of T-cell recognition (20, 68) and, subsequently, formulated differently, as a theory of determinant selection (2, 53). Although the possibility that MHC products determine the quality of antigen presentation and thus the degree of antigenicity is not formally excluded (and may explain some phenomena), currently this proposal is not accepted as a general explanation. The fact that recognition of self-H is acquired independently of foreign antigen X in the thymus is more readily compatible with a model in which T-cells have two receptor sites.

Within a two-receptor site model of T-cell recognition, it is proposed that the *Ir* defect is not expressed at the level of antigen presentation, but rather reflects a defect in the T-cell receptor repertoire for foreign antigen X. Since this defect is determined by the MHC this means that thymic selection of a receptor for a particular self-H limits this T-cells' receptor repertoire for X [several possible models have been proposed by Langman (34), Cohn & Epstein (13), and von Boehmer et al (9) and have been widely discussed or reviewed (68)].

For the present argument it is not really crucial which of the T-cell receptor models is correct. However, to link MHC polymorphism with T-cell restriction and the receptor repertoire, I prefer to define MHC-linked *Ir* defects as holes in the receptor repertoire and explain them as a direct consequence of T-cells being MHC restricted. Therefore, MHC polymorphism is essentially linked to the size of the T-cell receptor repertoire of the species and distributes the holes in the repertoire randomly in the population. In addition, gene duplication (e.g. *K* and *D* in H-2 or *A* and *B* in HLA) guarantees that in each individual at least two overlapping T-cell receptor repertoires are generated, thus minimizing the danger that a hole becomes apparent in the repertoire. MHC polymorphism, together with gene duplication, maximizes overall responsiveness in the species population and in the individual, minimizing the chance that the population (or any individual) is a nonresponder to, for example, a highly pathogenic virus. The extent of polymorphism (and duplication) of MHC products and the size of the T-cell receptor repertoire in a given population therefore must be linked and, probably, have co-evolved. The two following sets of experimental observations illustrate these arguments and are crucial for our explanation of MHC-associated disease. One set of observations concerns the role of T-cell-mediated immunity and the MHC products in handling intracellular parasites, and the second elucidates *Ir* gene functions in this context.

MHC-RESTRICTED T-CELL-MEDIATED IMMUNITY AGAINST INTRACELLULAR PARASITES: A MECHANISTIC FUNCTION FOR MHC PRODUCTS

Infectious diseases are dealt with here briefly and in terms of natural selection. Infections by extracellular bacteria or viruses and intracellular bacteria are among the most acute and life-endangering episodes of infancy and childhood, a fact easily forgotten in the Western world shaped by hygiene, preventive vaccinations, and antibiotics (10, 16, 22). Other infections, particularly parasitic diseases such as malaria, trypanosomiasis, leishmaniasis, filariasis, etc, are more chronic and, even when fatal, usually allow the patient to survive long enough to reproduce. From this point of view, the finding that T-cell-mediated immunity is often crucial for overcoming viral infections or infections with intracellular bacteria (4–6, 33, 37, 38, 49, 50) whereas antibodies and complement are essential for overcoming infections with extracellular bacteria such as pneumo-, staphylo-, gono-, or streptococci is very revealing. That is, the most polymorphic systems known in higher vertebrates are MHC products and Ig allotypes (34), and this diversity is apparently intimately linked to the fact that the species and the individual can respond to and rid themselves of the widest possible range of infectious agents. This discussion deals with cellular immune responsiveness in relation to the MHC and proposes that MHC restriction and MHC polymorphism have evolved because T-cells control against acute intracellular parasites. However, the fact that antibody-mediated responsiveness (particularly to polysaccharides as encountered on bacterial capsules) is linked to the Ig allotype indicates that polymorphism of Ig allotypes may have evolved under a similar selective pressure exerted by extracellular bacteria (reviewed in 24).

Over the last few years the following picture has emerged for T-cells involved in recovery from infections by intracellular parasites. Cytotoxic T-cells specific for viral antigens are also specific for self-H; thus, T-cells generally express this dual specificity when assayed in vitro in ^{51}Cr release tests or in vivo for adoptive transfer of protection (reviewed in 18, 68). The self-H involved is coded by *H-2K* or *D* (HLA-*A* or *B* in man). Clearly, recovery from viral infections is not solely promoted by cytotoxic T-cells, but rather in concert with recruited inflammatory cells such as macrophages, and with antibodies (4, 6, 50). However, cytotoxic T-cells may function critically early in viral infection by slowing the replication and spread of virus. T-cells destroy infected target cells during the eclipse phase of virus infection and eliminate the virus-producing cell before viral progeny are assembled. The important fact to keep in mind here is that viruses are eliminated by destruction of host cells, i.e. via immunological autoaggression (19, 68, 69).

Interestingly, T-cells involved in recovery from intracellular bacteria (e.g. *Listeria monocytogenes*) are also MHC-restricted, but to H-2I (70). These T-cells are not obviously cytotoxic, but act specifically to activate macrophages to increased bactericidal activity (37, 38). A similar mechanism may allow some T-cells to react against some viruses via activated macrophages.

Conceptually, these findings fit the following explanation for the function of MHC products (67): Viruses that infect phagocytic as well as non-phagocytic cells may be eliminated during the eclipse phase of the infectious cycle by cytotoxic T-cells. To fulfill this function, polymorphic K,D determinants, which are expressed universally on all cells, seem to have evolved (presumably from cell surface molecules involved in cell interactions or mediating differentiation signals) as receptors for lytic signals on a parallel course with cytotoxic T-cells. In contrast, polymorphic I region determinants are expressed on selected cells of mainly lymphohemopoietic origin (including macrophages). These determinants have evolved to function as receptors of nonlytic differentiation signals on macrophages to cause enzyme activation and on B-cells to cause antibody production or the switch from IgM to IgG production (67).

MHC-LINKED IR GENES

The fact that MHC genes influence immune responsiveness has been known for at least 10 years (3, 36, 40–43, 53, 68). These Ir genes have been studied most extensively with respect to their role in the antibody response and have the following characteristics: (a) Their regulatory role is antigen specific, dose dependent, and MHC haplotype (H-$2I$ region) dependent; (b) responsiveness phenotype is dominant (but nonresponder interaction cannot be rescued); and (c) the genes probably exert their effect at the level of T helper cells (either at the level of repertoire or at the level of antigen presentation and induction). Some similar effects have been mapped to H-$2I$ for T-cell responses measured by proliferation or delayed-type hypersensitivity (reviewed in 45, 53).

Recently, similar Ir regulation of expression and/or generation of cytotoxic effector T-cells has been detected for cytotoxic T-cell responses against trinitrophenyl (reviewed in 58), the male H-Y antigen (8, 60), as well as for viral antigens (17, 71). The latter types of Ir genes act antigen specifically (to a certain degree), MHC haplotype dependently, and map to K or D [i.e. to the same MHC regions that code for the restricting self-H (K,D) for cytotoxic T-cells]. In these reactions a nonresponsiveness linked to a nonresponder K or D gene cannot be rescued and has a dominant character.

Thus, MHC-linked Ir genes that regulate responsiveness of T-cells and the genes coding for the restricting self-H determinant are apparently identical or very closely linked. This conclusion is strengthened by the recent finding that T-cell specificity for self-H is selected in the thymus and by the thymic MHC. Similarly, the Ir-phenotype of maturing T-cells is determined by the MHC of the thymus rather than that of the precursor T-cells (9, 28, 68). Therefore, selection of the restriction specificity for thymic self-H also automatically determines the *Ir* phenotype. Although not proven, the idea that the *Ir* gene product and the restricting self-H are identical is very attractive indeed, because this concept would reduce some *Ir* gene phenomena to a direct consequence of the MHC restriction of T-cells (68).

WHY MHC POLYMORPHISM?
MHC POLYMORPHISM IS LINKED
TO THE MHC RESTRICTION OF T-CELLS

The extreme polymorphism of MHC products has been explained in many different ways. Most hypotheses assume that the interest of viruses in K,D products of H-2 may stem from the fact that the latter have evolved from cell and organ growth-regulating differentiation antigens (18, 31, 61, 61a, 68). The theories differ mainly in that some imply immunologic reasons for polymorphism and other do not. Arguments that polymorphism is not related to immunity are that polymorphism may serve as a marker system of individuality that prevents mutual fusion or parasitism between members of the same or other species (12, 64), or that when coupled with the immune system, polymorphism may prevent the spread of infectious tumors (11). Alternatively, polymorphism may have developed as a pure accident of nature and is maintained only because relatively closely linked loci are polymorphic (e.g. *T/t* in the mouse) (see 1, 7, 30). A different hypothesis is that since many viruses replicate best in multiplying cells, interaction of a virus with cell-surface antigens (e.g. 25, 51, 61) involved in cell differentiation and proliferation may influence susceptibility to infections. However, this argument (see 51, 61, 62) does not really explain why the MHC products are polymorphic. None of these mechanisms can be disproven, and some in fact may operate partially and simultaneously. Nevertheless, as developed in a previous section, the most compelling idea is that MHC polymorphism and MHC-restricted cell-mediated immunity to intracellular parasites are intimately linked; therefore, because T-cell effector function is determined by self-MHC products, size of the species' T-cell receptor repertoire for foreign antigens is directly dependent on the polymorphism of the MHC products (20, 27, 34, 68).

The inbred mice infected with any of the viruses tested so far generate strong cytotoxic T-cell responses. If this immune activity is separated into an H-2K-restricted response and an H-2D-restricted response, and one tests T-cell activity against self-K plus virus and against self-D plus virus, great differences are detected. For example, K^k is associated with very high response to poxvirus but rather weak response to lymphocytic choriomeningitis virus. In contrast, D^k is associated with high response to lymphocytic choriomeningitis virus, but no measurable response to poxvirus. Similar examples may be found for I-restricted T-cell function as exemplified in the H-Y model (9), but not for I-restricted virus-specific T-cells (71).

Although the present example deals only with expression of virus-specific cytotoxic T-cells, it is understood that I-restricted T-cell responsiveness parallels this. If the species mouse possessed only one single self-H marker as a receptor for lytic signals delivered by specific T-cells, for example D^k, the consequences would be disastrous for the species' survival. The first poxvirus pandemic would eliminate all mice. Polymorphism of self-H alone would reduce this chance substantially, but not eliminate it entirely, since deaths would accumulate as one after another of many possible highly mutable viruses attacks. Only duplication of self-H together with polymorphism deals effectively with the problem, because it becomes difficult for any virus to mutate in such a way as to mimic two or four self-H markers at the same time or otherwise escape MHC-restricted immune surveillance.

This concept implies that MHC products presently functioning in T-cell-mediated immunity fulfilled other but related functions earlier during phylogeny. In fact, duplication of these original MHC loci may have allowed some of them to be sequestered functionally to co-evolve with T-cell immunity and become highly polymorphic, whereas others have remained with original functions as markers for cell interactions, cell differentiation, organ formation, etc. Some of the many MHC-linked *Tl, Qa, T, L*, etc, loci may well represent points in case (32a).

In essence, the fact that MHC-coded self-H defines the effector function of T-cells, and because T-cells are MHC restricted, with the MHC influencing the T-cell receptor repertoire, implies that development of MHC polymorphism is intimately linked to T-cell-mediated immunity, both having formed under selective pressure by intracellular parasites.

A SPECULATION: MHC-ASSOCIATED DISEASES ARE OF IMMUNOPATHOLOGICAL ORIGIN AND CAUSED BY AUTOAGGRESSIVE MHC-RESTRICTED T-CELLS

As the introduction states, the association between MHC and disease relates not to acute infectious diseases but to chronic diseases with an aura of autoaggressiveness. From this starting point the concept was developed (*a*) T-cell mediated immunity is intimately tied to MHC products, because effector T-cells function via MHC-coded cell surface receptors. (*b*) T-cell effector functions—that is, lytic functions, which lead to host cell destruction or inflammation (but not lysis) via recruitment and activation of macrophages—result in recovery from intracellular parasites. (*c*) *Ir* gene products and restricting self-H are probably identical. *Ir* gene phenomena therefore are a direct consequence of MHC restriction. Whether T-cells recognize self-H and foreign antigen X as a complex neoantigen via a single receptor site or as two distinct entities via two separate recognition sites is irrelevant here.

Recovery from infectious diseases caused by intracellular bacteria and viruses, therefore, can be viewed as resulting from the balance between the viruses' ability to destroy cells (cytopathic effect) and the T-cells' ability to kill cells and destroy tissue (cytotoxicity and/or recruitment of inflammatory cells) (reviewed in 4, 6, 19, 46, 50, 65). Lymphocytic choriomeningitis in the mouse (14, 19, 26, 54) and autoaggressive hepatitis in humans (39) may serve as examples of the latter case. This balance is obviously influenced on one hand by the viruses' cytopathogenicity, tropism, rapidity of spread, generation time, and susceptibility to other factors such as antibody-mediated modulation, and on the other hand by the host's degree of immunocompetence and MHC linked *Ir* gene-dependent immune responsiveness.

In response to acute infection by highly cytopathic viruses that most commonly afflict young individuals who may die before reproducing, the host's only alternative to death is to eliminate the virus. Therefore, life-threatening infectious intracellular agents to which a population is exposed normally will eliminate low responders. Survivors will consist only of phenotypic high responders, and no associations between MHC and susceptibility to disease are noticeable. The finding that all mice are high responders to pox, lymphocytic choriomeningitis virus, or parainfluenza virus, three of the most prevalent infectious agents of the species, fits this concept very well indeed.

Therefore I propose that MHC-associated diseases are generally found only in relation to noncytopathic or poorly cytopathic agents that cause chronic infections and do not usually interfere with reproduction. Only these types of infections leave a certain leeway for the balance of immunoprotection versus damage caused either by the infectious agents or more importantly by the ensuing immune response. From this point of view we would consider MHC-associated diseases to be autoaggressive diseases and vice versa.

The association between susceptibility to disease and the MHC may develop as follows, depending again on the viruses' characteristics, its susceptibility to immune modulation, and the host's immunocompetence at the time of contact. (*a*) MHC-linked low responsiveness to a poorly cytopathogenic virus may magnify the spread of virus and subsequent extensive and chronic cell-mediated destruction of host tissue. Here, low-responder MHC alleles are associated with increased susceptibility when compared with high responder MHC alleles. (*b*) MHC-linked low responsiveness to a poorly cytopathogenic virus that has already spread widely (under cover of prenatal immunoincompetence, for example, or because of temporary immune modulation by passive maternal immunity or concurrent infection with cross-reactive agents) may be associated with decreased susceptibility to disease. The latter example would fit the fact that many MHC disease associations are dominant.

An important characteristic of the association between MHC type and susceptibility to disease is that it involves often entire haplotype configurations rather than single MHC alleles. Perhaps this is best explained by the following proposal: Since MHC-restricted T-cell activities are interconnected (e.g. I-restricted interactions between T helper cells and other lymphocytes or between T-cells and macrophages may ultimately generate K,D-restricted cytotoxic T-cells), certain combinations of K plus I or D plus I or various I region alleles may influence the overall result of immune responsiveness (9, 29, 68). Also, intergenic complementation in MHC may influence T-cell responsiveness (21, 56, 66). Whether the few examples known indicate that the MHC codes for more than only restricting self-H (e.g. parts of the T-cell receptors?) is unknown. Either mechanism may cause linkage with haplotype rather than single loci. The significance is that T-cell responses may be subject to far more complicated influences than was originally thought.

CONCLUSION

Diseases whose susceptibility is associated with certain alleles of MHC reflect (a) T-cell effector function determined by the restricting MHC products, (b) an intimate link between MHC polymorphism and size of the T-cell receptor repertoire, and (c) immunopathologic effects of T-cells. Autoaggressive T-cell-dependent diseases, therefore, are likely to be associated with the MHC, and MHC association indicates T-cell-mediated autoaggressive disease.

What are the consequences of such a proposal? As mentioned above, immunopathology may be favored by various mechanisms and only some individuals may profit from immunosuppressive therapy, although at this time no guidelines are at hand.

The present speculation also implies a caveat concerning the use of attenuated live vaccines. These viruses may shift the balance of immune protection versus immune destruction in favor of the latter because of the attenuated character (e.g. a poorer cytopathogenicity) of the virus. Fortunately, the general high responder status to most of the wild-type viruses is probably also valid for the attenuated virus, and genetic selection of low responders protected by vaccination may require some time and many generations. In contrast, if the hypothetical infectious agent causing an autoaggressive disease becomes known, development of appropriate vaccines could induce efficient elimination of this agent before widespread immunologic autoaggression occurs. On the other hand, tolerization of individuals to these particular agents may be an attractive therapeutic alternative possibility. Ultimately, to understand autoaggressive disease and its linkage to MHC and to devise treatment, we must have at hand a comprehensive biochemical analysis of T-cell receptors and a refined knowledge of viral physiology and of the interaction between virus and vertebrate host.

ACKNOWLEDGMENTS

I thank Andrea Rothman and Phyllis Minick for their invaluable editorial assistance and Annette Parson for her devoted help in preparing this manuscript. Part of this work was supported by USPHSG 13779 and AI-00273. This is Publication no. 1703 of the Immunology Departments of Scripps Clinic and Research Foundation and was completed on January 11, 1979.

Literature Cited

1. Amos, D. B., Bodmer, W. F., Ceppellini, R., Condliffe, P. G., Dausset, J., Fahey, J. L., Goodman, H. C., Klein, G., Klein, J., Lilly, F., Mann, D. L., McDevitt, H., Nathenson, S., Palm, J., Reisfeld, R. A., Rogentine, G. N., Sanderson, A. R., Shreffler, D. C., Simonsen, M., Van Rood, J. J. 1972. *Fed. Proc.* 31:1087–104
2. Benacerraf, B. 1978. *J. Immunol.* 120:1809–12
3. Benacerraf, B., Germain, R. 1978. *Immunol. Rev.* 38:70–119
4. Blanden, R. V. 1974. *Transplant. Rev.* 19:56–88
5. Blanden, R. V., Langman, R. E. 1972. *Scand. J. Immunol.* 1:379–91
6. Bloom, B. R., Rager-Zisman, B. 1975. In *Viral Immunology and Immunopathology,* ed. A. L. Notkins, pp. 113–136. New York: Academic
7. Bodmer, W. F. 1972. *Nature* 237:139
8. Boehmer, H. von, 1977. *The Cytotoxic Immune Response Against Male Cells: Control by Two Genes in the Murine Major Histocompatibility Complex,* pp. 1–18. Basel: Inst. Immunol.
9. Boehmer, H. von, Haas, W., Jerne, N. K. 1978. *Proc. Natl. Acad. Sci. USA* 75:2439–42
10. Burnet, F. M. 1962. In *Natural History of Infectious Disease,* 3rd ed. Cambridge: Cambridge Univ. Press
11. Burnet, F. M. 1971. In *Immunological Surveillance.* Sidney, Aust: Pergamon
12. Burnet, F. M. 1973. *Nature* 245:359–65
13. Cohn, M., Epstein, R. 1978. *Cell. Immunol.* 39:125–53
14. Cole, G. A., Nathanson, N. 1975. *Prog. Med. Virol.* 18:94
15. Dausset, J., Svejgaard, A. 1977. In *HLA and Disease,* ed. J. Dausset, A. Svejgaard, pp. 1–316. Copenhagen: Munksgaard
16. Defoe, D. 1722. In *A Journal of the Plague Year Written by a Citizen Who Continued All the While in London,* ed. E. Rhys. New York: Dutton. (1908)
17. Doherty, P. C., Biddison, W. E., Bennink, J. R., Knowles, B. B. 1978. *J. Exp. Med.* 148:534–43
18. Doherty, P. C., Blanden, R. V., Zinkernagel, R. M. 1976. *Transplant. Rev.* 29:89–124
19. Doherty, P. C., Zinkernagel, R. M. 1974. *Transplant. Rev.* 19:89–20
20. Doherty, P. C., Zinkernagel, R. M. 1975. *Lancet* 1:1406–9
21. Dorf, M. E., Benacerraf, B. 1975. *Proc. Natl. Acad. Sci. USA* 72:3671–75
22. Fenner, F. 1968. In *The Biology of Animal Viruses,* Vol. III. New York: Academic
23. Festenstein, H., Demant, P. 1978. *Curr. Top. Immunol.* 9:1–150. London: Arnold
24. Heidelberger, M. 1956. In *Lectures in Immunochemistry.* New York: Academic
25. Helenius, A., Morein, B., Fries, E., Simons, K., Robinson, P., Schirrmacher, V., Terhorst, C., Strominger, J. L. 1978. *Proc. Natl. Acad. Sci. USA* 75:3846–50
26. Hotchin, J. 1963. *Cold Spring Harbor Symp. Quant. Biol.* 27:479–99

27. Jerne, N. K. 1971. *Eur. J. Immunol.* 1:1–11
28. Kappler, J. W., Marrack, P. 1978. *J. Exp. Med.* 148:1510–22
29. Katz, D. H., Benacerraf, B. 1975. *Transplant. Rev.* 22:175–95
30. Klein, J. 1975. In *Biology of the Mouse Histocompatibility-2 Complex.* New York: Springer
31. Klein, J. 1976. *Curr. Top. Immunobiol.* 5:297–336
32. Klein, J. 1978. *Springer Semin. Immunopathol.* 1:31–39
32a. Klein, J. 1979. *Science* 203:516–21
33. Lane, F. C., Unanue, E. R. 1972. *J. Exp. Med.* 135:1104–12
34. Langman, R. E. 1978. *Rev. Phys. Biochem. Pharmacol.* 81:1
35. Lawrence, H. S. 1959. *Physiol. Rev.* 39:811–59
36. Levine, B. B., Ojeda, A. P., Benacerraf, B. 1963. *J. Exp. Med.* 118:953–57
37. Mackaness, G. B. 1964. *J. Exp. Med.* 120:105–20
38. Mackaness, G. B. 1969. *J. Exp. Med.* 129:973–92
39. Mackay, I. R. 1974. *NY Acad. Sci.* 52:453
40. McDevitt, H. O., Bodmer, W. F. 1974. *Lancet* 1:1269–75
41. McDevitt, H. O., Chinitz, A. 1969. *Science* 163:1207–8
42. McDevitt, H. O., Deak, B. D., Shreffler, D. C., Klein, J., Stimpfling, J. H., Snell, G. D. 1972. *J. Exp. Med.* 135:1259–78
43. McDevitt, H. O., Sela, M. 1965. *J. Exp. Med.* 122:517–31
44. McMichael, A. J., Ting, A., Zweerink, H. J., Askonas, B. A. 1977. *Nature* 270:524–26
45. Miller, J. F. A. P., Vadas, M. A. 1977. *Scand. J. Immunol.* 6:771–78
46. Mims, C. A. 1964. *Bacteriol. Rev.* 28:30
47. Morris, P. 1974. *Contemp. Top. Immunobiol.* 3:141
48. Munro, A. J., Bright, S. 1976. *Nature* 264:145–52
49. North, R. J. 1973. *Cell. Immunol.* 7:166–76
50. Notkins, A. L. 1975. In *Viral Immunology and Immunopathology,* ed. A. L. Notkins. New York: Academic
51. Ohno, S. 1977. *Transplant. Rev.* 33:59–69
52. Paul, W. E., Benacerraf, B. 1977. *Science* 195:1293–300
53. Rosenthal, A. S. 1978. *Immunol. Rev.* 40:136–52
54. Rowe, W. P. 1954. *Naval Med. Res. Inst. Res. Rep.* 12:167–220
55. Ryder, L. P., Svejgaard, A. 1976. *Report from the HLA and Disease Registry of Copenhagen.* Copenhagen: Ryder & Svejgaard. 34 pp.
56. Schwartz, R. H., David, C. S., Dorf, M. E., Benacerraf, B., Paul, W. E. 1978. *Proc. Natl. Acad. Sci. USA* 75:2387–91
57. Shearer, G. M. 1974. *Eur. J. Immunol.* 4:257
58. Shearer, G. M., Schmitt-Verhulst, A. M. 1977. *Adv. Immunol.* 25:55–91
59. Shreffler, D. C., David, C. S. 1975. *Adv. Immunol.* 20:125
60. Simpson, E., Gordon, R. D. 1977. *Immunol. Rev.* 35:59–75
61. Snell, G. D. 1968. *Folia Biol.* 14:335
61a. Snell, G. D. 1978. *The Harvey Lectures.* In press
62. Snell, G. D., Dausset, J., Nathenson, S. 1976. In *Histocompatibility.* New York: Academic
63. Svejgaard, A., Platz, P., Ryder, L. P., Nielsen, L. S., Thomsen, M. 1975. *Transplant. Rev.* 22:1–43
64. Theodor, J. L. 1970. *Nature* 227:690–702
65. Thomas, D. W., Clement, L., Shevach, E. M. 1978. *Immunol. Rev.* 40:181–204
66. Warner, C. M., McIvor, J. L., Maurer, P. H., Merryman, C. F. 1977. *J. Exp. Med.* 145:766
67. Zinkernagel, R. M. 1977. *Transplant. Proc.* 9:1835–38
68. Zinkernagel, R. M. 1978. *Immunol. Rev.* 42:224–70
69. Zinkernagel, R. M. 1979. *Transplant. Proc.* 11:624–27
70. Zinkernagel, R. M., Althage, A., Adler, B., Blanden, R. V., Davidson, W. F., Kees, U., Dunlop, M. B. C., Shreffler, D. C. 1977. *J. Exp. Med.* 145:1353–67
71. Zinkernagel, R. M., Althage, A., Cooper, A. A. S., Kreeb, G., Klein, P. A., Sefton, B., Flaherty, L., Stimpfling, J., Shreffler, D., Klein, J. 1978. *J. Exp. Med.* 148:592–606
72. Zinkernagel, R. M., Doherty, P. C. 1974. *Nature* 248:701–2
73. Zinkernagel, R. M., Doherty, P. C. 1977. In *HLA and Disease,* ed. J. Dausset, A. Svejgaard, pp. 256–68. Copenhagen: Munksgaard

Ann. Rev. Microbiol. 1979. 33:267–307

DYNAMICS OF THE MACROPHAGE PLASMA MEMBRANE

❖1755

Steven H. Zuckerman and Steven D. Douglas

Departments of Medicine and Microbiology, University of Minnesota
Medical School, Minneapolis, Minnesota 55455

CONTENTS

0066-4227/79/1001-0267$01.00 267

INTRODUCTION

The mononuclear phagocyte system (MNP) includes the circulating blood monocytes and tissue macrophages present in different anatomical sites and in various stages of differentiation. MNP have several important functions not directly related to their phagocytic activity, recognized since Metchnikoff. The general properties of MNP (38, 92), role in the immune response (215, 260, 261), secretory products (183), changes during activation (6, 129, 130, 151) and antigen presentation (260, 261), and endocytosis and cytolysis (7, 37, 69, 73, 79, 177, 179, 236) have been reviewed. These MNP functions are all related to primary events that occur at the plasma membrane. In this review we consider the structure and composition of the MNP plasma membrane and its functional components and relate MNP functions to the plasma membrane.

The MNP plasma membrane has major functions in macrophage-lymphocyte recognition and interaction (215, 216), target cell cytolysis (69, 73, 79, 234), cellular movement (240, 289), endocytosis (7, 34, 179, 192, 236, 268), and adherence to various substrata (1, 198, 267), and it is capable of antigen and lectin binding (86, 88, 260, 261) and transport of electrolytes and nonelectrolytes (20, 180). The fluidity of the macrophage membrane has been demonstrated by cell fusion (89–93), electron spin resonance (229), and ligand-induced redistribution of surface components (227).

The MNP carries out extensive phagocytosis and pinocytosis, resulting in interiorization of large portions of the membrane surface (20, 236, 242, 256). The macrophage microtubule-microfilament cytoskeletal network is important for the constraints and movement of membrane components (16, 180, 205).

Most studies of membrane function have focused on murine peritoneal macrophages (MPM), or rabbit pulmonary alveolar macrophages (PAM). The membrane properties of rabbit, rat, and guinea pig peritoneal macrophages and human peripheral blood monocytes are also considered. Transformed murine cell lines with macrophage-like properties have also been used for comparative membrane studies (52).

An important consideration in the interpretation of studies of MNP membranes is the procedure by which the macrophages are obtained. Peritoneal or alveolar macrophages obtained from the animal without the addition of an external irritant are defined as resident, nonstimulated, or nonelicited macrophages. Macrophages obtained by the introduction of an irritant such as proteose peptone, thioglycollate broth, adjuvant, sodium caseinate, or mineral oil are defined as stimulated or elicited macrophages. Macrophages obtained from animals immunologically sensitized to specific antigens or following bacterial infection are defined as activated macrophages (149–151). The distinction between activated and stimulated macrophages is important, yet the terms unfortunately are often used interchangeably. These three macrophage populations have distinct biologic properties which are considered in relationship to their plasma membrane properties.

MEMBRANE COMPOSITION

Membrane Morphology

MNP have a typical trilaminar plasma membrane when visualized by transmission electron microscopy. In close proximity to the plasma membrane are frequent endocytic vesicles that may contain acid hydrolases and variable numbers of coated vesicles with 20-nm-long radiating bristles (32). There are numerous submembranous contractile and cytoskeletal elements which include microtubules, microfilaments, and 10-nm intermediate filaments (vide infra) (Figure 1). Cytochemical studies of MPM (33) demonstrate the presence of an 8- to 16 nm-thick cell coat that stains with ruthenium red, colloidal iron, thorotrast, and acid mucopolysaccharide stains, and less readily with neutral mucopolysaccharide stains. The regeneration of surface anionic groups using cationized ferritin required 3 hr of incubation in the absence of ligand (237).

Plasma membrane folding and ruffling is observed by scanning electron microscopy of unstimulated and thioglycollate- and endotoxin-stimulated

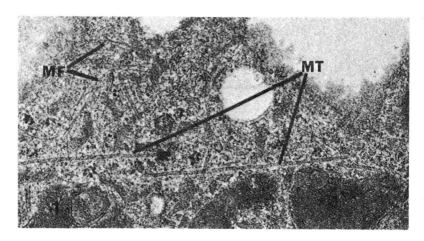

Figure 1   Electron micrograph of adherent human blood monocyte maintained in vitro for 40 days. Note the numerous microfilaments (MF) and microtubules (MT). X 42,000.

MPM (188), and in human monocyte cultures in the presence of *Candida* spores (184) or during cytoplasmic spreading (28) (Figure 2). Stimulated cells had more prominent ruffled membranes and extensive cytoplasmic pits.

Scanning electron microscopy studies of MPM interaction with opsonized erythrocytes have shown engulfment both by multiple pseudopodia and by single cuplike or funnel-like pseudopods (182). Kaplan et al (127, 128) reported that endotoxin-stimulated MPM internalized immunoglobulin (Ig) G-coated erythrocytes by enclosing them in a cuplike pseudopod protruding from the surface. In contrast, cells coated with IgM and complement were interiorized without involvement of membrane extensions (127, 128). Microvillus projections between IgG-coated erythrocytes and human monocytes have also been observed by transmission electron microscopy (59).

Plasma membrane immunoreceptors have been detected with ferritin-labeled antibody and with horseradish peroxidase-antiperoxidase complexes on human monocytes and rabbit peritoneal and alveolar macrophages (59, 157–159). These sites were more abundant on the cytoplasmic veils and pseudopodia in the perinuclear region of minimally spread cells. Recent freeze fracture studies by Douglas have demonstrated changes in the distribution of intramembrane particles in rabbit PAM following the binding of antibody-coated erythrocytes (58). Receptor-ligand interaction results in a redistribution of intramembrane particles from a random to an aggregated arrangement (Figure 3*A* and *B*).

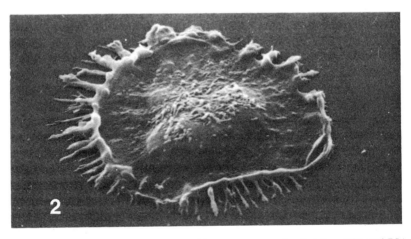

Figure 2   Scanning electron micrograph of human monocyte incubated on BSA-anti-BSA complexes for 1 hr. There is prominent thickening of the membrane and numerous microextensions. X 3,750.

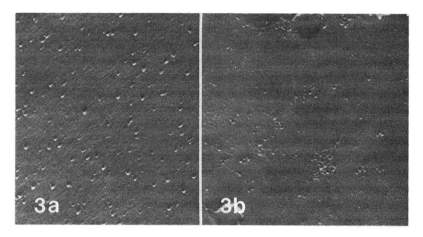

Figure 3   (*A*) Electron micrograph of freeze fracture replica of rabbit PAM incubated with sheep erythrocytes for 1 hr. Intramembrane particles are randomly distributed. X 94,000. (*B*) Freeze fracture replica of rabbit PAM incubated with IgG-coated sheep erythrocytes; intramembrane particles are aggregated in clusters. X 94,000.

Fractionation and Membrane Protein Studies

The composition of macrophage plasma membranes have been based on analysis of fractions prepared by hypotonic shock, homogenization, and sucrose gradient enrichment from bacille Calmette-Guérin (BCG)-elicited rabbit PAM (172, 173, 278). Phagolysosomes, prepared by the isolation of latex or paraffin oil-containing phagocytic vesicles, have also been investigated (155, 172, 173, 286). Wang et al (178) reported a 10-fold enrichment in plasma membrane alkaline phosphodiesterase I activity. Nachman et al (172, 173) reported a 40-fold enrichment of 5'-nucleotidase in a membrane preparation that was 46% protein, 41% lipid, 8% carbohydrate, and 3% RNA. These membranes derived following 1% glutaraldehyde and aqueous hypotonic shock had only limited solubility: 25% in sodium dodecyl sulfate (SDS) and 60–70% in phenol-urea-acetic acid. SDS gel electrophoresis revealed seven to nine bands with molecular weights between 70,000 to 140,000. Two bands co-stained for lipid and one co-stained for carbohydrate. Pulse-chase experiments with stimulated PAM followed by membrane fractionation and SDS gels indicated the uptake of tritiated choline in two bands and also glucosamine into two different bands. Although the rate of leucine incorporation in the individual bands differed, the estimated half-life for membrane protein was 7–8 hr. These observations suggest the rapid turnover of membrane protein components. Gel patterns from phagolysosomes were similar to those from plasma membranes (173). In a novel approach Scott et al induced plasma membrane vesiculation in mineral oil-elicited guinea pig peritoneal macrophages by the addition of 25 mM formaldehyde, and the phenomenon was potentiated with 2 mM dithiothreitol (232, 233). Greater vesiculation occurred with increased cytoplasmic spreading. These vesicles retained sites for lectin binding and Fc and C3 receptors and were capable of forming antigen-independent rosettes with thymic lymphocytes (233).

Recently, Pearlstein et al have compared the surface membrane proteins accessible by lactoperoxidase-catalyzed iodination of starch-elicited, spread and nonelicited, nonspread MPM (185). Stimulated macrophages by autoradiography had a band with molecular weight of 195,000, which was absent in the nonstimulated cells; the latter showed a 180,000-dalton band not detectable in the stimulated cells. Trypsinization of both adherent cell populations prior to iodination did not alter these bands. Neither stimulated nor nonstimulated macrophages had fibronectin as determined by gels or with fluorescein labeled anti-fibronectin.

Membrane Lipid

At least 95% of the total cholesterol in the macrophage is membrane associated (283–285). The plasma membrane contains two thirds of the total cholesterol and undergoes a rapid exchange with the environment. The lysosomal fraction contains the remaining cholesterol and is characterized by a slow rate of exchange. BCG-stimulated rabbit PAM and thioglycollate-induced MPM had greater cholesterol and phospholipid content than the nonstimulated cells (285). Increases in membrane cholesterol and total cell protein occur during culture in nonstimulated MPM (284). The ratio of cholesterol to membrane protein was constant, 12 μg of cholesterol/mg of protein (284). The rate of cholesterol exchange between macrophage cultures and the environment increases with increasing serum concentration. Maximal exchange of tritiated cholesterol was observed by 4 hr. Cholesterol exchange was temperature dependent, occurred in the presence of inhibitors of protein synthesis and pinocytosis, and was depressed by trypsin or by latex ingestion (284, 285). Recovery of cholesterol exchange rates to control values required approximately 8 hr and was dependent on protein synthesis (285).

Membrane lipid content can also be altered by phagocytosis. BCG-elicited rabbit PAM had increased uptake of tritiated oleic acid in membrane phospholipids 5–6 hr after phagocytosis (279).

The increased synthesis of phospholipids does not occur with phagocytosis, but only after a lag period of several hours. Similar observations were reported by Werb & Cohn (286), and membrane lipid synthesis was dependent on the presence of exogenous cholesterol. The changes observed following phagocytosis may be related to the activity of macrophage enzymes involved in lipid metabolism. Elsbach reported that rabbit PAM contain enzymes that convert lysolecithin into lecithin; the rate of this incorporation increased following phagocytosis (68). Wang et al reported a membrane-associated CDP choline phosphotransferase that catalyzed the last step in de novo synthesis of diacylglycerophosphocholine (277). BCG-stimulated rabbit PAM had twice the specific activity as did nonstimulated controls. The demonstration of this membrane-associated enzyme suggests an in situ mechanism for membrane phospholipid reconstitution following phagocytosis.

Mason et al have performed comparative studies on the phospholipid composition of phagolysosomes isolated from adjuvant-stimulated rabbit PAM (155). In contrast to the similar membrane protein profiles reported for plasma membranes and phagolysosomes (172, 173), these workers found distinct differences in the lipid composition. The cholesterol-to-phospholipid ratio was higher, and phagolysosome preparations had greater sphingomyelin and phosphatidylserine and less phosphatidylethanolamine, lecithin, and phosphatidylinositol than intact cells. These phagolysosomes contained lipid peroxides and generated malondialdehyde when incubated with ADP, $FeCl_3$, and NADH, suggesting peroxidation of endogenous lipids during phagocytosis. Arachidonic acid accounted for 20% of the total fatty acid content. In addition, phagolysosomes contained more saturated and less unsaturated fatty acids than intact cells. The differences in phospholipid composition, fatty acid saturation, and the appearance of lipid peroxides may be related to metabolic changes during phagocytosis or to selective interiorization of saturated fatty acids in phagolysosomes (155).

Changes in the fatty acid composition of the plasma membrane alter the phagocytic properties of both stimulated (229) and nonstimulated (152) MPM. The incubation of MPM in serum-less media with 19:0 or trans 18:1 fatty acids results in a twofold increase in the ratio of saturated to unsaturated fatty acids. The increase in saturated fatty acids resulted in a decreased rate of endocytosis with increased activation energy required for phagocytosis (152). In addition, cells with a higher content of cis unsaturated fatty acids (oleate enriched) are more phagocytic than cells incubated with a higher concentration of trans unsaturated fatty acids (elaidate enriched) (22). Although incorporation of select fatty acids can modulate phagocytic activity, differences in membrane fluidity could not be detected by electron spin resonance (229).

These findings demonstrate that both the fatty acid composition and membrane-related processes can be modulated by changes in the fatty acid content of the environment.

Membrane-Associated Contractile Proteins

The cytoskeletal microtubule-microfilament system is important in several membrane-associated processes, including cell locomotion, endocytosis, spreading, cell adherence, and membrane organization (8, 16, 22, 205, 236, 289). Reaven & Axline described the subplasmalemmal microtubule, microfilament organization of adherent nonstimulated MPM in a 400- to 600-Å layer subadjacent to the plasma membrane (16, 205). This cytoskeletal matrix could be divided into two regions, a random oriented matrix consisting of 40- to 50-Å microfilaments in an area 400–600 Å from the membrane, and immediately below this region, a zone of oriented bundles of microfilaments and microtubules (205). The random microfilament region is not altered by cytochalasin B and is evident at the substratum-associated region of the plasma membrane and associated with the nonadherent upper surface of the membrane. In contrast, the oriented microfilament region is sensitive to cytochalasin B and is found only at the substratum-associated region of the plasma membrane (16). Oriented bundles of microfilaments are also identified during phagocytosis in nonsubstratum-associated membrane regions surrounding latex particles (205). In addition, microtubule-associated microchannels were present at the sites of glass adherence. These sites may reflect specialized regions of membrane invagination that function in cell adhesion.

The macrophage actin-myosin system has been studied by Stossel and co-workers from homogenates of stimulated rabbit PAM (106–108, 246–249). The PAM contractile system can be reconstructed in vitro by four proteins isolated from these cells, which include actin (45,000 daltons), myosin with subunits of 200,000, 20,000, and 15,000 daltons, an actin binding protein (220,000 daltons), and an additional protein co-factor (107, 248). Macrophage F-actin binds to rabbit skeletal muscle myosin and activates its Mg^{2+} ATPase (107). However, neither macrophage nor rabbit skeletal muscle F-actin activates the Mg^{2+} ATPase activity of purified macrophage myosin without the addition of a protein co-factor (107, 248). The macrophage actin binding protein has no detectable ATPase activity and does not form filaments in the presence of KCl, but it binds to actin at physiologic pH and ionic strength. The actin binding protein could serve as a possible transducer between a stimulus at the plasma membrane and contraction of the cytoskeletal actin-myosin system.

The isolated macrophage actin, myosin, protein co-factor, and actin binding protein act in a cooperative manner and produce a gel in warm 0.34 M sucrose containing Mg^{2+}, ATP, and dithiothreitol. The actin binding protein binds with actin forming a gel and the myosin then contracts the gel into an aggregate in an ATP-dependent process. The rate of aggregation can be accelerated by the addition of the protein co-factor. Sucrose-containing extracts derived from macrophages undergoing phagocytosis gel more rapidly than extracts from non-phagocytosing cells (107). The distribution of actin binding protein is altered and two- to sixfold more protein is soluble in phagocytosing macrophages. Cytochalasin B inhibits the temperature-dependent assembly and gelation of actin in macrophage extracts and the gelation of purified actin by actin binding protein (108). In addition, cytochalasin B dissolves gels previously formed by actin plus actin binding protein, but it does not depolymerize actin filaments. The effect of cytochalasin B was reversible, and specific; it did not inhibit macrophage myosin Mg^{2+} ATPase activity (108).

The location and relationship of the macrophage contractile proteins within the plasma membrane during pseudopodial extension in rabbit PAM has also been studied (51, 106). Hyaline ectoplasm containing vesicles, podosomes, were isolated by sonication of PAM and ultracentrifugation of membrane-derived vesicles. These vesicles had a threefold enrichment of adenylate cyclase, contained myosin-like ATPase activity, and were capable of glucose oxidation, which increased with latex ingestion. SDS gels revealed bands that co-migrated with actin, actin binding protein, and myosin. The concentration of actin binding protein and myosin was higher in podosomes than in intact cells. The actin concentrations were similar (51). Podosomes were also obtained from rabbit PAM spread on nylon wool fibers. Podosomes and cell bodies were separated by shearing (106). Cell bodies were deficient in gelation and contained between 60–70% less actin binding protein and myosin, and 20% less actin than the podosomes. This suggests a selective redistribution of cytoskeletal elements in the advancing pseudopod. The major portion of the actin binding protein, myosin, and some actin moves with the peripheral portion of advancing pseudopods during cell spreading. Actin filaments behind the advancing pseudopods are actively disaggregated by the egress of actin binding protein and myosin and reassembled at the advancing front. The rapid gelation and dissolution of the cortical gel during pseudopod extension could explain the exclusion of cytoplasmic organelles from the pseudopod and the resulting lysosomal fusion with interiorized phagosomes (51, 106).

The function of the microtubule, microfilament cytoskeleton in macrophage movement, spreading, adherence, and endocytosis has been investigated with colchicine or vinblastine or by disruption of oriented microfilaments with cytochalasin B. Colchicine-treated nonstimulated (9, 21, 22) or stimulated (35) MPM exhibit an altered form of locomotion from directional gliding to a random amoeboid pattern. These cells fail to respond to a chemotactic gradient and have increased random mobility. This effect was not observed with lumicolchicine (35). Cytoplasmic spreading, cell adherence, and pinocytosis have been reported to be depressed by colchicine (21, 35). However, Allison et al reported that phagocytosis of opsonized bacteria was not affected by colchicine (9). Pretreatment of human monocytes with colchicine has been reported both to inhibit chemotaxis and random movement (212) and to enhance random movement (43). The basis for these discrepancies is unknown. Pretreatment of nonstimulated or stimulated MPM (9, 16, 35), human monocytes (212), or stimulated rabbit PAM (108) with cytochalasin B results in an inhibition of phagocytosis and pinocytosis to varying extents (9, 16, 108, 212), and an inhibition of cytoplasmic spreading (16, 35), cell movement, and membrane ruffling (9, 22, 212). The reversibility of the cytochalasin B-mediated effects were demonstrated in two of these studies (9, 22). The doses required to observe maximal inhibition of each of these processes differs. Cytochalasin B inhibited latex ingestion by 50% in nonstimulated MPM at a concentration between $2–5 \times 10^{-6}$, whereas it inhibited 2-deoxy-D-glucose transport by 50% at $2–3 \times 10^{-7}$ M concentration (16). In addition, cytochalasin B at 2×10^{-5} M does not affect the random microfilament 400- to 600-Å layer, but it does result in disruption of the oriented microfilament bundles (16).

FUNCTIONAL COMPONENTS OF THE MEMBRANE

Membrane Enzymes

Several enzymes have been localized to the macrophage plasma membrane, including adenylate cyclase (83, 84, 163, 207, 208, 282), alkaline phosphodiesterase I (64, 278), aminopeptidase (270–273), ATPase (89, 90, 171), proteolytic enzymes capable of degrading serum amyloid (134), and 5'-nucleotidase (62, 63, 120, 137, 286).

Increased adenylate cyclase activity resulting in increases in intracellular cAMP have been demonstrated in nonstimulated rabbit PAM (293), elicited and nonelicited MPM (163, 282), and rat and guinea pig peritoneal macrophages (83, 84, 207, 208). Although a detailed kinetic analysis of macrophage adenylate cyclase has not been reported, this enzyme is responsive to agents that enhance adenylate cyclase activity in other cell systems. Incubation of rabbit PAM with cholera toxin for 3 hr resulted in a twofold increase in cAMP. With further incubation or in the presence of 10^{-3} M aminophylline, cholera toxin induced a seven- to eightfold increase in intracellular cAMP (293). Elicited MPM respond to isoproterenol with a 3- to 3.5-fold increase in cAMP after 20 sec. As in the previous study, the increase in intracellular cAMP could be potentiated in the presence of phosphodiesterase inhibitors (282).

The adenylate cyclase response of elicited MPM differs from nonstimulated MPM following binding of calcitonin or parathyroid hormone

(163). Both macrophage cell populations had adenylate cyclase activity that could be stimulated 5- to 10-fold by sodium fluoride. Incubation of homogenates derived from elicited MPM with epinephrine, parathyroid hormone, or calcitonin resulted in a twofold increase in enzyme activity. Incubation of nonelicited MPM homogenates under identical conditions fail to result in stimulation of adenylate cyclase. Maximal increases in enzyme activity in intact cells was observed after 3 min (163).

Guinea pig peritoneal macrophages incubated with culture supernatants derived from sensitized lymphoid cells demonstrate an increase in adenylate cyclase activity after 24 and 48 hr of incubation (208). The incubation period required for increase in activity contrasts with those found in previous studies (83, 84, 163, 282, 293). Enzyme activity in stimulated guinea pig peritoneal macrophage homogenates in a separate study was responsive to β adrenergic catecholamines and the prostaglandins PGE_1 and PGE_2 (207). However, pretreatment of macrophages for 2 hr with PGE_2 or epinephrine resulted in enzyme desensitization. Adenylate cyclase activity from homogenates derived from PGE_2 pretreated cells was unresponsive to PGE_2, although these same homogenates could be stimulated by epinephrine. The homogenates from epinephrine-treated cells were unresponsive to epinephrine but were stimulated by PGE_2. Desensitization was dose dependent, which suggests that the macrophage membrane may become unresponsive during chronic exposure to agents that elevate adenylate cyclase activity (207). Gemsa et al reported that although neither Concanavalin A or colchicine affected intracellular cAMP levels, they greatly enhanced the cAMP elevation induced by PGE_1, isoproterenol, or cholera toxin in elicited rat peritoneal macrophages (84). Maximal elevation of cAMP by PGE_1 plus colchicine was observed by 15 min; lumicolchicine was equally effective. Phagocytosis of latex or zymosan also enhanced the elevation of intracellular cAMP in response to suboptimal concentrations of PGE_1, PGE_2, isoproterenol, or cholera toxin (83). Increased response to PGE_1 was detected by 10 min after latex addition. The extent of cAMP increase was related to the number of ingested particles: the greater the ingestion, the higher the PGE_1-induced cAMP increase. This increase was not apparent in the absence of PGE_1 (83).

Alkaline phosphodiesterase I has been demonstrated in nonstimulated and stimulated MPM and in rabbit PAM (64, 278). Most (80%) of the enzyme activity can be inactivated by a presumed membrane-impenetrable diazonium salt of sulfanilic acid. Enzyme activity is also sensitive to papain digestion. The specific activity of alkaline phosphodiesterase I was two- to fourfold greater in thioglycollate-stimulated MPM. The half-life of the enzyme was 14.1, 8.2, and 5.7 hr in nonstimulated, endotoxin-stimulated, or thioglycollate-stimulated macrophages, respectively (64). The difference in enzyme half-life at the membrane surface is consistent with the rates of pinocytosis by these cell populations (66).

Aminopeptidase has been localized to the plasma membrane of MPM (270–273). Membrane localization was based on immunofluorescent staining with rabbit anti-aminopeptidase and the sensitivity of the enzyme to papain digestion (270, 272). Aminopeptidase activity was papain sensitive and recovered to control values after 3 days in culture (273). Thioglycollate, but not endotoxin, adjuvant, or proteose peptone-stimulated macrophages had 10- to 15-fold the activity of nonstimulated cell (272). Nonstimulated MPM exhibit increased activity with culture. Maximal activity was observed by 13 days and following this time both enzyme activity and cell viability decreased (271). Increases in aminopeptidase activity were related to increased enzyme levels (270, 272). K_m and V_{max} values remained constant and were similar to those reported for aminopeptidase from kidney brush border membrane (270, 272). However, single cell determination of aminopeptidase antigenic sites and enzyme activity suggested heterogeneity in the amount of enzyme present (273).

Lavie et al have reported the presence of a membrane-associated enzyme on human monocytes that is capable of cleaving serum-associated amyloid protein (134). Diisopropyl fluorophosphate inhibited enzyme activity, which suggests a serine protease; the chloromethyl ketones tosyl phenylalanine chloromethyl ketone and tosyl lysine chloromethyl ketone had no effect.

Macrophage cell populations have also been demonstrated to have a membrane-associated Na^+-K^+ stimulated Mg^{2+}-dependent ATPase. The effect of divalent cations on ATPase activity was studied in sheep PAM. Cadmium, cobalt, copper, iron, mercury, lead, tin, and zinc inhibited enzyme activity to varying extents (171). ATPase activity was used to study the redistribution of MPM membrane components in macrophage-melanoma cell heterokaryons (90). The rapid mixing of the macrophage ATPase activity in the heterokaryon provided evidence supporting the fluid nature of the macrophage plasma membrane.

The enzyme 5'-nucleotidase has also been identified as a membrane-associated enzyme on human monocytes (120) and murine macrophages (62, 63, 137, 286). However, it has not been detected on stimulated rabbit PAM (278). Inhibition of 80% of the enzyme activity by the diazonium salt of sulfanilic acid suggests the association of 5'-nucleotidase with the plasma membrane (63). However, proteolysis of MPM failed to reduce enzyme activity (62). In contrast with the findings of alkaline phosphodiesterase I (64) and aminopeptidase (272), stimulated MPM have less 5'-nucleotidase activity than nonstimulated cells (62). Nonstimulated peritoneal macrophages had threefold greater enzyme activity than endotoxin-stimulated macrophages, whereas thioglycollate-stimulated cells had no detectable activity. Decreased activity reflects the surface half-life, approximately 14 hr in nonstimulated and 7 hr in endotoxin-stimulated cells (62). Werb & Cohn (286) demonstrated that phagocytosis of latex by MPM resulted in decreased 5'-nucleotidase activity, and the appearance of enzyme in phagolysosome vesicles. Return of 5'-nucleotidase activity after latex ingestion required 10–12 hr of incubation and was dependent on protein and RNA synthesis and on exogenous cholesterol. 5'-Nucleotidase activity increases during culture of human monocytes (120) or nonstimulated murine macrophages (62). The addition of AMP, ADP, or ATP to MPM cultures resulted in further increases in enzyme activity (137).

Transport Systems

Studies on membrane transport with rabbit PAM and murine and guinea pig peritoneal macrophages have demonstrated the presence of distinct transport systems for hexoses, amino acids, and nucleosides (19, 20, 26, 27, 213, 250, 251, 255–257). These transport systems exhibit specificity and saturation kinetics and are mediated by facilitated diffusion. Amino acid transport in rabbit PAM had specificity for amino acids with a positive charge and a long lipophilic side chain. L-Lysine transport was mediated by a single saturable system with a K_m of 0.1mM and a V_{max} of 0.44 nmol per 45 sec per 10^6 cells (255). L-Lysine transport was competitively inhibited by neutral amino acids, such as L-leucine, noncompetitively inhibited by Na^+ and K^+ ions, and depressed by low concentrations, 0.5 or 1%, of serum (251, 255). Transport was also inhibited by the sulfhydryl inhibitor p-chloromercuribenzene sulfonic acid (256) and depressed by trypsinization, which increased amino acid efflux (257). Amino acid transport by guinea pig peritoneal macrophages was mediated by a carrier transport system with a K_m of 0.05 mM for L-lysine and 0.1 mM for L-leucine. Double reciprocal plot analysis suggested the existence of two transport systems for amino acids with distinct K_m values (250).

Nucleoside transport by rabbit PAM exhibits a temperature dependence in carrier specificity directed at the 3'-ribose position (19). Arrhenius plots for both adenosine and lysine transport indicated inflections at approximately 25°C. This suggests that the carrier moieties for amino acids and nucleosides can exist in two or more conformations (19). Colchicine treatment results in a linear Arrhenius plot with no apparent transition temperature. Adenosine transport in colchicine-treated cells exhibits the specificity and activation energy of untreated cells below 25°C. In contrast to lysine, adenosine transport is stimulated by low concentrations of serum (251), is not affected by trypsin (257), and is less sensitive to p-chloromercuribenzene sulfonic acid (256).

Changes in transport rates following phagocytosis or during macrophage activation have been studied. Tsan & Berlin demonstrated that although latex ingestion resulted in interiorization of approximately 35–50% of the membrane, there was no reduction in adenosine or lysine transport by rabbit PAM (20, 256). This is in contrast to the loss of 5'-nucleotidase activity following latex ingestion (63, 286). Similar studies performed in the presence of cycloheximide indicated that the retention of nucleoside and amino acid transport systems during phagocytosis was independent of protein synthesis. This suggests that exclusion of transport systems from phagosomes rather than synthesis of new carrier molecules is responsible for the lack of effect of phagocytosis on membrane transport (256). Straus et al have also observed that ingestion of latex or staphylococci by elicited guinea pig peritoneal macrophages failed to affect amino acid transport rates (250). Studies by Ukena & Berlin suggest that the selective exclusion of membrane transport systems from phagocytic vesicles is due to the microtubule system (258). Rabbit neutrophils undergoing phagocytosis in the presence of colchicine had decreased lysine and adenosine transport. Whether colchicine-sensitive proteins have a similar role in the exclusion of transport systems from phagosomes in the macrophage is not clear. Straus et al did not observe a decrease in transport following phagocytosis for colchicine-treated guinea pig peritoneal macrophages (250). In contrast with amino acid and nucleoside transport, ingestion of latex or staphylococci resulted in increased uptake of 2-deoxy-D-glucose (26, 27, 250). Transport kinetics for 2-deoxy-D-glucose uptake after 90 sec revealed no effect on the K_m, although the V_{max} was increased (250). That this increase was observed shortly after the addition of latex suggests modifications of existing sites, but it does not exclude the possible synthesis and insertion of additional carrier molecules. Similar increases in transport were observed in activated macrophages or when nonstimulated peritoneal macrophages were incubated with supernatants from sensitized lymphoid cell cultures for 48 hr (27). Increased transport was related to an increased V_{max} with no effect on the K_m.

In contrast to the facilitated diffusion carrier systems for hexoses, amino acids, and nucleosides, transport of sodium occurs by an active transport system (213). It will be of interest to determine the effect of membrane interiorization on the kinetics of sodium transport.

Receptors

HORMONES   Macrophage plasma membrane receptors for insulin (17, 25, 170, 211, 230), glucagon (25), calcitonin (163), and parathyroid hormone have been reported (163). Calcitonin and parathyroid hormone increase adenylate cyclase activity in thioglycollate-stimulated MPM (163). Insulin inhibits antibody-dependent cell cytotoxicity by the murine macrophage cell line P388D$_1$ (17), depresses increased Fc receptor activity in cultured guinea pig peritoneal macrophages (211), and inhibits Fc-mediated ingestion in both stimulated MPM and the macrophage cell line J774.2 (170). However, whether or not inhibition is related to conventional insulin receptors on the membrane surface has not been clearly determined.

Murine macrophages, P388D$_1$, and human mononuclear cells exhibit nonlinear Scatchard kinetics for insulin binding (17, 230). Insulin binding to human monocytes has been demonstrated by autoradiography (230) and is unaffected by latex ingestion, or by sodium azide or iodoacetamide (230). In contrast, Blecher & Goldstein reported that insulin interaction with human monocytes did not alter the kinetics of glucose or α-aminoisobutyrate transport (25). Furthermore, iodoacetamide or sodium azide significantly inhibited insulin binding, suggesting that the major mode of insulin-monocyte interaction is by endocytosis (25). The basis for the discrepancy between these two studies is unclear.

Glucagon has also been reported to bind to human monocytes. This binding was not inhibited by iodoacetamide or sodium azide (25). Glucagon binding only slightly elevated intracellular cAMP levels.

MIGRATION INHIBITION FACTOR   Migration inhibition factor (MIF) is derived from the supernatants of sensitized lymphoid cultures (49). MIF binding to macrophages is assayed by the inhibition of macrophage migration from capillary pipettes. Elicited guinea pig peritoneal macrophages are sensitive to the effects of MIF and are capable of adsorbing MIF activity from lymphocyte culture supernatants (49, 142). Adsorption of MIF is dependent on concentration, time, and temperature. Trypsinization of macrophages abrogated the response to MIF (142). Guinea pig PAM did not respond to MIF and failed to adsorb activity from culture supernatants (142). The addition of 0.1 M α-L-fucose, but not other sugars, reversibly inhibited the MIF-mediated effect on stimulated guinea pig peritoneal macrophages (206). Treatment of macrophages with α-L-fucosidase rendered them nonresponsive; response was restored with culture. Incubation of nonsensitized guinea pig peritoneal macrophages with sensitized lymphoid cell culture supernatants results in increased adenylate cyclase activity by 24 to 48 hr (208). By 72 hr these cells have increased spreading, ingestion, and glucose oxidation (174).

Fc RECEPTORS   The Fc receptor can be defined as a site on the plasma membrane that is capable of binding the Fc portion of IgG. The properties of this receptor have been reviewed (55, 254, 294). Fc receptors on non-stimulated MPM that bind 19S IgM mouse anti-sheep erythrocyte complexes (136), and on guinea pig peritoneal macrophages that bind monomeric 8S IgM (210), have also been identified. Fc receptors are detected by the binding of soluble immune complexes, opsonized bacteria or erythrocytes, and aggregated or monomeric IgG.

Fc receptors exhibit both class and subclass specificity for immunoglobulin. The human monocyte binds IgG_1 and IgG_3 (3, 115–117, 135), murine macrophages and macrophage cell lines bind IgG_{2a} and IgG_{2b} (54, 110, 265, 266, 275), and guinea pig peritoneal macrophages bind IgG_1 and IgG_2 subclass proteins (3, 141). The CH_2 and CH_3 domains of the immunoglobulin molecule are necessary for receptor binding (3, 55). Although the Fc receptor exhibits subclass specificity, there is less requirement for species specificity. MPM, macrophage cell lines and human monocytes and alveolar macrophages will bind 7S rabbit antiserum immune complexes (47, 60, 115, 209, 266). These cells have a finite number of high affinity receptors that exhibit saturation kinetics at high ligand concentration (12, 55). Quantitative binding studies have been performed using monomeric immunoglobulin or immune complexes of defined size (Table 1). The number of Fc receptors is between 10^5–10^6 sites per cell. Stimulated macrophages bind increased amounts of ligand compared to nonstimulated cells (11, 12, 165).

Studies with murine macrophages and macrophage cell lines suggest the presence of separate Fc receptors for IgG_{2a} and IgG_{2b} (54, 110, 265, 266, 275). IgG_{2a} was capable of binding to a murine macrophage cell line, IC-21,

Table 1 Quantitative studies on Fc receptor

Cell type[a]	Ligand[b]	Receptors/cell $(\times 10^5)$	Binding affinity (L/M) $(\times 10^6)$	Ref.
P–388D$_1$	IgG_{2a} (UPC–10)	1.4–3.9	2.3–8.1	233a
	IgG_{2a} (LPC–1)	0.84–2.1	110–130	266
	IgG_{2b} (MPC–11)	1.1	7.5	265
	DNP-anti-DNP (R)	4.6–8.7	17–33	266
	IgG^+ (R)	2.1–3.9	110–130	233a
MPM	IgG_{2a} (LPC–1)	1.1–4.4	130–140	266
	IgG_{2b} (MPC–11)	0.5–2.9	6.8–9.0	266
RPAM	IgG (R)	12.1–21	0.76–0.9	11
GPPM	IgG_1 (GP)	13	0.61	141
	IgG_2 (GP)	26.5	1.44	141
HM	IgG_1	0.31	107	3
	IgG_3	0.34	78	3

[a] RPAM, Rabbit PAM; GPPM, guinea pig peritoneal macrophages; HM, human monocytes.
[b] Proteins used were monomeric (7S) unless otherwise indicated. +, Dimers, trimers; (R), rabbit; (GP), guinea pig.

in either an aggregated or nonaggregated form, whereas IgG_{2b} bound only as aggregated complexes (275). The inability of these two proteins to competitively displace each other suggests independent receptor sites. A separate receptor for monomeric IgG_{2a} has also been reported for MPM and the macrophage cell line, $P388D_1$ (110, 265, 266). Binding of monomeric IgG_{2a} was trypsin sensitive, whereas binding of aggregated IgG was trypsin insensitive. Furthermore, binding of IgG_{2a} was inhibited by fluid phase-aggregated IgG_{2a}, but not by other subclass proteins. Unkeless has reported the isolation of a variant line from $P388D_1$ that bound normal amounts of IgG_{2a} but had only 10% the number of sites (although with increased binding affinity) for rabbit immune complexes (266). Recently, Diamond and co-workers developed IgG_{2a} and IgG_{2b} monoclonal antibodies against sheep erythrocytes (54). These reagents detected separate Fc receptors for IgG_{2a} and IgG_{2b} on nonstimulated and stimulated MPM and on J774.2 and FC-1 murine macrophage cell lines (54). Binding of IgG_{2a}-coated erythrocytes was inhibited by fluid phase-aggregated IgG_{2a}. Fluid phase-aggregated IgG_{2a} did not inhibit the binding of IgG_{2b}-coated erythrocytes. Likewise, IgG_{2b}-coated erythrocytes could be displaced by fluid phase-aggregated IgG_{2b}, but not by IgG_{2a}. Both receptors bound rabbit immune complexes and mediated ingestion of either IgG_{2a}- or IgG_{2b}-coated erythrocytes. IgG_{2a} receptor activity was inhibited by trypsin and cytochalasin B and was depressed at 4°C, whereas the IgG_{2b} receptor was not affected. Diamond and coworkers have also selected a variant from the FC-1 macrophage cell line that binds both IgG_{2a}- and IgG_{2b}-coated erythrocytes, but only phagocytoses the latter (54)

The composition of the Fc receptor has been investigated on intact cells and following solubilization. The receptor(s) is trypsin sensitive or insensitive depending on the receptor subclass (48, 54, 266, 275). Phospholipase A treatment of guinea pig peritoneal macrophages inhibited Fc receptor activity (48).

Solubilization of the Fc receptor by Nonidet P-40 has been reported from the murine macrophage cell line $P388D_1$ (10, 97, 147). The Fc receptor in one study exhibited the physical properties of a lipoprotein and was bound to but not eluted from an aggregated IgG affinity column (10, 97). Loube and co-workers reported that Nonidet P-40-solubilized Fc receptor activity could be bound and eluted from a human IgG_1- or mouse IgG_{2a}-linked affinity column (147). SDS gels of the eluted material indicated a major protein band with a molecular weight of 57,000 and two minor bands at 28,000 and 24,000. This decrepancy is difficult to reconcile.

Fc receptor-ligand interaction can result in target cell cytolysis and in Fc-mediated phagocytosis of opsonized bacteria or erythrocytes and may play a role in macrophage-lymphocyte interaction (55, 118, 276, 294). Fc receptor-ligand interaction induces the release of lysosomal enzymes in MPM (8, 15a, 31).

Modulation of Fc receptor activity has been observed with MPM heterokaryons (89, 91, 93) and in the J774.2 macrophage cell line (169, 170). Gordon et al (89, 91, 93) demonstrated the loss of Fc receptor expression in heterokaryons derived from fusion of MPM with L cells, melanoma cells, and Ehrlich ascites tumor cells, but not with chicken erythrocytes. Receptor activity was unmasked by trypsin, but this effect was reversible with further culture. Furthermore, if macrophages were fused with ultraviolet-irradiated melanoma cells, no receptor masking was observed (91). Muschel and co-workers have selected variants of the J774.2 macrophage cell line capable of binding but not ingesting antibody-coated ligand; the ability of these cells to ingest latex was unaltered (169).

Fc receptor activity can also be modulated by agents that alter cAMP levels. Insulin inhibits Fc-mediated phagocytosis by J774.2 (170), and by murine and guinea pig peritoneal macrophages (170, 211). This inhibitory effect by insulin on J774.2 and in variants deficient in Fc-mediated phagocytosis was reversed with the addition of 8-bromoadenosine-3'5'-cyclic monophosphoric acid (170). Maximal recovery of Fc-mediated phagocytosis required 5–10 hr of incubation. Zuckerman & Douglas observed that cholera toxin plus aminophylline diminished Fc receptor activity in nonstimulated PAM (293). This effect was observed by 1 hr, although the degree of inhibition did not directly reflect intracellular cAMP levels.

Fc receptor expression is also inhibited by cytochalasin B (15, 109) and by corticosteroids (226). The effect of cytochalasin B was reversible in rabbit PAM. Cytochalasins A and E were more potent inhibitors; however, their effect was not reversible (15).

C3 RECEPTORS   Studies of the specificity and properties of the macrophage C3 receptor have demonstrated its independence from the Fc receptor. The macrophage binds 19S antibody-coated erythrocytes in the presence of complement (24, 67, 98, 153, 281). Binding is associated with a trypsin labile receptor for C3b (24, 67, 98). Human monocytes and stimulated guinea pig peritoneal macrophages also bind C3d-coated ligand (67, 281). However, C3d binding was not detected in MPM or human PAM (98, 209). Quantitative studies on the amount of 7S antibody required on erythrocytes to mediate attachment and ingestion by macrophages demonstrated that Fc and C3 receptors act in a synergistic fashion and reduce the concentration of antibody required for opsonization (67, 98, 153). Although the C3 receptor facilitates ligand attachment, C3-coated erythrocytes are not usually phagocytosed by MPM or human peripheral blood monocytes.

This property was utilized by Griffin and co-workers (98) in studies concerned with the extent of membrane involvement during phagocytosis. C3b-coated erythrocytes were bound but not interiorized by nonstimulated MPM. If these cells were incubated with latex or opsonized pneumococci, significant ingestion of the test particles was observed. However, the C3b-coated erythrocytes were retained on the membrane, and ingested only if a 7S anti-C3 serum was added to the rosette-bearing macrophages. These studies provide evidence that the macrophage membrane can respond to an external phagocytic stimulus in a specific fashion and limit the extent of membrane involvement.

Stimulated, in contrast to nonstimulated, MPM exhibit significant ingestion of C3-coated erythrocytes (24, 167). Both C3-mediated binding and ingestion in stimulated MPM are inhibited by macrophage trypsinization (24, 98). Ingestion of C3b- or C3d-coated erythrocytes was also reported in starch-elicited guinea pig peritoneal macrophages (281). Thus, although both stimulated and nonstimulated macrophages ingest 7S antibody-coated ligand, only stimulated macrophages ingest C3-coated ligands. However, human monocytes have been demonstrated to ingest complement-coated sheep erythrocytes if the erythrocytes are neuraminidase treated prior to antibody and complement fixation (46).

Murine macrophage C3 receptor activity during culture is dependent on the presence of serum. In the absence of serum, C3 receptor activity is no longer expressed (194). In contrast, Fc receptor activity was not dependent on serum during culture (194). Finally, C3b receptors on rabbit PAM can be inhibited by cytochalasins B and D in a reversible fashion and irreversibly by cytochalasins A and E. Colchicine and vinblastine also resulted in irreversible inhibition of rosette formation (14). Human monocyte C3 receptor activity was inhibited by corticosteroids (226).

DETERMINANTS   Cell surface Ia-like antigens associated with the HLA-D region have been observed on human macrophages (2, 113). Human peripheral blood monocytes in culture for 8 days were capable of stimulating allogeneic lymphocytes in an in vitro mixed lymphocyte-macrophage culture by determinants coded for by the HLA-D locus (113). HLA-D-like determinants were also detected in a subpopulation of human monocytes after 48 hr in culture. Although antisera against HLA-A or HLA-B determinants plus complement were capable of causing 100% lysis, anti-HLA-D plus complement was cytotoxic for 30–70% of the cells (2). Ia-like antigens have also been identified on murine (42, 175, 222, 231) and stimulated guinea pig peritoneal macrophage subpopulations (291). Membrane-associated lymphocyte-activating determinants were stable during culture of nonstimulated MPM for 10 days (222). These activating determinants were related to differences between macrophages and allogeneic lymphocytes at both the M and H-2 locus (222). [M locus is a genetic region outside of the H-2 locus that codes for determinants responsible for a mixed leukocyte response between H-2 compatible donors. The M locus has been reviewed by Festenstein (75a) and is not discussed in this review.] Ia antigens precipitated from murine macrophages consisted of two polypeptide chains with a combined molecular weight of 58,000 (231). Using microcytotoxicity assays and the fluorescence-activated cell sorter, the percentage of Ia-positive cells was determined for splenic and peritoneal macrophages (42, 231). Between 8–15% of stimulated or nonstimulated MPM and greater than 50% of splenic macrophages had Ia antigens. Ia expression in splenic macrophages decreased with culture, and by 7 days these cells resembled peritoneal macrophages in the expression of Ia antigens (42).

The role of Ia antigens in macrophage function has been investigated (175, 231, 291). Anti-Ia serum does not inhibit the binding of aggregated IgG to Fc receptors (231). However, anti-Ia treatment of splenic macrophages inhibited the in vitro IgM plaque-forming cell response to burro erythrocytes (175). Furthermore, lysis of the 15–25% positive Ia-bearing guinea pig peritoneal macrophages resulted in a viable macrophage population capable of latex ingestion, but which failed to induce lymphocyte stimulation in antigen-dependent macrophage lymphocyte clusters (291).

Finally, Kaplan et al have described the presence of a pronase-labile membrane-associated determinant(s) on activated MPM (125, 126). This determinant was not detected on stimulated or nonstimulated macrophages by a rabbit anti-macrophage serum. These determinants provide further evidence that intrinsic differences between stimulated and activated macrophages exist.

MEMBRANE-RELATED PROCESSES

Endocytosis

Macrophages are capable of ingesting extracellular particles (phagocytosis) and soluble substances (pinocytosis). The mechanism of endocytosis, its specificity, energy requirements, and related cellular changes have been reviewed (7, 37, 130, 177, 179, 192, 218, 236, 268).

The process of interiorization of particulate or soluble substances by macrophages is preceded by attachment of the ligand to the membrane surface. Under certain circumstances it is possible to dissociate attachment from subsequent interiorization. Attachment to MPM without ingestion has been observed with mycoplasma (122–124), *Toxoplasma gondii* in the presence of cytochalasin D (219), glutaraldehyde-treated sheep erythrocytes, surface immunoglobulin-capped lymphocytes, and F(ab')$_2$ cross-linked erythrocytes (98–102). Concanavalin A binding can also result in attachment of bacteria (5), yeast (18), and erythrocytes (86) to the macrophage surface without interiorization. Attachment of ligand does not require serum, is less dependent on temperature than ingestion, and occurs in the presence of metabolic inhibitors. Ingestion of one ligand by macrophages does not result in the ingestion of other membrane-associated ligands (98–102). Neither mouse erythrocytes attached to MPM by F(ab')$_2$ rabbit antisera nor complement-coated sheep erythrocytes are interiorized during ingestion of latex or opsonized pneumococci (98, 101). Furthermore, B lymphocytes coated with 7S anti-IgG under capping conditions are bound to the macrophage but are not interiorized during ingestion of 7S antibody-coated erythrocytes (100). Rabinovitch studied binding of glutaraldehyde-treated erythrocytes to macrophages and also concluded that ligand attachment was insufficient to initiate ingestion (190–192). The addition of heat-killed staphylococci to MPM binding glutaraldehyde-treated erythrocytes, however, resulted in ingestion of both ligands (199). Thus, the selectivity exhibited by the macrophage between ligand binding and ingestion of an unrelated particle in part is dependent on the ligand.

Ingestion is dependent on temperature and metabolism and can be subdivided into phagocytosis and pinocytosis. Pinocytosis can be further divided into macropinocytosis and micropinocytosis. These processes are distinguished by the size of the ingested ligand and phagocytic vesicle, by agents able to induce or inhibit ingestion, and by the sensitivity to metabolic inhibitors (7, 8, 34, 36, 181, 236). Phagocytosis is defined as the ingestion of particles 1 μm or greater in diameter. Phagocytosis in peritoneal macrophages or human monocytes is sensitive to inhibitors of glycolysis, iodoacetate, and sodium fluoride, and less sensitive to inhibitors or uncouplers of oxidative phosphorylation (6, 7, 36–38, 122, 156, 181, 236). In contrast, phagocytosis by guinea pig PAM is more sensitive to inhibitors of oxidative phosphorylation (181). Phagocytosis is enhanced with culture (269), activation (129, 130, 151), in the presence of calcium or magnesium (245), and by the tetrapeptide tuftsin (41) and is inhibited by cytochalasin B and sulfhydryl reactive agents (9, 156).

The macrophage can mediate phagocytosis of immunologic and nonimmunologic ligands by distinct independent processes (Table 2). Ingestion but not attachment of 7S antibody-coated erythrocytes, or complement-coated erythrocytes by MPM, can be reversibly inhibited by 50 mM 2-deoxy-D-glucose (161). Latex and zymosan ingestion, however, is not affected. The inhibitory effect of 2-deoxy-D-glucose can be dissociated from its ATP depletion effect (161). Incubation of macrophages with anti-macro-

Table 2 Properties of immunologic (Fc mediated) and non-immunologic (latex phagocytosis

Properties	Fc mediated	Latex	Ref.
Phagocytic variants cloned in vitro	yes	no	169
Adherent cells more active	yes	no	170
Engulfment	membrane flow	direct inter- iorization	128
Induction of lysosomal enzymes	yes	no	15a
Enhanced by 8–Br–cAMP	yes	no	170
Inhibited by			
Anti-macrophage sera	yes	no	114
Spreading on immune complexes	yes	no	57, 200
Corticosteroids	yes	no	226
2–deoxy–D–glucose	yes	no	161

phage serum also inhibits Fc-mediated phagocytosis but not ingestion of latex (114). In addition, although ingestion of zymosan- or formalin-treated erythrocytes in nonelicited MPM results in lysosomal enzyme secretion and increased glucose oxidation, latex ingestion failed to elicit a similar cellular response (15a).

Griffin and co-workers have demonstrated that phagocytosis of immunoprotein-coated ligand requires a circumferential interaction of macrophage immunoreceptors with the ligand-coated particles, the "zipper" hypothesis (99, 100). Thus, although macrophages ingest B lymphocytes coated with 7S anti-immunoglobulin under noncapping conditions, only binding occurs if the immunoglobulin anti-immunoglobulin is capped to one pole of the cell (100). Furthermore, ingestion of complement-coated erythrocytes by stimulated MPM is inhibited if these cells are trypsinized following attachment (99). Trypsin did not affect the phagocytic capacity of the macrophages and the addition of 7S anti-C3 antibody resulted in ingestion (99). Although phagocytosis of immunoprotein-coated ligand by MPM occurs by a limited segmental response, studies of human peripheral blood monocytes have demonstrated generalized loss of Fc receptor activity following latex ingestion (223). Recovery of Fc receptor activity was observed after 6 hr of incubation. The effects of phagocytosis on other membrane-related processes is summarized in Table 3.

The metabolic changes that occur concomittant with phagocytosis include release of lysosomal enzymes, increased oxygen consumption, glucose oxidation, H_2O_2, and superoxide anion production and chemiluminescence (36, 121, 130, 162, 181, 218, 220, 225). Several of these effects were induced in rabbit PAM with phospholipase C (218, 220) in nonelicited murine and guinea pig peritoneal macrophages following exposure to endotoxin, deoxycholate, or digitonin (96) and by contact of human mono-

Table 3 Effects of phagocytosis on macrophage membrane components

Process	Ligand	Effect	Ref.
Cholesterol exchange	latex	decreased	285
5'-Nucleotidase	latex	decreased	63, 286
2-deoxy-D-glucose transport	latex; heat killed staphylococci	increased	250
Lysine, adenosine transport	latex	no effect	256
Fc receptor activity	latex	decreased	223
Con A binding	latex	decreased	148
Attachment of complement coated erythrocytes	latex; opsonized pneumococci	no effect	98
Additional latex ingestion	latex	decreased	286
Ingestion of glutaraldehyde treated erythrocytes	heat killed staphylococci	increased	199
Spreading	latex	decreased	286
PGE_1-induced cAMP elevation	latex, zymosan	increased	83

cytes with aggregated immunoglobulin linked to micropore filters (121). Thus, several of the early metabolic changes detected during phagocytosis may be related to perturbation of the macrophage plasma membrane.

Macropinocytosis is similar to phagocytosis and results in membrane invagination and the formation of intracellular vacuoles 0.3–2 μm in diameter. This process is temperature dependent, sensitive to cytochalasin B, stimulated by serum and other inducers, and inhibited by inhibitors of glycolysis and of oxidative phosphorylation (7, 8, 37, 39, 40, 61, 66, 179, 236, 290).

Pinocytosis can be enhanced with increased serum concentration and induced by anionic molecules including albumin, fetuin, polyglutamic acid, aspartic and glutamic acids, hyaluronic acid, chondroitin sulfate, dextran sulfate, DNA, and RNA. Neutral or cationic molecules are poor inducers of pinocytosis (39). Steinman and co-workers quantified pinocytosis of horseradish peroxidase in nonstimulated MPM (242–244). Macrophages form greater than 125 vesicles per cell per min, resulting in interiorization of approximately 3.1% of the cell surface area. Thus, through pinocytosis, the macrophage interiorizes the equivalent of the total cell surface area every 33 min (242). Thioglycollate-stimulated MPM pinocytosed horseradish peroxidase at a three- to fourfold greater rate than nonstimulated cells (66). Endotoxin-stimulated MPM were intermediate in the rate of pinocytosis. Pinocytic activity by these cells remained constant over a 3-day culture period. Pinocytosis by thioglycollate-stimulated macrophages was enhanced by Concanavalin A (66).

Horseradish peroxidase uptake occurs with little adsorption of protein to the macrophage membrane (243, 244). This observation is at variance with the finding of adsorption of protein to the macrophage membrane prior to pinocytosis (264). These differences suggest that the properties of the protein can influence the mechanism of pinocytosis. Macropinocytosis of aggregated albumin and ferritin can be inhibited by proteolysis of nonelicited rat peritoneal macrophages (132). Pinocytic activity could be recovered after 6 hr in culture. Thus, pinocytosis of certain molecules requires membrane binding and can be inhibited by modification of the cell surface.

Macrophage binding of B lymphocytes capped with surface immunoglobulin-7S anti-immunoglobulin was characterized by the absence of ingestion of lymphocytes. The surface immune complexes, however, were interiorized without any apparent damage to the lymphocytes (100). Feldman & Pollock reported that Keyhole limpet hemocyanin bound to rat erythrocytes by chromic chloride or to Bio-Gel beads with carbodiimide was pinocytosed by stimulated rat peritoneal macrophages to a larger extent, 18- to 70-fold, than was free Keyhole limpet hemocyanin (75). However, the erythrocyte or Bio-Gel bead itself was not interiorized. These studies further demonstrate the selectivity of the membrane response during endocytosis.

Micropinocytosis can be distinguished from macropinocytosis by the formation of vacuoles 70–100 nm in diameter. Alterations in the rate of micropinocytosis are usually evaluated by the uptake of radioactive gold (50, 94, 95). Micropinocytosis is temperature dependent and is not sensitive to cytochalasin B. Furthermore, micropinocytosis can occur in low serum concentrations, whereas macropinocytosis requires higher serum concentrations (7, 8, 50). The pinocytosis of colloidal gold in rabbit peritoneal macrophages has been divided into two phases. The first is the reversible adsorption of colloidal gold to the macrophage surface, and the second step is irreversible and results in ingestion (94, 95). Micropinocytosis in MPM increases at a linear rate with time for several hours (50). At 37°C, between 2–20% of the surface-bound colloidal gold is pinocytosed per minute (94).

Activation

Macrophages obtained from the peritoneal cavity following infection with various microorganisms, including *Listeria monocytogenes, Brucella abortus,* and *Mycobacterium tuberculosis,* or from animals sensitized against allogeneic cells have distinct morphologic, metabolic, and functional properties (149–151). These include increases in spreading, phagocytic and bactericidal capacity, lysosome number, lysosomal enzyme content, and increased ability to lyse target cells by a nonphagocytic mechanism. Activated macrophages also have increased pinocytotic rates, increased glucose oxidation, and decreased 5'-nucleotidase activity and are capable of ingesting complement-coated erythrocytes (65, 105, 129, 202). The process of activation requires the presence of sensitized lymphoid cells. As demonstrated by adaptive transfer experiments, nonsensitized macrophages can be activated by the transfer of viable sensitized splenic cells plus antigen (150). The process of activation can be simulated in vitro by incubation of macrophage cultures with supernatants from antigen-sensitized lymphoid cells (49, 138, 166, 174, 208, 253). Incubation of sodium caseinate-elicited guinea pig peritoneal macrophages with supernatants from sensitized guinea pig lymphoid cells resulted in increased adenylate cyclase activity after 24–48 hr (208). Increased adherence, spreading, membrane ruffling, mobility, phagocytosis, bactericidal capacity, and glucose oxidation were observed by 72 hr (49, 174). The increased phagocytic activity was selective; activated macrophages showed increased phagocytosis of mycobacteria, but decreased uptake of aggregated hemoglobin (49). A similar pattern of activation was observed for rabbit peritoneal macrophages incubated with supernatants from tuberculin-sensitized rabbit lymph node cells plus antigen. Incubation for 24–48 hr led to increased cell adherence, spreading, and mobility (166). Hammond & Dvorak reported that maximal uptake of tritiated glucosamine by macrophages during activation was observed between 48–72 hr in the presence of sensitized lymphocytes (104).

Thrasher et al (253) have detected changes in the macrophage plasma membrane 1 hr after incubation with antigen-sensitized lymphoid culture supernatants. Incubation resulted in a 16% reduction in the contact angle of guinea pig peritoneal macrophages or PAM (253). Macrophages will phagocytose objects that have a higher contact angle than themselves, reflecting the hydrophobicity of the test particles (253, 268). Thus, the lowering of the macrophage contact angle results in increased phagocytic capacity.

Cytoplasmic Spreading

The classic studies by Fenn (76) demonstrated that rat peritoneal exudate cells preferentially adhere to wetable substrata and that adhesion and spreading occur both in the presence or absence of serum. Fenn demonstrated that phagocytic events require the spreading of cell cytoplasm over the surface of particles. MNP undergo spreading in the presence of various inducers (Table 4) (23, 57, 178, 193, 195, 196).

Spreading is related to the force of adhesion between cells and substrate and is inversely related to the resistance of cells to deformation. Two classes of cell spreading are distinguishable. "Fast" spreading can be induced with various stimuli and is inhibited by serum (193). "Slow" spreading requires a longer period and occurs in the presence of serum enriched medium (252).

Table 4 Inducers of fast macrophage spreading

Inducers	Ref.
Isoimmune serum	193
ATP	178
Proteolytic enzymes (e.g. subtilisin)	195
Dithiothreitol	195
Interferon inducers (e.g. Newcastle disease virus, lipopolysaccharide)	201
Manganese chloride	196
Complement-dependent system	23
Coagulation (contact phase) dependent system	23
Low ionic strength	195
pH 5.5–6.0	195
Antigen-antibody complexes	57, 178, 196
Substrate modification (poly–L–lysine, con A)	193

Rabinovitch & DeStefano have reported that induced spreading of MPM occurs optimally at pH 7 or below (195, 196). Spreading is magnesium dependent but does not require calcium. Magnesium can be replaced by manganese or other transition metals. These workers have also demonstrated that subtilisin-induced spreading is inhibited by inhibitors of oxidative phosphorylation and by local anesthetics and cytochalasin B (195, 197). Phospholipase C inhibited spreading of human monocytes on glass and immune complexes without affecting latex phagocytosis and Fc receptor activity (29).

Fast spreading on glass has been demonstrated to be functionally and morphologically distinguishable from spreading on immune complexes. Fc but not C3 receptor activity is inhibited in MNP undergoing spreading on immune complexes, whereas receptor activity was unaffected by spreading on glass (57, 200). Using scanning electron microscopy, Bumol & Douglas have demonstrated that human monocytes spread on glass coverslips show symmetrical spreading with membrane ruffling (28). In contrast, when monocytes are spread on immune complexes, a peripheralized specialization occurs with prominent microadhesion points to the substrate (Figure 2).

Spreading can be correlated with changes in macrophage functional activity. Macrophages activated in vitro by lymphokines show increased ability to spread (174). However, studies by Dekaris et al (53) have demonstrated that spreading is inhibited when cells are incubated with supernatants of antigen-stimulated lymphocytes for short periods, 2–6 hr. The spreading of MPM from mice treated with interferon inducers is increased (201). An age-related decline in the spreading ability of mouse peritoneal macrophages has also been reported (119).

Cell Adherence

Cell adhesion involves a complex series of events which have been reviewed by Grinnel (103). Macrophage adherence to glass or plastic substrates is temperature dependent. Adherent macrophages are not detached in significant number by trypsinization or chelation of divalent cation (198). These differences from other cell types are consistent with the lack of detectable fibronectin or other high-molecular-weight trypsin-sensitive proteins (185). Rabinovitch & DeStefano have observed that adherent MPM incubated with cationic local anesthetics undergo cell rounding characterized by cell contraction, withdrawal of cellular processes, and increased numbers of retraction fibrils (198). This process is temperature dependent, less effective at 5°C, and reversed by removal of the anesthetic. Macrophages could be detached from their substratum and replated in new vessels. Primary, secondary, and tertiary amine anesthetics were capable of inducing rounding up of macrophages, whereas quaternary amines had little activity. The concentration of anesthetic required for cell rounding correlated with their lipophilic nature, as determined by their octanol-water partition coefficient (198). Ackerman & Douglas have demonstrated that human peripheral blood monocytes and murine macrophages can be detached from baby hamster kidney-21 microexudate coated tissue culture flasks by ethylenediaminetetraacetic acid chelation (1). Peritoneal macrophages and macrophage cell lines fail to adhere to teflon- (267) or agarose-coated surfaces (77). Murine peritoneal and bone marrow macrophages, as well as the macrophage cell lines P388D$_1$, J774–1, and N6H1–3, can be maintained in suspension on teflon-coated surfaces with high viability after 24 hr (267). These studies suggest that macrophage adherence can be altered by changing the properties of the substratum.

Chemotaxis

Macrophages respond to a chemotactic stimulus, resulting in the directional migration of these cells toward the chemotactic gradient (240, 289). Chemotactic stimuli include alkali-denatured serum albumin, C5a, kallikrein, plasminogen activator, collagen, bacterial products, N-formylmethionyl di- and tripeptides, and supernatants from mitogen-stimulated lymphocytes or from resorbing bone cultures (140, 168, 189, 221, 239, 241, 280, 288). In addition, pyran-elicited MPM when co-cultured, but not in direct contact, with carcinoma cells had increased rates of lateral movement relative to nonstimulated macrophages (238). Chemotaxis is inhibited by pretreatment of the cells with serine esterase inhibitors (13, 280). The potency of N-formylmethionyl peptides as chemoattractants was related to their rate of hydrolysis. This conclusion, largely derived from neutrophil studies, is that the more potent N-formylmethionyl dipeptides had greater rates of hydrolysis (13). These studies led to the postulate that directional migration by macrophages and neutrophils is related to the binding of the peptide to the cell surface, with subsequent cleavage by membrane-associated proteases. The observation that increasing hydrophobicity of the second and third amino acids in the N-formylmethionyl peptides correlates with more potent chemotaxis supports this hypothesis (221).

Interaction of chemotactic agents with the macrophage results in membrane spreading, ruffling, and pseudopod formation, as well as in lysosomal enzyme release (81, 289). Directional but not random migration of macrophages can be inhibited by colchicine, whereas colchicine plus cytochalasin B inhibits total cell movement (9, 21, 22, 35). Macrophage movement can also be blocked by inhibitors of glycolysis (289) and by agents that alter the plasma membrane. Migration by stimulated guinea pig peritoneal macrophages can be inhibited by sodium periodate oxidation, and this inhibition was reversible with sodium borohydride reduction (78). Phospholipase C has been reported to inhibit the chemotactic response of human blood monocytes to casein (289). Human monocytes maintained in culture for 3 weeks migrate toward C5a, endotoxin-activated serum, and N-formylmethionine leucine-phenylalanine (81). These chemotactic agents added to macrophage cultures induced within seconds a membrane hyperpolarization with decreased membrane resistance that lasted over 30 sec. Repeated exposure of macrophages to the chemotactic agent resulted in desensitization and no further hyperpolarization to that stimulus. Magnesium-ethyleneglycol-bis(βaminoethyl ether)-N,N'-tetraacetic acid (EGTA) blocked hyperpolarization whereas cytochalasin B or colchicine had no effect on membrane hyperpolarization (81). These changes in membrane potential preceeded morphologic alterations in response to chemotactic agents. Thus, changes in membrane potential, related to ion fluxes, reflect early events that occur following interaction of a chemotactic stimulus with the macrophage plasma membrane.

Membrane Hyperpolarization

Membrane hyperpolarization has been observed in macrophage cultures as a spontaneous event and can also be induced by mechanical stimulation or by chemotactic agents (56, 81, 82). Membrane hyperpolarization is related to increases in potassium permeability. The potassium ionophore valinomycin produces a rapid and permanent hyperpolarization in elicited MPM (56). Tetraethyl ammonium chloride, an inhibitor of potassium current in excitable cells, reduces the amplitude of hyperpolarization (56). Calcium may play a regulatory role in hyperpolarization (56, 82). Magnesium-EGTA inhibits both spontaneous and induced hyperpolarization of guinea pig, murine, and human macrophage cultures. The calcium ionophore A23187 sustains this hyperpolarization (56, 81, 82). The functional significance of macrophage membrane hyperpolarization is not clear. The spontaneous hyperpolarization in macrophage cultures, however, suggests that potassium ion permeability may be in a constant state of flux due to changes in intracellular calcium concentration. The observation by Levy et al (143) that murine macrophage cultures exhibit cytoplasmic bridging and electrotonic coupling, together with the observation of spontaneous and induced hyperpolarization, provides further evidence for the dynamic nature of the macrophage plasma membrane.

Anti-Macrophage Sera

The effects of antibodies bound to the macrophage plasma membrane have been investigated using polyclonal rabbit antisera against murine and guinea pig peritoneal macrophages (24, 80, 114, 154, 227–229). Antimacrophage sera (AMS) inhibits the phagocytosis of shigella, opsonized mycoplasma, and the attachment and ingestion of 7S antibody-coated erythrocytes. AMS also inhibited C3 receptor activity, although the effect was less significant than that observed for Fc receptor interaction (24, 114). In contrast, no significant reduction occurred in the ingestion of latex, formalin-treated erythrocytes, or yeast cell walls (114). The inhibitory effect of AMS on Fc-mediated phagocytosis was only partially reversible with further culture. After 48 hr, AMS-treated macrophages had 50% of the phagocytic activity of untreated controls (114). The inhibitory effect of AMS on phagocytosis of shigella was observed with $F(ab')_2$ or Fab fragments of AMS, but not with Fc fragments (227). AMS has also been reported to decrease macrophage adherence to glass (80). Studies with spin label probes, however, failed to demonstrate an effect of AMS binding on membrane fluidity (229). At 4°C AMS binding to MPM as detected by a fluorescein-labeled goat anti-rabbit immunoglobulin sera was characterized by diffuse ring fluorescence. After incubation at 37°C fluorescence is capped to one pole of the cell. Binding studies with I^{125}-labeled AMS detected between $4–8 \times 10^5$ antigenic sites (227). AMS activity can be adsorbed with culture supernatants from stimulated MPM (80, 228). The recent development of techniques for the preparation of monoclonal antibodies against antigenic determinants should permit a more precise analysis of the effect of antibody binding on macrophage function.

Lectin Binding

Concanavalin A (conA) and wheat germ agglutinin stimulate pinocytosis, resulting in extensive vacuole formation (61, 86, 88). Other lectins such as soybean agglutinin and peanut agglutinin bind to neuraminidase-treated macrophages, but they do not stimulate vacuolation (88). The ability of lectins to induce cytoplasmic vacuole formation appears to be related to lectin valency. Succinylated conA failed to induce vacuolation, whereas glutaraldehyde cross-linked soybean or peanut agglutinin was capable of inducing vacuolation in neuraminidase treated macrophages (87, 88). Both succinylated conA and tetravalent conA were interiorized by pinocytosis (88).

ConA binding increases glucose oxidation and oxygen consumption in rabbit PAM and guinea pig peritoneal macrophages (214, 292). Both succinylated and tetravalent conA were capable of increasing oxygen consumption in guinea pig peritoneal macrophages, whereas only the latter stimulated vacuolation in MPM (88, 292). This suggests that conA-stimulated vacuolation is more dependent on receptor cross-linking than is conA-stimulated oxygen consumption. ConA vacuolation is enhanced by the local anesthetic chlorpromazine, yet phagocytosis of heat-killed yeast is reduced. The binding of tritiated conA as well as the rate of interiorization by pinocytosis is not affected by chlorpromazine (203, 204). Approximately one third of the cell-associated conA could not be removed with α-methyl mannoside after 30 min of incubation at 24°C (87). The process of vacuolation can also be increased by colchicine and inhibited by cytochalasin B (85). ConA stimulates lysosomal enzyme activity. Increased acid phosphatase activity was observed 1 hr after conA binding. ConA-treated macrophages had twice the acid phosphatase activity of nontreated cultures after 48 hr (87). Other studies however, have failed to show lysosomal fusion with conA pinocytic vesicles and the induction of lysosomal enzymes (61, 186).

ConA binding to nonelicited MPM results in a 3.5- to 4.5-fold increase in pinocytosis (61). This effect was apparent by 15 min and the number of pinocytic vesicles increased linearly for at least 60 min at 37°C. Pinocytosis was not observed at 4°C or in the presence of α-methyl mannoside. ConA-induced pinocytosis had no effect on the rate of latex- or Fc-mediated phagocytosis and did not alter 5'-nucleotidase activity observed in macrophage homogenates (61).

The effect of phagocytosis and spreading on the number of conA binding sites in stimulated or nonstimulated MPM was investigated using I^{125}-labeled conA (148). Macrophages induced to undergo spreading bound similar amounts of conA as nonspread or suspension macrophages. In contrast, ingestion of inert particles decreased conA binding by 25–35%. Recovery of conA binding sites was observed after 8 hr of incubation and was inhibited by cycloheximide. Therefore, the behavior of membrane associated conA binding sites differs in cells undergoing spreading from cells undergoing phagocytosis. Thus lectin binding can be used to dissociate ligand attachment from ingestion (86). ConA binding to the macrophage surface also results in increased pinocytosis, metabolic activity, and vacuolation.

Antigen Interaction

The kinetics and qualitative aspects of antigen uptake (164, 224, 260–262), the localization of antigen (30, 44, 263), and its immunogenicity at the membrane surface have been demonstrated (45, 259, 264, 274). Antigen uptake by macrophages occurs in vivo and in vitro and is not reduced by prior irradiation of the cells (164, 260–262). Both autologous and heterologous albumin and immunoglobulin are ingested by nonsensitized murine macrophages at comparable rates (44, 224). A more critical factor involves the form of antigen presentation; aggregated horse and mouse albumin are more rapidly ingested than the nonaggregated forms (224). Although the majority of ingested antigen [80–95% for keyhole limpet hemocyanin (KLH)] is catabolized and eliminated from the cell, a fraction is retained by the macrophage in an immunologically recognizable form. Unanue & Cerottini have reported the localization of I^{125}-labeled KLH and *Maia squinado* hemocyanin to the macrophage membrane surface and to lysosomes and pinocytic vacuoles (263). The amount of antigen retained on the macrophage membrane is between 1–5%. Activated macrophages have greater quantities of membrane-associated antigen than nonactivated cells (133, 261–262, 264). Surface replicas of hemocyanin binding revealed clusters of hemocyanin molecules on the membrane surface. Incubation of these cells for 3 hr at 37°C resulted in loss of most detectable membrane-associated hemocyanin (262).

The role of membrane-associated antigen in the generation of an immune response has been investigated. Macrophage-bound KLH or sheep erythrocytes are highly immunogenic in adaptive transfer experiments. Treatment of these macrophages with trypsin or Fab preparations of rabbit anti-KLH or rabbit anti-erythrocyte sera abrogated immunogenicity (45, 264). Binding of the synthetic random polymer L-glutamic acid, L-alanine, and L-tyrosine to macrophages rendered the molecule more highly immunogenic, 6000-fold over the soluble form in an in vitro splenic assay (187). Enhanced immunogenicity of membrane-associated antigen has been demonstrated to be specific for the sensitizing antigen. Macrophage-bound 2,4-dinitrophenol (DNP)-KLH was more effective than the soluble form in eliciting an immune response by splenic cultures sensitized to DNP-KLH, but it had no effect on cultures sensitized to DNP-BCG (131). Waldron et al reported that macrophages incubated with purified protein derivative at

37°C were more immunogenic than macrophages incubated at 4°C (274). Immunogenicity was trypsin sensitive if antigen adsorption was at 4°C and trypsin insensitive at 37°C (274).

Lymphocyte Interaction

Macrophage-lymphocyte interaction in vitro is characterized by the formation of clusters, usually with a central macrophage surrounded by lymphocytes (215, 216). This process can be divided into two stages. The first stage is antigen-independent binding of macrophages to lymphocytes. The second stage is dependent on the presence of the sensitizing antigen. The result of this interaction is the induction of DNA synthesis and lymphocyte proliferation (145, 215).

In vitro antigen-independent binding of guinea pig peritoneal macrophages to lymphocytes requires metabolically active macrophages, but not lymphocytes. Binding can be inhibited by metabolic inhibitors such as sodium azide and 2-deoxy-D-glucose. Splenic and alveolar macrophages were also capable of forming antigen-independent clusters with thymocytes or lymph node cells. PAM consistently bound fewer thymocytes than other macrophage populations (144). Macrophages bound both T and B lymphocytes and binding did not require histocompatible lymphocytes. Allogeneic lymphocytes could be demonstrated to form antigen-independent clusters (144, 146, 215, 216). Maximal binding by peritoneal macrophages occurred by 1 hr at 37°C and was not dependent on serum or exogenous antigen. Binding was dependent on divalent cations, with calcium the most effective, and was reversibly inhibited by cytochalasin B or by trypsinization of macrophages (144, 216). Electron microscopy studies of antigen-independent clusters revealed broad zones of close contact between macrophage and lymphocytes. There was no evidence for specialization of subplasmalemmal filaments or of cytoplasmic bridging.

Macrophages pulsed with the sensitizing antigen exhibit a distinct form of macrophage-lymphocyte interaction (145, 176, 215–217, 287). Antigen-dependent binding requires both viable macrophages and lymphocytes, is not sensitive to cytochalasin B, and exhibits specificity, forming clusters between histocompatible cells (145, 215–217, 287). The kinetics of cluster formation differ during antigen-dependent binding; maximal numbers of clusters form between 8–20 hr (145, 215, 287). Allogeneic nonimmune lymphocytes or cells sensitized with a different antigen than that used to pulse macrophage cultures develop fewer clusters (145, 176, 215, 287). As a consequence of antigen-dependent macrophage-lymphocyte cluster formation, uptake of tritiated thymidine by lymphoid cells can be detected by 48 hr (145, 215). As determined by autoradiography, a greater proportion of lymphocytes directly bound to macrophages exhibit thymidine uptake than the nonadherent lymphocytes in the same culture. Lymphocyte proliferation requires a viable macrophage population and is dependent on cell-cell contact. The histocompatibility requirement suggests that the initial antigen-independent macrophage-lymphocyte interaction is not as specific as the subsequent antigen-dependent process.

Target Cell Cytolysis

Macrophages exhibit target cell cytolysis or cytostasis by nonphagocytic mechanisms in an antibody-dependent Fc-mediated process, ADCC (276), and in the absence of detectable antibody. Non-antibody-dependent cytolysis of tumor cells or erythrocytes has been reviewed (69, 73, 79, 234). Activated macrophages derived from allograft or immunized syngeneic mice will kill allogeneic, syngeneic, or xenogeneic tumor cells by a process dependent on cell contact (4, 69, 73, 111, 112, 139, 160, 234). Target cell destruction may occur rapidly or require more than 24 hr before target cells are irreversibly damaged (4, 139).

Macrophages stimulated in vitro by endotoxin, double-stranded RNA, poly(I)·poly(C), or peptidoglycan kill lymphoma cells by a contact-dependent process (4, 73, 112). Lymphoma cells incubated with these macrophages for 4, 12, and 24 hr were capable of cell growth when transferred to a new culture vessel. By 48 hr, macrophage-lymphoma contact resulted in irreversible damage to the target cells. The mechanism of target cell cytolysis is not known, although membrane fusion between macrophages and target cells may be involved (111). Activated macrophages, or macrophages activated in vitro, are capable of target cell cytolysis. Thioglycollate-stimulated or nonstimulated macrophages are not capable of cytotoxicity unless further stimulated in vitro with endotoxin (4, 73, 112).

Macrophage target cell cytotoxicity may be specific or nonspecific depending on the activation procedure (69–74). Thymus-derived lymphoid cells immunized against an allogeneic tumor release a soluble factor between 50,000 and 60,000 molecular weight, specific macrophage arming factor (SMAF) (73, 74). Incubation of nonstimulated macrophages with SMAF results in the activation of these cells and the cytolysis of target cells in an immunologically specific pattern (73, 74).

Nonstimulated MPM and human monocytes lyse mouse erythrocytes during culture (160, 234, 235). MPM cultured overnight in fetal calf serum were capable of cytolysis of syngeneic or allogeneic erythrocytes. Freshly isolated macrophages exhibit limited cytotoxicity in the presence of zinc ions or conA (160). Cytolysis required cell contact and was inhibited if erythrocytes were separated from macrophages by a membrane filter. Fur-

thermore, cytolysis required viable macrophages, was not inhibited by cytochalasin B or colchicine, and occurred with little morphologic evidence of
phagocytosis (160, 234, 235).

CONCLUSIONS

The biochemical properties and immunologic role of the macrophage
plasma membrane have been considered. Membrane fluidity has been demonstrated by electron spin resonance, by cell fusion, and by receptor-ligand
studies (89, 90, 227, 229). Studies on endocytosis have revealed membrane
events that occur during phagocytosis and pinocytosis. Membrane internalization is selective and involves the exclusion of membrane transport systems (20, 26, 250, 256) with the interiorization of other membrane
components, including conA binding sites (148), Fc receptors (223), and
5'-nucleotidase activity (63, 286). That the ingestion of latex can occur with
the retention of complement-coated erythrocytes on the membrane surface
provides further evidence for the segmental or localized response to a
specific ligand (99, 101, 236). Although the response is segmental with
respect to interiorization, freeze fracture studies have demonstrated the
generalized redistribution of intramembrane particles following binding of
immunoprotein-coated ligand (58). The possible association between these
membrane components, plasma membrane movement, and the cytoskeletal
microtubule-microfilament system has been considered. Attachment of ligand to the membrane surface can evoke independent cellular responses
presumably through distinct forms of surface interaction. Furthermore, the
effect of proteases on various membrane processes further demonstrates the
complexity of the macrophage cell surface (Table 5).

The macrophage membrane undergoes distinct changes during in vitro
culture. In addition, the properties of the membrane and cellular responses
observed in nonstimulated, stimulated, and activated macrophages differ.
Distinct properties and functions of the macrophage are apparent in com-
parisons between peritoneal, peripheral blood, splenic, and alveolar macrophage cell populations.

The interaction of macrophages with other cell types is also informative
in considering the dynamic nature of the membrane. At least four distinct macrophage membrane-related events follow cell-cell interaction:
Phagocytosis of 7S antibody-coated or complement-coated erythrocytes or
lymphocytes occurs (24, 59, 115, 153); the selective endocytosis of substances such as KLH or immune complexes from the surface of erythrocytes or lymphocytes occurs (75, 100); the macrophage is capable of
interaction with Ia-compatible lymphocytes in an antigen-dependent process, resulting in the induction of proliferation of the adherent lymphocytes

Table 5 Effects of proteases on macrophage membrane processes

Process	Effect	Ref.
Spreading	increased	195
Adherence	no effect	185
Con A binding	no effect	148
C3b receptor	decreased	24, 98
Fc IgG$_{2a}$ receptor	decreased	
Fc IgG$_{2b}$ receptor	no effect	54, 266
Cholesterol exchange	decreased	285
Binding of glutaraldehyde-treated erythrocytes	decreased	192
Pinocytosis	decreased	132
Antigen-independent macrophage lymphocyte cluster	decreased	144
Immunogenicity of membrane-bound antigen	decreased	264
Target cell cytolysis	decreased	112
Lysine transport	decreased	257
Adenosine transport	no effect	257
Response to MIF	decreased	142
Aminopeptidase, alkaline phosphodiesterase I activity	decreased	64, 273
5′-Nucleotidase activity	no effect	62

(145, 176, 215, 216); and macrophages activated in vivo or in vitro interact with target cells, resulting in cytolysis (4, 69–74, 160).

Our understanding of the detailed molecular basis by which a membrane-associated stimulus evokes a cellular response requires further investigation. Study of the physiologic and genetic regulatory mechanisms involved in the expression of various plasma membrane components will be an important area of research. Knowledge of macrophage plasma membranes should yield new insights into the molecular and cell biology of the immune response.

ACKNOWLEDGMENTS

The research in our laboratory is supported by the United States Public Health Service, USPHS grant AI-12478-05 from the National Institute of Allergy and Infectious Disease, the Kroc Foundation, Santa Ynez, California, and the Arthritis Foundation, Minnesota Chapter.

SHZ is an American Lung Association Postdoctoral fellow.

Literature Cited

1. Ackerman, S. K., Douglas, S. D. 1978. *J. Immunol.* 120:1372–74
2. Albrechtsen, D. 1977. *Scand. J. Immunol.* 6:907–12
3. Alexander, M. D., Andrews, J. A., Leslie, R. G. Q., Wood, N. J. 1975. *Immunology* 35:115–23
4. Alexander, P., Evans, R. 1971. *Nature New Biol.* 232:76–78
5. Allen, J. M., Cook, G. M. W., Poole, A. R. 1972. *Exp. Cell Res.* 68:466–71
6. Allison, A. C. 1978. *Int. Rev. Exp. Pathol.* 18:303–46
7. Allison, A. C., Davies, P. 1974. *Symp. Soc. Exp. Biol.* 28:419–46
8. Allison, A. C., Davies, P. 1975. In *Mononuclear Phagocytes in Immunity Infection and Pathology,* ed. R. Van Furth, pp. 487–504. Oxford: Blackwell Sci. 1062 pp.
9. Allison, A. C., Davies, P., DePetris, S. 1971. *Nature New Biol.* 232:153–55
10. Anderson, C. L., Grey, H. M. 1974. *J. Exp. Med.* 129:1175–88
11. Arend, W. P., Mannik, M. 1973. *J. Immunol.* 110:1455–63
12. Arend, W. P., Mannik, M. See Ref. 8, pp. 303–14
13. Aswanikumar, S., Schiffmann, E., Corcoran, B. A., Wahl, S. M. 1976. *Proc. Natl. Acad. Sci. USA* 73:2439–42
14. Atkinson, J. P., Michael, J. M., Chaplin, H., Parker, C. W. 1977. *J. Immunol.* 118:1292–99
15. Atkinson, J. P., Parker, C. W. 1977. *Cell Immunol.* 33:353–63
15a. Axline, S. G., Cohn, Z. A. 1970. *J. Exp. Med.* 131:1239–60
16. Axline, S. G., Reaven, E. P. 1974. *J. Cell Biol.* 62:647–59
17. Bar, R. S., Kahn, C. R., Koren, H. S. 1977. *Nature* 265:632–34
18. Bar-Shavit, Z., Goldman, R. 1976. *Exp. Cell Res.* 99:221–36
19. Berlin, R. D. 1973. *J. Biol. Chem.* 248:4724–30
20. Berlin, R. D. See Ref. 8, pp. 547–55
21. Bhisey, A. N., Freed, J. J. 1971. *Exp. Cell Res.* 64:419–29
22. Bhisey, A. N., Freed, J. J. 1975. *Exp. Cell Res.* 95:376–84
23. Bianco, C., Eden, A., Cohn, Z. A. 1976. *J. Exp. Med.* 144:1531–43
24. Bianco, C., Griffin, F. M., Silverstein, S. C. 1974. *J. Exp. Med.* 141:1278–90
25. Blecher, M., Goldstein, S. 1977. *Mol. Cell. Endocrinol.* 8:301–15
26. Bonventre, P. F., Mukkada, A. J. 1974. *Infect. Immun.* 10:1391–96
27. Bonventre, P. F., Straus, D., Baughn, R. E., Imhoff, J. 1977. *J. Immunol.* 118:1827–35
28. Bumol, T. F., Douglas, S. D. 1977. *Cell. Immunol.* 34:70–78
29. Bumol, T. F., Douglas, S. D. 1978. *J. Reticuloendothel. Soc.* 24:49–55
30. Calderon, J., Unanue, E. R. 1974. *J. Immunol.* 112:1804–14
31. Cardella, C. J., Davies, P., Allison, A. C. 1974. *Nature* 247:46–48
32. Carr, I. 1973. *The Macrophage. A Review of Ultrastructure and Function,* pp. 10–18. London: Academic. 154 pp.
33. Carr, I., Everson, G., Rankin, A., Rutherford, J., Zellforsch, Z. 1970. *Mikrosk. Anat.* 105:339–49
34. Casley-Smith, J. R. 1969. *J. Microsc.* 90:15–30
35. Cheung, H. T., Cantaron, W. D., Sundharadas, G. 1978. *Exp. Cell Res.* 111:95–103
36. Cline, M. J., Lehrer, R. I. 1968. *Blood* 32:423–35
37. Cohn, Z. A. 1970. In *Mononuclear Phagocytes,* ed. R. Van Furth, pp. 121–32. Philadelphia: Davis. 654 pp.
38. Cohn, Z. A. 1975. *Fed. Proc.* 34:1725–29
39. Cohn, Z. A., Parks, E. 1967. *J. Exp. Med.* 125:213–34
40. Cohn, Z. A., Parks, E. 1967. *J. Exp. Med.* 125:1091–104
41. Constantopoulos, A., Najjar, V. A. 1972. *Cytobios* 6:97–100
42. Cowing, C., Schwartz, B. D., Dickler, H. B. 1978. *Immunology* 120:378–84
43. Crispe, I. N. 1976. *Exp. Cell Res.* 100:443–47
44. Cruchaud, A., Berney, M., Balant, L. 1975. *J. Immunol.* 114:102–9
45. Cruchaud, A., Unanue, E. R. 1971. *J. Immunol.* 107:1329–40
46. Czop, J. K., Fearon, D. T., Austin, K. F. 1978. *Proc. Natl. Acad. Sci. USA* 75:3831–35
47. Daughaday, C. C., Douglas, S. D. 1976. *J. Reticuloendothel. Soc.* 19:37–45
48. Davey, M. J., Asherson, G. L. 1967. *Immunology* 12:13–20
49. David, J. R. 1975. *Fed. Proc.* 34:1730–36
50. Davies, P., Allison, A. C., Haswell, A. D. 1972. *Biochem. Biophys. Res. Commun.* 52:627–34
51. Davies, W. A., Stossel, T. P. 1977. *J. Cell Biol.* 75:941–55
52. Defendi, V. 1976. In *Immunobiology of the Macrophage,* ed. D. S. Nelson, pp. 275–90. New York: Academic. 633 pp.
53. Dekaris, D., Smerdel, S., Vesche, B. 1971. *Eur. J. Immunol.* 1:402–4
54. Diamond, B., Bloom, B. R., Scharff, M. 1978. *J. Immunol.* 121:1329–33

55. Dorrington, K. J. 1976. *Immunol. Commun.* 5:263-80
56. DosReis, G. A., Oliveira-Castro, G. M. 1977. *Biochim. Biophys. Acta* 469: 257-63
57. Douglas, S. D. 1976. *Cell Immunol.* 21:344-49
58. Douglas, S. D. 1978. *J. Immunol.* 120:151-57
59. Douglas, S. D., Huber, H. 1972. *Exp. Cell Res.* 70:161-72
60. Douglas, S. D., Schmidt, M. E., Siltzbach, L. E. 1972. *Immunol. Commun.* 1:25-38
61. Edelson, P. J., Cohn, Z. A. 1974. *J. Exp. Med.* 140:1364-86
62. Edelson, P. J., Cohn, Z. A. 1976. *J. Exp. Med.* 144:1581-95
63. Edelson, P. J., Cohn, Z. A. 1976. *J. Exp. Med.* 144:1596-608
64. Edelson, P. J., Erbs, C. 1978. *J. Exp. Med.* 147:77-86
65. Edelson, P. J., Erbs, C. 1978. *J. Immunol.* 120:1532-36
66. Edelson, P. J., Zwiebel, R., Cohn, Z. A. 1975. *J. Exp. Med.* 142:1150-64
67. Ehlenberger, A. G., Nussenzweig, V. 1977. *J. Exp. Med.* 145:357-71
68. Elsbach, P. 1967. *J. Clin. Invest.* 46:1052
69. Evans, R. See Ref. 8, pp. 827-41
70. Evans, R., Alexander, P. 1970 *Nature New Biol.* 228:620-22
71. Evans, R., Alexander, P. 1972. *Immunology* 23:615-26
72. Evans, R., Alexander, P. 1972. *Immunology* 23:627-36
73. Evans, R., Alexander, P. See Ref. 52, pp. 535-76
74. Evans, R., Grant, C. K., Cox, H., Steele, K., Alexander, P. 1972. *J. Exp. Med.* 136:1318-22
75. Feldman, J. D., Pollock, E. M. 1974. *J. Immunol.* 113:329-42
75a. Festenstein, H. 1973. *Transplant Rev.* 15:62
76. Fenn, W. O. 1922. *J. Gen. Physiol.* 4:373-85
77. Folger, R., Weiss, L., Glaves, D., Subjeck, J. R., Harlos, J. P. 1978. *J. Cell Sci.* 31:245-57
78. Fox, R. A., Fernandez, L. A., Rajaraman, R. 1977. *Scand. J. Immunol.* 6:1151-57
79. Gallily, R. See Ref. 8, pp. 895-908
80. Gallily, R., Schroit, A. J. See Ref. 8, pp. 363-67
81. Gallin, E. K., Gallin, J. I. 1977. *J. Cell Biol.* 75:277-89
82. Gallin, E. K., Wiederhold, M. L., Lipsky, P. E., Rosenthal, A. S. 1975. *J. Cell Physiol.* 86:653-62

83. Gemsa, D., Seitz, M., Kramer, W., Till, G., Resch, K. 1978. *J. Immunol.* 120: 1187-94
84. Gemsa, D., Steggemann, L., Till, G., Resch, K. 1977. *J. Immunol.* 119: 524-29
85. Goldman, R. 1976. *Exp. Cell Res.* 99:385-94
86. Goldman, R., Bursuker, I. 1976. *Exp. Cell Res.* 103:279-94
87. Goldman, R., Raz, A. 1975. *Exp. Cell Res.* 96:393-405
88. Goldman, R., Sharon, N., Lotan, R. 1976. *Exp. Cell Res.* 99:408-22
89. Gordon, S. See Ref. 8, pp. 387-403
90. Gordon, S., Cohn, Z. 1970. *J. Exp. Med.* 131:981-1003
91. Gordon, S., Cohn, Z. 1971. *J. Exp. Med.* 134:947-62
92. Gordon, S., Cohn, Z. 1973. *Int. Rev. Cytol.* 36:171-214
93. Gordon, S., Ripps, C. S., Cohn, Z. 1971. *J. Exp. Med.* 134:1187-200
94. Gosselin, R. E. 1956. *J. Gen. Physiol.* 39:625-49
95. Gosselin, R. E. 1967. *Fed. Proc.* 26: 987-93
96. Graham, R. C., Karnovsky, M. J., Shafer, A. W., Glass, E. A., Karnovsky, M. L. 1967. *J. Cell Biol.* 32:629-47
97. Grey, H. M., Anderson, C. L., Heusser, C. H., Borthistile, B. K., von Eschen, K. B., Chiller, J. M. 1976. *Cold Spring Harbor Symp. Quant. Biol.* 41:315-21
98. Griffin, F. M., Bianco, C., Silverstein, S. C. 1975. *J. Exp. Med.* 141:1269-77
99. Griffin, F. M., Griffin, J. A., Leider, J. E., Silverstein, S. C. 1975. *J. Exp. Med.* 142:1263-82
100. Griffin, F. M., Griffin, J. A., Silverstein, S. C. 1976. *J. Exp. Med.* 144:788-809
101. Griffin, F. M., Silverstein, S. C. 1974. *J. Exp. Med.* 139:323-36
102. Griffin, F. M., Silverstein, S. C. See Ref. 8, pp. 283-86
103. Grinnel, F. 1978. *Int. Rev. Cytol.* 53:65-144
104. Hammond, M. E., Dvorak, H. F. 1972. *J. Exp. Med.* 136:1518-32
105. Hard, G. C. 1970. *Br. J. Exp. Pathol.* 51:97-105
106. Hartwig, J. H., Davies, W. A., Stossel, T. P. 1977. *J. Cell Biol.* 75:956-67
107. Hartwig, J. H., Stossel, T. P. 1975. *J. Biol. Chem.* 250:5696-705
108. Hartwig, J. H., Stossel, T. P. 1976. *J. Cell Biol.* 71:295-303
109. Herskovitz, B., Guerry, D., Cooper, R. A., Schreiber, A. D. 1977. *Blood* 49:245-57
110. Heusser, C. H., Anderson, C. L., Grey, H. M. 1977. *J. Exp. Med.* 145:1316-27

304   ZUCKERMAN & DOUGLAS

111. Hibbs, J. B. 1974. *Science* 184:468–71
112. Hibbs, J. B., Taintor, R. R., Chapman, H. A., Weinberg, J. B. 1977. *Science* 197:279–82
113. Hirschberg, H., Kaakinen, A., Thorsby, E. 1976. *Nature* 263:63–64
114. Holland, P., Holland, N. H., Cohn, Z. A. 1972. *J. Exp. Med.* 135:458–75
115. Huber, H., Douglas, S. D., Fudenberg, H. H. 1969. *Immunology* 17:7–21
116. Huber, H., Douglas, S. D., Huber, C., Goldberg, L. S. 1971. *Int. Arch. Allergy Appl. Immunol.* 4:262–67
117. Huber, H., Douglas, S. D., Nusbacher, J., Kochwa, S., Rosenfield, R. E. 1971. *Nature* 229:419–21
118. Huber, H., Holm, G. See Ref. 8. pp. 291–301
119. Johnson, D. R., Fernandes, G., Douglas, S. D. 1978. *Devel. Comp. Immunol.* 2:347–54
120. Johnson, W. D., Mei, B., Cohn, Z. A. 1977. *J. Exp. Med.* 146:1613–26
121. Johnston, R. B., Lehmeyer, J. E., Guthrie, L. A. 1976. *J. Exp. Med.* 143:1551–56
122. Jones, T. C. See Ref. 8, pp. 269–82
123. Jones, T. C., Hirsch, J. G. 1971. *J. Exp. Med.* 133:231–59
124. Jones, T. C., Yeh, S., Hirsch, J. G. 1972. *Proc. Soc. Exp. Biol. Med.* 139:464–70
125. Kaplan, A. M., Bear, H. D., Kirk, L., Cummins, C., Mohanakumar, T. 1978. *J. Immunol.* 120:2080–85
126. Kaplan, A. M., Mohanakumar, T. 1977. *J. Exp. Med.* 146:1461–66
127. Kaplan, G. 1977. *Scand. J. Immunol.* 6:797–807
128. Kaplan, G., Gaudernack, G., Seljelid, R. 1975. *Exp. Cell Res.* 95:365–75
129. Karnovsky, M. L., Lazdins, J., Drath, D., Harper, A. 1975. *Ann. NY Acad. Sci.* 256:266–74
130. Karnovsky, M. L., Lazdins, J., Simmons, S. R. See Ref. 8, pp. 423–38
131. Katz, D. H., Unanue, E. R. 1973. *J. Exp. Med.* 137:967–90
132. Lagunoff, D. 1971. *Proc. Soc. Exp. Biol. Med.* 138:118–23
133. Lane, F. C., Unanue, E. R. 1973. *J. Immunol.* 110:829–34
134. Lavie, G., Zucker-Franklin, D., Franklin, E. C. 1978. *J. Exp. Med.* 148:1020–31
135. Lawrence, D. A., Weigle, W. D., Spiegelberg, H. L. 1975. *J. Clin. Invest.* 55:368–76
136. Lay, W. H., Nussenzweig, V. 1969. *J. Immunol.* 102:1172–78
137. Lazdins, J., Karnovsky, M. L. 1978. *J. Cell Physiol.* 96:115–22
138. Lazdins, J. K., Kühner, A. L., David, J. R., Karnovsky, M. L. 1978. *J. Exp. Med.* 148:746–58
139. Lejeune, F., Evans, R. 1972. *Eur. J. Cancer* 8:549–55
140. Leonard, E. J., Skeel, A. 1976. *Exp. Cell Res.* 102:434–38
141. Leslie, R. G. Q., Cohen, S. 1976. *Eur. J. Immunol.* 6:848–55
142. Leu, R. W., Eddleston, A. L. W. F., Hadden, J. W., Good, R. A. 1972. *J. Exp. Med.* 136:589–603
143. Levy, J. A., Weiss, R. M., Dirksen, E. R., Rosen, M. R. 1976. *Exp. Cell Res.* 103:375–85
144. Lipsky, P. E., Rosenthal, A. S. 1973. *J. Exp. Med.* 138:900–924
145. Lipsky, P. E., Rosenthal, A. S. 1975. *J. Exp. Med.* 141:138–54
146. Lipsky, P. E., Rosenthal, A. S. 1975. *J. Immunol.* 115:440–45
147. Loube, S. R., McNabb, T. C., Dorrington, K. J. 1978. *J. Immunol.* 120:709–14
148. Lutton, J. D. 1973. *J. Cell Biol.* 56:611–17
149. Mackaness, G. B. 1964. *J. Exp. Med.* 120:105–20
150. Mackaness, G. B. 1969. *J. Exp. Med.* 129:973–92
151. Mackaness, G. B. See Ref. 37, pp. 461–77
152. Mahoney, E. M., Hamill, A. L., Scott, W. A., Cohn, Z. A. 1977. *Proc. Natl. Acad. Sci. USA* 74:4895–99
153. Mantovani, B., Rabinovitch, M., Nussenzweig, V. 1972. *J. Exp. Med.* 135:780–92
154. Marsman, A. W. J., van der Hart, M., van Loghem, J. J. 1970. *Clin. Exp. Immunol.* 6:899–903
155. Mason, R. J., Stossel, T. P., Vaughan, M. 1972. *J. Clin. Invest.* 51:2399–407
156. Mazur, M. T., Williamson, J. R. 1977. *J. Cell Biol.* 75:185–99
157. McKeever, P. E., Garvin, A. J., Hardin, D. H., Spicer, S. S. 1976. *Am. J. Pathol.* 84:437–56
158. McKeever, P. E., Garvin, A. J., Spicer, S. S. 1976. *J. Histocytochem.* 24:948–55
159. McKeever, P. E., Spicer, S. S., Brissie, N. T., Garvin, A. J. 1977. *J.*
160. Melsom, H., Seljelid, R. 1973. *J. Exp. Med.* 137:807–20
161. Michl, J., Ohlbaum, D. J., Silverstein, S. C. 1976. *J. Exp. Med.* 144:1465–83
162. Miles, P. R., Lee, P., Trush, M. A., Dyke, K. V. 1977. *Life Sci.* 20:165–70
163. Minkin, C., Blackman, L., Newbrey, J., Pokress, S., Posek, R., Walling, M. 1977. *Biochem. Biophys. Res. Commun.* 76:875–81

164. Mitchison, N. A. 1969. *Immunology* 16:1–14
165. Montarroso, A. M., Myrvik, Q. N. 1978. *J. Reticuloendothel. Soc.* 24: 93–99
166. Mooney, J. J., Waksman, B. H. 1970. *J. Immunol.* 105:1138–45
167. Morland, B., Kaplan, G. 1977. *Exp. Cell Res.* 108:279–88
168. Mundy, G. R., Varani, J., Orr, W., Gondek, M. D., Ward, P. A. 1978. *Nature* 275:132–35
169. Muschel, R. J., Rosen, N., Bloom, B. R. 1977. *J. Exp. Med.* 145:175–86
170. Muschel, R. J., Rosen, N., Rosen, O. M., Bloom, B. R. 1977. *J. Immunol.* 119:1813–20
171. Mustafa, M. G., Cross, C. E., Munn, R. J., Hardie, J. A. 1971. *J. Lab. Clin. Med.* 77:563–71
172. Nachman, R. L., Ferris, B., Hirsch, J. G. 1971. *J. Exp. Med.* 133:785–806
173. Nachman, R. L., Ferris, B., Hirsch, J. G. 1971. *J. Exp. Med.* 133:807–20
174. Nathan, C. F., Karnovsky, M. L., David, J. R. 1971. *J. Exp. Med.* 133: 1356–76
175. Niederhuber, J. E., Shreffler, D. C. 1977. *Transplant. Proc.* 9:875–79
176. Nielsen, M., Jensen, H., Braendstrup, O., Werdelin, O. 1974. *J. Exp. Med.* 170:1260–72
177. North, R. J. 1968. *J. Reticuloendothel. Soc.* 5:203–29
178. North, R. J. 1969. *Exp. Cell Res.* 54:267–78
179. North, R. J. 1970. *Semin. Hematol.* 7:161 71
180. Oliver, J. M., Berlin, R. D. See Ref. 52, pp. 559–73
181. Oren, R., Farnham, A. E., Saito, K., Milofsky, E., Karnovsky, M. L. 1963. *J. Cell Biol.* 17:487–501
182. Orenstein, J. M., Shelton, E. 1977. *Lab. Invest.* 36:363–74
183. Page, R. C., Davies, P., Allison, A. C. 1978. *Int. Rev. Cytol.* 52:119–57
184. Parakkal, P., Pinto, J., Hanifin, J. M. 1974. *J. Ultrastruct. Res.* 48:216–26
185. Pearlstein, E., Dienstman, S. R., Defendi, V. 1978. *J. Cell Biol.* 79: 263–67
186. Pesanti, E. L., Axline, S. G. 1975. *J. Exp. Med.* 142:903–13
187. Pierce, C. W., Kapp, J. A., Wood, D. D., Benacerraf, B. 1974. *J. Immunol.* 112:1181–89
188. Polliack, A., Gordon, S. 1975. *Lab. Invest.* 33:469–77
189. Postlethwaite, A. E., Kang, A. H. 1976. *J. Exp. Med.* 143:1299–307

190. Rabinovitch, M. 1967. *Exp. Cell Res.* 46:19–28
191. Rabinovitch, M. 1967. *J. Immunol.* 99:232–37
192. Rabinovitch, M. 1968. *Semin. Hemat.* 5:134–55
193. Rabinovitch, M. See Ref. 8, pp. 369–83
194. Rabinovitch, M., DeStefano, M. J. 1973. *J. Immunol.* 110:695–701
195. Rabinovitch, M., DeStefano, M. J. 1973. *Exp. Cell Res.* 77:323–34
196. Rabinovitch, M., DeStefano, M. J. 1973. *Exp. Cell Res.* 79:423–30
197. Rabinovitch, M., DeStefano, M. J. 1974. *Exp. Cell Res.* 88:153–62
198. Rabinovitch, M., DeStefano, M. J. 1976. *J. Exp. Med.* 143:290–303
199. Rabinovitch, M., Gary, P. P. 1968. *Exp. Cell Res.* 52:363–69
200. Rabinovitch, M., Manejias, R. E., Nussenzweig, V. 1975. *J. Exp. Med.* 142: 827–38
201. Rabinovitch, M., Manejias, R. E., Russo, M., Abbey, E. E. 1977. *Cell Immunol.* 29:86–95
202. Ratzan, K. R., Musher, D. M., Keusch, G. T., Weinstein, L. 1972. *Infect. Immunol.* 5:499–504
203. Raz, A., Goldman, R. 1976. *Biochim. Biophys. Acta* 433:437–42
204. Raz, A., Goldman, R. 1976. *Biochim. Biophys. Acta* 455:226–40
205. Reaven, E. P., Axline, S. G. 1973. *J. Cell Biol.* 59:12–27
206. Remold, H. G. 1973. *J. Exp. Med.* 138:1065–76
207. Remold-O'Donnell, E. 1974. *J. Biol. Chem.* 249:3615–21
208. Remold-O'Donnell, E., Remold, H. G. 1974. *J. Biol. Chem.* 249:3622–27
209. Reynolds, H. Y., Atkinson, J. P., Newball, H. H., Frank, M. M. 1975. *J. Immunol.* 114:1813–19
210. Rhodes, J. 1973. *Nature* 243:527–28
211. Rhodes, J. 1975. *Nature* 257:597–99
212. Rinehart, J. J., Boulware, T. 1977. *J. Lab. Clin. Med.* 90:737–43
213. Robin, E. D., Smith, J. D., Tanser, A. R., Adamson, J. S., Millen, J.E., Packer, B. 1971. *Biochim. Biophys. Acta* 241:117–28
214. Romeo, D., Zabucchi, G., Rossi, F. 1973. *Nature New Biol.* 243:111–12
215. Rosenthal, A. S., Blake, J. T., Ellner, S. J., Greineder, D. K., Lipsky, P. E. See Ref. 52, pp. 131–60
216. Rosenthal, A. S., Lipsky, P. E., Shevach, E. M. 1975. *Fed. Proc.* 34: 1743–48
217. Rosenthal, A. S., Shevach, E. M. 1973. *J. Exp. Med.* 138:1194–212

218. Rossi, F., Zabucchi, G., Romeo, D. See Ref. 8, pp. 441–60
219. Ryming, F. W., Remington, J. S. 1978. *Infect. Immunol.* 20:739–43
220. Sachs, F. L., Gee, J. B. L. 1973. *J. Reticuloendothel. Soc.* 14:52–58
221. Schiffmann, E., Corcoran, B. A., Wahl, S. M. 1975. *Proc. Natl. Acad. Sci. USA* 72:1059–62
222. Schirrmacher, V., Peña-Martinez, J., Festenstein, H. 1975. *Nature* 255: 155–56
223. Schmidt, M. E., Douglas, S. D. 1972. *J. Immunol.* 109:914–17
224. Schmidtke, J. R., Unanue, E. R. 1971. *J. Immunol.* 107:331–38
225. Schnyder, J., Baggiolini, M. 1978. *J. Exp. Med.* 148:1449–57
226. Schreiber, A. D., Parsons, J., McDermott, P., Cooper, R. A. 1975. *J. Clin. Invest.* 56:1189–97
227. Schroit, A. J., Gallily, R. 1974. *Immunology* 26:971–81
228. Schroit, A. J., Geiger, B., Gallily, R. 1973. *Eur. J. Immunol.* 3:354–59
229. Schroit, A. J., Rottem, S., Gallily, R. 1976. *Biochim. Biophys. Acta* 426:499–512
230. Schwartz, R. H., Bianco, A. R., Handwerger, B. S., Kahn, C. R. 1975. *Proc. Natl. Acad. Sci. USA* 72:474–78
231. Schwartz, R. H., Dickler, H. B., Sachs, D. H., Schwartz, B. D. 1976. *Scand. J. Immunol.* 5:731–43
232. Scott, R. E., Maercklein, P. B. 1977. *Lab. Invest.* 37:430–36
233. Scott, R. E., Rosenthal, A. S. 1977. *J. Immunol.* 119:143–48
233a. Segal, D. M., Hurwitz, E. 1977. *J. Immunol.* 118:1338–47
234. Seljelid, R. See Ref. 8, pp. 911–22
235. Seljelid, R., Munthe-Koos, A. 1973. *Exp. Cell Res.* 80:473–76
236. Silverstein, S. C., Steinman, R. M., Cohn, Z. A. 1977. *Ann. Rev. Biochem.* 46:669–722
237. Skutelsky, E., Hardy, B. 1976. *Exp. Cell. Res.* 101:337–45
238. Snodgrass, M. J., Harris, T. M., Geeraets, R., Kaplan, A. M. 1977. *J. Reticuloendothel. Soc.* 22:149–57
239. Snyderman, R., Altman, L. C., Hausman, M. S., Mergenhagen, S. E. 1972. *J. Immunol.* 108:857–60
240. Snyderman, R., Mergenhagen, S. E. See Ref. 52, pp. 323–48
241. Snyderman, R., Shin, H. S., Hausman, M. H. 1971. *Proc. Soc. Exp. Biol. Med.* 138:387–90
242. Steinman, R. M., Brodie, S. E., Cohn, Z. A. 1976. *J. Cell Biol.* 68:665–87
243. Steinman, R. M., Cohn, Z. A. 1972. *J. Cell Biol.* 55:186–204

244. Steinman, R. M., Cohn, Z. A. See Ref. 8, pp. 743–51
245. Stossel, T. P. 1973. *J. Cell Biol.* 58:346–56
246. Stossel, T. P., Hartwig, J. H. 1975. *J. Biol. Chem.* 250:5706–12
247. Stossel, T. P., Hartwig, J. H. See Ref. 8, pp. 533–44
248. Stossel, T. P., Hartwig, J. H. 1976. *J. Cell. Biol.* 68:602–19
249. Stossel, T. P., Mason, R. J., Pollard, T. A., Vaughan, M. 1972. *J. Clin. Invest.* 51:604–14
250. Straus, D. C., Imhoff, J. G., Bonventre, P. F. 1977. *J. Cell. Physiol.* 93: 105–16
251. Strauss, P. R., Berlin, R. D. 1973. *J. Exp. Med.* 137:359–68
252. Territo, M. C., Cline, M. J. 1977. *J. Immunol.* 118:187–92
253. Thrasher, S. G., Yoshida, T., van Oss, C. J., Cohen, S., Rose, N. R. 1973. *J. Immunol.* 110:321–26
254. Tizard, I. R. 1971. *Bacteriol. Rev.* 35: 365–78
255. Tsan, M.-F., Berlin, R. D. 1971. *Biochim. Biophys. Acta* 241:155–69
256. Tsan, M.-F., Berlin, R. D. 1971 *J. Exp. Med.* 134:1016–35
257. Tsan, M.-F., Taube, R. A., Berlin, R. D. 1973. *J. Cell Phys.* 81:251–56
258. Ukena, T. E., Berlin, R. D. 1972. *J. Exp. Med.* 136:1–7
259. Unanue, E. R. 1969. *J. Immunol.* 102:893–98
260. Unanue, E. R. 1972. *Adv. Immunol.* 14:95–165
261. Unanue, E. R. See Ref. 8, pp. 721–38
262. Unanue, E. R., Calderon, J. 1975. *Fed. Proc.* 34:1737–42
263. Unanue, E. R., Cerottini, J. C. 1969. *Nature* 222:1193–95
264. Unanue, E. R., Cerottini, J. C. 1970. *J. Exp. Med.* 131:711–25
265. Unkeless, J. C. 1975. *J. Exp. Med.* 142:1520–33
266. Unkeless, J. C. 1977. *J. Exp. Med.* 145:931–47
267. Van der Meer, J. W. M., Bulterman, D., Van Zwet, T. L., Elzenga-Claasen, I., Van Furth, R. 1978. *J. Exp. Med.* 147:271–76
268. Van Oss, C. J. 1978. *Ann. Rev. Microbiol.* 32:19–39
269. Viken, K. E., Odegaard, A. 1974. *Acta Pathol. Microbiol. Scand. Sect. B* 82:235–44
270. Wachsmuth, E. D. 1975. *Exp. Cell Res.* 96:409–12
271. Wachsmuth, E. D., Staber, F. G. 1977. *Exp. Cell Res.* 109:269–76
272. Wachsmuth, E. D., Stoye, J. P. 1977. *J. Reticuloendothel. Soc.* 22:469–83

273. Wachsmuth, E. D., Stoye, J. P. 1977. *J. Reticuloendothel. Soc.* 22:485–97
274. Waldron, J. A., Horn, R. G., Rosenthal, A. S. 1974. *J. Immunol.* 112:746–55
275. Walker, W. S. 1976. *J. Immunol.* 116:911–14
276. Walker, W. S., Demus, A. 1975. *J. Immunol.* 114:765–69
277. Wang, P., Dechatelet, L. R., Waite, M. 1976. *Biochim. Biophys. Acta* 450:311–21
278. Wang, P., Shirley, P. S., Dechatelet, L. R., McCall, C. E., Waite, B. M. 1976. *J. Reticuloendothel. Soc.* 19:333–45
279. Wang, P., Waite, M., Dechatelet, L. R. 1977. *Biochim. Biophys. Acta* 487:163–74
280. Ward, P. A. 1968. *J. Exp. Med.* 128:1201–21
281. Wellek, B., Hahn, H. H., Opferkuch, W. 1975. *J. Immunol.* 114:1643–45
282. Welscher, H. D., Cruchaud, A. 1978. *Eur. J. Immunol.* 8:180–84
283. Werb, Z. See Ref. 8, pp. 331–45

284. Werb, Z., Cohn, Z. A. 1971. *J. Exp. Med.* 134:1545–69
285. Werb, Z., Cohn, Z. A. 1971. *J. Exp. Med.* 134:1570–90
286. Werb, Z., Cohn, Z. A. 1972. *J. Biol. Chem.* 247:2439–46
287. Werdelin, O., Braendstrup, O., Pedersen, E. 1974. *J. Exp. Med.* 140:1245–59
288. Wilkinson, P. C. 1973. *Nature* 244:512–13
289. Wilkinson, P. C. See Ref. 52, pp. 349–65
290. Wills, E. J., Davies, P., Allison, A. C., Haswell, A. D. 1972. *Nature New Biol.* 240:58–60
291. Yamashita, U., Shevach, E. M. 1977. *J. Immunol.* 119:1584–88
292. Yasaka, T., Kambara, T. 1978. *Biochim. Biophys. Acta* 408:306–12
293. Zuckerman, S. H., Douglas, S. D. 1977. *Immunology* 32:247–53
294. Zuckerman, S. H., Douglas, S. D. 1979. *Crit. Rev. Microbiol.* 7:1–26

Ann. Rev. Med. 1977. 28:425–52

THE ASSOCIATION BETWEEN GENES IN THE MAJOR HISTOCOMPATIBILITY COMPLEX AND DISEASE SUSCEPTIBILITY

♦7253

Takehiko Sasazuki, M.D. and Hugh O. McDevitt, M.D.
Division of Immunology, Department of Medicine, Stanford University School of Medicine, Stanford, California 94305

F. Carl Grumet, M.D.
Department of Pathology, Stanford University School of Medicine, Stanford, California 94305

INTRODUCTION

During the past four years, there has been an extraordinarily rapid accumulation of evidence showing that genes of the human major histocompatibility system have a marked effect on susceptibility to a wide variety of diseases. The human major histocompatibility system is a cluster of genes on the VIth human chromosome that determine the structure of cell-surface glycoproteins found on all the cells of the body. These glycoproteins differ from individual to individual and form a complex set of antigenic determinants that constitute the strongest (major) antigenic barrier to tissue transplantation between genetically nonidentical individuals. In addition, by analogy to the major histocompatibility system in several animal species, other genes in the same chromosomal region have marked regulatory effects on immune responsiveness to a wide variety of antigens. Indeed, it appears that almost all of the genes that have been identified in this chromosomal region have some effect upon, or relation to, the immune system, as is shown below.

Perhaps the first demonstration of an association between the major histocompatibility system and susceptibility or resistance to disease was reported by Lilly (1), who showed that genes linked to the mouse major histocompatibility system, the H-2 system, determined resistance to Gross virus–induced leukemia. The mechanism of action of this genetic factor for resistance to viral leukemogenesis was not

8243-2502/80/0310-0297$01.00   425

apparent, but Lilly speculated that it might be due to some type of effect on the immune response to the virus.

In 1967 Amiel (2) reported a moderate increase in the incidence of one particular human transplantation antigenic specificity (at that time designated 4c) in patients with Hodgkin's disease over that in a normal control population. The search for associations between genes in the human major histocompatibility system and disease susceptibility or resistance was given fresh impetus by the demonstration that immune response (*Ir*) genes, controlling the immune response to a wide variety of antigens, were linked to the murine major histocompatibility complex (3). Immune response genes were first described by Benacerraf and his colleagues in studying the immune response of guinea pigs to hapten-substituted synthetic polypeptides such as poly-L-lysine (4). Genetic control of the immune response to other synthetic polypeptides in mice was analyzed by McDevitt (5), in collaboration with Sela and Humphrey.

Ir genes have been reviewed extensively (4–6). The major class of *Ir* genes are those closely linked to the species' major histocompatibility system. These genes control the cellular and humoral response to specific antigens and have been described in the mouse, guinea pig, rat, and monkey. The precise mechanism of *Ir* gene action is not yet known, but they appear to control the ability of immunocompetent lymphocytes to recognize an antigen as foreign, and to initiate both a cellular and humoral response to the antigen. Much of the evidence indicates that *Ir* genes are expressed in thymus-derived lymphocytes (T cells) and may function as a new class of foreign-antigen receptor on the surface of these T lymphocytes. It seems clear that this type of *Ir* gene-controlled antigen recognition does not involve any known immunoglobulins, since none of the structural genes for immunoglobulins have been found to be linked to the major histocompatibility system in any mammalian species. Current evidence [presented in detail in (6)] indicates that genes mapping in the *I*, or immune response region of the mouse major histocompatibility system (see below), determine the structure and/or function of cell-surface receptors for foreign antigens on the surface of T lymphocytes, and possibly also on the surface of macrophages and B lymphocytes (the precursors of antibody-producing cells).

The demonstration that genes in the major histocompatibility system have a profound effect on determining the ability to respond well or poorly to specific antigens suggested that genes in the major histocompatibility system might have a major effect on resistance to those diseases in which the immune system was protective, or in autoimmune diseases, in which the immune system itself might initiate the disease process. The possibility of such a functional relationship, as well as the earlier demonstrations of associations between the major histocompatibility system and disease, led to a series of studies in many laboratories around the world, searching for associations between the human major histocompatibility system, the *h*uman *l*eukocyte *a*ntigen (HLA) system—and disease susceptibility.

During the past four years, this search has been extraordinarily productive and has led to the discovery that a number of rheumatic, autoimmune, neurologic, endocrine, gastrointestinal, and dermatologic diseases show definite associations with particular genetic variants (alleles) of several genes in the human major his-tocompatibility system. Before discussing the human major histocompatibility sys-tem and the disease associations in detail, a brief description of the genetic structure of the murine major histocompatibility system—the H-2 system—will permit us to indicate some of the functional relationships between this complex genetic region and the immune system.

THE H-2 SYSTEM

Figure 1 is a schematic diagram of the H-2 system. [For a detailed discussion of the genetic fine structure of the murine H-2 system, its gene products, and some of their functions, the reader is referred to a comprehensive review by Shreffler & David (7).] The H-2 system is bounded by *H-2K* and *H-2D,* which are the initially described, classical transplantation antigens that can be detected by cytotoxic T cells as well as by alloantisera. The *H-2K* and *H-2D* gene products are 45,000-MW cell-surface glycoproteins found on all the tissues of the body, with the possible exception of sperm and very early embryonic tissues. The human counterparts are the *HLA-B* and *-A* genes, respectively (see Figure 2).

The true function of the *H-2K* and *H-2D* gene products is not known; however, recently it has become apparent that these genes are intimately involved in the induction and effector phases of T-cell–mediated cytotoxicity, or T-cell killer func-tion. In several systems it has been shown that cytotoxic T cells specific for viruses, and for minor transplantation antigens such as the H-Y or male-transplantation antigen, recognize not only the antigen to which they have been sensitized, but also the *H-2K* and/or *D* gene product on the immunizing cells. Thus, after an animal is immunized with foreign cells carrying a particular virus, its T cells will only recognize virus on the surface of cells of the same foreign transplantation antigen type as those originally used for immunization. Even though the animal has been

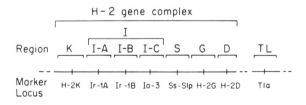

Figure 1   A schematic diagram of the H-2 complex. The H-2 system is bounded by the *H-2K* and *H-2D* loci. The *I* region of the H-2 system includes *Ir-1A, Ir-1B,* and *Ir-1C.* The corresponding Ia regions are *I-A, I-B,* and *I-C.* Earlier genetic maps of the *I* region included only the *Ir-1A, B,* and *C* regions, but recent analysis of several *H-2* recombinants has indicated that a new region, *I-J,* must be intercalated between *Ir-1B* and *Ir-1C,* and that another region exists between *I-J* and *Ir-1C,* which has been given the preliminary designation of *I-E* (13). The *S* locus or region of the H-2 system determines at least two genes, one of which determines the structure of a component of the C4 molecule. There is also evidence that the *S* region determines the levels of C1, 2, and 3.

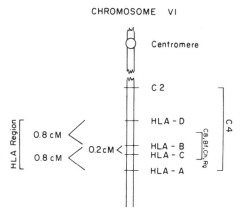

Figure 2   A schematic diagram of the HLA system on human chromosome VI. *HLA-B* and *A,* which are analogous to *H-2K* and *D,* are separated by 0.8 recombination units or centimorgans (cM). The *HLA-C* locus does not have a counterpart in the mouse. The *HLA-D* locus or region determines the structure of lymphocyte cell-surface antigens eliciting the mixed-culture reaction, and therefore may be analogous to the *I* region of the mouse. The genes for C4 deficiency, C8 deficiency, Bf (properdin factor B) and for the Chido (Ch) and Rogers blood-group antigen have not been precisely mapped, but are within the *HLA* system.

immunized to these virus-bearing cells, it will not kill cells of its own transplantation antigen type that carry the same amount of virus on their cell surface (8). It is thus clear that the *H-2K* and *H-2D* gene products have a major effect on the development and specificity of cell-mediated killer functions. It is not yet known whether this is the primary or even a major function of these gene products. There has been considerable speculation that these gene products, because of their ubiquitous tissue distribution, must play a more fundamental role in cellular interaction and tissue morphogenesis. As yet, however, there is no definite evidence for these latter postulated functions.

The *I* region was originally defined because genetic control of specific immune response to several polypeptides was shown to map in the chromosomal region lying between the *H-2K* and *S* genes of the H-2 system (9). Within a short time, it became apparent that in addition to genetic control of specific immune responses, this region also determined the structure of cell-surface antigens that elicited the mixed-lymphocyte-culture reaction and the graft-versus-host reaction. Studies designed to produce antisera against *I*-region gene products resulted in the identification of a new class of cell-surface alloantigens, the *I*mmune-response region–*a*ssociated antigens, or Ia antigens. These cell-surface allo-antigens are also glycoproteins that fall into two molecular-weight ranges, 25,000 and 33,000, and are found predominantly on the surface of lymphocytes, macrophages, sperm, and epidermal cells. A systematic analysis of a number of different inbred mouse strains, and of recombinant H-2 chromosomes derived by crossing over between the *H-2K* and *H-2D* loci, led to the subdivision of the *I* region into the *I-A, I-B,* and *I-C* subregions. Genes controlling the immune response to particular foreign antigens were mapped in the *I-A, I-B,* or *I-C* regions and were designated *Ir-1A, Ir-1B,* and *Ir-1C.* In several instances it also became apparent that two *I*-region genes were required to develop a high response to a particular antigen (10).

It is now apparent that the Ia antigens are the primary cell-surface alloantigens that stimulate in the mixed-lymphocyte-culture reaction in vitro and that elicit the graft-versus-host reaction in vivo. A major research effort now centers on determining the relationship of the Ia antigens to *Ir* gene function. During the past year, it has been shown that factors can be isolated from thymus-derived lymphocytes that appear to be capable of regulating specific immune responses. These factors mimic the effects of helper thymus-derived lymphocytes and thus potentiate the immune response to a particular antigen (11), or they mimic the effects of suppressor thymus-derived lymphocytes (12) and suppress the specific immune response to a particular antigen.

Both types of factor have a number of interesting properties in common. They have a molecular weight in the 40,000–50,000 range; they bind specifically to antigen-immunoabsorbent columns; they lack all immunoglobulin antigenic determinants; and they possess Ia antigenic specificities. Preliminary evidence indicates that helper factors bear Ia determinants mapping in the *I-A* subregion (12) and suppressor-factor Ia determinants map in a new *I* subregion that has tentatively been placed between *I-B* and *I-C*, and has been given the preliminary designation of *I-J* (13). These preliminary findings are important because they indicate that Ia antigens may be part of structures derived from T cells that have the ability to recognize specific antigenic determinants. If these results are borne out, they indicate that the *I* subregion of the H-2 system contains a number of genes that are in some way involved in the structure of a new class of antigen-specific receptors found on the surface of immunocompetent T lymphocytes.

Ir genes have not yet been conclusively demonstrated in man, so that a precise human counterpart to the murine *I* region does not yet exist. However, the Ia antigens elicit the mixed-lymphocyte reaction [MLR (see below)] and lymphocyte antigens determined by the *HLA-D* locus have a similar function (see Figure 2). By analogy, it is presumed that the *HLA-D* region may be the human *I* region.

The major histocompatibility system has yet another intimate relationship with the immune system. As is shown below, structural genes for several complement components (the second, fourth, and eighth complement components) are linked to the human major histocompatibility system, the HLA system. In the mouse, recent studies (7) have shown that the *S* gene of the H-2 system, which had been known to control the structure and serum levels of a serum β-globulin, is in fact the structural gene for one of the polypeptide chains of the fourth component of complement C4 (7). (The human C4 gene has not been accurately mapped as yet, cf Figure 2.) Thus, in addition to being intimately involved in the specificity of T-cell–mediated cytotoxicity, and in regulating both the potentiation (help) and the inhibition (suppression) of the immune response, the major histocompatibility system also determines the structure of several complement components.

It is not yet known whether the close linkage of all of these genes, which regulate cellular, humoral, and effector arms of the immune response, indicates a functional interrelationship and an underlying structural homology between these three genetic regions of the major histocompatibility system. However, the extraordinary finding that all three classes (the K and D genes, the I-region genes, and the S-region genes) of the major histocompatibility system are involved in particular functional aspects of the immune response suggests that regulation of the immune response is a major function of the major histocompatibility system and that the different genes in this complex system may be both functionally and structurally interrelated (14).

In many ways, the H-2 system has served as a prototype for extending our understanding of the human major histocompatibility system, the HLA system. This system is described in detail in the following section.

THE HLA SYSTEM

Background

Studies of the human major histocompatibility (HLA) system began in the late 1950s, when it was reported that leukoagglutinating antibodies could be detected in the sera of multiply transfused patients, and also of parous women (15, 16). Because these antibodies reacted with some, but not all, leukocytes from normal individuals, it was recognized that the leukocyte antigens involved belonged to a genetic polymorphic system. As many more such sera became identified during the early 1960s, studies of families, and computer-assisted analyses of population studies with these antisera, provided the first examples of the allelic nature of the antigens detected (17–19), i.e. that these antigens were variant, or allelic, products of the same gene (or genes). During that same time, it was shown that the leukocyte antigens could also be detected by lymphocyte cytotoxicity.

The development of a microtechnique soon led to the general acceptance of the antibody- and complement-mediated lymphocyte microcytotoxicity assay as the standard in the field (20). This technique, which has changed little over the succeeding decade, basically consists of a 1–2-hr incubation of approximately 2000 viable lymphocytes with each of a selected series of antisera, plus fresh-frozen rabbit serum as a source of complement. At the end of the incubation period, each test is read for residual viable cells using a vital dye. Although additional techniques have been developed, the antibody-mediated, lymphocyte microcytotoxicity technique remains the most widespread and accepted standard. As data concerning this system began to accumulate, the need for closer collaboration among investigators in the field was realized and a series of international workshops, held approximately every two years, was initiated in 1964. A well-documented model of the very complex genetic system we now refer to as HLA emerged from those workshops, as well as from a great deal of work carried on in the laboratories of many independent investigators. [For general reviews see (21–23).]

Serologically Detectable Antigens

The genetic determinants of all the HLA antigens reside in a segment of chromosome VI that is estimated to be approximately 1000 genes long and is referred to as the HLA region (21–27). Within this region lie the four currently defined HLA loci, *HLA-A, HLA-B, HLA-C,* and *HLA-D.* Antigens determined by the *A, B,* and *C* loci are present on the surfaces of all nucleated cells (also on blood platelets) and are detectable by serological techniques such as the lymphocyte cytotoxicity method described above. Each locus has its own series of unique antigens that are the products of the allelic genes belonging to that particular locus. Antigens that can be identified by presently available antisera are shown in Table 1. Antigens written with an A, B, or C followed by an arabic numeral are those acknowledged by the International Workshops and the World Health Organization to be clearly defined. Those written with a w preceding the arabic numeral are less clearly defined and are the subject of further workshop evaluation, whereas those antigens without an A, B, or C prefix have been reported by only a few laboratories and remain to be confirmed at an International Workshop. There are currently 19 well-characterized *A* locus antigens and 24 *B* locus antigens, accounting for over 95% of the *A* and *B* locus genes (28, 29). The more recently defined *C* locus has only six antigens agreed upon, accounting for only about half of the alleles at this locus.

HLA typings are written as in Table 2. Each individual possesses two HLA regions, one paternally and one maternally derived. Because the HLA antigens are

Table 1   HLA antigens

A Locus	B Locus	C Locus	D Locus
HLA-A1	HLA-B5		
-A2	-B7		
-A3	-B8		
-A9	-B12		
-A10	-B13		
-A11	-B14		
-A28	-B18		
-A29	-B27		
HLA-Aw23	HLA-Bw15	HLA-Cw1	HLA-Dw1
-Aw24	-Bw16	-Cw2	-Dw2
-Aw25	-Bw17	-Cw3	-Dw3
-Aw26	-Bw21	-Cw4	-Dw4
-Aw30	-Bw22	-Cw5	-Dw5
-Aw31	-Bw35		-Dw6
-Aw32	-Bw37		
-Aw33	-Bw38	-T7	
	-Bw39		
-Aw36	-Bw40		-LD-107
-Aw43	-Bw41		-LD-108
	-Bw42		
	TT		
	KSO		
	Hs		
	407*		

codominantly expressed and there are no known silent or amorphic alleles, each individual is characterized by two antigens from each of the loci (i.e. a set of six serologically determined antigens). Because of the close linkage between the loci, the entire HLA region is inherited intact in approximately 99% of offspring. Within any given family, then, a particular haplotype (i.e. a fixed combination of HLA antigens determined by the HLA region of a single chromosome VI) will be inherited so that a specific set of A, B, and C antigens will always appear together. Because the crossover frequency is finite, however, hundreds of generations of random human matings have resulted in every possible combination of *A, B,* and *C* genes. In the random population, therefore, the presence of a particular antigen at one of the loci generally does not affect the probability of finding any particular antigens at the other loci.

An illustration of the transmission of HLA haplotypes is given in the pedigree shown in Table 3. In six of the seven children, the haplotypes have been inherited intact as would be expected. One child (#6), however, demonstrates a rare (<1% of offspring) event defined as an HLA crossover. During meiosis a recombination between maternal chromosomes has occured so that a new haplotype has been

Table 2 Common genetic terminology

Haplotype =	A combination of antigens determined by the HLA region of a single chromosome, e.g. A1, B8, Cw3, Dw5
Genotype =	A pair of haplotypes possessed by a particular individual, e.g. A1, B8, Cw3, Dw5; A2, B12, Cw4, Dw3
Phenotype =	The antigens possessed by a particular individual regardless of haplotype assignment e.g. A1, A2; B8, B12; Cw3, Cw4; Dw3, Dw5

Table 3 Transmission of HLA haplotypes in a family

Individual	HLA genotype
Father (a/b)	A1, B8, C-, D-; A3, B18, C-, D-
Mother (c/d)	A2, B27, Cw1, Dw1; A29, B12, C-, D-
Child #1 (a/d)	A1, B8, C-, D-; A29, B12, C-, D-
Children #2, 3, 5, 7 (b/d)	A3, B18, C-, D-; A29, B12, C-, D-
Child #4 (b/c)	A3, B18, C-, D-; A2, B27, Cw1, Dw1
Child #6 (b/cd)[a]	A3, B18, C-, D-; A2, B12, C-, D-
	c d

[a] Child #6 possesses the recombinant chromosome (cd). The designations C- and D- represent as yet unidentified antigens at the *C* and *D* loci. Data kindly provided by Dr. Rose Payne, Department of Medicine/Division of Hematology, Stanford University School of Medicine, Stanford, California 94305).

created. The A2 from the c chromosome is now combined with the B12, C-, and D- of the d chromosome. This new haplotype can now be passed on intact to future descendants of child #6.

As with other polymorphic genetic markers, the frequency of each antigen will depend upon the ethnic group studied (28). For example, the HLA-A1 antigen appears in 33% of Caucasians, but is absent from Chinese, whereas the Hs antigen occurs in 25% of Chinese, but is absent from Caucasians (30). This marked ethnic variability is, of course, an important consideration in selecting appropriate controls for any population study utilizing the HLA system.

The chemical structure of the HLA antigens is an area of active research at present. The serologically detectable antigens have been solubilized from the cell surface and consist of a dimer with a heavy glycoprotein chain (MW 44,000) containing the antigenic specificity, and a β_2 microglobulin chain (MW 12,000) (31). The β_2 microglobulin does not possess HLA antigenic markers and the locus for the β_2 chain has been located on chromosome XV (32).

The D Locus and Mixed Leukocyte Cultures (MLC)

Unlike the serologically defined A, B, and C antigens, D-locus markers can at present be recognized only by an in vitro lymphocyte culture test. Although some variations of technique are now used, the basic test consists of several days of culture of lymphocytes of one individual (the responder) with X-irradiated or mitomycin-C–treated lymphocytes of a second individual (the stimulator). If the stimulator possesses D-locus antigens not present in the responder, the lymphocytes of the latter undergo transformation, resulting in DNA synthesis that can be quantified as an index of response. (The X-irradiation or mitomycin-C prevents the stimulator cells from reacting similarly.) Through careful selection of individuals homozygous for D-locus alleles (e.g. offspring of first-cousin marriages), it is possible to obtain "typing cells," which may then be used to test others for the presence or absence of a particular D-locus antigen (33). D-locus typing is technically difficult and has only recently been developed, so that only six allelic types are generally agreed upon for this locus (34). Because MLC nonstimulation between random individuals is such a rare event, it is anticipated that many D-locus alleles exist and are yet to be identified. The problem is further complicated by the likelihood that the D locus is several (or many) loci, as is the case for the analogous I region in the mouse.

Linked Loci and Linkage Disequilibrium

Through the studies of families with recombinant haplotypes, it has been possible to map not only the HLA loci, but also a number of other loci as well. A graphic presentation of the HLA region is shown in Figure 2. It is particularly interesting to note that three components of the complement system are linked to the HLA loci, thus defining yet another important function (in addition to transplantation antigenicity, disease susceptibility linkage, and probably human immune-response genes) for this segment of chromosome VI.

Based on the principle of random human matings over hundreds of generations, with small but finite recombination frequencies within the region, almost all possible haplotype combinations should appear at a frequency proportional to the product of the frequencies of the individual component genes. Although this rule is generally valid, some exceptions do occur such that certain combinations of alleles at different loci appear together on the same chromosome more frequently than would be predicted. When this occurs, the genes are said to be in linkage disequilibrium. For example, in Danes, the frequency of the haplotype containing both the A1 and B8 antigens is 0.099, whereas its predicted frequency (if no linkage disequilibrium existed between those two antigens) is 0.022 (23). Among Caucasians of the Middle East or Asia, however, the linkage disequilibrium between those same two antigens is not significant, i.e. A1 and B8 do not occur together more frequently than predicted by random matings.

No mechanism has yet been proven to account for the observed linkage disequilibrium between HLA antigens; however, several may be postulated. For example, some unknown survival value might accrue in some environments from certain combinations of antigens, some combinations might affect chromosomal stability and therefore have relatively lower recombination frequencies, or some combinations might derive from relatively new mutants that have not yet had time to dissociate to a state of linkage equilibrium.

Regardless of mechanism, the phenomenon of linkage disequilibrium exists sufficiently frequently in the HLA system to suggest that some biological function may underlie the associations observed (see below).

B-Cell Antigens

In several animal species the existence of immune response (*Ir*) genes linked to the species' major histocompatibility region has been clearly documented, and preliminary evidence to support the existence of similar genes in man has also been gathered (5, 35). In the best-studied model, that of the mouse, loci for the *Ir* genes map within the *H-2* region, closer to the *K* than to the *D* locus. Also mapping at the same (or as yet genetically indistinguishable) loci as the *Ir* genes are a series of immune response–associated *Ia* genes (36). The products of the *Ia* genes are antigens present in greatest concentration on the surface of B lymphocytes (and also in small quantities on T lymphocytes) and detectable by antibody-mediated lymphocyte cytotoxicity.

The exact function of Ia antigens and their relation to the functionally defined *Ir* genes is not yet known. It is reasonable to postulate that Ia markers may represent the serologically detectable *Ir* gene cell-surface receptors for antigen recognition. For this reason, a great deal of research activity has recently centered upon a search for human B-cell antigens as possible murine Ia analogs [several such antigens have already been described (37–39)] and as possible serologically detectable *D* locus gene products.

A number of methods for testing for human B-cell antibodies are available, and one of the most common is to first remove HLA-A, B, or C antibodies from antisera by their absorption onto platelets (which lack "Ia" antigens). The absorbed sera are then tested for residual antibodies against purified B cells obtained either from patients with chronic lymphocytic leukemia (a disease characterized by proliferation of a clone of B cells) or from normal B cells separated from T cells by virtue of differential adherence to sheep cells or anti-immunoglobulin columns. Preliminary studies reporting the identification of B-cell antigens in man have already been published, and the next (1977) International HLA Workshop will focus on this aspect of HLA serology, particularly the clarification of B-cell antigens and their genetic mapping and probable correlations with D-locus genes.

SPECIFIC ASSOCIATIONS BETWEEN HLA AND DISEASE

The first association between HLA and disease was reported by Amiel in 1967 (2) involving Hodgkin's disease and an HLA-B locus antigen then designated 4c. Over the next 10 years a progressively larger number of diseases has revealed association or linkage with HLA-A, B, or C antigens. The most striking of these is still the association between B27 and ankylosing spondylitis (AS), an association so strong that it has been utilized as an aid to clinical diagnosis.

In 1973, Jersild et al (40) reported the first association of a disease with a D-locus antigen, multiple sclerosis and Dw2. These findings suggested that the less impressive, but earlier reported association of HLA-B7 with multiple sclerosis was possibly secondary to the existence of strong linkage disequilibrium between B7 and Dw2. More recently Terasaki et al (41) reported an even stronger association of multiple sclerosis with a serologically defined B-cell alloantigen type, Group II, which is linked to HLA and may be related to the HLA-D antigen Dw2. As finer genetic mapping of the HLA region evolves, it may be possible to define even closer markers of disease-susceptibility genes, and eventually even to test directly for the disease-susceptibility genes themselves.

Although rapid progress is being made in analyzing other HLA and disease associations, as is shown below, a number of precautions must be observed in studying these associations. First, proper control populations must be selected for each new patient population, particularly with respect to racial background. Second, diagnostic classification is critical. For example, if diabetes mellitus was taken as a single disease, it would not have been possible to detect an association with any HLA type. Only when juvenile-onset, insulin-dependent diabetes was considered separately was an association with HLA-B8 evident. Similarly, if psoriasis vulgaris is not differentiated from pustulosis palmaris et plantaris, the associations of B13, Bw17, and Bw37 with the former disease would be masked or diluted out. This type of problem is called "dilution" and may obscure a true association.

Third, quantitative measures of the strength of HLA and disease associations must be considered carefully. An accepted measure of the intensity of an association is the relative risk (RR):

$$ RR = \frac{(\# \text{ patients with the HLA antigen}) \times (\# \text{ controls without the antigen})}{(\# \text{ controls with the antigen}) \times (\# \text{ patients without the antigen})} $$

a calculated term that represents the risk of developing a disease in an individual possessing a particular HLA antigen as compared to an individual lacking that antigen. In determining the statistical significance of the associations it is also important to be aware that p values (or X^2) may be misleading unless the number of variables examined in any comparison of populations is also taken into account. Thus, if one is studying the association of 20 different *HLA-B* alleles with a given disease, it is likely that one of these 20 will show a significant difference (uncorrected $p < 0.05$) in frequency from the control population by chance alone. Multiplying an uncorrected p value by the number of HLA antigens tested for provides a roughly "corrected p," and ensures that probability values observed are not artificially elevated simply because of the large number of variables studied.

Finally, a distinction must be made between association and linkage. Association is demonstrated in population studies of unrelated individuals when two particular traits (e.g. a selected HLA antigen and expression of a specific disease) occur together at a frequency different from that predicted by chance alone. Linkage cannot be proven by population studies, but rather must be shown by studies in families in which segregation of two traits (e.g. an HLA antigen and C4 deficiency, or an HLA antigen and a specific disease) can be demonstrated in a consistent pattern. Linked traits do not necessarily show association, and vice versa.

Despite the difficulties of performing and analyzing population studies, approximately 40 diseases have already been shown to be associated with HLA antigens, and several others demonstrate linkage. The majority of these associations, arranged into categories according to medical specialty, are listed in Tables 4–10 and are briefly discussed below. [Because of space limitation, primary references have been given only for those diseases not already cited in (42) and (43).]

Rheumatology (Table 4)

The strongest HLA and disease association observed is that found between AS and HLA-B27. This association is so strong that B27 typing has become a clinically useful aid in the diagnosis of this disease at an early stage, i.e. prior to the appearance of characteristic X-ray findings. More than 90% of Caucasian patients with AS possess B27, whereas only 5–9% of controls have this specificity. This strong association is also prominent in other ethnic groups. For example, among some Canadian Indians, 100% of AS patients had B27. These data are significant even though the number of patients tested was small and the normal frequency of B27 in this ethnic group is extremely high compared with that of Caucasians. In Japanese, in whom B27 is extremely rare, AS again has a strong association with B27.

Population surveys have revealed that roughly 20% of the B27(+) population has radiologically detectable sacroiliitis, which is frequently symptomatic and previously undetected (44). The sex incidence is equal in these undetected cases. Thus, some manifestations of AS are ten times more frequent than previously thought in males, and many, many times more frequent than previously thought in females. The total number of such cases in the US population would thus approach two million. [250×10^6 population $\times 0.05$ B27 (+) frequency $\times 0.20$ frequency of AS findings in B27(+) individuals.]

Table 4 Rheumatology

Disease	HLA antigen	% Antigen frequency		Relative risk	p Value
		patient	control		
Ankylosing spondylitis					
Caucasians	B27	90	8	87.8	1.0×10^{-10}
Haida Indians	B27	100	51	34.4	0.17×10^{-4}
Bella Coola Indians	B27	100	26	20.2	0.19×10^{-1}
Japanese	B27	67	0	305.7	1.0×10^{-10}
Reiter's syndrome	B27	78	8	35.9	1.0×10^{-10}
Yersinia arthritis	B27	79	9	24.3	1.0×10^{-10}
Salmonella arthritis	B27	67	9	17.6	0.36×10^{-9}
Psoriasis arthropatica					
peripheral	B13	10	6	2.2	0.95×10^{-2}
	B27	16	9	2.5	0.35×10^{-3}
	Bw17	25	6	5.8	1.0×10^{-10}
	Bw38	13	3	4.5	0.32×10^{-3}
central	B13	20	6	4.8	0.76×10^{-7}
	B27	40	9	8.6	1.0×10^{-4}
	Bw17	12	6	2.5	0.46×10^{-2}
	Bw38	23	3	9.1	0.56×10^{-6}
Psoriasis arthropatica					
unspecified	B27	42	8	7.1	0.25×10^{-9}
	Bw17	25	8	3.9	0.73×10^{-3}
Juvenile					
rheumatoid arthritis	B27	26	9	4.7	1.0×10^{-10}
Rheumatoid arthritis	Dw4	36	16	3.0	0.5×10^{-2}

Reiter's syndrome, defined strictly by the triad of arthritis, nongonococcal ure-thritis, and conjunctivitis, also has a strong association with B27. Available evidence suggests that this syndrome can appear as a complication of Shigellosis (flexneri) occurring primarily in B27-positive persons (45, 46). It is also of interest to note that patients with gonococcal arthritis rarely possess the B27 antigens, raising questions about an etiologic relationship between gonococci and Reiter's syndrome (47, 48).

Reactive arthritis following exposure to infectious agents such as *Yersinia en-terocolitica* and *Salmonella* has also shown an association with B27. Psoriatic arthritis on the other hand, has a weaker association with B27 and significant associations with B13, Bw17, and Bw37. These latter associations are similar to those of all psoriasis vulgaris patients, as seen in Table 6. Juvenile rheumatoid arthritis (JRA) also has a weaker association with B27. The observation that each of these types of arthritis is associated with the same HLA antigen, B27, strongly suggests that they may share some combination of common determinants of suscep-tibility, pathogens, or pathogenic process.

Unlike the preceding forms of arthritis, classical adult rheumatoid arthritis (RA) is not associated with B27, but rather is associated with the HLA-D specificity Dw4 (or R, r) (49, 50). The absence of an association of RA with B27 raises the possibility that this disease is pathogenetically distinct from the B27-associated forms of arthritis. RA is the first disease to show an association only with an *HLA-D* locus type, in the absence of any *HLA-A, B,* or *C* association. This is potentially a very important observation, and is discussed in the section on Mechanisms.

Rheumatic fever and gout have not shown any significant associations.

Neurology—Psychiatry (Table 5)

Multiple sclerosis (MS) was first reported to have a slight but significant association with HLA-A3, and later, a stronger association with B7. Subsequently, HLA-Dw2 was shown to be even more strongly associated. These data suggest that the *D* locus may be the closest of the *HLA* loci to the actual locus determining MS susceptibility, and that the disease associations of B7 and even A3 may merely arise because of the linkage disequilibrium of B7 with Dw2, and of A3 with B7. More recently, a B-lymphocyte alloantigen has been shown to be more strongly associated with multiple sclerosis than Dw2, suggesting that the locus for this new B-cell alloantigen may be yet closer to the actual MS disease-susceptibility locus.

Myasthenia gravis (MG) has a strong association with B8, and a weaker association with A1, presumably secondary to the strong linkage disequilibrium between A1 and B8. In a preliminary study of a small group, an association of MG with Dw3 also appears (30% of patients versus 9% of controls). Manic-depression has been reported to be associated with Bw16, and for both schizophrenia and paralytic poliomyelitis conflicting reports have appeared describing the presence or absence of HLA associations. Each of these diseases must be further studied before any conclusion should be drawn regarding the validity of their HLA associations.

Table 5 Neurology

Disease	HLA antigen	% Antigen frequency		Relative risk	*p* Value
		patient	control		
Multiple sclerosis	A3	36	26	1.5	0.94×10^{-8}
	B7	34	25	1.6	0.76×10^{-9}
	Dw2	67	18	6.9	0.17×10^{-5}
	Group 4[a]	84	33		$0.3 \ \times 10^{-2}$
Myasthenia gravis	A1	45	26	2.5	0.87×10^{-9}
	B8	52	23	4.4	$1.0 \ \times 10^{-10}$
Paralytic poliomyelitis	B7	21	21	1.0	0.65×10^{-3}
	B7	38	19	2.6	
Schizophrenia	A28	19	6	3.5	0.28×10^{-5}
	A28	4	7	0.7	
Manic-depression	Bw16	13	5	2.8	0.79×10^{-4}

[a] Proposed B-cell alloantigen

Dermatology (Table 6)

Psoriasis vulgaris has an association with three different *HLA-B* locus antigens, B13, Bw17, and Bw37. Psoriasis (nonspecific) is associated with Bw16, as well as with B13 and Bw17. Psoriasis pustulosis, on the other hand, has been associated with B27.

Dermatitis herpetiformis (DH) is associated with Dw3, B8, and A1. As with some other HLA and disease associations involving more than one HLA antigen, the primary association of DH may be with the B8 antigen, and the weaker association with A1 may arise as a result of the linkage disequilibrium between B8 and A1. More recently, it has been reported that an antiserum obtained from the parous wife of a patient with dermatitis herpetiformis reacted with the B lymphocytes from 15 of 15 patients with this disorder, but none of 37 healthy controls (51). The relation of this apparent B-cell–specific antigen to the HLA region is not yet known.

Behçet's disease, rare in both Europe and America, but fairly common in the eastern Mediterranean and in northern parts of Japan, has an association with B5 in both Caucasians and Japanese. Recrudescent herpes labialis has been reported to be associated with A1 and B8, and pemphigus is associated with A10. Scleroderma, acne conglobata and recurrent aphthous stomatitis show no HLA associations in Caucasians, and other ethnic groups have not yet been studied.

Table 6 Dermatology

Disease	HLA antigen	% Antigen frequency		Relative risk	p Value
		patient	control		
Psoriasis vulgaris	B13	20	5	4.7	1.0×10^{-10}
	Bw17	26	8	5.0	1.0×10^{-10}
	Bw37	8	1	6.4	0.73×10^{-7}
Psoriasis nonspecificata	B13	15	5	3.9	1.0×10^{-10}
	Bw16	16	3	4.3	0.21×10^{-10}
	Bw17	28	7	5.4	1.0×10^{-10}
Psoriasis pustulosis	B27	28	9	3.8	0.18×10^{-3}
Dermatitis herpetiformis	A1	69	30	4.4	1.0×10^{-10}
	B8	77	25	9.2	1.0×10^{-10}
	A10	39	13	3.1	0.12×10^{-3}
Behçet's disease					
Caucasian	B5	35	11	4.3	0.81×10^{-4}
Japanese	B5	75	31	6.5	0.24×10^{-5}
Recrudescent herpes labialis	A1	56	25	3.7	0.13×10^{-7}
	B8	33	17	2.5	0.35×10^{-3}

Endocrinology (Table 7)

Juvenile-onset, insulin-dependent diabetes is associated with B8 and Bw15. It is also interesting that both B8- and Bw15-positive persons have a much higher relative risk than persons with only B8 or Bw15, but individuals homozygous for B8 or Bw15 do not differ in relative risk from individuals heterozygous for B8 and Bw15. These data indicate that there is no gene dose effect for either B8 or Bw15 alone, but that the two genes together yield a complementary or additive effect and therefore each may affect disease susceptibility in a different manner. No significant deviation of HLA specificities was found in maturity-onset diabetes mellitus. Because one subgroup of diabetics (juvenile-onset) are characterized by an increased frequency of a specific genetic marker (B8 and/or Bw15), and another subgroup (adult-onset) is not, it is entirely possible that the syndrome of diabetes may arise from distinct pathogenetic mechanisms in each of these disease subgroups. Further subdivision of diabetes into even more homogeneous groups might yield still additional associations, suggesting the existence of still other pathogenetic mechanisms.

Thyrotoxicosis, particularly Graves's disease, is associated with B8 in Caucasian and with Bw35 in Japanese patients.

Subacute thyroiditis (de Quervain type) also has an association with Bw35 in Caucasians. Hashimoto's disease, on the other hand, lacks any significant HLA associations.

Idiopathic Addison's disease has an association with Dw3 and also with B8, an antigen that is in linkage disequilibrium with Dw3.

It should also be noted that several autoimmune diseases with organ-specific autoantibodies, such as juvenile-onset, insulin-dependent diabetes, Graves's disease, Addison's disease, and MG each have associations with B8 and many have even

Table 7 Endocrinology

Disease	HLA antigen	% Antigen frequency		Relative risk	p Value
		patient	control		
Diabetes (juvenile-onset, insulin-dependent only)	B8	37	22	2.1	1.0×10^{-10}
	Bw15	23	15	2.1	1.0×10^{-10}
	Dw3	50	18	4.5	0.7×10^{-2}
Thyrotoxicosis					
Caucasian	B8	42	24	2.5	1.0×10^{-10}
Japanese	Bw35	57	21	5.0	0.46×10^{-4}
Addison's disease	B8	50	23	3.9	0.73×10^{-5}
	Dw3	70	18	10.5	0.3×10^{-2}
Subacute thyroiditis (de Quervain type)	Bw35	77	13	22.2	1.0×10^{-10}

stronger associations with Dw3. These findings suggest the possibility that these syndromes may share some common step in their pathogenesis.

Gastroenterology (Table 8)

Chronic active hepatitis is associated with B8 and A1, with the latter antigen association possibly due to the linkage disequilibrium between A1 and B8. An increased frequency of homozygosity for B8 was reported (28.5% in the patient group compared to 2.8% in the control group), indicating that the susceptibility gene for chronic active hepatitis might be recessive with linkage disequilibrium with B8. It was also reported that healthy carriers of the hepatitis-associated antigen HB_sAg have an increased frequency of Bw41.

Idiopathic hemochromatosis, a disease with an increased familial incidence, but without any clear-cut immunologic abnormalities in its pathogenesis, has been associated with A3 and B14. These antigens are not in linkage disequilibrium with each other.

Celiac disease has strong associations with A1 and B8. The relative risk for Bw35 in this disease is substantially less than 1.0 (0.47), indicating a possible disease resistance in Bw35 persons.

Ulcerative colitis and Crohn's disease are reported to have no significant associations with any HLA specificities, and pernicious anemia has had conflicting reports relating to a weak association with B7.

Oncology (Table 9)

Hodgkin's disease was the first reported association of an HLA specificity and disease. In the ten years subsequent to that report, intensive studies have been done

Table 8 Gastroenterology

Disease	HLA antigen	% Antigen frequency		Relative risk	p Value
		patient	control		
Chronic active hepatitis	A1	42	28	1.8	0.64×10^{-4}
	B8	44	20	3.0	1.0×10^{-10}
Idiopathic hemochromatosis	A3	78	27	9.5	0.21×10^{-10}
	B14	26	3	9.2	0.53×10^{-5}
Celiac disease	A1	64	30	4.2	1.0×10^{-10}
	B8	71	23	8.9	1.0×10^{-10}
	Bw35	7	17	0.5	0.39×10^{-3}
HB_sAg	Bw41	12	1	11.2	0.72×10^{-3}
Pernicious anemia	B7	36	22	2.2	0.12×10^{-3}

Table 9   Oncology

Disease	HLA antigen	% Antigen frequency		Relative risk	p Value
		patient	control		
Hodgkin's disease	A1	39	31	1.4	1.0×10^{-6}
	B5	16	11	1.6	1.0×10^{-6}
	B8	29	24	1.3	1.0×10^{-4}
	B18	13	7	1.9	1.0×10^{-6}
Acute lymphocytic leukemia	A2	60	54	1.3	1.0×10^{-2}
Retinoblastoma	B12	10	25	0.3	0.27×10^{-3}
	Bw35	25	11	2.8	0.38×10^{-3}
Nasopharyngeal cancer	Hs(Sin-2)	44	21	3.0	0.7×10^{-2}
	Sin-2a[a]	100	10	–	0.1×10^{-2}

[a] Proposed D-locus antigen

to confirm this association. In the 1972 International Histocompatibility Workshop, more than 1500 patients were tested and it was shown that in the patient group there were slight increases in frequencies of A1, B5, B8, and B18.

Among the other malignant diseases, retinoblastoma has the highest relative risk with the HLA specificity Bw35. Individuals with B12 may have some resistance to this disease, as seen by the low relative risk of 0.3. Nasopharyngeal cancer, a disease that is rare outside of the Chinese population, was reported to have an association with the recently described HLA-B specificity Hs (or Sin-2) (52). Multiple myeloma, Burkitt's lymphoma, malignant melanoma, mammary carcinoma, and trophoblastic neoplasia did not show significant associations with any HLA specificities.

In childhood acute lymphocytic leukemia, the A2 antigen is increased if a patient population is tested at the time of diagnosis and is even more substantially increased among long-term survivors. These data suggest that individuals with the A2 antigen are at a questionably higher risk of developing the disease, but that patients with A2 have a better prognosis than those without A2 (53).

Chronic lymphocytic leukemia has not shown any association with specific HLA antigens; however, in family studies susceptibility to this disease seems to be linked to the *HLA* locus (54).

Miscellaneous (Table 10)

Sjögren's syndrome has an association with B8, and systemic lupus erythematosus has conflicting reports of an association with Bw15.

No significant associations were observed for sarcoidosis, chronic glomerulonephritis, polycystic kidney disease, acquired hemolytic anemia and idiopathic thrombocytopenic purpura. In family studies, hay fever (ragweed pollen allergy) was reported to be linked to the *HLA* locus; however, population studies fail to show any significant associations (55). Also linked to the *HLA* locus are genes regulating quantitative levels of several of the components of the complement system (56, 57).

Table 10 Miscellaneous

Disease	HLA antigen	% Antigen frequency		Relative risk	p Value
		patient	control		
Sjögren's syndrome	B8	51	24	3.3	0.19×10^{-6}
Congenital heart malformation	A2	80	44	4.9	0.13×10^{-5}
Acute anterior uveitis	B27	57	8	15.4	1.0×10^{-10}
Vogt-Koyanagi– Harada's disease	LD AH[a]	67	16	10.5	0.3×10^{-6}
Open-angle glaucoma	Bw35	47	23	3.0	0.48×10^{-3}

[a] Proposed D-locus antigen

Among congenital deformities, congenital heart malformation was associated with A2, but spina bifida and cleft lip had no HLA associations. Despite the lack of an association with any specific antigen, in one family study spina bifida did appear to be linked to the *HLA* locus (58).

Acute anterior uveitis has a strong association with B27, possibly because this disorder is so frequently found as a complication of the B27-associated forms of arthritis. In contrast, patients with aortic insufficiency, another frequent complication of AS, do not have an increased B27 frequency (59). Diffuse bilateral granulomatous uveitis associated with poliosis, vitiligo, alopecia, dysacusis, and vertigo is called Vogt-Koyanagi-Harada's disease. This disease is extremely rare in Caucasians, but fairly common in Japanese. A recent report from Japan associated this disease with Bw22J, a Japanese-specific W22-related *HLA-B* locus antigen, and even more strongly with a Japanese-specific new D-locus antigen LD AH (60). Finally, open-angle glaucoma has been shown to have an association with Bw35 (61).

Clinical Implications

In the preceding subheadings of this section, we have done little more than list the specific associations between HLA-antigenic specificities and particular diseases. The detailed analysis of many of these associations is just beginning, and the reader interested in a particular disease category is urged to read the source references for further details. Thus, several of the references describing the association between MS and HLA-Dw2 indicate that Dw2-positive patients with MS have a more severe, unremitting course than those patients who are Dw2-negative. Further analysis of this finding may permit subclassification of patients with MS.

In psoriasis vulgaris there is a well-known biphasic curve seen when plotting the age of onset of the disease, with peaks at about 15 years of age and again in the 30s and 40s. However, those patients who are HLA-B13- and B17-positive fall almost exclusively under the first peak, with the peak age at onset in the mid-teens. Analysis of families in which both psoriasis and B13 or B17 are segregating indicates linkage between the HLA complex and susceptibility to psoriasis. Other genetic factors not linked to HLA also have a major effect on susceptibility, since in these kindreds numerous individuals can be identified who have the disease but are HLA-B13- or B17-negative. These findings indicate that multiple genetic factors determine susceptibility to psoriasis, and that there may well be several types. This conclusion is further supported by the finding, noted earlier, that other types of psoriasis, such as pustular psoriasis, are not associated with a particular HLA type.

Analysis of a number of "autoimmune" diseases, including idiopathic Addison's disease, chronic active hepatitis, MG, Sjögren's syndrome and possibly celiac disease, dermatitis herpetiformis, Graves's disease, and insulin-dependent, juvenile-onset diabetes mellitus are all associated with HLA-B8, and many of them show an even stronger association with HLA-Dw3. It is not yet clear whether each of these diseases is associated with a particular allele of different genes, all of which are in linkage disequilibrium with HLA-B8 and HLA-Dw3, or whether all of these diseases are associated with the same allele of the same gene and there is a common initiating pathogenetic event in this very diverse list of diseases. These are but a few of the clinical correlations and questions that have been raised by an analysis of HLA and disease associations, that promise to provide important new insights into diagnostic and prognostic classification and to studies of etiology and pathogenesis.

At present, the mechanism underlying the association between HLA and specific diseases has not yet been worked out for any of the known disease associations. A knowledge of the mechanism of HLA and disease association is obviously of central importance in understanding the way in which the HLA system regulates disease susceptibility, as well as in understanding the pathogenesis of each of the associated diseases. In the absence of specific information, we are forced to deal with theoretical possibilities, and these are taken up in the next section.

POSSIBLE MECHANISMS OF HLA AND DISEASE ASSOCIATIONS

In exploring the possible mechanisms that might explain the numerous associations between the HLA system and disease, we are of necessity forced to rely partly on guesswork, and partly on our fragmentary knowledge of the known functions of genes within the major histocompatibility system in both animal and human studies. Since the function of the H-$2K$ and D, and HLA-A, B, and C loci are as yet unknown, and since it is not certain that all of the functions of genes in the I and S regions of the mouse or in the HLA-D and complement-determining genes of man are known, it is unlikely that any theoretical list of possible mechanisms will include all the actual mechanisms yet to be discovered. On the contrary, it is quite probable that a detailed analysis of the mechanism of HLA and disease associations will lead to the discovery of new functions of the major histocompatibility system. The following is a list of the theoretical mechanisms for HLA and disease association:

1. HLA antigens may function as cell-surface receptors for viruses or for toxins.
2. HLA antigens may be incorporated into the protein coat of viruses budding from the cell surface. If this were the case, viruses from one individual would more readily infect another individual sharing the same major histocompatibility antigen.

3. A virus or toxin might share antigenic configurations with histocompatibility antigens, thus rendering the host with a particular allele of a histocompatibility antigen tolerant to those determinants on the virus or toxin.

4. *H-2K* and *D*, and *HLA-A* and *B* are known to be intimately involved in the specificity of cytotoxic T cells sensitized to viruses, minor transplantation antigens, or chemical haptens conjugated to the cell surface. It is theoretically possible that particular H-2K or D or HLA-A or B antigens might lead to more or less effective T-cell–mediated cytotoxicity against a particular virus, thus affecting the immune response to that virus.

5. Associations between HLA and disease might reflect the effect of a linked immune response (*Ir*) or immune suppression (*Is*) gene that is in linkage disequilibrium with the *HLA-A, B,* or *D* allele associated with the disease in question.

6. Abnormalities in structural genes for complement components may affect disease susceptibility. There is a very strong association between the haplotype A10-Bw18-Dw2 and C2 deficiency. While many individuals who are C2-deficient may be normal, there appears to be a high frequency of a disease resembling systemic lupus erythematosus in these individuals (62). There may also be a higher incidence of lupus-like disease in heterozygotes. While the mechanism is unknown, it seems clear from these findings that complement deficiency may predispose to certain types of "autoimmune" disease.

7. The associations between HLA and disease may be due to other linked genes, in linkage disequilibrium with particular *HLA-A, B,* or *D* alleles, but unrelated to these genes. For example, it has been shown in mice that cyclic AMP levels and testosterone levels are correlated with *H-2* type (63, 64). It is also possible that the function of a wide variety of cell-surface receptor molecules for hormones, neurotransmitters, etc is affected by different alleles of the *HLA-A, B,* or *D* regions.

Finally, it is possible that the major histocompatibility antigens have a fundamental effect on cell-cell recognition and interaction in both early development and the maintenance of normal cell interactions in the adult. Different alleles of these cell-surface proteins might permit normal development and cell-cell interaction, but, in a way as yet unsuspected, predispose to disease upon exposure to particular viruses, toxins, or environmental agents such as gluten, the factor in wheat initiating the intestinal damage in celiac disease.

With this background of theoretical possibilities, we can now examine the general characteristics of HLA and disease associations. First, there are virtually no instances in which the HLA type associated with the disease is found in all of the patients with that disease, or confers a 100% probability of contracting the disease. On the contrary, almost all of the associations are ones in which a particular allele of one of the genes in the HLA system is found in a markedly increased incidence in the patient population, but not in 100% of the patients, and the majority of individuals in the population bearing the specified allele of the *HLA* gene being studied are normal and do not have the disease. In many cases, this can be shown in family studies to be due to the fact that other genetic factors also predispose to the disease in question. In some situations (e.g. ankylosing spondylitis, where 95%

of patients have HLA-B7), it is possible that the actual disease-susceptibility gene is found in only 20% of B27-positive haplotypes, and all of these individuals develop some manifestations of the disease. Controlled family studies will be required to resolve this point.

The second major generalization is that almost all of the HLA and disease associations are for susceptibility rather than resistance, and the susceptibility effect is dominant, since most individuals are heterozygous at all of the known genetic loci in the HLA system. This generalization turns out to be of little value in analysis, since all of the genes in the HLA system appear to be codominantly expressed (i.e. the heterozygote expresses both alleles of the gene) and since almost all of the theoretical mechanisms described above, with the exception of complement deficiency, would be dominant in the heterozygote.

The third generalization is that many, if not most, of the HLA and disease associations appear to be due to genes in the *HLA-D* region, or to genes that show the strongest linkage disequilibrium with genes in the *HLA-D* region. Table 11 classifies HLA and disease associations as being due to associations with a *B* locus; with the *B* locus, but reflecting a stronger association with a *D*-locus allele; or as an association with the *D* locus only. Most of these associations either show a stronger association with an *HLA-D* allele or the patient populations have not yet been typed for their *HLA-D* type. This table reflects what has developed as a general trend over the past several years. Frequently, initial studies have reported a disease as being associated with an *HLA-A*- or *B*-locus antigen. Further study has shown that the association is stronger with the *HLA-B* antigen, and where studies have

Table 11   HLA and disease associations

Disease	B–Locus association	B– and D– association	D–Locus association only
Ankylosing spondylitis	X		
Reiter's disease	X		
Rheumatoid arthritis			X
Diabetes mellitus		X	
Addison's disease		X	
Hyperthyroidism		X	
Multiple sclerosis		X	
Myasthenia gravis		X	
Gluten-sensitive enteropathy	X	?	
Dermatitis herpetiformis	X	?	
Psoriasis	X	?	
Chronic active hepatitis	X	?	
Sjögren's syndrome	X·	?	

been carried out using homozygous MLC-typing cells, the association with *HLA-B* has been found to be a function of a stronger association with an *HLA-D* allele in linkage disequilibrium with the *HLA-B* allele. Before turning to the significance of this trend, it should be noted that ankylosing spondylitis, Reiter's disease, and hemochromatosis appear to be exceptions to this generalization. Controlled family studies will be required to resolve the reason for these exceptions, but if they are due to stronger associations with *HLA-A* or *HLA-B* antigens, it would seem clear that there must be several different mechanisms underlying HLA and disease associations.

Since most HLA and disease associations appear to be due to the effect of genes either in the *HLA-D* region, or showing strongest linkage disequilibrium with this region, we must, for the moment, assume that an understanding of the function of genes in the *HLA-D* region will permit us to understand the mechanism of this type of association. Unfortunately, our knowledge of the function of the *HLA-D* gene(s) is fragmentary. At present, it is clear that these genes determine the structure of lymphocyte cell-surface antigens, eliciting a mixed-lymphocyte-culture reaction. Preliminary evidence indicates that this genetic region also determines the structure of lymphocyte cell-surface antigens analogous to the murine Ia antigens. It is probable that these antigens are the same ones that elicit the mixed-lymphocyte-culture reaction.

Beyond this, we are forced to rely on analogy with the murine model, where genes determining the structure of the Ia antigens are genetically inseparable from genes determining immune responsiveness (*Ir*) and immune suppression (*Is*), as well as cellular interaction between T lymphocytes and B lymphocytes, and T lymphocytes and macrophages. The evidence that Ia antigens are intimately involved in antigen-specific, T-cell–derived, "receptor" molecules has been cited earlier. By extrapolation, we can then postulate that many of the HLA and disease associations may be due to the effects of specific *Ir* or *Is* genes that result in hypernormal response to environmental agents, or conversely, to suppression of the normal response to environmental agents. Thus, suppression of the normal cell-mediated immune response to a virus, toxin, or environmental antigen might predispose to disease, even though superficial measurement of antibody response to the virus in question reveals no significant differences.

Although all of the available evidence indicates that HLA-linked *Ir* and *Is* genes are major factors in HLA and disease associations, it must be emphasized that *Ir* genes have not yet been conclusively demonstrated in man. In addition, the several HLA-linked complement genes have not yet been precisely mapped. It is quite possible that the genetic organization of the HLA system shows considerable differences from the H-2 system, a possibility underlined by the existence of the *HLA-C* locus, which does not yet have a murine counterpart. The different recombination rates between *HLA-A* and *B,* and *H-2K* and *D,* and the different position of the *HLA-D* gene(s) and the *I*-region genes emphasizes the possibility that the genetic organization of the HLA system may show important differences from the H-2 system, despite the very close overall analogy in the structure and molecular weight of the gene products of both of the systems. Noting these cautions, the actual and potential analogies are still impressive. Thus, in the mouse it has been demonstrated (see Section 2) that two genes in the *I* region are required for immune responsiveness to some antigens. This finding offers a potential explanation for the marked linkage disequilibrium seen in the HLA system and postulated to account for the association between particular *HLA-B* or *D* alleles and disease. Thus, a particular *HLA* haplotype might be selected for because it carried two genes required for immune response (or conversely, suppression of the immune response) to a particular foreign antigen.

Study of this possibility will require identification of the numerous genes postulated to exist in the *HLA-D* region of the HLA system. It is probable that the *HLA-D* region is as complex as the *I* region in the mouse, and that particular combinations of alleles of different genes in the *HLA-D* region have marked selective survival advantage. While these haplotype combinations may have conferred a survival advantage during the course of evolution, it is also possible that particular alleles of one or more genes within the *HLA-D* region predispose to a particular disease. (In this respect, it is important to note that most of the HLA-associated diseases do not affect the individual until after the peak reproductive period, and would thus not function as semilethals.)

CONCLUSIONS AND PROSPECTS

It is now clear that the HLA system plays a major role in determining susceptibility to a wide variety of diseases. Many, but not all of these HLA-disease associations are due to genes in the *HLA-D* region, the human analog of the murine *I* region. It seems clear that many of these disease associations are due to the effect of immune response (*Ir*) or immune suppression (*Is*) genes determining hyper- or hyponormal responsiveness to viruses, toxins, or environmental antigens. It seems equally clear that this extraordinarily complex genetic system has other functions, and that derangements in some of these other functions underlie some of the observed HLA-disease associations.

Our knowledge of the genetic organization of the HLA system is presently very incomplete, particularly with respect to genes other than those determining the serologically detectable antigens (*HLA-A, B, C*). Because of the importance of the *HLA-D* region in disease association, and because of the complexity of the analogous *I* region in the mouse, the next major step in analyzing the function of the HLA system and its disease associations will involve development of techniques for detecting particular alleles of the multiple genes in the *HLA-D* region, which presumably code for cell-surface proteins analogous to murine Ia antigens. The demonstration that some pregnancy sera contain antibodies that react primarily with B lymphocytes, and which also identify a set of cell-surface alloantigens on B lymphocytes of approximate molecular weight 33,000, indicates that specific sera are available. Analysis of this alloantigenic system may permit subdivision and identification of alleles at closely linked loci in a manner analogous to the analysis of the *HLA-A, B,* and *C* loci.

The ability to detect different alleles of the multiple genes that almost certainly exist in the *HLA-D* region offers great promise in further analyzing and understanding associations between the HLA system and disease. First, correlation of these postulated genes with immune responsiveness to a wide variety of antigens should permit conclusive demonstration and mapping of human *Ir* and *Is* genes. Second, it is likely that identification of multiple genes within the *HLA-D* region will result in demonstration of extremely strong associations between particular alleles of genes in this region and particular diseases. Thus, if adequate reagents were available, it might be possible to demonstrate that all or nearly all patients with a particular autoimmune disease such as Sjögren's syndrome or chronic active hepatitis carried a particular allele of one or two genes in the *HLA-D* region, whereas current methods of *HLA-D* locus typing (MLC typing) can detect only those patients who share all genes in the *HLA-D* region.

If such strong associations can be detected for those diseases known to be associated with the HLA system, it is also likely that new associations between particular genes in the *HLA-D* region and other diseases will be discovered. The list of candidate diseases is large (e.g. polyarteritis nodosa, scleroderma, dermatomyositis, Guillain-Barré syndrome, Wegner's granulomatosis, polymyalgia rheumatica, etc). If new and stronger associations are discovered with *HLA-D* region genes, then HLA typing, and in particular *HLA-D* typing, may well be extremely important diagnostic and prognostic tools. For those diseases showing strong associations with *HLA-D* region genes, abnormalities in immune responsiveness, either hyper- or hyponormal, may well be major predisposing factors, and it will be important to identify the environmental agent—virus, toxin, or environmental antigen—responsible for initiating the pathogenic process.

Finally, we hope that studies of the function of the *H-2K* and *H-2D*, and *HLA-A, B,* and *C* gene products, as well as a study of their structure, will lead to an understanding of the function of these gene products, their polymorphism, and their relationship to other cell-surface molecules, such as receptor molecules. This in turn should permit an understanding of the way in which different alleles of these genes might predispose to diseases such as ankylosing spondylitis and hemochromatosis. The recent findings that diseases such as hemochromatosis and primary open-angle glaucoma show an association with genes in the HLA system underlines the extraordinarily broad effects of this system, and emphasizes the probability that the major histocompatibility system plays a major role in the function of cell-surface molecules and in cellular interaction. Unraveling all of these complex functions promises to make major contributions to our understanding of the pathogenesis of a wide variety of diseases.

ACKNOWLEDGMENTS

This work was supported in part by National Institutes of Health Grants AI 07757 and AI 11313.

450 SASAZUKI, GRUMET & MCDEVITT

1. Lilly, F., Boyse, E. A., Old, L. J. 1964. Genetic basis of susceptibility to viral leukaemogenesis. *Lancet* ii:1207–9
2. Amiel, J. L. 1967. In *Histocompatibility Testing*, ed. E. S. Curtoni, P. L. Mattius, R. M. Tosi, pp. 79–81. Copenhagen: Munksgaard. 458 pp.
3. McDevitt, H. O., Tyan, M. L. 1968. Genetic control of the antibody response in inbred mice: Transfer of response by spleen cells and linkage to the major histocompatibility (H-2) locus. *J. Exp. Med.* 128:1–11
4. McDevitt, H. O., Benacerraf, B. 1969. Genetic control of specific immune responses. *Adv. Immunol.* 11:31–74
5. Benacerraf, B., McDevitt, H. O. 1972. The histocompatibility-linked immune response genes. *Science* 175:273–79
6. Katz, D. H., Benacerraf, B. 1976. *The Role of Products of the Histocompatibility Gene Complex in Immune Responses.* New York: Academic. 780 pp.
7. Shreffler, D. C., David, C. S. 1975. The *H-2* major histocompatibility complex and the *I* immune response region: Genetic variation, function, and organization. *Adv. Immunol.* 20:125
8. Zinkernagel, R. M., Doherty, P. C. 1976. See Ref. 6, pp. 203–12
9. McDevitt, H. O., Deak, B. D., Shreffler, D. C., Klein, J., Stimpfling, J. H., Snell, G. D. 1972. Genetic control of the immune response: Mapping of the *Ir-1* locus. *J. Exp. Med.* 135:1259–78
10. Benacerraf, B. 1976. See Ref. 6, pp. 225–48
11. Taussig, M. J., Munro, A. J., Luzzati, A. L. 1976. See Ref. 6, pp. 541–52
12. Tada, T., Taniguchi, M. 1976. See Ref. 6, pp. 506–12
13. Murphy, D. B., Okumura, K., Herzenberg, L. A., Herzenberg, L. A., McDevitt, H. O. 1976. Selective expression of separate *I* region loci in functionally different lymphocyte subpopulations. *J. Exp. Med.* In press
14. McDevitt, H. O. 1976. The evolution of genes in the major histocompatibility complex. *Fed. Proc.* 35:2168–73
15. Dausset, J. 1954. Leuco-agglutinins. IV. Leuco-agglutinins and blood transfusion. *Vox Sang.* 4:190–98
16. Payne, R. 1957. Leukocyte agglutinins in human sera. *Arch. Intern. Med.* 99:587–606
17. van Rood, J. J., van Leeuwen, A., Schippers, A., Vooys, W. H., Frederiks, H., Balner, H., Eernisse, J. G. 1965. in *Histocompatibility Testing*, ed. D. B. Amos, J. J. van Rood, pp. 37–50. Copenhagen: Munksgaard. 288 pp.
18. Payne, R., Tripp, M., Wigle, J., Bodmer, W., Bodmer, J. 1964. A new leukocyte isoantigen system in man. *Cold Spring Harbor. Symp. Quant. Biol.* 29:285–95
19. Dausset, J., Ivanyi, P., Ivanyi, D. 1965. See Ref. 17, pp. 51–62
20. Terasaki, P. I., McClelland, J. D. 1964. Microdroplet assay of human serum cytotoxins. *Nature* 204:998–1000
21. Kissmeyer-Nielsen, F., Thorsby, E. 1970. Human transplantation antigens. *Transplant. Rev.* 4:1–176
22. Thorsby, E. 1974. The human major histocompatibility system. *Transplant. Rev.* 18:51-129
23. Svejgaard, A., Hauge, M., Jersild, C., Platz, P., Ryder, L. P., Staub-Nielsen, L., Thomsen, M. 1975. The HLA system: An introductory survey. *Monogr. Hum. Genet.* 7:3–102
24. Lammn, L. U., Friedrich, U., Petersen, G. B., Jorgenson, J., Nielsen, J., Therkelsen, A. M., Kissmeyer-Nielsen, F. 1974. Assignment of the major histocompatibility complex to chromosome No. 6 in a family with pericentric inversion. *Hum. Hered.* 24:243–84
25. Kissmeyer-Nielsen, F., Svejgaard, A., Hauge, M. 1968. Genetics of the human HL-A transplantation system. *Nature* 219:1116–19
26. Low, B., Messeter, L., Mansoon, S., Lindholm, T. 1974. Crossing-over between the SD-2 (four) and SD-3 (AJ) loci of the human major histocompatibility chromosomal region. *Tissue Antigens* 4:405
27. Dupont, B., Staub-Nielsen, L., Svejgaard, A. 1971. Relative importance of four and LA loci in determining mixed-lymphocyte reaction. *Lancet* ii:1336–40
28. Bodmer, J. G., Colombani, J., Rocques, P., Degos, L., Bodmer, W. F., Dausset, J., Piazza, A. 1972. In *Histocompatibility Testing*, ed. J. Dausset, J. Colombani, pp. 621–67. Copenhagen: Munksgaard. 778 pp.
29. Bodmer, J. 1975. In *Histocompatibility Testing.* ed. F. Kissmeyer-Nielsen, pp. 21–99. Copenhagen: Munksgaard. 1035 pp.
30. Payne, R., Radvany, R., Grumet, F. C. 1975. A new second locus HL-A antigen in linkage disequilibrium with HL-

A2 in Cantonese Chinese. *Tissue Antigens* 5:69–71
31. Strominger, J. L., Chess, L., Herrmann, H. C., Humphreys, R. E., Malenka, D., Mann, D., McCune, J. M., Parham, R., Robb, R., Springer, T. A. Terhorst, C. 1975. See Ref. 29, pp. 719–30
32. Goodfellow, P., Jones, E., van Heyningen, V., Solomon, E., Bobrow, M., Miggiano, V., Bodmer, W. F. 1975. The β-2 microglobulin gene is on chromosome #15 and not in the HL-A region. *Nature* 254:267–69
33. van den Tweel, J. G., Blusse van Oud Alblas, A., Keuning, J. J., Goulmy, E., Termijtelen, A., Bach, M. S., van Rood, J. J. 1973. Typing for MLC (LD): I. Lymphocytes from cousin-marriage offspring as typing cells. *Transplant. Proc.* 5:1535–49
34. Thorsby, E., Piazza, A. 1975. See Ref. 29, pp. 414–58
35. Haverkorn, M. J., Hofman, B., Masurel, N., van Rood, J. J. 1975. HL-A linked genetic control of immune response in man. *Transplant. Rev.* 22:120–24
36. McDevitt, H. O., Delovitch, T. L., Press, J. L., Murphy, D. B. 1976. Genetic and functional analysis of the Ia antigens: Their possible role in regulating the immune response. *Transplant. Rev.* 30:197–235
37. Wernet, P. 1976. Human Ia-type alloantigens: Methods of detection, aspects of chemistry and biology, markers for disease states. *Transplant. Rev.* 30:270–98
38. Walford, R. L., Gosset, T., Troup, G. M., Gatti, R. M., Mittal, K. K., Robbins, A., Ferrara, G. B., Zeller, E. 1976. The Merritt alloantigenic system of human B-lymphocytes. Evidence for 13 possible factors including one six member segregant series. *J. Immunol.* 116:1704–10
39. Ting, A., Mickey, M. R., Terasaki, P. I. 1976. B-lymphocyte alloantigens in Caucasians. *J. Exp. Med.* 143:981–86
40. Jersild, C., Fog, T., Hansen, G. S., Thomsen, M., Svejgaard, A., Dupont, B. 1973. Histocompatibility determinants in multiple sclerosis with special reference to clinical course. *Lancet* ii:1221–25
41. Terasaki, P. I., Park, M. S., Opelz, G., Ting, A. 1976. Multiple sclerosis and high incidence of a B lymphocyte antigen. *Science.* In press
42. Ryder, L. P., Svejgaard, A. 1976. In *Report from the HLA and Disease Reg-*

istry of Copenhagen 1976, pp. 1–34 Copenhagen: Ryder & Svejgaard. 34 pp.
43. Svejgaard, A., Platz, P., Ryder, L. P., Staub-Nielsen, L., Thomsen, M. 1975. HLA and disease associations—A survey. *Transplant. Rev.* 22:3–44
44. Calin, A., Fries, J. F. 1975. Striking prevalence of ankylosing spondylitis in "Healthy" W27 positive males and females. A controlled study. *N. Engl. J. Med.* 293:835–39
45. Sairanen, E., Tiilikinan, A. 1975. HL-A27 in Reiter's Disease following shigellosis. *Scand. J. Rheumatol.* 4:30–41
46. Calin, A., Fries, J. F. 1976. An "experimental" epidemic of Reiter's syndrome revisited. Follow-up evidence on genetic and environmental factors. *Ann. Intern. Med.* 84:564–66
47. Wagner, L. P., Fessel, W. J. 1975. HL-A27 (W27) absent in gonococcal arthritis. *Lancet* i:1094–95
48. Morris, R., Metzger, A. L., Bluestone, R., Terasaki, P. I. 1974. HL-A W27— A clue to the diagnosis and pathogenesis of Reiter's syndrome. *N.Engl. J. Med.* 290:554–56
49. Stastny, P. 1975. See Ref. 29, pp. 797–804
50. McMichael, A. J., Sasazuki, T., McDevitt, H. O., Payne, R. O. Manuscript in preparation
51. Mann, D. L., Katz, S. J., Nelson, D. L., Abelson, L. D., Strober, W. 1976. Specific B cell antigens associated with gluten-sensitive enteropathy and dermatitis herpetiformis. *Lancet* i:110–11
52. Simons, N. J., Chan, S. H., Ho, J. H. C., Chan, J. C. W., Day, N. E., de The, G. B. 1975. See Ref. 29, pp. 809–12
53. Rogentine, G. N., Trapani, R. J., Yankee, R. A., Henderson, E. S. 1973. HL-A antigens and acute lymphocytic leukemia: The nature of the HL-A2 association. *Tissue Antigens* 3:470–76
54. Delmas-Marsalet, Y., Hors, J., Colombani, J., Dausset, J. 1974. Study of HL-A genotypes of a case of familial chronic lymphocytic leukemia (CLL). *Tissue Antigens* 4:441–45
55. Levine, B. B., Stember, R. H., Fotino, M. 1972. Ragweed hayfever: Genetic control and linkage to HLA haplotypes. *Science* 178:1201–3
56. Fu, S. M., Kunkel, H. G., Brusman, H. P., Allen, F. H., Fotino, M. 1975. Evidence for linkage between HL-A histocompatibility genes and those involved in the synthesis of the second

component of complement. *J. Exp. Med.* 140:1108–12

57. Rittner, C., Hauptman, G., Grosse-Wilde, H., Grosshaus, E., Tongio, M. M., Mayer, S. 1975. See Ref. 29, pp. 945–54
58. Amos, D. B., Ruderman, R., Mendell, N. R., Johnson, A. H. 1975. Linkage between HL-A and spinal development. *Transplant. Proc.* 7:93–95
59. Calin, A., Fries, J. F., Stinson, E. B., Payne, R. 1976. Normal frequency of HL-A B27 in aortic insufficiency. *N. Engl. J. Med.* 293:397–99
60. Tagawa, Y., Sugiura, S., Yakura, H., Wakisaka, A., Aizawa, M., Itakura, K. 1976. In *HLA and Disease* ed. J. Dausset, A. Svejgaard, p. 263 Paris: Inst. Natl. Sante Rech. Med. 333 pp.
61. Aviner, Z., Henley, W. L., Fotino, M., Leopold, I. H. 1976. Histocompatibility

(HLA) antigens and primary open angle glaucoma. *Tissue Antigens* 7:193–200
62. Stem, R., Fu, S. M., Fotino, M., Agnello, V., Kunkel, H. G. 1976. Hereditary C2 deficiency associations with skin lesions of systemic lupus erythematosus. *Arthritis Rheum.* 19:517–19
63. Meruelo, D., Edidin, M. 1975. Association of mouse liver adenosine 3':5'-cyclic monophosphate (cyclic AMP) levels with histocompatibility-2 genotype. *Proc. Natl. Acad. Sci. USA* 72:2644–48
64. Ivanyi, P., Hampl, R., Starka, L., Mickova, M. 1972. Genetic association between H-2 gene and testosterone metabolism in mice. *Nature New Biol.* 283:280–81

Ann. Rev. Med. 1977. 28:37–42
Copyright © 1977 by Annual Reviews Inc. All rights reserved

IgA-ASSOCIATED GLOMERULONEPHRITIS

♦7220

John J. McPhaul, Jr., M.D.

Clinical Research Laboratory, Wilford Hall USAF Medical Center (AFSC), Lackland AFB, Texas 78236, and the Department of Internal Medicine, University of Texas, Southwestern Medical School and Veterans Administration Hospital, Dallas, Texas 75216

INTRODUCTION

Experimental immunopathologic studies in laboratory animals have defined the principal pathogenetic mechanisms causing glomerulonephritis: nephrotoxic (glomerular basement membrane) antibody and immune-complex diseases (1). Although these mechanisms have been confirmed in man (2), numerous clinicopathologic groups of human glomerulonephritis are incompletely defined and understood. Conspicuous among the latter is immunoglobulin A (IgA)-associated glomerulonephritis.

First described by Berger in 1969 (3), the salient immunohistochemical features constitute its most enigmatic facets: (*a*) diffuse and generalized involvement of every glomerulus with IgA deposits, usually with other immunoglobulins; (*b*) primary mesangial localization; and (*c*) indolent and persistent clinical disease, usually with hematuria, unassociated with other obvious systemic signs.

The apparent incidence of this glomerulonephropathy varies in different series from 5–20% of patients biopsied—the variation is probably related to different patient populations and indications for renal biopsy. Males are more frequently affected than females, and most patients are adolescents and young adults below 30 years of age. Although there is no unanimity regarding familial incidence of this disorder, there is unexpectedly frequent reference to clinical renal disease among family members in several reports (4–6).

IgA-ASSOCIATED GLOMERULONEPHRITIS

Clinical Syndrome: Clinical Features, Epidemiology, and Natural History

IgA-associated glomerulonephritis is diagnosed most frequently by renal biopsy undertaken to define the cause of macroscopic hematuria, with often recurrent

8243-2502/80/0310-0325$01.00   37

and/or persistent microhematuria not explicable by other techniques. Although several reports suggest that this disorder is the most frequent cause of idiopathic hematuria, other reports find more varied immunopathologic bases for this syndrome (7, 8). It is important to stress that the diagnosis is established only by immunohistochemical staining of renal tissue positive for IgA.

At the time of diagnostic studies, most patients have normal renal function, trivial to modest proteinuria, and no signs of systemic disease, although 10–15% may have elevated serum creatinine concentrations and progress to renal failure. Nephrotic syndrome, arterial hypertension, and recurrent urinary-tract infections have been described in patients with this nephropathy, but are not usual. Several patients with IgA-associated nephropathy and renal failure have received renal allografts, and in numerous grafts recurrent IgA deposition has been observed (9).

Etiology and epidemiology of this clinical entity are obscure. Although an occasional patient has been documented to have intercurrent or recent streptococcal infection with first signs of disease, most give no discrete history of antecedent respiratory or skin infection. Nevertheless, gross hematuria, the single most frequent sign and symptom, often occurs within 24–72 hr of common respiratory infections, fever, unusual exercise, or trauma; an inciting event cannot be suggested in many cases. Although IgA-associated glomerulonephritis was reported first from France, subsequent studies have detected it worldwide.

Histopathology

The histopathology of renal biopsies in this disorder is varied. Although some biopsies are relatively normal or show only mild glomerular stalk thickening by light microscopy, most reports characterize the glomerular changes as a focal and segmental proliferative glomerulonephritis, primarily involving mesangial cells and matrix (10). In 20–30% of such cases, adhesions to Bowman's capsule, segmental glomerulosclerosis, and/or small fibrocellular crescents may be seen; focal necrosis of glomerular tufts is uncommon but has been reported. Diffuse and generalized mesangial proliferative glomerulonephritis has predominated in some series; tubulointerstitial changes that are noted are usually found in this group (3) and in patients with end-stage glomerulonephritis with extensive glomerular sclerosis. Patterns more typical of membranoproliferative and lupus nephritis are rare (11).

Electron Microscopy

Ultrastructural analyses by electron microscopy almost uniformly show mesangial deposits, commonly just below the glomerular basement membrane reflecting over the mesangial region, as well as mild mesangial hypercellularity and hypertrophy of mesangial matrix. In general, the number and size of mesangial electron-dense deposits correlate with the extent and intensity of mesangial staining of immunoglobulins seen by immunofluorescence. Although deposits along peripheral capillary loops are unusual, both subepithelial and subendothelial glomerular deposits have been reported; the dense deposits seen rarely in Bowman's capsule are of uncertain significance (12).

Immunofluorescent Findings

By definition, immunohistochemical stains show the characteristic mesangial staining of host IgA, usually accompanied by IgG and sometimes by other immunoglobulins; distribution of IgA is generalized and diffuse, and surprisingly intense
even in biopsies that show no substantial abnormality by light microscopy. Stains
for serum-complement components usually indicate deposition of C'3 and properdin, rarely C'$_1$q or C'4. Fibrinogen/fibrin is found often in a focal and segmental
mesangial location, with much more variability between glomeruli than other proteins. Mounting evidence indicates that secretory IgA is not present in affected
glomeruli.

FEATURES OF SPECIAL INTEREST

Interest in IgA-associated glomerulonephritis is directed toward three intriguing
facets of its immunopathogenesis that have not been explained completely: (a) the
role of IgA, (b) involvement primarily of renal mesangium, and (c) relationship of
this syndrome to Henoch-Schönlein purpura (H.S.P.) and other systemic diseases
with glomerular IgA deposition.

Role of IgA

IgA, a major component of the serum Ig pool, exists in two subclasses: IgA$_1$ is the
major component of total serum IgA, whereas IgA$_2$ is in much greater concentration
in external secretions (tears, nasal secretions, saliva, succus entericus, etc). IgA
functions as the principal antibody class in these secretions, particularly against viral
antigens, whereas the immune function of serum IgA is not as well specified.
Although discrete antibody activities have been measured in the IgA class, including
autoantibodies such as antinuclear and anti–gamma globulin factors, predominantly
IgA systemic serologic response is not characteristic of usual immunogens (13). This
disparity has prompted the suggestion that an antigen may diffuse from the gut and
excite a preferential IgA response with resulting deposition of immune complexes
in the kidney. In fact, several patients with IgA-associated glomerulonephritis have
a history of chronic or recurrent sinus infections, and onset of hematuria in many
patients seems triggered by common respiratory infections. Thus far, no evidence
has been adduced in support of the alimentary antigen(s) or route of immunization,
and the weight of present data does not favor significant participation of secretory
IgA in this disorder.

Renal Mesangium

Important immunologic and ultrastructural studies have addressed the functional
role of renal mesangium and factors contributory to the localization and deposition
of circulating immune complexes; they have been reviewed recently (14, 15). Mesangial function in transport and disposition of a variety of macromolecules, including
colloids and protein aggregates, has been shown to be a dynamic process, with

apparent preferential collection along subendothelial aspects of glomerular basement membrane, uptake into the mesangium, and movement in channels between mesangial cells towards the hilum and vascular pole of the glomerulus. The loss of electron-dense, fluorescent, or radioactive markers in these experiments is interpreted to result from degradation of the test materials and transport into hilar lymphatics.

Immune complexes formed in vitro and administered passively, as well as complexes formed in vivo in response to soluble protein and viral antigens, may localize preferentially to the mesangium. Such mesangial deposition is characteristic of larger complexes with very high molecular weight antigens or complexes formed in relative antibody excess. Corticosteroids can influence this localization by altering antibody synthesis and affecting antigen:antibody ratios, by affecting metabolism of complexes, or by direct effects on GBM and/or the mesangium (16).

Although the renal mesangium functions in the handling and ultimate fate of a variety of macromolecules that may not be immunologically active, it clearly is an important site—even a primary site—of immune-complex localization.

Relationship to Systemic Diseases with IgA Deposits

Primary mesangial deposition of serum immunoglobulins, including IgA, has been noted in systemic diseases, particularly in H.S.P., systemic lupus erythematosus, viral hepatitis, and hepatic cirrhosis. In many cases the glomerular immunoglobulin is predominantly IgA, such as in H.S.P. and hepatic cirrhosis; the putative antigen(s) involved that elicits presumed IgA antibodies is not evident.

Significant elevations of serum IgA concentrations have been noted in hepatic cirrhosis and H.S.P., particularly early in the disease (17). The frequent clinical involvement of gastrointestinal tract in H.S.P., increased serum IgA concentration, and renal deposition of IgA has focused attention on the GI tract as source of antigen and/or antibodies in this presumed immunological disease. While serum IgA concentrations have been reported to be high in IgA-associated glomerulonephritis without systemic disease, not all series are in agreement.

Further data linking IgA nephropathies with or without systemic disease have been offered in reports that IgA and other immunoreactive proteins can be seen in walls of cutaneous capillaries of uninvolved skin of patients with IgA-associated glomerulonephritis and patients with H.S.P. (18, 19). Confirmation of these observations would add to the likelihood that IgA deposits in both sites resulted from circulating immune complexes, although systematic use of tests for detecting such complexes in IgA-associated glomerulonephritis have not been rewarding thus far. Moreover, the similarities of IgA-associated nephropathy to the nephritis of H.S.P. are so striking that it is not clear whether there is only a quantitative difference between the two disorders, or more fundamental differences.

IMMUNOPATHOGENETIC HYPOTHESIS

The primary hypothesis regarding immunopathophysiology operative in IgA-associated glomerulonephritis suggests that the nephropathy results from renal deposition of circulating immune complexes containing IgA. The preferential renal mesangial site of deposition is thought to result from the size of the circulating immune complexes; the indolent clinical pace of the nephritic lesion and its frequently unimpressive morphologic response probably result from a slower rate of immune-complex deposition and the faster turnover and disposal of complexes localized to the mesangium. In the absence of systematic data, it has not been demonstrated conclusively whether IgA is present as antigen or antibody; one study has indicated that the renal IgA does not have antiglobulin activity and that sera from these patients do not have anti-IgA antibodies (20). Cryoglobulins have been found infrequently in IgA-associated glomerulonephritis and have not always contained IgA. Although it is not likely in the usual case, anti-mesangial antibody participation has not been ruled out (20).

Aggregates of IgA are known to initiate complement activation through the "alternate" pathway (21). Numerous studies of renal biopsies from patients with IgA-associated glomerulonephritis attest to the high frequency of $C'3$ (Beta 1C) and properdin deposition in these glomeruli, although C'_1q and $C'4$ have rarely been seen; serum concentrations of classical and alternate pathway components as a rule are normal in these patients. The data are compatible with activation of the complement seen in these lesions through the alternate pathway. The majority of tests performed for cold activation of complement (22) and $C'3$ "nephritic factor" have been negative (23).

SUMMARY

In summary, IgA-associated glomerulonephritis is an interesting clinical problem. The immunohistochemical identification of renal IgA deposits is the sine qua non of its diagnosis, although most of the patients reported have had hematuric syndromes, particularly recurrent gross hematuria. The importance of this immunopathologic entity devolves from the crucial use of special stains to identify IgA, the enigmatic role of IgA, the usual mesangiopathic expression of histologic response, and the ill-defined relationship of this clinical problem to nephropathies associated with systemic diseases that also have glomerular IgA deposits.

Although still unproven, it is likely that the usual instance of IgA-associated glomerulonephritis is due to deposition of circulating immune complexes containing IgA. The nature of the exciting antigen(s), quantitative measures and characteristics of such complexes, and the role of mediating systems, including coagulation, have not yet been elucidated.

Literature Cited

1. Unanue, E. R., Dixon, F. J. 1967. Experimental glomerulonephritis: immunological events and pathogenetic mechanisms. *Adv. Immunol.* 6:1–90
2. Dixon, F. J. 1968. The pathogenesis of glomerulonephritis. *Am. J. Med.* 44:493–98
3. Berger, J. 1969. IgA glomerular deposits in renal disease. *Transplant. Proc.* 1:939–44
4. deWerra, P., Morel-Maroger, L., Leroux-Robert, C., Richet, G. 1973 Glomérulites à dèpôts d'IgA diffus dans le mésanguim. *Schweiz Med. Wochenschr.* 103:797–803
5. Sessa, A., Cioffi, A., Allaria, P., Conte, F., D'Amico, G. 1973. Hereditary nephritis with immunofluorescent mesangial deposits. *Lancet* 2:853
6. Sissons, J. G. P., Woodrow, D. F., Curtis, J. R., Evans, D. J., Gower, P. E., Sloper, J. C., Peters, D. K. 1975. Isolated glomerulonephritis with mesangial IgA deposits. *Br. Med. J.* 3:605–6
7. van de Putte, L. B. A., de la Riviere, G. B., van Breda Vriesman, P. J. C. 1974. Recurrent or persistent hematuria: sign of mesangial immune complex deposition. *N. Engl. J. Med.* 290:1165–70
8. Kupor, L. R., Mullins, J. D., McPhaul, J. J. Jr. 1975. Immunopathologic findings in idiopathic renal hematuria. *Arch. Intern. Med.* 135:1204–11
9. Berger, J., Yaneva, H., Nabarra, B., Barbanel, C. 1975. Recurrence of mesangial deposition of IgA after renal transplantation. *Kidney Int.* 7:232–41
10. Levy, M. Beaufils, H., Gubler, M. C., Habib, R. 1972. Idiopathic recurrent macroscopic hematuria and mesangial IgA-IgG deposits in children (Berger's Disease). *Clin. Nephrol.* 1:63–69
11. Finlayson, G., Alexander, R., Juncos, L., Schlein, E., Teague, P., Waldman, R., Cade, R. 1975. Immunoglobulin A glomerulonephritis: a clinicopathologic study. *Lab. Invest.* 32:140–48
12. McCoy, R. C., Abramowsky, C. R., Tisher, C. C. 1974. IgA nephropathy. *Am. J. Pathol.* 76:123–44

13. Vodopick, H., Chaskes, S. J., Solomon, A., Stewart, J. A. 1974. Transient monoclonal gammopathy associated with cytomegalovirus infection. *Blood* 44:189–95
14. Vernier, R. L., Mauer, S. M., Fish, A. J., Michael, A. F. 1971. The mesangial cell in glomerulonephritis. *Adv. Nephrol.* 1:31–46
15. Germuth, F. G. Jr., Rodriguez, E. 1975. Focal mesangiopathic glomerulonephritis: prevalence and pathogenesis. *Kidney Int.* 7:216–23
16. Haakenstad, A. O., Case, J. B., Mannik, M. 1975. Effect of cortisone on the disappearance kinetics and tissue localization of soluble immune complexes. *J. Immunol.* 114:1153–60
17. Trygstad. C. W., Stiehm, E. R. 1971. Elevated serum IgA globulin in anaphylactoid purpura. *Pediatrics* 47:1023–28
18. de la Faille-Kuyper, E. H. B., Kater, L., Kuijten, R. H., Kooiker, C. J., Wagenaar, S. S., van der Zouven, P., Dorhout Mees, E. J. 1976. Occurrence of vascular IgA deposits in clinically normal skin of patients with renal disease. *Kidney Int.* 9:424–29
19. Tsai, C. C., Giangiacomo, J., Zuckner, J. 1975. Dermal IgA deposits in Henoch-Schönlein purpura and Berger's nephritis. *Lancet* 1:342–43
20. Lowance, D. C., Mullins, J. D., McPhaul, J. J. Jr. 1973. Immunoglobulin A (IgA) associated glomerulonephritis. *Kidney Int.* 3:167–76
21. Götze, O., Müller-Eberhard, H. J. 1971. The C_3-activator system: An alternate pathway of complement activation. *J. Exp. Med.* 134:90s–108s(Suppl.)
22. Day, N. K., Geiger, H., McLean, R., Resnick, J., Michael, A., Good, R. A. 1973. The association of respiratory infection, recurrent hematuria, and focal glomerulonephritis with activation of the complement system in the cold. *J. Clin. Invest.* 52:1698–1706
23. Zimmerman. S. W., Burkholder, P. M. 1975. Immunoglobulin A nephropathy. *Arch. Intern. Med.* 135:1217–23

Ann. Rev. Med. 1978. 29:191–203

IMMUNOLOGICAL ASPECTS OF RENAL TUBULAR AND INTERSTITIAL DISEASES[1]

♦7276

Robert T. McCluskey, M.D. and Robert B. Colvin, M.D.

Department of Pathology, Massachusetts General Hospital, Boston, Massachusetts 02114

Considerable effort over the last 25 years has been directed at the elucidation of the immunological basis of glomerular diseases. As a result, two major forms of antibody-mediated glomerular injury have been recognized; that due to immune complexes and that due to antibodies reactive with the glomerular basement membrane. Only recently have investigations focussed on immunologic mechanisms in tubulointerstitial nephritis, which comprises a large, diverse group of clinically important renal diseases. Already it is clear that analogous immunological mechanisms may cause tubulointerstitial damage.

Two types of antibody-mediated tubulointerstitial nephritis have been described in experimental animals (1, 2). One is mediated by autoantibodies reactive with the tubular basement membrane (anti-TBM disease) and is characterized by continuous (linear) accumulation of immunoglobulin along the TBM, as seen by immunofluorescence. The second is mediated by accumulation of immune complexes along the TBM or in the interstitium, and is manifested by granular deposits of immunoglobulins and complement. Evidence has been obtained, principally through immunofluorescence, that these mechanisms cause renal disease in man. Experimental studies also indicate that cell-mediated reactions can occur in the renal interstitium; however, the importance of cell-mediated sensitivity in human renal disease is uncertain, except in allografts. We review here experimental models of immunologically mediated tubulointerstitial disease and what appear to be corresponding lesions in man. In addition, drug-induced interstitial nephritis (for which there is no model) is discussed.

[1]Supported in part by a National Institutes of Health Grant 1 R01 AM 18729-01.

191

TUBULOINTERSTITIAL IMMUNE-COMPLEX LESIONS

Renal tubulointerstitial immune-complex deposits have been described in rabbits or rats sensitized with homologous renal tissue in adjuvant, and in rabbits with renal allografts (3–5). After several weeks, rabbits repeatedly injected with a soluble extract of renal cortex in adjuvant developed tubulointerstitial nephritis, with interstitial fibrosis, interstitial mononuclear cell infiltration, and tubular damage (5). The glomeruli were generally normal. Granular deposits of IgG and C3 were seen along the TBM of proximal tubules. After many months the deposits were sometimes no longer present, although tubulointerstitial damage remained. Anti-TBM antibodies were not demonstrable in the serum or in eluates of renal tissue, but there were antibodies directed against antigens in the cytoplasm of proximal tubular cells. We therefore suggested that the immune complexes were formed in situ, as a result of antigens exiting from tubular cells and meeting autoantibodies at the level of the TBM.

Tubulointerstitial immune-complex deposits also may form in situ in rats immunized with Tamm-Horsfall protein, a glycoprotein found in the distal nephron and a major constituent of casts (6). The deposits were found along the ascending thick limb of the loops of Henle, the macula densa, and part of the distal tubule; these are believed to be the sites of Tamm-Horsfall production. Mild interstitial mononuclear infiltration occurred in the vicinity of the deposits. Rats immunized with homologous kidney tissue in Freund's adjuvant sometimes developed broad deposits of IgG along the basal portions of Henle's loops and distal tubules (7), but the antigen was not identified. Local formation of complexes could probably occur only if the antigens are released into the extracellular space. Most tissue-specific autoantibodies directed against intracellular antigens do not have access to their corresponding antigen, and do not therefore cause local immune-complex formation.

Recently Brentjens et al (8), in a study of chronic serum sickness in rabbits induced by multiple daily injections of bovine serum albumin (BSA), found that immune-complex deposition occurs in various extraglomerular sites as well as in glomeruli. Immunofluorescence showed deposits of BSA, IgG, and IgM along the TBM, in Bowman's capsule, and around peritubular capillaries; electron microscopy showed dense deposits in these locations. Interstitial fibrosis, accumulation of mononuclear cells and neutrophils, as well as tubular cell damage, were present. The findings in this model indicate that the extraglomerular deposition occurs because very large amounts of circulating complexes are formed, which suggests that saturation of the usual removal mechanisms is involved. It is also possible, as noted above, that the complexes are formed locally, or that special receptors are involved in their localization.

In most models with tubulointerstitial immune deposits, interstitial inflammation and fibrosis occur, as well as tubular cell damage. In the study of Brentjens et al (8) a positive correlation was found between deposits and tubulointerstitial damage, which supports a pathogenic role of the complexes. No direct evidence exists concerning the secondary mechanisms by which the complexes mediate the injury. Moreover, even though complexes are present, other pathogenetic mechanisms (immunologic or nonimmunologic) may also contribute to the damage. A role for the infiltrating cells has been suggested in NZB/W mice, which develop severe interstitial nephritis in addition to glomerular lesions (9, 10). Although immunoglobulin deposition in glomeruli correlates with glomerular damage, a similar association is not found between the extent of tubulointersitital deposits and interstitial inflammation (9, 10). The tubular cell damage occurs near areas of mononuclear cell accumulation, which suggests that the infiltrating cells contribute to the cell injury (10). However, it is possible even here that immune complexes initiate the damage, but are present only intermittently or in undetectable amounts.

Following observations in experimental models, tubulointerstitial immunoglobulin and complement deposits were identified in man (11–13). The deposits had apparently previously been overlooked, or perhaps had been misinterpreted as reabsorption droplets, or as proteins present in peritubular capillaries. Even now, there may occasionally be such difficulties in interpretation. Electron microscopic studies may help by revealing dense deposits along or within tubular and capillary basement membranes or in the interstitium; however, because of the focal nature of the deposits, this is of limited usefulness.

The condition in which tubulointerstitial deposits are most often found is lupus nephritis (11–13). The deposits are often quite focal, but may be very widespread. By immunofluorescence, they appear to be located either along or within TBMs, around peritubular capillaries, or free in the interstitium; electron microscopic observations have substantiated these interpretations. The deposits invariably contain IgG and C3, and often IgM and/or IgA. In a few instances DNA has been demonstrated in the deposits, which provides additional evidence that they are immune complexes (13). In two reports, deposits were present in about half or more of the cases studied (12, 13). In general, interstitial inflammation and fibrosis and tubular cell damage appear to correlate with the abundance of the extraglomerular deposits. However, interstitial mononuclear cell infiltrates are sometimes found in the kidneys of patients with lupus nephritis with few if any tubulointerstitial deposits, similar to NZB/W mice. In most cases of lupus nephritis, the severity of the tubulointerstitial damage also parallels that of the glomerular disease. However, prominent tubulointerstitial nephritis has been observed with only mild glomerular involvement in a patient with renal failure (14, 15). Even when associated with glomerular lesions, the tubulointerstitial damage probably contributes to renal functional impairment.

Tubulointerstitial deposits have been described in the absence of glomerular disease in only a few other situations, namely in renal allografts (16), in a patient with Sjögren's syndrome (17), and in several patients with idiopathic interstitial nephritis (11). Tubulointerstitial deposits are sometimes much more abundant than glomerular deposits, which suggests that special factors are involved in their localization, rather than mere saturation of the sites in which complexes usually deposit.

Other forms of glomerulonephritis in which tubulointerstitial deposits have been described include glomerulonephritis with mixed cryoglobulinemia, membranoproliferative glomerulonephritis, and "rapidly progressive" (crescenteric) glomerulonephritis (11, 12). With the exception of mixed cryoglobulinemia, extraglomerular deposits are uncommon. In some cases of mixed cryoglobulinemia, widespread tubulointerstitial deposits are found, containing IgM, IgG, and C3. Rheumatoid factor activity has been found in the deposits (R. B. Colvin, unpublished), which is consistent with the interpretation that IgM–anti-IgG complexes are important.

Aside from systemic lupus erythematosus, where antigen (DNA) has been demonstrated in deposits, and in mixed cryoglobulinemia, where anti-IgG antibodies and IgG have been identified, there is no evidence concerning the identity of the antigen presumed to be present in the tubulointerstitial deposits, so that direct proof that they represent immune complexes is lacking (as is true in most glomerular diseases believed to be mediated by immune complexes).

ANTI-TUBULAR BASEMENT MEMBRANE ANTIBODY DISEASE

In 1971 Steblay & Rudofsky (18) reported that guinea pigs developed a fatal tubulointerstitial nephritis after immunization with the insoluble fraction of rabbit renal cortex, rich in tubules, in complete Freund's adjuvant. Light microscopy revealed interstitial mononuclear cells, multinucleated peritubular giant cells, and tubular cell damage. Immunofluorescence revealed linear deposition of IgG along most of the cortical TBMs. High titers of anti-TBM antibodies were detected in the sera by indirect immunofluorescence. Similar lesions occur in guinea pigs sensitized with bovine TBM (19, 20) and in certain strains of rats immunized with homologous or heterologous TBM (21, 22). In both species, transfer of serum containing anti-TBM antibodies to normal recipients results in renal lesions with the same immunofluorescence and histologic features as in actively immunized animals (20, 21, 23).

Precisely how the anti-TBM antibodies bring about tubular damage is not known. Guinea pigs genetically deficient in C4 are as susceptible to anti-TBM disease as normal animals (24). Although C3 is sometimes seen along the TBM, it may be absent, even in animals with severe disease (18–20). Because guinea pigs depleted of C3 by cobra venom factor are resistant to passively transferred disease, a pathogenic role of complement has been suggested (25), but cobra venom has other effects that might inhibit the development of renal lesions.

A recent study indicates that anti-TBM antibodies may amplify the disease by stimulating the production of further autoantibodies (C. L. Hall, R. B. Colvin, K. Carey, R. T. McCluskey, *J. Exp. Med.,* in press). This conclusion was reached in passive transfer studies in strain XIII guinea pigs. We began the investigation to determine whether IgG_1 or IgG_2 anti-TBM antibodies (or both) mediated the disease. Recipients of either IgG_1 or IgG_2 developed typical anti-TBM disease, as seen on day 14. This was surprising, in view of the known differences in the biological effects of the two isotypes. Analysis of the recipients' sera 14 days after they had received either IgG_1 or IgG_2 showed unexpectedly high levels of anti-TBM antibodies in both IgG_1 and IgG_2 fractions. In contrast, in recipients of similarly fractionated control IgG_1 and IgG_2 anti–bovine γ-globulin (BGG) antibodies, the titers declined markedly and anti-BGG activity was found only in the IgG fraction that had been transferred. These findings indicated that the recipients of antibodies were actually stimulated to produce their own anti-TBM antibodies. These experiments also showed that the autoantibodies produced by the recipient participated in the renal damage. It is not known whether the stimulation of autoantibodies by autoantibodies (which we call autoimmune amplification) is a common phenomenon; in most situations it would be difficult or impossible to detect. However, when it does occur, it may provide a mechanism for the intensification or perpetuation of autoimmune diseases.

A central question in anti-TBM disease is the pathogenic significance of the infiltrating mononuclear cells. In the guinea pig a majority of the infiltrating cells appear to be monocytes or macrophages, although numerous lymphocytes are also present. Macrophages have a wide assortment of digestive enzymes, and presumably have the potential to destroy the TBM, but whether they initiate the destruction of the TBM or merely ingest already-damaged membranes is not known. Electron microscopic observations suggest that the giant cells are formed by fusion of macrophages, which envelop fragments of TBM (21). However, giant cells are not an essential feature of anti-TBM disease in guinea pigs (19).

The nature of the infiltrating cells in anti-TBM disease has been studied by a rosetting technique that permits identification of B cells and monocytes in tissue sections (20). Many of the mononuclear cells bound IgG-coated red cells, which indicates they were monocytes or macrophages bearing Fc receptors (B cell Fc receptors do not bind in this assay). No C3 receptor–bearing lymphocytes were detected, which suggests that many of the lymphocytes were T cells or null cells. However, some B cells must have participated, because small numbers of plasma cells appeared later in the reaction. In lethally radiated guinea pigs reconstitution with normal bone marrow cells is essential for the development of disease after passive transfer of anti-TBM serum, which indicates that the bone marrow is a major source of the infiltrating cells (26). Since recipients of anti-TBM antibodies produce their own autoantibodies (see above), the protective effect of radiation may be attributable in part to suppression of antibody production rather than simply to elimination of cells that infiltrate the kidneys. Although the mononuclear nature of the infiltrate suggests a cell-mediated reaction, attempts to produce lesions by transfer of lymphoid cells have been unsuccessful (20, 27). Furthermore, lesions comparable to those in actively immunized animals can be produced by transfer of serum as early as three days, which indicates that antibodies alone are capable of initiating the process (5, 7). Nevertheless, it is conceivable that the combination of antibody with the TBM results in the formation of a conjugate that stimulates the development of delayed reactivity (as well as antibody production), and that this plays a role in the later stages of the disease.

Anti-TBM disease can be produced only in certain rat strains (21, 22). The resistant strains (Lewis, Wistar-Furth, and Maxx) lack the pertinent TBM antigens, as demonstrated by the failure of anti-TBM sera to bind their kidneys. This allotypic specificity is not determined by the major histocompatibility locus in the rat (Ag-B); Fisher 344 and Lewis are Ag-B identical, yet discordant in the expression of the TBM antigen. The same anti-TBM antibodies that fail to react with the resistant strains of rats do react with the TBM of a variety of other species.

Another recently appreciated aspect of anti-TBM disease is the genetic influence of the immune response to TBM antigen (28, 29). Strain XIII guinea pigs develop much more severe anti-TBM disease when immunized with rabbit TBM than strain II guinea pigs (28). Strain II animals produce little or no antibody reactive with guinea pig TBM, in contrast with strain XIII guinea pigs. The strain II kidneys possess the TBM antigen(s) that bind anti-TBM antibodies from strain XIII animals; thus, their failure to develop disease is not caused by the absence of the pertinent TBM antigen. Strain II animals also fail to develop disease even when given anti-TBM antibodies; this is probably due to a failure of the recipients to produce their own anti-TBM antibodies. Certain rat strains also are low responders to TBM (22). In the guinea pig a dominant immune-response (Ir) gene(s) linked to the major histocompatibility locus controls the auto-immune anti-TBM response (28).

Since the demonstration of anti-TBM disease in animals, small numbers of cases of human anti-TBM disease have been recognized. The evidence for anti-TBM antibodies consists of finding linear accumulation of IgG and C3 along cortical tubules, primarily proximal tubules, as well as demonstrating anti-TBM activity by indirect immunofluorescence in the sera and in eluates of kidneys. (Irregular linear deposits of C3 alone are sometimes seen in normal kidneys). In all instances there has been interstitial inflammation, often with fibrosis, and tubular cell damage. However, multinucleated giant cells have been reported in only one case (2).

A majority of patients with anti–glomerular basement membrane (anti-GBM) disease with Goodpasture's syndrome (or, less commonly, rapidly progressive glomerulonephritis) have associated anti-TBM disease (12). Moreover, eluates of renal tissue have exhibited anti-TBM activity, in addition to antibodies that react with glomerular and often pulmonary basement membranes.. Absorption of eluates with solubilized GBM has been shown to remove the anti-TBM activity (30). These results indicate that the responsible antigenic determinants are present both in the TBM and GBM.

Anti-TBM antibodies have also been reported in several situations in the absence of anti-GBM antibodies, including immune-complex glomerulo-nephritis (31–33), drug-induced interstitial nephritis (see below) (34–36), id-iopathic interstitial nephritis (37), and renal allografts (38, 39). The explanation for the association of immune-complex glomerular disease and anti-TBM antibodies (which has been observed in more instances than would appear likely on a chance basis) is not clear. Possibly the glomerular disease, which in at least one case clearly preceded the anti-TBM disease (33), brings about secondary tubular damage, which in turn triggers an autoimmune response. It may also be that damage to the GBM stimulates autoantibodies that are directed primarily against cross-reacting antigens in the TBM.

Allotypes of TBM antigens have been detected in man (39), and some human anti-TBM sera react with the Brown Norway (BN) but not the Lewis TBM (34, 37). The anti-TBM antibodies found in a patient with a renal allograft reacted with the TBM in the allograft and all other human kidneys tested, but not with the patient's own kidneys (38). However, another human renal allograft recipient developed anti-TBM antibodies that reacted with his own kidneys as well as the transplanted and other kidneys (39), which indicates that allografts may sometimes stimulate antibody production to autologous TBM antigens.

CELL-MEDIATED TUBULOINTERSTITIAL DISEASE

The possibility that delayed hypersensitivity directed against autologous antigens can produce interstitial nephritis is supported by the observation that some rats injected with homologous kidney preparations develop interstitial mononuclear cell infiltrates; the fact that these infiltrates often occur early, before evidence of autoantibody production, favors a cell-mediated mechanism (T. Sugisaki, J. Klassen, G. A. Andres, R. T. McCluskey, unpublished). In addition, Grupe (40) found that lymphocytes from rats immunized with kidney tissue produced macrophage-migration inhibitory factor in the presence of renal antigens. Furthermore, renal antigens also elicit delayed skin reactions and provoke lymphocyte blast transformation (41). However, early interstitial nephritis following immunization with kidney homogenates does not occur consistently and conclusive evidence that the lesions can be transferred with cells has not been obtained.

It has only recently been shown that delayed hypersensitivity can be elicited in renal tissue with exogenous antigens (42). Guinea pigs and rats were sensitized to BGG using methods that favor the development of delayed hypersensitivity. Direct injection of aggregated BGG into the renal cortex resulted in a mononuclear interstitial infiltrate, with focal tubular destruction. Reactivity could be transferred with lymph node cells, but not with serum. Although reactions were consistently produced with heat-aggregated BGG, soluble BGG generally failed to elicit reactions, presumably because it rapidly diffused from the injection site. In contrast, soluble BGG was fully as effective as aggregated material in eliciting delayed reactions in the skin. These findings show that the conditions required for the development of delayed reactions are not the same in all tissues, and suggest that in the kidney only those antigens that are aggregated, particulate (such as bacteria), or fixed (such as autologous antigens) are highly effective in eliciting delayed reactions.

Some effort has been made to relate cellular reactivity to bacterial antigens to the pathogenesis of pyelonephritis (43). In experimental models mononuclear cells appear very rapidly in the infiltrate. Furthermore, Cotran (43) showed that rats with pyelonephritis induced by streptococci developed cellular reactivity to the bacteria, as indicated by lymphocyte stimulation in vitro. In addition, bacterial antigens were shown by the immunofluorescence in amorphous and particulate form, both within leukocytes and free in the interstitium. Obviously, if bacterial antigens do elicit delayed reactions in the kidney, this would be only one aspect of the pathogenesis of pyelonephritis. Other mechanisms by which bacteria produce tissue damage might be of greater importance. Furthermore, the delayed reaction might be important in defense, as well as in tissue injury. It seems unlikely that delayed reactivity against bacterial antigens could provide a mechanism for perpetuation of pyelonephritis beyond the period when viable organisms are present in the kidney, since this would require persistence of bacterial antigen in sufficient amounts and in appropriate physical form. Indeed, in both human and experimental pyelonephritis, bacterial antigens are usually not demonstrable in kidneys after eradication of bacteria, and when present are found only within macrophages (43). There is no substantial evidence that bacterial infections of the kidney induce an autoimmune response against renal antigens (43).

In many forms of renal disease in man, with or without associated glomerular lesions, interstitial mononuclear cell infiltrates are conspicuous. To what extent these infiltrates represent delayed hypersensitivity reactions is unknown. This uncertainty stems largely from the lack of reliable criteria for the identification of cell-mediated reactions. Histologic features do not provide a reliable guide. Mononuclear cell infiltrates can be seen in certain antibody-mediated reactions (as in anti-TBM disease), as well as in nonimmunological reactions. Even the use of newer techniques that permit the identification of different types of mononuclear cells in tissue sections has not yet made it possible to identify delayed reactions, nor to assess the functional activity of the cells. The in vitro demonstration of cell-mediated reactivity against a particular antigen does not establish an in vivo role for this mechanism in the production of disease. The most reliable evidence for a pathogenic role of delayed sensitivity—transfer of disease with lymphocytes—obviously cannot be obtained in man. It is apparent that new approaches to the recognition of delayed reactions and for evaluation of their significance are needed. Nevertheless, there are reasons to suspect that cell-mediated reactions occur in human renal disease and that they may be directed against either autologous or exogenous antigens.

Rocklin, Lewis & David (44) demonstrated production of migration inhibition factor by lymphocytes from some patients with anti-GBM disease when their lymphocytes were incubated with preparations of GBM (which undoubtedly included a variety of renal antigens). Others made similar observations in patients with focal or diffuse proliferative glomerular disease, as well as in some patients with renal vascular disease (45). Delayed hypersensitivity to bacterial antigens may play a role in the pathogenesis of pyelonephritis (see above). Some forms of drug-induced interstitial nephritis may be due, at least in part, to cell-mediated mechanisms, as discussed below.

DRUG-INDUCED TUBULOINTERSTITIAL NEPHRITIS

A variety of drugs are known to induce acute tubulointerstitial nephritis in man, characterized histologically by interstitial edema, tubular cell damage, and irregular interstitial leucocytic infiltration. The infiltrate usually consists principally of mononuclear phagocytes and lymphocytes, but eosinophils are generally present, often in large numbers, and plasma cells and small numbers of basophils are sometimes also found. Tubules are invaded by mononuclear cells and eosinophils. The blood vessels and glomeruli appear normal. Clinically the renal disease is manifested by hematuria, proteinuria, enlargement of the kidneys, and in severe cases acute renal failure. Mild cases may go unrecognized. The drugs most frequently incriminated are methicillin, ampicillin, rifampicin, and phenindione [for complete list, see (46)]. With certain agents, especially methicillin and related antibiotics, there is considerable evidence that the lesions result from immunological mechanisms, rather than from toxic effects (46–48). Thus, only a small proportion of patients receiving the antigen develop interstitial nephritis, and this is not dose related. Moreover, most of the patients show evidence of hypersensitivity, with fever, rash, arthralgia, and eosinophilia. Repeated exposure to the same drug, or a closely related agent, sometimes brings about recurrence of the interstitial nephritis.

Certain infections, notably scarlet fever and diphtheria, are sometimes complicated by acute interstitial nephritis (presumably not due to bacterial invasion of the kidney). The possibility that the infection caused the interstitial nephritis seen in some patients receiving antibiotic treatment is therefore worth considering. However, the same renal lesions have been observed in patients treated for a variety of infections, most of which have not in the past been associated with interstitial nephritis; moreover, severe interstitial nephritis has been observed to develop in some patients given methicillin prophylactically (35).

In an individual patient it is often difficult to determine whether renal damage is due to toxic effect of the drug, an immunological reaction initiated by the drug, an infectious process, or some other unknown cause. Moreover, in patients receiving multiple drugs, it may be difficult to identify the offending agent. Identification of the cause of renal damage is usually easier when renal tissue is available for pathological studies, but even these studies are not always conclusive. In instances in which hypersensitivity is responsible, there is usually conspicuous interstitial leucocytic infiltration and edema, features that are generally lacking or mild in toxic injury. There are probably no criteria for identification of acute interstitial nephritis associated with infection. In addition, especially with small samples, it is sometimes uncertain whether one is dealing with interstitial nephritis at all, rather than simply an unimportant interstitial infiltrate, as may be seen around areas of ischemia or other forms of damage.

The immunological mechanisms usually responsible for drug-induced inter-stitial nephritis have not been elucidated. Probably several mechanisms are involved and vary in importance from one case to another. In some cases of methicillin- or penicillin-associated interstitial nephritis, a derivative of the antibiotic is bound to certain sites in renal tissue, in particular to the TBM (34, 47, 48). Assuming that renal fixation is important, two general possibilities can be considered: (a) The drug hapten binds to renal tissues in all patients receiving the drug, and the development of lesions depends on an unusual immune response (either humoral or cell-mediated); or (b) The binding of hapten occurs only in those patients who develop interstitial nephritis. There is conflicting evidence concerning this point. Border et al (34) were unable to find methicillin antigen in the kidneys of animals given methicillin; however, they did not provide information concerning the dosage or time of administration. In contrast, Colvin et al (48) described binding of antipenicillin antibodies to the TBM and interstitium in autopsy specimens of histologically normal kidneys from patients who received large amounts of penicillin shortly before death.

Several observations indicate that cell-mediated reactivity (presumably direc-ted against a conjugate of the drug and a structural renal protein) may be important: the predominance of mononuclear cells in the infiltrate, the scarcity or absence of immunoglobulins and C3 deposits in the kidneys in many cases, and the presence of cellular reactivity to drug. However, as noted above, none of these findings proves that the lesions are due to delayed sensitivity.

The presence of eosinophils points to an antibody-mediated component. Increased levels of IgE in the serum (49), IgE-containing plasma cells (in a case of interstitial nephritis associated with phenobarbital) (50), and the presence of basophils (48) all suggest a role for reaginic antibodies in some cases.

Anti-TBM antibodies were present in a case of drug-induced interstitial nephritis reported by Border et al (34). Linear accumulation of IgG and C3 was found along the TBM, together with a methicillin-derived antigen. Circulating anti-TBM antibodies were found. It was suggested that dimethoxyphenyl pen-icillin, which is largely secreted by the proximal tubules, binds to the TBM and results in the formation of a methicillin-TBM conjugate that stimulates anti-TBM autoantibody production. It is also possible, however, that anti-TBM antibodies result from tubular damage produced in some other way. In any case, anti-TBM antibodies have been reported in only a few cases and would appear to be an uncommon and secondary pathogenetic mechanism.

CONCLUSION

Four general conclusions can be stated. First, renal tubulointerstitial immune-complex deposition has been described in several models, and is associated with tubulointerstitial damage. Similar deposits have been described in man. They appear to be common in lupus nephritis, probably in the renal disease associated with mixed cryoglobulinemia, and possibly in renal allografts. The role of extraglomerular deposits in Sjögren's syndrome deserves further study, since otherwise unexplained interstitial nephritis is often found in these patients. It seems unlikely that future studies will reveal tubulointerstitial deposits in an appreciable percentage of cases of most forms of glomerulonephritis or in idiopathic interstitial nephritis. However, the remote possibility remains that immune complexes do account for certain forms of unexplained tubulointerstitial damage, even though they are not detectable by immunofluorescence. Second, anti-TBM antibodies cause severe tubulointerstitial nephritis in animals. Anti-TBM antibodies have been found in man in small numbers of patients, most often in association with anti-GBM diseases. In view of the resemblance of the findings in man to the experimental models, it seems probable that the anti-TBM antibodies are of pathogenetic significance. Third, delayed hypersensitivity reactions can occur in the kidneys of animals. It is quite likely that the interstitial mononuclear cell infiltrates seen in some human renal diseases represent cell-mediated reactions; however, proof will require the development of methods to identify such reactions in vivo. Fourth, a common form of acute interstitial nephritis is believed to be caused by hypersensitivity to a variety of drugs. Cellular reactivity, IgE, and rarely anti-TBM antibodies may participate in this form of renal injury.

Literature Cited

1. McCluskey, R. T., Klassen, J. 1973. Immunologically mediated glomerular, tubular and interstitial renal disease. *N. Engl. J. Med.* 288:564–70
2. Andres, G. A., McCluskey, R. T. 1975. Tubular and interstitial renal disease due to immunologic mechanisms. *Kidney Int.* 7:271–89
3. Unanue, E. R., Dixon, F. J., Feldman, J. D. 1967. Experimental allergic glomerulonephritis induced in the rabbit with homologous renal antigens. *J. Exp. Med.* 125:163–75
4. Klassen, J., Milgrom, F. 1969. Autoimmune concomitants of renal allografts. *Transplant. Proc.* 1:605–8
5. Klassen, J., McCluskey, R. T., Milgrom, F. 1971. Nonglomerular renal disease produced in rabbits by immunization with homologous kidney. *Am. J. Pathol.* 63:333–50
6. Hoyer, J. R. 1976. Autoimmune tubulointerstitial nephritis induced in rats by immunization with rat Tamm-Horsfall (TH) urinary glycoprotein. *Kidney Int.* 10:544 (Abstr.)
7. Klassen, J., Suqisaki, T., Milgrom, F., McCluskey, R. T. 1971. Studies on multiple renal lesions in Heymann nephritis. *Lab. Invest.* 25:577–85
8. Brentjens, J. R., O'Donnell, D. W.,

Pawlowski, I. B., Andres, G. A. 1974. Extra-glomerular lesions associated with deposition of circulating antigen-antibody complexes in kidneys of rabbits with chronic serum sickness. *Clin. Immunol. Immunopathol.* 3:112–22
9. Hurd, E. R., Ziff, M. 1977. Quantitative studies of immunoglobulin deposition in the kidney, glomerular cell proliferation and glomerulosclerosis in NZB/NZW F. hybrid mice. *Clin. Exp. Immunol.* 27: 261–68
10. Hurd, E. R., Ziff, M. 1977. Influence of interstitial infiltration on tubule cells in kidneys of NZB/NZW FI (B/W) hybrid mice and the effect of cyclophosphamide. *Arthritis Rheum.* 20:122 (Abstr.)
11. Klassen, J., Andres, G. A., Brennan, J. C., McCluskey, R. T. 1972. An immunologic renal tubular lesion in man. *Clin. Immunol. Immunopathol.* 1:69–83
12. Lehman, D. H., Wilson, C. B., Dixon, F. J. 1975. Extraglomerular immunoglobulin deposits in human nephritis. *Am. J. Med.* 58:765–86
13. Brentjens, J. R., Sepulveda, M., Baliah, T., Bentzel, C., Erlanger, B. F., Elwood, C., Montes, M., Hsu, K. C., Andres, G. A. 1975. Interstitial immune complex neph-

ritis in patients with systemic lupus erythematosus. *Kidney Int.* 7:342–50

14. Case Records of the Massachusetts General Hospital. Case 2-1976. *N. Engl. J. Med.* 294:100–5

15. Nicastri, A. D., Chen, C. K., Rao, T. K. S., Ginzler, E. M., Kaplan, D., Friedman, E. A. 1975. Renal disease with tubular immunofluorescence deposits. *Kidney Int.* 8:452 (Abstr.)

16. Andres, G. A., Accinni, L., Hsu, K. C., Penn, I., Porter, K. A., Randall, J. M., Seegal, B. C., Starzl, T. E. 1970. Human renal transplants: III. Immunopathologic studies. *Lab. Invest.* 22:588–604

17. Sawhney, A. S., Winer, R. L., Cohen, A. H., Gorman, J. T. 1975. Sjogren's syndrome with immune complex tubulointerstitial renal disease. *Kidney Int.* 6:453 (Abstr.)

18. Steblay, R. W., Rudofsky, U. 1971. Renal tubular disease and autoantibodies against tubular basement membrane induced in guinea pigs. *J. Immunol.* 107:589–94

19. Lehman, D. H., Marquardt, H., Wilson, C. B., Dixon, F. J. 1974. Specificity of autoantibodies to tubular and glomerular basement membranes induced in guinea pigs. *J. Immunol.* 112:241–48

20. Van Zwieten, M. J., Bhan, A. K., McCluskey, R. T., Collins, A. B. 1976. Studies on the pathogenesis of experimental anti-tubular basement membrane nephritis in the guinea pig. *Am. J. Pathol.* 83:531–46

21. Sugisaki, T., Klassen, J., Milgrom, F., Andres, G. A., McCluskey, R. T. 1973. Immunopathologic study of an autoimmune tubular and interstitial renal disease in Brown Norway rats. *Lab. Invest.* 28:658–71

22. Lehman, D. H., Wilson, C. B., Dixon, F. J. 1974. Interstitial nephritis in rats immunized with heterologous tubular basement membrane. *Kidney Int.* 5:187–95

23. Steblay, R. W., Rudofsky, U. 1973. Transfer of experimental autoimmune renal cortical tubular and interstitial disease in guinea pigs by serum. *Science* 180:966–68

24. Rudofsky, U. H., McMaster, P. R. B., Ma, W., Steblay, R. W., Pollara, B. 1974. Experimental autoimmune renal cortical tubulointerstitial disease in guinea pigs

lacking the fourth component of complement (C4). *J. Immunol.* 112:1387–93

25. Rudofsky, U. H., Steblay, R. W., Pollara, B. 1975. Inhibition of experimental autoimmune renal tubulointerstitial disease in guinea pigs by depletion of complement with cobra venom factor. *Clin. Immunol. Immunopathol.* 3:396–402

26. Rudofsky, U. H., Pollara, B. 1976. Studies on the pathogenesis of experimental autoimmune renal tubulointerstitial disease in guinea pigs. II. Passive transfer of renal lesions by anti-tubular basement membrane autoantibody and nonimmune bone marrow cells to leukocyte-depleted recipients. *Clin. Immunol. Immunopathol.* 6:107–14

27. Lehman, D. H., Wilson, C. B. 1976. Role of sensitized cells in antitubular basement membrane interstitial nephritis. *Int. Arch. Allergy Appl. Immunol.* 51:168–74

28. Hyman, L. H., Steinberg, A. D., Colvin, R. B., Bernard, E. F. 1977. Immunopathogenesis of autoimmune tubulointerstitial nephritis. II. Role of an immune response gene linked to the major histocompatibility locus. *J. Immunol.* 117:1894–97

29. Hyman, L. R., Colvin, R. B. Steinberg, A. D. 1976. Immunopathogenesis of autoimmune tubulointerstitial nephritis. I. Demonstration of differential susceptibility in strain II and strain XIII guinea pigs. *J. Immunol.* 116:327–35

30. McPhaul, J. J., Dixon, F. J. 1970. Characterization of human anti-glomerular basement membrane antibodies eluated from glomerulonephritic kidneys. *J. Clin. Invest.* 49:308–17

31. Levy, M., Gagnadoux, M. F., Habib, R. 1974. An immunologic Fanconi syndrome. *Int. Symp. Pediatr. Nephrol., 3rd,* Washington, DC

32. Harner, M. H., Nolte, M., Wilson, C. B., Talwalkar, Y. B., Musgrave, J. E., Brooks, R. E., Campbell, R. A. 1974. Anti-TBM antibody and nephrotic syndrome associated with milk allergy. See Ref. 31

33. Morel-Maroger, L., Kourilsky, O., Mignon, F., Fichet, G. 1974. Anti-tubular basement membrane antibodies in rapidly progressive post-

streptococcal glomerulonephritis: Report of a case. *Clin. Immunol. Immunopathol.* 2:185–94

34. Border, W. A., Lehman, D. H., Egan, J. D., Sass, H. J., Glade, J. E., Wilson, C. B. 1974. Antitubular basement membrane antibodies in methicillin associated interstitial nephritis. *N. Engl. J. Med.* 291:381–84

35. Olsen, S., Asklund, M. 1976. Interstitial nephritis with acute renal failure following cardiac surgery and treatment with methicillin. *Acta Med. Scand.* 199:305–10

36. Hyman, L. R., Ballow, M., Knieser, M. R. 1975. Diphenylhydantoin nephropathy: Evidence for an autoimmune pathogenesis. *Kidney Int.* 8:450 (Abstr.)

37. Bergstein, J. M., Litman, N. 1975. Interstitial nephritis with antitubular basement membrane antibody. *N. Engl. J. Med.* 292:875–78

38. Wilson, C. B., Lehman, D. H., McCoy, R. C., Gunnelli, C. J., Stickel, D. L. 1974. Antibular basement membranes after renal transplantation. *Transplantation* 18:447–52

39. Klassen, J., Kano, K., Milgrom, F., Menno, A. B., Anthone, S., Anthone, R., Sepulveda, M., Elwood, C. M., Andres, G. A. 1973. Tubular lesions produced by autoantibodies to tubular basement membrane in human renal allografts. *Int. Arch. Allergy Appl. Immunol.* 45:674–89

40. Grupe, W. E. 1968. An "in vitro" demonstration of cellular sensitivity in experimental autoimmune nephrosis in rats. *Proc. Soc. Exp. Biol. Med.* 127:1217–22

41. Litwin, A., Adams, L. E., Levy, R., Cline, S., Hess, E. B. 1971. Cellular immunity in experimental glomerulonephritis of rats: I. Delayed hypersensitivity and lymphocyte stimulation studies with renal tubular antigens. *Immunology* 20:755–66

42. Van Zweiten, M. J., Leber, P. D., Bhan, A. K., McCluskey, R. T. 1977. Experimental cell mediated interstitial nephritis induced with exogenous antigens. *J. Immunol.* 118:589–93

43. Cotran, R. S., Piessens, W. F. 1976. Pathogenesis of chronic pyelonephritis. *Proc. Int. Congr. Nephrol., 6th,* pp. 509–23. Basel: Karger

44. Rocklin, R. E., Lewis, E. J., David, J. R. 1970. *In vivo* evidence for cellular hypersensitivity to glomerular basement membrane antigens in human glomerulonephritis. *N. Engl. J. Med.* 283:497–501

45. Mahieu, P., Dardenne, M., Bach, J. F. 1972. Detection of humoral and cell-mediated immunity to kidney basement membranes in human renal diseases. *Am. J. Med.* 53:185–92

46. Mery, J. P., Morel-Moroger, L. 1976. Acute interstitial nephritis. A hypersensitivity reaction to drugs. *Proc. Int. Congr. Nephrol., 6th,* pp. 524–29. Basel: Karger

47. Baldwin, D. S., Levine, B. B., McCluskey, R. T., Gallo, G. R. 1968. Renal failure and interstitial nephritis due to penicillin and methicillin. *N. Engl. J. Med.* 279:1245–52

48. Colvin, R. D., Burton, N. E., Hyslop, N. E. Jr., Spitz, L., Lichtenstein, N. S. 1974. Penicillin-associated interstitial nephritis. *Ann. Int. Med.* 81:404–5

49. Ooi, B. S., First, M. R., Pesce, A. J., Pollak, V. E., Bernstein, I. L., Jao, W. 1974. IgE levels in interstitial nephritis. *Lancet* 1:1254–56

50. Faarup, P., Christensen, E. 1974. IgE containing plasma cells in acute tubulointerstitial nephropathy. *Lancet* 2:718

Ann. Rev. Med. 1979. 30:375–404

IMMUNOBIOLOGY OF THE ◆7330
MATERNAL-FETAL RELATIONSHIP

Ross E. Rocklin, M.D. [1]

Department of Medicine, Harvard Medical School, Robert Breck Brigham
Hospital, Boston, Massachusetts 02120

John L. Kitzmiller, M.D.

Department of Obstetrics and Gynecology, Harvard Medical School,
Boston Hospital for Women, Boston, Massachusetts 02115

Michael D. Kaye, Ph.D.

Department of Obstetrics and Gynecology, Sydney University,
Sydney, Australia

INTRODUCTION

The fetuses of all outbred mammalian species present an immunogenetic set
of paternal antigens that are foreign to the mother. Yet the fetus will survive
the period of intrauterine gestation without rejection despite the fact that
its mother will reject fetal or paternal tissues grafted at any other site. This
apparent paradox of transplantation immunology still remains an enigma
today even though it has been the focus of active research over the past
twenty years. Medawar (1) hypothesized many years ago that the success
of the fetus as an allograft could be explained as follows: (a) the conceptus
was not immunogenic and therefore did not invoke a maternal immunologic
response; (b) pregnancy altered the maternal immunologic response; (c) the
uterus was an immunologically privileged site; (d) the placenta was an
effective immunologic barrier; and (e) the fetus was not yet immunologically competent. While many of these hypotheses did not withstand the test
of time, they provided investigators with the opportunity to critically analyze, and as a result enhance understanding of, this very complex phenome-

[1]Present address: Department of Medicine, Box 30, T-NEMC, 171 Harrison Avenue, Boston,
Massachusetts 02111.

0066-4219/79/0401-0375$01.00

375

non. In this chapter we review the immunobiology of the maternal-fetal relationship, including the factors that lead to maternal sensitization, the maternal responses to fetal antigens, the factors that alter these responses, the fetal responses to maternal antigens, and a summary of the mechanisms that might allow fetal survival.

MATERNAL EXPOSURE AND LOCAL RESPONSE TO ANTIGENS RELATED TO CONCEPTION

Antigens of Semen and Sperm: Local and Systemic Responses

Semen contains many antigenic components from the testis and accessory glands of the male reproductive tract as well as spermatozoa (2). There is haploid expression of the major histocompatibility antigens on spermatozoa in man (3) and the mouse (4). An enzyme, lactic dehydrogenase-X (LDH-X), appears to be specific for spermatozoa (5), while the carbohydrate ABO antigens on spermatozoa are probably the result of adsorption rather than haploid expression (4). Seminal plasma or "sperm-coating antigens" are present in the acrosomes of ejaculated spermatozoa, and their removal may have something to do with the process of capacitation within the female genital tract (2).

Female immune responses to semen and sperm can be arbitrarily divided into antibody production and lymphocyte reactivity. The plasma cells of the cervix appear to be the major producers of immunoglobulin (Ig) in the female genital tract. Cervical mucus contains IgA and SIgA (two serum IgA molecules plus a secretory component), and IgG and small amounts of IgM and complement factors. Mucus also exhibits antibacterial and phagocytic activities caused by lysozymes and opsonizing antibodies (2). Sperm recovered from the uterus in the mouse and rabbit have antibodies attached, while those from the oviduct do not (6). This suggests that sperm populations may differ in their immunologic interaction with the female genital tract. That "selection" by the female genital tract occurs is amply demonstrated by the observation that only 5% of sperm migrate upwards from the vagina in mammals. In the uterus, most spermatozoa undergo phagocytosis by leukocytes within a few hours. The concept that spermatozoal selection may be the result of errors in spermatogenesis (7) has been refuted (8).

The introduction of allogeneic washed epididymis spermatozoa into the uterus of rats sensitizes the animals to later intradermal injection of lymphoid cells of the same strain, and also produces a marked local inflammatory response 24–48 hours after reexposure to the spermatozoa. Subsequent mating with allogeneic males enhances the reproductive efficiency of the sensitized uterine horn. Inoculation of virgins with allogeneic sperm produces enlargement of the uterine regional nodes when compared with inoculation by syngeneic sperm. The results suggest a local cellular response to spermatozoa within the uterus (9).

Infertility due to humoral factors has been ascribed to women with otherwise unexplained inability to conceive, is controversial, and has been reviewed elsewhere (2).

The Blastocyst

The ovum is surrounded by a mucoprotein coat, the zona pellucida. Contact of the sperm with the zona pellucida in the fallopian tube is species specific and depends on the interaction of terminal sugars on the cell surface glycoproteins of both (10). Once fertilization occurs, the zona pellucida becomes impenetrable to further spermatozoa because of the active mucoids or glycoproteins released from the cortical granules and diffused through the perivitelline space to the zona (11). The zona may protect the blastocyst during passage through tube and uterus, although zona-free eggs will survive and implant in the uterus of sensitized recipients (12). In the mouse, immunoglobulins coat the blastocyst by the time of implantation (13) and the zona pellucida is permeable to them (14). The source and biological role of these immunoglobulins are unknown.

There is ample evidence that preimplantation mouse blastocysts are immunogenic. They will be rejected upon transfer to ectopic sites in presensitized hosts (15), although the presence of the zona pellucida prolongs time to rejection (16). As an initial challenge in other recipients, blastocysts develop into trophoblast and induce specific unresponsiveness to later skin grafts from the donor strain (17). Trophoblast cells grown in culture from four-day mouse blastocysts somehow inhibit the in vitro growth of macrophage monolayers (18). Minor histocompatibility antigens (non–H-2) have been demonstrated on the trophectoderm surface of the 4–8-cell zygote, the morula, and the early murine blastocyst by immunoperoxidase labeling in the mouse (16). Other workers confirmed these results by cytotoxicity and immunofluorescence techniques (17, 19–21). Cleavage eggs and the inner cell mass also express tumor-related embryonic antigens (teratoma-like; SV-40), which may be lost at 4½ days. Most investigators could not identify major H-2 antigens on the outer trophectoderm of the blastocyst, but they are present on the inner cell mass (19, 22, 23), which differentiates to embryo, yolk sac, and amnion.

The Placenta

IMPLANTATION   As implantation nears, the zona pellucida is lost, and the outer trophectoderm seems to lose its non–H-2 antigenic determinants along with a decrease in concanavalin A and colloidal iron binding (22, 24). It is interesting that this occurs at the time of first intimate contact with maternal tissues, and in conjunction with the development of polyploidy of the outer trophoblast cells and the appearance of their phagocytic and secretory properties. Trophoblast differentiation in vitro also leads to loss of surface antigens, so it is not dependent on the maternal environment (22).

At implantation in the mouse, trophectoderm penetrates the uterine epithelium and further differentiates mural trophoblast to primary giant cells, polar trophoblast to secondary giant cells and ectoplacental cone. Trophoblast invasion of decidua probably occurs through a combination of cytoplasmic penetration around maternal cells, phagocytosis, and diffusion of cytolytic enzymes. In hemochorial placentation common to primates and laboratory rodents, maternal capillaries are tapped and the trophoblast villi or labyrinths are bathed with maternal blood. Cytotrophoblast migrates up uterine arteries to or beyond the myometrium, which induces dramatic structural changes that lead to expansion of the vessels. Giant cells also migrate through decidua and myometrium.

In primates the proliferative core cells (cytotrophoblast) undergo cytoplasmic differentiation, and the cell membranes break down to form a syncytium, the outer syncytiotrophoblast. The microvilli and glycocalyx of this layer of trophoblast are in contact with maternal blood.

Contact of the blastocyst with the uterine wall begins the process of decidualization whereby the uterine and stromal cells undergo rapid DNA synthesis and mitosis (25). In the mouse the decidual cells increase their DNA content by endoreduplication (26), and the trophoblast cells cease dividing as they move away from the influence of the inner cell mass (27) but continue their DNA synthesis by endoreduplication (28).

Whether or not there is cell fusion between trophoblast and uterine cells is controversial. The process was first noted in the Australian marsupial Native cat (29) and bandicoot (30, 31). This was confirmed in woman (32, 33) by light microscopy, and at the electron microscope level in the bandicoot (34), rabbit (35, 36), and hamster (37). Other investigators noted fine decidual cytoplasmic protrusions approaching human trophoblast cells, but no evidence of cell fusion (38). The trophoblast cells are phagocytic, and they will incorporate labeled maternal nuclear material from the uterus of rats (39) or mice (40). Decidual cells similarly incorporate label from the nuclei of mouse blastocysts labeled in vitro with ^{3}H-thymidine prior to their transfer to pseudopregnant recipients (41). These observations may have important implications in the development of a barrier between fetal and maternal tissues. When the cells of different species hybridize in vitro and nuclear mixing occurs, the resultant hybrid cell undergoes a marked alteration in its cell surface antigens (42, 43). Other investigators believe the high DNA count of giant cells arises from endoreduplication rather than from cell fusion (27). Studies of artificially implanted embryos did not reveal hybrid enzymes, which would be expected if maternal cells fused with trophoblast (28, 44).

PLACENTAL ANTIGENS   A variety of methods have been employed to determine whether postimplantation trophoblast is immunogenic. Since some of these methods disrupt the normal anatomical arrangements of the placental tissue, one should bear in mind that conclusions about trophoblast antigens may be artifactual. Extracts of mouse and rat placentae have been used to raise antisera that will then cause placental damage and abortions in pregnant animals of the same strain (45, 46). The antisera are absorbed with somatic cells or tissues prior to injection, which suggests that there are organ-specific antigens in the placenta. These techniques, however, cannot determine which type of placental cell is contributing the antigens. Youtananukorn et al (47) applied the papain digest method of preparing soluble, surface histocompatibility antigens to the human placenta, and determined that autologous lymphocytes were sensitized (migration inhibitory factor production) to the "placental antigens." Finally, placental fraction with enzyme specificities of plasma membrane exhibited only 5% of the HLA-A and B and β_2-microglobulin titers found in spleen cells (48).

Transplantation of murine ectoplacental cone trophoblast to ectopic sites revealed that trophoblast growth is not affected by prior sensitization with donor-strain skin grafts or injections of spleen cells (49, 50). The conclusion that implanted, differentiated trophoblast is not immunogenic is supported by more recent studies in which antibody binding to H-2 and non–H-2 determinants on ectoplacental cone derivatives was negative, while antibody binding to embryonic sacs was strongly positive (21, 22). Beer et al (51) showed, however, that rat ectoplacental cone trophoblast transplanted to renal capsules of allogeneic females (a) induces hypertrophy of draining lymph nodes, (b) induces production of paternal-strain hemagglutinins, and (c) slightly impairs subsequent alloimmune responses of the hosts.

Since there is a highly sulfated sialomucoprotein substance on the surface of murine trophoblast cells (52), many have suggested that this coat may render trophoblast nonimmunogenic by masking antigenic sites or repelling lymphocytes by the high electronegative charge. Currie et al (53) reported that treatment with neuraminidase to remove sialic residues enabled ectoplacental cone trophoblast to induce transplantation reactions, but this result was not confirmed by Simmons et al (54). Billington (17) cautions that experiments with explants of ectoplacental cones may be misleading, since all of the trophoblasts become multinucleate, polyploid cells.

Immunologic studies of trophoblast cells in tissue culture are fraught with similar difficulties concerning the origin and nature of the reacting cells. Anti-HLA sera and complement were cytotoxic to human placental cells from early pregnancy, although the density of HLA antigenic sites was much less than on fetal skin cells (55). Two groups of investigators observed that autologous leukocytes (but not purified lymphocytes) were cytotoxic to trypsinized human placental cells in culture, and that trophoblast cells induced a blastogenic response in the lymphocytes (56, 57). The leukocytotoxic effects on the placental cells were blocked by autologous serum (57). Using the immunoperoxidase-labeling technique, Jenkinson & Billington (58) showed that early embryonic cells grown in culture were certainly positive for histocompatibility antigens as compared to placental cells. However, Billington and co-workers (21) most recently studied postimplantation trophoblast in culture with a mixed hemadsorption technique, and they found that *some* trophoblast cells were positive for non–H-2 antigens. They present a cogent discussion of possible reasons for trophoblast cells to shed antigens after implantation, and point out that inner diploid cells may remain antigen positive, while outer differentiated polyploid cells are negative (17, 21).

Frozen sections of intact human placentae have been studied by immunohistologic techniques, and many immunoproteins have been identified (59). In late pregnancy, IgG is primarily localized in the trophoblast basement membrane, while IgM and C3 are found in deposits of intervillous fibrin (60–63). HLA-reactive sites and β_2-microglobulin were present in mesenchymal and fetal endothelial cells, but not on the surface or basement membrane of trophoblast cells (64). In conclusion, it is perhaps useful to recall Billington's statement that a weakly antigenic trophoblast, despite its failure to induce a state of transplantation immunity in the host, still may be responsible for the induction of circulating antibodies (17).

THE UTERUS AS AN IMMUNOLOGICALLY PRIVILEGED SITE   A question has been raised concerning whether or not the uterus is an immunologically privileged site similar to the anterior chamber of the eye and the hamster cheek pouch, where poor lymph drainage is related to failure of graft rejection (65). This would imply that the reason the conceptus thrives within the uterus is that either the afferent or efferent arms (or both) of the expected allograft response are ineffective at that site. The concept does not explain, of course, the rare human abdominal pregnancy that proceeds to term. The idea of a protective intrauterine environment is suggested by experiments in which blastocysts transplanted to ectopic sites in presensitized mice are destroyed, while blastocysts transferred to the uterus develop normally (49).

Beer & Billingham (9) carried out an elegant series of experiments demonstrating that the decidual response produced by pseudopregnancy or hormone injections leads to prolongation of a graft of allogeneic skin within the uterus, but that decidua were not enough to prevent rapid rejection of intrauterine skin grafts in presensitized hosts (9). The possible role of decidua in limiting recognition of the conceptus as an allograft remains unclear, since there is lymphatic drainage of the decidua and myometrium, and lymphocytic infiltration near the trophoblast is observed in human pregnancy (66, 67). Recent ultramicroscopic studies demonstrate intermingling of human decidual and trophoblastic cells without structural elements as a barrier between them (38, 68). Fibrillar deposits were distributed randomly around the deciduotrophoblastic complexes, and there is some evidence this material is produced by the maternal decidual cells (38, 68). A close association of small developing decidual cells with lymphoblasts around precapillary arterioles was also noted (38).

A variety of local immune responses can be induced within the uterus of laboratory animals. Transfer of allogeneic skin, leukocytes, or lymph node cells to one uterine horn stimulates ipsilateral hypertrophy of the para-aortic lymph nodes, sensitizes the host for accelerated rejection of a subsequent skin graft, and *locally* sensitizes the uterus for a delayed inflammatory reaction to a second inoculum of lymphoid cells (9). Thus, the uterus does not seem to be protected from participation in immune reactions. Interestingly, allogeneic trophoblast also induces hypertrophy of the para-aortic nodes in rats, mice, and hamsters (9), while in contrast a decrease in size and cellularity of germinal centers of the pelvic and para-aortic lymph nodes in human mid- and late pregnancy has been described (69, 70). More recent experiments in rats indicate that removal of para-aortic nodes prior to allogeneic pregnancy preserves maternal responses to paternal antigens subsequent to pregnancy, which are otherwise impaired after control pregnancies (51). Adoptive transfer of para-aortic node cells (or serum) from multiparas suppresses host antibody response to paternal-strain skin grafts. Based on these experiments and others (71), Beer suggests that lymph nodes draining the uterus may be the site of generation of immunosuppressive T cells or blocking antibody (see below).

THE PLACENTA AS AN IMMUNOLOGIC BARRIER   Undoubtedly, a major factor in the immunological coexistence of gravida and fetus is their ordinarily complete vascular separation. Interposed is the placenta, which conceivably could prevent immunogenic fetal cells from reaching the maternal circulation or protect the fetus from maternal lymphocyte attack. However, the placenta is an incomplete barrier in this respect, and it is well known that small amounts of fetal blood containing red cells, leukocytes, and lymphoid cells enter the maternal circulation prior to termination of pregnancy (72–75). Occasionally, an Rh-negative gravida will be sensitized to Rh-positive fetal red cells during her first pregnancy, although this is much more likely following the larger fetal-to-maternal transfusion associated with labor and delivery. The passage of maternal lymphocytes to the fetus is apparently a much rarer event, but is not unheard of (73). Besides cellular material (including deportation of syncytiotrophoblast fragments to maternal lungs), placental glycoprotein hormones, which are at least immunogenic across species (xenogeneic), also pass to the maternal circulation. However, in primates the cross reactivity of human chorionic gonadotropin (hCG) with maternal gonadotropins (FSH and LH) and of human placental lactogen (hPL) with growth hormone may be protective.

The placenta probably acts as a selective filter for maternal immunoglobulins reaching the fetus. Fc receptors are identified on placental cells. IgG is transported across the placenta, but not IgM or IgA. In rodents, immunoglobulin transport across the yolk sac is also important (76). Cytotoxic antibodies to fetal antigens are absent in neonatal blood (77), perhaps because of sequestration in the placenta (78, 79). Johnson, Trenchev & Faulk (80) also suggested that immune complexes might be removed from fetal blood by deposition in the placental stem vessels (80).

Embryonic Antigens and Fetal Blood Cells

As noted above, the earliest appearance of the major histocompatibility (H-2) antigens was found on cells of the inner cell mass of mouse embryos by the late blastocyst stage (96 hours after fertilization) (23) or slightly later (19, 81). As development proceeds, antigenicity increases at different rates in various embryonic organs (82).

The red cell carbohydrate antigens of the ABO system are present from 5–6 weeks of gestation but are not fully mature until 2–4 years of life. These antigens are present on all somatic cells as well as on certain intestinal gram-negative bacteria, which accounts for the presence of isoagglutinins in O-positive, six-month-old infants. These facts also account for the observation that firstborn infants may be affected by ABO incompatibility, and that increasing severity with subsequent children may not occur since the fetal red cells are poorly immunogenic and the fetal somatic cells compete with the red cells for the maternal IgG (83).

The major histocompatibility antigens are present on red cells in rats, but not in man. These antigens are present on human fetal leukocytes, and antibodies are found in the serum of 25% of multiparous women (84, 85). Maternal exposure to allogeneic fetal leukocytes may not be obligatory for the production of anti-HLA antibodies, however, since they have been detected in maternal sera after molar pregnancies (86). Women exposed to sperm do not develop anti-HLA antibodies prior to their first pregnancies (87).

MATERNAL RESPONSES TO THE FETUS

General Maternal Immunocompetence

An important issue concerning survival of the fetus is focused on the ability of the mother to mount an immunologic response to foreign (paternal) antigens. Is the mother immunocompetent in this regard throughout the period of gestation, and if not, does her inability to respond reflect a specific or more generalized defect? The answers to these questions are complex and the data incomplete.

The morphology and histology of lymphoid tissue and the enumeration of T and B cells in pregnancy has been evaluated in man as well as in animals. There is an involution of the thymus during pregnancy (69) and a decrease in the size and cellularity (B cells) of germinal centers present in para-aortic lymph nodes (70). However, the weight and proportion of T cells within the spleen and mesenteric lymph nodes is apparently increased. The overall percentage of, and total lymphocyte count is essentially unchanged. However, there are fewer circulating T cells early in pregnancy (up to 20 weeks gestation) with a compensatory increase in B cells (88, 89). This reversal of the normal T:B cell ratio is gradually corrected after 20 weeks of gestation. It is quite possible that the apparent reduction in circulating T cells in early pregnancy represents not a "loss" of these cells but rather their redistribution or transfer to another lymphoid compartment. Data quantifying the various subsets of T cells would be extremely valuable in determining whether populations of helpers or suppressors are being selectively affected.

Humoral and cellular immune responses to a variety of antigens have been measured. In most studies, the plasma concentrations of IgG, IgM, and IgA in pregnancy are normal compared to those in the nonpregnant state (90). However, IgG levels decrease somewhat late in pregnancy, possibly because of placental transfer (91). Little information is available concerning IgD and IgE levels, although the former has been reported to be elevated at term (92). The production of specific antibodies to environmental antigens is normal, which suggests that these aspects of T and B cell function in general are intact during pregnancy (93). Tuberculin skin reactivity is either normal (94) or slightly depressed (25% of cases) in the last trimester of pregnancy (95). Graft rejection, another in vivo manifestation of cellular immunity, is marginally impaired during pregnancy. The rejection of primary ("first set") skin grafts is abnormal, but the secondary rejection of a graft from the same donor is normal (96). Two other components of the immune system, complement, and phagocytosis and bactericidal activity, have also been evaluated during pregnancy. The total complement level (CH_{50}) and the third component (C3) are progressively elevated during the course of pregnancy although it is not clear whether this reflects inflammatory changes or, more likely, is hormonally related (97). Leukocytes from pregnant women show markedly increased rates of phagocytosis and bactericidal activity (98). Whether the latter finding is also a result of hormonal influences remains to be clarified. Thus, during pregnancy the various components of immunity per se are basically intact with only minor alterations.

Humoral Antibody Responses

A wide range of antibodies are produced against fetal antigens. The production of anti-Rh antibody by Rhdd women carrying RhD fetuses is a well known example of this response (83). Furthermore, mothers whose red cells lack A or B red cell antigens and who carry a fetus possessing these antigens usually exhibit a rise in anti-A or anti-B titers.

The gravida also develops antibodies to paternal HLA-A, B, and C series antigens. These antibodies will be detected in 20–30% of primagravid women, and the incidence and titers increase with succeeding pregnancies (99, 100). Titers of antibody rise during pregnancy and decrease slightly after delivery. However, in some subjects these antibodies persist for months to many years after the last pregnancy. In addition, non–anti-HLA cytotoxic antibodies can be detected in maternal sera and exhibit different kinetics. These antibodies decrease during the third trimester and reappear after delivery. It is tempting to attribute the disappearance of these antibodies to the combination of antibody with fetal antigen that is shed into the maternal bloodstream.

Recently, IgG antibodies have been described that are not directed against HLA (ABC) antigens, are noncytotoxic, and are directed against HLA-D antigens (101). These antibodies are of particular interest because they identify antigens present on paternal cells that are thought to be involved in initiating the mixed lymphocyte reaction in vitro and presumably in vivo as well. That is, these antigens are important for triggering sensitized effector lymphocytes, and the presence of these antibodies in vitro blocks the reaction. The latter may be analogous to the anti-Ia antibodies described in the mouse (102). Their role in the survival of the fetus is discussed more fully in the section on specific immunosuppression.

Cellular Immune Responses

Through use of a variety of in vitro assays to measure maternal lymphocyte responses, including proliferation, cytotoxicity, and lymphokine production, it has been demonstrated that maternal cells are clearly reactive against paternal antigens. In the presence of normal serum (but not autologous serum), cells from pregnant women proliferate as well as cells from nonpregnant females when mixed together in vitro with paternal cells (103–106). The maternal response is somewhat stronger, however, against third-party cells. The reasons for this disparity will also be discussed in the section on specific immunosuppression. Furthermore, when fetal lymphocytes are used to stimulate maternal cells, a weak proliferative response is observed (107). The mechanism for the latter observation is not clear but may relate to the ability of fetal mononuclear cells to secrete soluble factors that have inhibitory effects on proliferation (108).

Cells that are directly cytotoxic (killer T cells) against fetal cells, and to a lesser extent against paternal cells as well, are also found in the maternal circulation (109). These cytotoxic lymphocytes are rarely found circulating in the blood of normal individuals, since they are usually only generated in vitro during the course of a mixed lymphocyte reaction (MLR). Therefore, the presence of these cells in the blood of pregnant women, as well as the finding that these cells exhibit cytotoxicity toward fetal/paternal but not third-party cells, suggests that an active sensitization to paternal antigens is occurring in vivo. Of further interest, maternal lymphocytes also exhibit cytotoxicity toward trophoblast tissue from their own pregnancies and, to a lesser extent, for trophoblast cells from other pregnancies (57). Since trophoblast cells bind large amounts of IgG, even after vigorous washing, this phenomenon may be mediated by lymphocytes (K cells) capable of binding IgG through their Fc receptor, which activates them for killing (antibody-dependent cellular cytotoxicity).

Further evidence of a state of maternal sensitization to paternal antigens was demonstrated in studies in which lymphokine production was measured. Lymphocytes from pregnant women cultured in vitro with cord blood or paternal mononuclear cells or placental antigens produce macrophage migration inhibitory factor (MIF) within 24 hours (110, 111). This maternal response is indicative of a state of specific presensitization since mononuclear cells from randomly mixed normal donors did not produce MIF within this period of culture, and maternal cells usually do not make MIF against third-party cells (112). In addition, there was a correlation between the presence of MIF production and the parity, which indicates that sensitization is progressive with repeated exposure to antigen (111). Taken together, these data imply that washed maternal lymphocytes, cultured in the absence of autologous serum, are perfectly capable of responding in a number of ways against cells bearing paternal antigens.

Nonspecific Immunosuppression

STEROID HORMONES   The placenta synthesizes estrogens from fetal and maternal precursors and secretes them into maternal and fetal circulations in increasing concentrations as pregnancy proceeds. Maternal serum levels of the most active estrogen, estradiol, are ~20 ng/ml at term, but the concentration is ~50 ng/ml in the intervillous blood (113).

Early studies failed to show an immunosuppressive effect of estradiol on experimental allograft rejection, but the tissue levels of estrogen may have been too low (114, 115). More recently, estradiol has been shown to prolong first- and second-set skin grafts in mice (116) and to inhibit the rejection of corneal grafts in preimmunized rabbits (117). In another study estradiol only prolonged first-set allogeneic skin grafts in sublethally irradiated mice (as compared to nonirradiated mice). The authors speculated that the estrogen impaired the development or proliferation of thymic stem cells during recovery from irradiation (118). Estradiol certainly involutes the thymus in adult experimental animals (69). Estrogen and hCG in combination produced a marked decrease in thymic weight and in the number of small lymphocytes in the thymus (118). As noted above, involution of the maternal thymus is well recognized in human pregnancy. The murine thymus is able to metabolize progesterone by 20-α-hydroxylation to a much greater degree than lung or kidney tissue (119). Isolated thymocytes have even greater specific activity, which suggests a role for progesterone in thymic function.

Progesterone is synthesized and secreted by trophoblast cells into the maternal blood, and thus is in much higher concentration in the intervillous blood (886 ng/ml) than in peripheral blood (160 ng/ml, late pregnancy) (120a). Placental concentration of progesterone is 3.1 μg/gm wet weight at term (120b). Injection of progesterone into experimental animals did not prolong allograft survival in several early studies (114, 116, 121). The dosage or route of administration may have been inadequate, since subsequent experiments showed that progesterone or a synthetic progestin extended viability of homologous skin grafts in rhesus monkeys or of heart grafts in rats, respectively (122, 123). Siiteri and colleagues (124) first studied the effects of progesterone released into local tissue in high concentrations from tubular Silastic® inserts. In these experiments, later confirmed by Beer & Billingham (125), tissue concentrations of 50–200 μg/ml progestorne suppressed the expected inflammatory reaction to cotton threads and prolonged the survival of skin xeno- and allografts in rats.

The effects of reproductive steroids on in vitro models of cellular immunity have been widely studied in recent years. Estradiol, progesterone, and diethylstilbestrol in the dose range of 10–50 μg/ml have all been shown to reduce the lymphocyte proliferative response to the mitogenic plant lectins phytohemagglutinin and concanavalin A (126–128). In human studies of the mixed lymphocyte reaction, doses as low as 0.2 μg/ml estradiol slightly stimulated lymphocyte reactivity, while higher doses of 20 μg/ml of estradiol or progesterone inhibited the uptake of tritiated thymidine by responding lymphocytes (128, 129). Washing lymphocytes removed the inhibitory effect of the reproductive steroids (129, 130). One study showed that estradiol must be present from the beginning of the five-day mixed lymphocyte culture in order to show its inhibitory effect (129); however, Siiteri and co-workers (130) demonstrated that progesterone (20 $\mu g/ml$) could be added to the end of the five-day mixed lymphocyte culture and it still would inhibit the uptake of tritiated thymidine, which is the marker for cellular proliferation. Thus, the latter suggests that progesterone is suppressing not cell activation but incorporation of labeled thymidine into DNA. Reproductive steroids do not produce cytotoxic effects on the lymphocytes at the effective dose ranges.

We have examined another model of cellular immunity, the production of migration inhibitory factor (MIF) by presensitized guinea pig lymphocytes. Neither estradiol nor progesterone in concentrations of 2–20 $\mu g/ml$ significantly inhibited either the production of MIF or the macrophage response to preformed MIF (131).

There are fewer studies of the effects of reproductive steroids on humoral immune responses. Treatment of mice with 2.5 μg of estradiol resulted in increased numbers of splenic antibody-producing cells in mice sensitized to *Escherichia coli* (132). Incubation of murine spleen and thymic cells with low doses of estradiol (500–5000 pg/ml) produced significant increases in numbers of antibody-producing cells and in the uptake of tritiated thymidine by the lymphoid cells (132). Much higher doses of estradiol slightly suppressed these aspects of the humoral and cellular immune systems. Beer's most recent studies indicated that the lowest dose of locally released progesterone (4 ng/ml serum, 100 ng/ml tissue) caused earlier initiation of antibody production in rats stimulated with dermal allografts (125). Higher doses of progesterone (186 ng/ml serum, 200 ng/ml tissue) significantly inhibited the formation of hemagglutinating antibodies in these experiments.

The plasma levels of transcortin, transcortin- and albumin-bound cortisol, and free unbound cortisol all increase progressively during pregnancy. The increased cortisol levels (5–20 $\mu g/ml$) probably result from reduced hepatic clearance of cortisol secondary to estrogen, independent of the increase in transcortin synthesis, also an estrogen effect (133). Maternal cells and tissues are thus exposed to an average daily concentration of cortisol at least twice normal. Cortisol was early shown to delay allograft rejection in animals (122), and corticosteroids are used clinically in human renal transplantation. Corticosteroids have cytolytic effects on lymphoid cells of some species (mouse, rabbit, rat) but not of guinea pigs or primates (134). Decreased circulating lymphocyte counts produced by phar-

368 of 480

388   ROCKLIN, KITZMILLER & KAYE

macologic doses of corticosteroids result from a redistribution of B and T cells (135). Low doses of cortisol may enhance lymphoid cell proliferation, but sufficiently high concentrations nonspecifically suppress DNA synthesis in basal and stimulated lymphoid cells (136). Cortisol inhibits MLC response (uptake of ^{3}H-thymidine) in the dose range of 1–20 μg/ml, but the effect is different from that of progesterone, in that cortisol must be present early in the five-day culture for maximum suppressive effect (130). Washing lymphocytes preincubated with cortisol does not reduce the MLC suppressive effect, as it does with progesterone (130).

Corticosteroids have pronounced effects on the macrophage. Aggregation or migration inhibition responses to lymphokines are suppressed (137, 138a), phagocytic activity is decreased, and the binding activity of membrane receptors for IgG and C3 is reduced (135). Corticosteroids may influence cell membrane function directly. It is probable that the effects of corticosteroids on allograft and delayed hypersensitivity reactions depend more on anti-inflammatory effects (decreased capillary permeability; increased vascular tone; decreased macrophage responses) than on direct suppression of lymphocyte function. Cortisol may be concentrated at the placental surface, since a transcortin-like protein with immunosuppressive effects has been demonstrated in trophoblast extracts (138b).

Several lines of experimental evidence thus indicate that the anti-inflammatory effects of steroid hormones may play a role in the immunologic coexistence of gravida and conceptus, especially considering the high placental concentrations of estrogen and progesterone. Even more intriguing is the conjecture that reproductive steroids may play a role in the shifting balance of thymic and lymphocyte proliferation and suppression as pregnancy evolves.

GESTATIONAL HORMONES   Human chorionic gonadotropin (hCG) and human placental lactogen (hPL) are glycoproteins synthesized by the syncytiotrophoblast. Peak secretion rate (10^5 IU/day) and blood levels (10 IU/ml peripheral, 600 IU/gm placenta wet weight) of hCG are reached at ten-weeks gestation, but there is a progressive rise in hPL secretion throughout pregnancy. There is no evidence for an immunosuppressive effect of hPL. Initial studies with commercially available hCG extracted from pregnancy urine suggested an immunosuppressive role for hCG. In vivo, injection of crude hCG was shown to diminish delayed hypersensitivity to PPD in guinea pigs (138c), but did not interfere with rejection of intrauterine skin grafts in rats (138d). Crude lots of hCG in the dose range 1,000–10,000 IU/ml were noted to inhibit lymphocyte mitogenic response to PHA (138d, 138e, 139) or to allogeneic lymphocytes in MLR (140, 141, 142a). The suppressive effect was lost by washing lymphocytes preincubated with crude hCG (140) or by increasing the dose of PHA (142b). Several investigators observed that low doses of crude or purified hCG (100–1000 IU/ml) enhanced the uptake of ^{3}H-thymidine by unstimulated lymphocytes in culture (142c, 143) or augmented lymphocyte responses to pokeweed mitogen (142c) or the MLR (142b, 143). However, hCG purified from the crude lots by Sephadex chromatography and gel filtration in higher doses of 10,000–15,000 IU/ml did not inhibit lymphocyte blastogenic responses to mitogens or allogeneic cells (142b, 143, 144).

Experiments have been carried out to define the immunosuppressive substances in the various preparations of crude hCG. Patillo et al (144) observed that concentrations of phenol equivalent to that in Organon hCG completely inhibited mitogenic responses to the plant lectins. Immunoabsorption of IgG removed the anticomplement activity from another preparation of crude hCG (145). Crude hCG can be separated by gel chromatography into fractions with biologic activity of hCG or inhibitory effects on lymphocyte transformation (146). Experiments with neuraminidase suggest that the inhibitory factors may be sialoglycoproteins found in pregnancy urine and distinct from hCG (143, 146).

ALPHA-FETOPROTEIN   Alpha-fetoprotein (AFP) is a normal component of amniotic fluid and fetal serum in many species and has structural and biochemical similarities to albumin (147, 148). It is present in high concentrations early in fetal life and reaches a maximum concentration of several milligrams per milliliter in the first trimester of human pregnancy, falling gradually to 20–50 μg/ml by birth (149). Murgita & Tomasi (150, 151) first reported that AFP isolated from mouse amniotic fluid was a potent inhibitor of in vitro mitogen-induced and mixed lymphocyte proliferation as well as primary and secondary humoral antibody responses. Since then a number of studies have presented conflicting findings (152–154). In these latter studies, lymphocyte proliferation to mitogens and antigens was either normal or abnormal, while the production of a lymphokine (macrophage migration inhibitory factor), E-rosette formation by T cells, and lymphocyte cytotoxicity were unaffected. Interestingly, AFP activates lymphocyte suppressor cells, and this finding may account in part for its inhibitory effects on cell function (155, 156). However, it is still unresolved whether this immunosuppressive property is due to AFP itself, a contaminant, or is an artifactual result of the process of purification, unrelated to its biologic effect in vivo (154).

PREGNANCY-SPECIFIC GLYCOPROTEINS   In addition to hCG, there are a number of other pregnancy-associated glycoproteins that may have immunosuppressive properties. These include ovamucoid, fetuin, α_2-macroglobulin and β_1-glycoprotein (SP$_1$). α_2-Macroglobulin isolated from maternal (not fetal) circulation has a molecular weight range of 3–7.5 $\times$ 10^5, as reported by several laboratories (157–159), and is present on the surface of lymphocytes (160). It has inhibitory effects on MIF production and lymphoproliferative responses to mitogens and antigens (157, 161–163). Of interest, the inhibitory effects of α_2-macroglobulin on mitogen responses have been attributed in part to its ability to bind to the lectin, thus limiting the quantity available to the cells (162). β_1-Glycoprotein is a product of the syncytial trophoblast. Its concentration in serum increases with advancing pregnancy and may reach levels as high as 30 mg% (162). It has an apparent molecular weight of 1.1×10^5 and has been reported to suppress PHA responses (164). Further studies using more purified preparations are required to discern the exact role of these glycoproteins in suppressing maternal lymphocyte responses during pregnancy.

Specific Immunosuppression

SERUM   While some studies show that maternal serum can nonspecifically inhibit cellular immune responses to several stimuli (165–167), many others demonstrate immunologic specificity. Such specific "enhancement" or "blocking" by maternal serum was first found in mice when the survival of paternal-strain tumors and skin grafts in females was increased by strain-specific pregnancies (168, 169). These effects became more profound with succeeding pregnancies but were usually detected with the first pregnancy. The latter findings prompted Kaliss & Dagg (170) to suggest that immunological enhancement, a phenomenon in which humoral antibodies facilitate the growth of antigenically foreign cells that are normally rejected in their absence, might be operative during pregnancy. This hypothesis was supported by the findings of Hellstrom et al (109), who showed that serum from BALB/C mice made pregnant by C3H males was able to prevent the in vitro inhibition of colony formation of C3H embryonic cells by presensitized BALB/C lymphocytes. Similar results were also obtained with tumors and could be passively transmitted (171).

In the in vitro systems, multiparous serum has been found to inhibit the MLR between maternal and paternal, maternal and newborn, and even between maternal and third-party cells with no absolute correlation with HLA type (105, 106, 172–174). Similar results have been obtained in other in vitro systems. As reported in the section on cellular immune responses, lymphocytes from multiparous women produce MIF in response to newborn or paternal cells and placental extracts (110, 111). This response can be specifically ablated by autologous maternal serum but not by serum from other multiparous women (175, 176). In addition, maternal lymphocytes can be prevented from exhibiting cytotoxicity toward trophoblast cells in vitro if the latter are grown in maternal serum (57).

The enhancing factor present in maternal serum that accounts for the effects described above has been partially characterized and studied for its possible biologic function in pregnancy. It has been described as belonging to the IgG class, since its elution pattern on gels is with 7S molecules and it can be removed by affinity chromatography with anti-IgG (57, 112, 174, 176). These antibodies can be absorbed by paternal cells but not by pooled human platelets, which suggests that they are not directed against the classical HLA-A, B, or C series antigens but against HLA-D antigens. Therefore, they may be analogous to the anti-Ia antibodies described in the mouse (102). These antibodies are cytotoxic to B cells (but not T cells), and their $F(AB^1)_2$ fragments suppress EA-rosette formation with Fc-bearing lymphocytes and inhibit the MLR (177).

A biologic role for these antibodies in the maintenance of a normal-term pregnancy has been suggested in clinical studies with women who have recurrent idiopathic spontaneous abortions. Rocklin et al (112) found that while lymphocytes from chronic aborters were presensitized to paternal antigens, their sera did not contain a blocking factor that could prevent their MIF response to paternal cells. In contrast, serum from normal multiparous women contained a blocking factor that did inhibit their MIF response to their mate. Of particular interest, blocking activity appeared in the serum of chronic aborters during subsequent successful pregnancies. In further studies, blocking activity has been detected in the serum of 80% of primagravid women between 16–24 weeks of pregnancy (131). Because blocking activity has not always been detected in the serum of normal primagravid women, one could question whether these antibodies play a significant role in fetal survival. One possible explanation for their absence from the serum of some normal women may be that they are attached to one possible target organ, the placenta, and are not present in high enough titer to be detected systemically by the available techniques. In fact, antibodies with blocking activity can be eluted from placentae, as is discussed below.

Although the data are suggestive, there is no objective proof that enhancing (blocking) antibodies play a major role in the in vivo survival of the mammalian embryo or fetus. However, in patients receiving allografts, a situation somewhat analogous to the fetal allograft, the presence of enhancing antibodies may improve graft survival. For example, hemodialysis patients who receive repeated blood transfusions develop blocking factors similar to those found in multiparous women (178). There is a better survival of future kidney grafts in these patients. Moreover, the administration of pooled IgG (obtained from retroplacental blood of multiparous women) to renal transplant patients has been associated with increased graft survival (compared to IgG obtained from normal serum) (179, 180).

IMMUNOGLOBULIN ELUTED FROM PLACENTAE   Immunoglobulin has been identified on human trophoblast membrane and mouse placentae by immunohistologic techniques (61, 181). Placental material has been eluted and the IgG fraction isolated and tested for its immunosuppressive and enhancing activity. IgG eluted from human term placentae was shown to inhibit in vitro mitogen, antigen, and MLR proliferative responses (62, 182). This effect was nonspecific because the eluate inhibited normal as well as maternal cells. However, in more recent studies IgG eluted from human placentae was found to specifically suppress MIF production by maternal cells in response to paternal antigens (131). Of particular interest in this latter study, blocking activity was detected in the placental eluate but not in the serum of a primagravid woman, which supports the suggestion made earlier that blocking antibodies may be in low titer with first pregnancies. IgG eluted from mouse placentae binds in vitro to paternal lymphocytes and if administered in vivo will enhance the take of paternal-strain sarcoma allografts in mice of the maternal strain (181).

Analysis of the IgG eluted from pooled human placentae revealed at least two antibody populations similar to that present in multiparous sera (177). One antibody exhibits lymphocytotoxicity in the presence of complement and has anti-HLA specificities. The other has been identified as having specificity for HLA-D antigens and is comparable to the anti-Ia antibodies described earlier. It is of interest that alloantisera directed against mouse Ia and rat Ia-like antigens enhance skin or kidney allografts, and in man a similar antisera can impair in vitro antibody-dependent cellular cytotoxicity and Ig synthesis (102, 183, 184).

ROLE OF SUPPRESSOR CELLS   In addition to their role as effector cells in cellular-immune reactions and as helper cells in antibody formation, T cells also play a regulatory role in the immune response (185). Both under in vivo and in vitro conditions, a subpopulation of T cells is capable of suppressing the function of killer cells, antibody-producing and lympho-kine-producing cells. These cells can be identified in the mouse as having the Ly 2, 3$^+$ phenotype (186) and in man as having Fc receptors for IgG (187) and histamine receptors (188a). Their role in pregnancy is being investigated (125).

HISTOCOMPATIBILITY AND PREGNANCY OUTCOME

The perhaps unwarranted model of the placenta as an allograft in the gravida naturally led to the proposition that antigenic differences between gravida and fetus might influence placental size. Billington first observed that F_1 hybrids produced larger placentae than within-strain matings in the mouse (188b), and that there was greater proliferation of allogeneic than syngeneic trophoblast when transplanted to the testis (189). However, better controlled investigations in mice and other species produced no evidence that placental size or outgrowths were affected by major histocompatibility antigen differences (190–194). The initial report that immunization of mice prior to pregnancy increased placental weights (195) was also unconfirmed by subsequent studies (196). McLaren points out in her review of these studies (197) that larger hybrid placentae could result from the genetic process of heterosis, in which greater reproductive vigor parallels a higher degree of heterozygosity.

The question of the role of histoincompatibility and maternal immunologic status in determining fetal and placental weights remains open, however, because of the careful studies of Beer and co-workers (198, 199). They observed that mean placental weights and litter sizes were increased in allogeneic compared to syngeneic matings in hamsters, mice, and rats, and were further increased by presensitization of the gravidas. Allogeneic pregnancies also produced enlargement of maternal para-aortic lymph nodes and spleens as another indicator of immune response. Excision of para-aortic nodes prior to mating in allogeneic pregnancies resulted in smaller fetal-placental units.

A few studies found decreased litter size from embryonic mortalities subsequent to maternal preimmunization to paternal antigens (196, 200). This result might be explained by the reduction in the maternal decidual reaction produced in mice by histoincompatible matings (201) or maternal immunization (202). The reduced decidual reaction was associated with smaller fetuses, but not placentae, in those studies.

There is little evidence of immunologic influences on fetal growth or placental size in human pregnancy, although large-scale systematic studies are yet to be performed. ABO incompatibility has not been confirmed as a determinant of placental growth (197). Maternal production of anti-IILA antibodies is not associated with adverse pregnancy outcome, except for an unconfirmed association of fetal congenital anomalies with maternal leukocytotoxic antibodies (203). Heightened maternal-fetal MLR was supposedly associated with larger placentae in one preliminary study (172). Since typing of cells and sera for minor histocompatibility loci is now possible, our knowledge of the immunogenetics of human reproduction should advance in the next few years.

Preeclampsia is a syndrome of acute hypertension and glomerular damage primarily arising in the latter half of first pregnancies. Since the cause(s) remains unknown, many have sought evidence (so far unsuccessfully) that some pathologic features of the syndrome are immunologically mediated.

These studies were recently reviewed (204). A greater number of histocompatible pairings among women with preeclampsia was found (205), but not confirmed elsewhere (206). In a preliminary study, Bodmer found that a surprising percentage of subjects with severe preeclampsia were homozygous at both HLA loci (207). The implications of this remain unknown.

FETAL IMMUNOLOGIC RESPONSES TO MATERNAL ANTIGEN

Despite the report in 1904 (208) of the ability of a fetal goat to produce antibodies to heterologous blood injected in utero, the fetus was considered to be immunologically incompetent until, in the early 1950s, Australian workers demonstrated that a fetal lamb could reject a skin allograft in utero (209). Recent work in the mouse, lamb, and primate has done much to quantify what the nineteenth century pathologists described in congenital infections of the newborn.

Competence of immune responses arises early in development, despite the small numbers of immunocompetent cells; this raises the possibility of multipotentiality of the cells. Immunocompetence develops in a controlled manner with humoral responses to certain antigens developing in a stepwise fashion. The maturation of immunologic competence occurs prior to maturation of lymph nodes, spleen, or gut-associated nodes. This presumably arises in the lymphoid cells of the fetal liver, the mammalian equivalent of the bursa of Fabricius of birds (210). The initial fetal immune responses are mature in quantity and quality of cellular responses and immunoglobulin titers with class sequences IgM, IgG_1 and IgG_2 (211).

A recent report suggests that one function of the thymus in the developing embryo may be its ability to alter bone-marrow–derived lymphocytes in such a way that on leaving the thymus, the lymphocytes will recognize their own "self" antigens (212). Interestingly, the thymus of mouse embryos will reconstitute the immune responses of their thymectomized mother following pregnancy (213).

The inability of neonates to respond to some antigens when challenged early appears to be the result of suppression by passively acquired maternal IgG rather than a defect in the neonatal immune system (214, 215).

SUMMARY

It is clear from the foregoing that no one simple mechanism can possibly explain the success of the fetus as an allograft. In fact, it would be surprising if there were just one, considering the importance of reproduction for the propagation and survival of the species. There appear to be an array of mechanisms that probably contribute to this process. Some may be specific in nature, while others are nonspecific.

The maternal immune system is challenged with paternal antigens through exposure to trophoblast tissue and fetal cells crossing the placenta into the maternal circulation. The dose of antigen, the manner of presentation (cellular, subcellular, or soluble), and the nature of the antigen all determine the type of response that will be elicited. It is also clear that complex maternal immunologic responses, including antibodies to red cell antigens, HLA-A, B, and C series and HLA-D antigens, and cell-mediated responses such as proliferation, lymphokines, cytotoxicity, and possibly suppressor cells, are generated to a variety of paternal antigenic determinants. The fact that some of these reactions are detected in vitro in the absence of maternal serum, but not in its presence, suggests that the local milieu is important in influencing their expression in vivo. For example, such factors as hormones (cortisol, progesterone, estrogen), pregnancy-associated glycoproteins (α_2-macroglobulin, β_1-glycoprotein), and AFP, which have immunosuppressive properties, may all serve to nonspecifically inhibit and decrease the general tone of maternal immunologic responses, particularly at the placental interface where many of these are present in high concentrations. However, these nonspecific factors may not be sufficient to prevent presensitized effector lymphocytes from continuing an ongoing rejection process, as is often the case in the chronic rejection of an allograft. For this purpose specific enhancing antibodies would play an important role.

There may be a subtle balance created on the trophoblast cell surface between specific antibodies and trophoblast or embryonic alloantigens resulting in a limited expression of antigens capable of inducing rejection reactions. This could favor the production of blocking antibodies and/or T suppressor cells as opposed to cytotoxic antibody and killer cells. In fact, low levels of antigen density on cell surface favor a blocking effect by IgG rather than cytotoxicity (216).

Blocking or enhancing antibodies might exert their effect on maternal immunologic responses in several ways. They could block the afferent limb by combining with antigen and preventing sensitization or increasing the level of sensitivity. An example of the latter would be the coating of fetal cells that enter the maternal circulation. Enhancing antibodies could work directly on the effector cells to suppress their function. The antibody itself, or more likely, antigen-antibody complexes, may be important in this regard. It is known that antigen-antibody complexes can suppress effector lymphocytes in tumor-bearing individuals (217), and have been detected in the circulation of pregnant mice and guinea pigs (218). The effector limb of the maternal response could also be regulated by enhancing antibodies.

Adsorption of the antibodies to trophoblast tissue could render it less susceptible to immunologic attack. Furthermore, paternal antigens could be "covered" or shed into the circulation, thus preventing the recognition of the tissue as foreign. Therefore, despite the presence of sensitized maternal cells, no reaction would ensue because they would not be triggered.

While the role of blocking antibodies is strongly suggested as a mechanism of fetal survival, formal proof is still lacking. There is an association between the presence of these antibodies in normal multigravid women and their absence in women who chronically abort. However, their presence in primagravid women is not consistent. Therefore, if they do play an important role one must explain a successful first pregnancy in their absence. As suggested previously, it is possible that the antibodies are fixed in the placenta but are not present in high enough titer to be detected systemically. In fact, IgG with blocking activity has been eluted from placentae. Under other circumstances the administration of these anti-Ia-like antibodies in vivo has also been shown to enhance allograft survival. Taken together, the data strongly implicate these antibodies as one mechanism of survival of the fetus. It would be of considerable interest to determine whether IgG obtained from normal multigravid women would provide protection to the fetus of women who chronically abort. However, further characterization of these antibodies must occur before such studies can be undertaken.

Literature Cited

1. Medawar, P. B. 1954. Some immunological and endocrinological problems raised by the evolution of viviparity in vertebrates. *Symp. Soc. Exp. Biol.* 7: 320–28
2. Jones, W. R. 1976. Immunological aspects of infertility. In *Immunology of Human Reproduction,* ed. J. S. Scott, W. R. Jones, pp. 375–413. London: Academic
3. Fellous, M., Daussett, J. 1970. Probable haploid expression of HLA antigens on human spermatozoa. *Nature* 225: 191–93
4. Erickson, R. P. 1977. Differentiation and other alloantigens of spermatozoa. In *Immunology of Gametes,* ed. M. Edidin, M. H. Johnson, pp. 85–107. London: Cambridge Univ. Press
5. Goldberg, E. 1974. Effects of immunization with LHH-X on fertility. In *Immunology Approaches to Fertility Control,* ed. E. Diezfalusy, pp. 202–22. Stockholm: Karolinska Institute
6. Cohen, J., Werrett, D. J. 1975. Antibodies and sperm survival in the female tract of the mouse and rabbit. *J. Reprod. Fertil.* 42:301–10
7. Cohen, J., McNaughton, D. C. 1974. Spermatozoa: the probable selection of a small population by the genital tract of the female rabbit. *J. Reprod. Fertil.* 39:297–310
8. Overstreet, J. W., Katz, D. F. 1977. In *Development in Mammals,* ed. M. H. Johnson, pp. 31–66. Amsterdam: North-Holland
9. Beer, A. E., Billingham, R. E. 1974. Host responses to intra-uterine tissue, cellular and fetal allografts. *J. Reprod. Fertil.* 21:59–88
10. Vacquier, V. D. 1977. Hooks and eyes of sperm and eggs. *Sci. News* 112:356
11. Yanagimachi, R. 1977. Specificity of sperm-egg interaction. See Ref. 4, pp. 255–89
12. Kirby, D. R. S. 1969. On the immunologic function of the zona pellucida. *Fertil. Steril.* 20:933–37
13. Bernard, O., Ripoche, M. A., Bennett, D. 1977. Distribution of maternal immunoglobulins in the mouse uterus and embryo in the days after implantation. *J. Exp. Med.* 145:58–75
14. Sellens, M. H., Jenkinson, E. J. 1975. Permeability of the mouse zona pel-

lucida to immunoglobulin. *J. Reprod. Fertil.* 42:153–57

15. Kirby, D. R. S. 1968. The immunological consequences of extra-uterine development of allogeneic mouse blastocysts. *Transplantation* 6:1005–9

16. Searle, R. F., Johnson, M. H., Billington, W. D. 1974. Investigation of H-2 and non-H-2 antigens on the mouse blastocyst. *Transplantation* 18:136–41

17. Billington, W. D. 1976. The immunobiology of trophoblast. See Ref. 2, pp. 81–102

18. Fauve, R. M., Hevim, B., Jacob, H. 1974. Anti-inflammatory effects of murine malignant cells. *Proc. Natl. Acad. Sci. USA* 71:4052–56

19. Heyner, S. 1973. Detection of H-2 antigens on cells of the early mouse embryo. *Transplantation* 16:675–78

20. Carter, J. 1976. The effect of progesterone, estradiol, and hCG on cell-mediated immunity in pregnant mice. *J. Reprod. Fertil.* 46:211–16

21. Billington, W. D., Jenkinson, J., Searle, R. F., Sellens, M. H. 1977. Alloantigen expression during early embryogenesis and placental ontogeny in the mouse: immunoperoxidase and mixed hemoadsorption studies. *Transplant. Proc.* 9:1371–77

22. Searle, R. F., Sellens, M. H., Elson, J., Jenkinson, E. J., Billington, W. D. 1976. Detection of alloantigens during preimplantation development and early trophoblast differentiation in the mouse by immunoperoxidase labelling. *J. Exp. Med.* 143:348–59

23. Webb, C. G., Gall, W. E., Edelman, G. M. 1977. Synthesis and distribution of H-2 antigens in pre-implantation mouse embryos. *J. Exp. Med.* 146:923–32

24. Hakansson, S., Heyner, S., Sundqvist, K. G., Bergstrom, S. 1975. The presence of paternal H-2 antigens on hybrid mouse blastocysts during experimental delay of implantation and the disappearance of their antigens after onset of implantation. *Int. J. Fertil.* 20:137–40

25. Ledford, B. E., Rankin, J. E., Froble, L., Serve, M. J., Markwald, R. R., Baggett, B. 1978. The decidual cell reaction in the mouse uterus: DNA synthesis and autoradiographic analysis of responsive cells. *Biol. Reprod.* 18:506–9

26. Ansell, J. D., Barlow, P. W., McLaren, A. 1974. Binucleate and polyploid cells in the decidua of the mouse. *J. Embryol. Exp. Morphol.* 31:223–27

27. Gardner, R. L. 1975. Origins and properties of trophoblast. In *Immunobiology of Trophoblast,* ed. R. G. Edwards, C.

W. S. Howe, M. H. Johnson, pp. 43–61. Cambridge Univ. Press

28. Chapman, V. M., Ansell, J. D., McLaren, A. 1972. Trophoblast giant cell differentiation in the mouse: expression of glucose phosphate isomerase (GP1-1) electrophoretic variants in transferred and chimeric embryos. *Dev. Biol.* 29:48–54

29. Hill, J. P. 1900. On the fetal membranes, placentation and parturition of the Native cat. *Anat. Anz.* 18:364–73

30. Hill, J. P. 1897. The placentation of Perameles (Contributions to the embryology of the Marsupialia I). *Q. J. Microsp. Sci.* 40:385–446

31. Hill, J. P. 1900. Contributions to the embryology of the Marsupialia II. On a further stage in the placentation of Perameles. *Q. J. Microsp. Sci.* 43:1–23

32. Park, W. W. 1968. Fetal maternal cellular interactions. *J. Reprod. Fertil.* 3:37–39

33. Enders, A. C. 1976. Cytology of human early implantation. *Res. Reprod.* 8:1

34. Padykula, H. A., Taylor, J. M. 1977. In *Reproduction and Evolution,* Proc. Int. Symp. Comp. Biol. Reprod., 4th, eds. J. H. Calaby, C. H. Tyndale-Biscoe, pp. 303–24. Australian Acad. Sci.

35. Larsen, J. F. 1961. Electron microscopy of the implantation site in the rabbit. *Am. J. Anat.* 109:319–25

36. Enders, A. C., Schlafke, S. 1971. Penetration of the uterine epethelium during implantation in the rabbit. *Am. J. Anat.* 132:219–40

37. McLennan, J. G. 1974. Ultrastructural studies of early nidation in pregnancy and pseudopregnancy. *Am. J. Obstet. Gynecol.* 120:319–34

38. Tekelioglu-Uysal, M., Edwards, R. G., Kisnisci, H. A. 1975. Ultrastructural relationships between decidua, trophoblast and lymphocytes at the beginning of human pregnancy. *J. Reprod. Fertil.* 42:431–38

39. Galassi, L. 1967. Reutilization of maternal nuclear material by embryonic trophoblastic cells in the rat for the synthesis of DNA. *J. Histochem. Cytochem.* 15:573–79

40. Ledoux, L., Charles, P. 1967. Uptake of exogenous DNA by mouse embryos. *Exp. Cell Res.* 45:498–501

41. Kaye, M. D. 1977. An autoradiographic study of the implantation of transferred mouse blastocysts. *Aust. J. Biol. Sci.* 30:577–82

42. Harris, H., Sidebottom, E., Grace, D. M., Bramwell, M. E. 1969. The expression of genetic information, a study

with hybrid animal cells. *J. Cell Sci.*
4:499–525
43. Croce, C. M., Kaprowski, H. 1978. The genetics of human cancer. *Sci. Am.* 238:117
44. Gearhart, J. D., Mintz, B. 1972. Glucose phosphate isomerase subunit-reassociation tests for maternal-fetal and fetal-fetal cell fusion in the mouse placenta. *Dev. Biol.* 29:55
45. Koren, Z. 1968. Antigenicity of mouse placental tissue. *Am. J. Obstet. Gynecol.* 102:340–46
46. Beer, A. E., Billingham, R. E., Yang, S. L. 1972. Further evidence concerning the autoantigenic status of the trophoblast. *J. Exp. Med.* 135:1177–84
47. Youtananukorn, V., Matangkasombut, P., Osathanondh, V. 1974. Onset of human maternal cell-mediated immune reaction to placental antigens during the first pregnancy. *Clin. Exp. Immunol.* 16:593–98
48. Goodfellow, P. N., Barnstable, C. J., Bodmer, W. F., Snary, D., Crumpton, M. J. 1976. Expression of HLA system antigens on placenta. *Transplantation* 22:595–603
49. Kirby, D. R. S., Billington, W. D., James, D. A. 1966. Transplantation of eggs to the kidney and uterus of immunized mice. *Transplantation* 4:713–18
50. Simmons, R. L., Russell, P. S. 1962. The antigenicity of mouse trophoblast. *Ann. NY Acad. Sci.* 99:717–32
51. Beer, A. E., Head, J. R., Smith, W. G., Billingham, R. E. 1976. Some immunoregulatory aspects of pregnancy in rats. *Transplant. Proc.* 8:267–73
52. Bradbury, S., Billington, W. D., Kirby, D. R. S., Williams, F. A. 1969. Surface mucin of human trophoblast. *Am. J. Obstet. Gynecol.* 104:416–18
53. Currie, G. A., Van Doorninck, W., Bagshawe, K. O. 1968. Effect of neuraminidase on the immunogenicity of early mouse trophoblast. *Nature* 219:191
54. Simmons, R. L., Lipschultz, M. L., Rios, A., Ray, P. K. 1971. Failure of neuraminidase to unmask histocompatibility antigens on trophoblast. *Nature* 231:111–12
55. Loke, Y. W., Josey, V. C., Borland, R. 1971. HLA antigens on human trophoblast cells. *Nature* 232:403
56. Douthwaite, R. M., Uhrbach, G. I. 1971. In vitro antigenicity of trophoblast. *Am. J. Obstet. Gynecol.* 109:1023–28
57. Taylor, P. V., Hancock, K. W. 1975. Antigenicity of trophoblast and possible

antigen-masking effect during pregnancy. *Immunology* 28:973–82
58. Jenkinson, E. J., Billington, W. D. 1974. Differential susceptibility of mouse trophoblast and embryonic tissue to immune cell lysis. *Transplantation* 18:286–88
59. Johnson, P. M., Faulk, W. P. 1978. Immunological studies of human placentae: identification and distribution of proteins in immature chorionic villi. *Immunology* 34:1027–35
60. Fox, H. 1968. Fibrinoid necrosis of placental villi. *J. Obstet. Gynaecol. Br. Commonw.* 75:448–52
61. McCormick, J. N., Faulk, W. P., Fox, H., Fudenberg, H. H. 1971. Immunohistological and elution studies of the human placenta. *J. Exp. Med.* 133:1–12
62. Faulk, W. P., Jeannet, M., Creighton, W. D., Carbonara, A., Hay, F. 1974. Immunological studies of the human placenta. *J. Clin. Invest.* 54:1011–19
63. Faulk, W. P., Johnson, P. N. 1977. Immunological studies of human placentae: identification and distribution of proteins in mature chorionic villi. *Clin. Exp. Immunol.* 27:365–75
64. Faulk, W. P., Sanderson, A., Temple, A. 1977. Distribution of MHC antigens in human placental chorionic villi. *Transplant. Proc.* 9:1379–84
65. Billingham, R. E. 1978. From transplantation biology to reproductive immunobiology. *Obstet. Gynecol. Ann.* 7:1–14
66. Park, W. V. 1971. In *Choriocarcinoma: A Study of Its Pathology.* London: Heineman
67. Edwards, R. G. 1975. Discussion. See Ref. 27, p. 149
68. Wynn, R. M. 1976. Foetomaternal cellular relations in the human basal plate. An ultrastructural study of the placenta. *Am. J. Obstet. Gynecol.* 97:832
69. Nelson, J. H., Hall, J. E., Manuel-Limson, G. 1967. Effect of pregnancy on the thymolymphatic system. *Am. J. Obstet. Gynecol.* 98:895
70. Nelson, J. H., Lo, T., Hall, J. E., Krown, S., Nelson, J. M., Fox, C. W. 1973. The effect of trophoblast on immune state of women. *Am. J. Obstet. Gynecol.* 117:689–99
71. Head, J. R., Hamilton, M. S., Beer, A. E. 1978. Maternal hamster immune response to alloantigens of fetus. *Fed. Proc.* 37:2054–56
72. Adinolfi, M. 1975. The human placenta as a filter for cells and plasma proteins. See Ref. 27, pp. 193–210

73. Schroder, J., De La Chapelle, A. 1972. Fetal lymphocytes in the maternal blood. *Blood* 39:153
74. Schroder, J. 1975. Are fetal cells in maternal blood mainly B lymphocytes? *Scand. J. Immunol.* 4:279–85
75. Walknowska, J., Conte, F. A., Grumbach, M. M. 1969. Practical and theoretical implications of fetal/maternal lymphocyte transfer. *Lancet* 1:1119–22
76. Brambell, F. W. R. 1966. The transmission of immunity from mother to young and the catabolism of immunoglobulins. *Lancet* 2:1087–93
77. Lanman, J. T., Herod, L. 1965. Homograft immunity in pregnancy. The placental transfer of cytotoxic antibody in rabbits. *J. Exp. Med.* 122:579–86
78. Carlson, G. A., Wegmann, T. G. 1978. Paternal-strain antigen excess in semiallogeneic pregnancy. *Transplant. Proc.* 10:403–7
79. Morisada, M., Yamaguchi, H., Iizuka, R. 1976. Immunobiological function of syncytiotrophoblast: a new theory. *Am. J. Obstet. Gynecol.* 125:3–16
80. Johnson, P. M., Trenchev, P., Faulk, P. W. 1975. Immunological studies of human placentae binding of complexed immunoglobulin by stromal endothelial cells. *Clin. Exp. Immunol.* 22:133–38
81. Jenkinson, E. J., Billington, W. D. 1977. Cell surface properties of early mammalian embryos. In *Concepts in Mammalian Embryogenesis*, ed. M. I. Sherman, pp. 235–66. Cambridge: MIT Press
82. Faulin, M. 1972. Histocompatibility genes in transplantation antigens and pregnancy. In *Transplantation Antigens: Markers of Biological Individuality*, ed. B. D. Kahan, R. A. Rensfeld, pp. 75–114. New York: Academic
83. Queenan, J. T. 1977. *Modern Management of the RH Problem*, p. 9. Hagerstown: Harper & Row. 2nd ed.
84. van Rood, J. J., van Leevmen, A., Eernisse, J. G. 1959. Leukocyte antibodies in sera of pregnant women. *Vox Sang.* 4:427–44
85. Payne, R. 1962. The development and persistence of leukogglutinins in parous women. *Blood* 19:411–24
86. Lawler, S. D., Klonda, P. T., Bagshawe, K. D. 1974. Immunogenicity of molar pregnancies in the HLA system. *Am. J. Obstet. Gynecol.* 120:857–61
87. Ahrons, S. 1971. Leukocyte antibodies: occurrence in primigravidae. *Tissue Antigens* 1:178–83
88. Finn, R. S., Hill, C. A., Gover, A. J., Rolfs, I. G., Gurney, I. J., Denye, V. 1972. Immunological responses in pregnancy and survival of fetal homograft. *Br. Med. J.* 111:150–53
89. Strelkauskas, A. J., Wilson, B. S., Dray, S., Dodsen, M. 1975. Inversion of human T and B cell levels in early pregnancy. *Nature* 258:331–33
90. Gudson, J. P. Jr. 1969. Fetal and maternal immunoglobulin levels during pregnancy. *Am. J. Obstet. Gynecol.* 103:895–900
91. Maroulis, G. B., Buckley, R. H., Younger, J. B. 1971. Serum immunoglobulin concentrations during normal pregnancy. *Am. J. Obstet. Gynecol.* 109:971–76
92. Gudson, J. P. Jr., Prichard, D. 1972. Immunoglobulin D in pregnancy. *Am. J. Obstet. Gynecol.* 112:867–73
93. Valquist, B., Lagecrantz, R., Nordbring, F. 1950. Maternal and fetal titres of antistreptolysin and antistaphtolysin at different stages of gestation. *Lancet* 2:851–53
94. Lichtenstein, M. R. 1942. Tuberculin reaction in tuberculosis during pregnancy. *Am. Rev. Tuberc.* 49:89–92
95. Montgomery, W. P., Young, R. C., Aller, M. D., Horden, K. A. 1968. The tuberculin test in pregnancy. *Am. J. Obstet. Gynecol.* 100:829–31
96. Peer, L. A. 1958. Behavior of skin grafts exchanged between parents and offspring. *Ann. NY Acad. Sci.* 73:854–59
97. Kitzmiller, J. L., Stoneburger, L., Yelenosky, P. F., Lucas, W. E. 1973. Serum complement in normal pregnancy and pre-eclampsia. *Am. J. Obstet. Gynecol.* 117:312–15
98. Mitchell, G. W., Jacobs, A. A., Haddad, V., Paul, B. B., Straus, R. R., Sbama, A. J. 1970. The role of the phagocyte in host-parasite interactions. XXV. Metabolic and bacterial activities of leukocytes from pregnant women. *Am. J. Obstet. Gynecol.* 108:805–13
99. Van der Werf, A. J. M. 1971. Are lymphocytotoxic iso-antibodies induced by early human trophoblast? *Lancet* 1:595–96
100. Doughty, R. W., Gelsthorpe, K. 1974. An initial investigation of lymphocyte antibody activity through pregnancy and in eluates prepared from placental material. *Tissue Antigens* 4:291–98
101. Winchester, R. J., Fu, S. M., Wernet, P., Kunke, H. G., Dupont, B., Jersild, C. 1975. Recognition by pregnancy serums of non-HLA alloantigens selectively expressed on B lymphocytes. *J. Exp. Med.* 141:924–29

102. Davies, D. A. L., Staines, N. A. 1976. A cardinal role for I-region antigens (Ia) in immunological enhancement, and the clinical implications. *Transplant. Rev.* 30:18–39

103. Lewis, J. L., Slang, L., Nagel, B., Oppenheim, J. J., Perry, S. 1966. Lymphocyte transformation in mixed leukocyte cultures in women with normal pregnancy or tumors of placental origin. *Am. J. Obstet. Gynecol.* 96:287–90

104. Cepellini, R., Bonnard, G. D., Coppo, F., Miggiano, V. D., Popisil, M., Curtoni, E. S., Pelligrino, M. 1971. Mixed leukocyte cultures and HLA antigens. I. Reactivity of young fetuses, newborns and mothers at delivery. *Transplant. Proc.* 3:58–63

105. Revillard, J. P., Robert, M., Betuel, H., Latour, M., Bonneau, M., Brochier, J., Trager, J. 1972. Inhibition of the mixed lymphocyte reaction by antibodies. *Transplant. Proc.* 4:173–76

106. Robert, M., Betuel, H., Revillard, J. P. 1973. Inhibition of the mixed lymphocyte reaction by sera from multipara. *Tissue Antigens* 3:39–56

107. Olding, L. B., Oldstone, M. B. A. 1974. Lymphocytes from human newborns abrogate mitosis of their mother's lymphocytes. *Nature* 249:161–63

108. Wolf, R. L., Lomnitzer, R., Rabson, A. R. 1977. An inhibition of lymphocyte proliferation and lymphokine production released by unstimulated fetal monocytes. *Cell. Immunol.* 27:464–68

109. Hellstrom, K. E., Hellstrom, I., Brown, J. 1969. Abrogation of cellular immunity to antigenically foreign mouse embryonic cells by a serum factor. *Nature* 224:914–15

110. Youtananukorn, V., Matangkasombu, P. 1972. Human maternal cell mediated immune reaction to placental antigens. *Clin. Exp. Immunol.* 11:549–56

111. Rocklin, R. E., Zuckerman, J. E., Alpert, E., David, J. R. 1973. Effect of multiparity on human maternal hypersensitivity to fetal antigen. *Nature* 241:130–32

112. Rocklin, R. E., Kitzmiller, J. L., Carpenter, C. B., Garovoy, M. R., David, J. R. 1976. Maternal-fetal relation: absence of an immunologic blocking factor from the serum of women with chronic abortions. *N. Engl. J. Med.* 295:1209–13

113. Tulchinsky, D. 1973. Placental secretion of unconjugated estrone, estradiol, and estriol into the maternal and the fetal circulation. *J. Clin. Endocrinol. Metab.* 36:1079–87

114. Krohn, P. L. 1954. The effect of steroid hormones on the survival of skin homografts in the rabbit. *J. Endocrinol.* 11:78–82

115. Hulka, J. F., Mohr, K. 1967. Interference of cortisone-induced homograft survival by progestins. *Am. J. Obstet. Gynecol.* 97:407–10

116. Simmons, R. L., Price, A. L., Ozerkis, A. J. 1968. The immunologic problems of pregnancy. V. The effect of estrogen and progesterone on allograft survival. *Am. J. Obstet. Gynecol.* 100:908–11

117. Waltman, S. R., Burde, R. M., Barrios, J. 1971. Prevention of corneal homograft rejection by estrogens. *Transplantation* 11:194–96

118. Thompson, J. S., Crawford, M. K., Reilly, R. W., Severson, C. D. 1967. The effect of estrogenic hormones on immune responses in normal and irradiated mice. *J. Immunol.* 98:331–35

119. Weinstein, Y., Lindner, H. R., Eckstein, B. 1977. Thymus metabolizes progesterone—possibly enzymatic marker for T lymphocytes. *Nature* 266:632–33

120a. Tulchinsky, D., Okada, D. M. 1975. Hormones in human pregnancy. IV. Plasma progesterone. *Am. J. Obstet. Gynecol.* 121:293–99

120b. Ferre, F., Janssens, Y., Tanguy, G., Breuiller, M., DePariente, D., Cedard, L. 1978. Steroid concentrations in human myometrial and placental tissues at week 39 of pregnancy. *Am. J. Obstet. Gynecol.* 131:500–2

121. Hulka, J. F., Mohr, K., Liberman, M. W. 1965. Effect of synthetic progestational agents on allograft rejections and circulating antibody production. *Endocrinology* 77:897–901

122. Munroe, J. S. 1971. Progesteroids as immunosuppressive agents. *J. Reticuloendothel. Soc.* 9:361–75

123. Pettirossi, H. A., Wechter, W. J., Kountz, S. L. 1976. Prolongation of rat heart allografts survival by a synthetic progestagen (melengestrol acetate and ara-cytidine acylates). *Transplantation* 21:408–11

124. Siiteri, P. K., Febres, F., Clemens, L. E. 1977. Progesterone in maintenance of pregnancy: is progesterone nature's immunosuppressant? *Ann. NY Acad. Sci.* 286:384–97

125. Beer, A. E., Billingham, R. E. 1979. Maternal immunological recognition mechanisms during pregnancy. In *Maternal Recognition Mechanisms.* CIBA Found. Symp., Vol. 64. In press

126. Ablin, R. M., Bruns, G. R., Guinan, P. 1974. The effect of estrogen on the incorporation of ³H-thymidine by PHA-stimulated human peripheral blood. *J. Immunol.* 113:705–7

127. Mori, T., Kobayashi, H., Nishimoto, H. 1977. Inhibitory effect of progesterone and 20α-hydroxypregn-4-en-3-one on the phytohemagglutinin-induced transformation of human lymphocytes. *Am. J. Obstet. Gynecol.* 127:151–57

128. Wyle, F. A., Kent, J. R. 1977. Immunosuppression by sex steroid hormones. *Clin. Exp. Immunol.* 27:407–15

129. Schiff, R. I., Mercier, D., Buckley, R. H. 1975. Inability of gestational hormones to account for the inhibitory effects of pregnancy plasma on lymphocyte responses in vitro. *Cell. Immunol.* 20:69–80

130. Clemens, L. E., Stites, D., Siiteri, P. K. 1977. In vitro suppression of human lymphocyte transformation by progesterone. *Gynecol. Invest.* 8:20

131. Kitzmiller, J. L., Rocklin, R. E. 1978. Unpublished data

132. Kenny, J. F., Pangburn, P. O., Trail, G. 1976. Effect of estradiol on immune competence: in vivo and in vitro studies. *Infect. Immun.* 13:448–56

133. Peterson, R. E., Imperato-McGinley, J. 1976. Cortisol metabolism in the perinatal period. In *Diabetes and Other Endocrine Disorders During Pregnancy and in the Newborn*, ed. M. I. New, R. H. Fiser, Jr., pp. 141–172. New York: Liss

134. Claman, H. N. 1972. Corticosteroids and lymphoid cells. *N. Engl. J. Med.* 287:388–97

135. Schreiber, A. D. 1977. Clinical immunology of the corticosteroids. *Prog. Clin. Immunol.* 3:103–14

136. Makman, M. H., Dvorkin, B., White, A. 1968. Influence of cortisol on the utilization of precursors of nucleic acids and protein by lymphoid cells in vitro. *J. Biol. Chem.* 243:1485–97

137. Balow, J. E., Rosenthal, A. S. 1973. Glucocorticoid suppression of macrophage migration inhibitory factor. *J. Exp. Med.* 137:1031–41

138a. Weston, W. L., Claman, H. N., Krueger, G. G. 1973. Site of action of cortisol in cellular immunity. *J. Immunol.* 110:880–83

138b. Werthamer, S. F., Govindaraj, S., Amaral, L. 1976. Placenta, transcortin, and localized immune response. *J. Clin. Invest.* 57:1000–8

138c. Han, T. 1975. Human chorionic gonadotropin. Its inhibitory effect on cell mediated immunity in vivo and in vitro. *Immunology* 29:509–15

138d. Kaye, M. D., Jones, W. R., Ing. R. M. Y., Markham, R. 1971. Effect of human chorionic gonadotropin on intrauterine skin allograft survival in rats. *Am. J. Obstet. Gynecol.* 110:640–43

138e. Kaye, M. D., Jones, W. R. 1971. Effect of hCG in vitro lymphocyte transformation. *Am. J. Obstet. Gynecol.* 109:1029–31

139. Contractor, S. F., Davies, H. 1973. Effect of human chorionic somatomammotrophin and hCG on phytohemagglutinin-induced lymphocyte transformation. *Nature* 243:284

140. Adcock, E. W. III, Teasdale, E., August, C. S., Cox, S., Meschia, G., Battaglia, F. C., Naughton, M. A. 1973. Human chorionic gonadotrophin: its possible role in material lymphocyte suppression. *Science* 181:845–47

141. Han, T. 1974. Inhibitory effect of human chorionic gonadotrophin on lymphocyte blastogenic responses: hCG and mitogen, antigen and allogenic human cells. *Clin. Exp. Immunol.* 18:529–35

142a. Jenkins, D. M., Acres, M. G., Peters, J., Riley, J. 1972. Human chorionic gonadotropin and the fetal allograft. *Am. J. Obstet. Gynecol.* 114:13–15

142b. Caldwell, J. L., Stites, D. P., Fudenberg, H. H. 1975. Human chorionic gonadotropin: effects of crude and purified preparations on lymphocyte responses to phytohemagglutinin and allogeneic stimulation. *J. Immunol.* 113:1249

142c. Beck, D., Ginsburg, H., Naot, Y. 1977. Modulating effect of human chorionic gonadotropin on lymphocyte blastogenesis. *Am. J. Obstet. Gynecol.* 129:14–20

143. Morse, J. H., Stearns, G., Arden, J. 1976. The effects of crude and purified human gonadotropin on in vitro stimulated human lymphocyte cultures. *Cell. Immunol.* 25:178–88

144. Pattillo, R. A., Shalaby, M. R., Hussa, R. O., Bahl, O. M. P., Mattingly, R. F. 1976. Effect of crude and purified hCG on lymphocyte blastogenesis. *Obstet. Gynecol.* 47:557–61

145. Loke, Y. W., Pepys, M. B. 1975. Effects of human chorionic gonadotropin preparations on complement in vitro. *Am. J. Obstet. Gynecol.* 121:37

146. Merz, W. E., Schmidt, W., Hilgenfeldt, U., Schackert, K., Lenhard, V. 1976. Isolation of substances from crude preparation of human chorionic gonadotro-

pin (hCG) which strongly inhibit the transformation of lymphocytes. *Z. Immunitaetsforsch.* 152:286–89

147. Alpert, E., Drysdale, J. W., Schur, P. H., Isselbacher, K. J. 1971. Human AFP: purification and physical properties. *Fed. Proc.* 30:246

148. Ruoslahti, E., Terry, W. D. 1976. Alpha-fetoprotein and serum albumin show sequence homology. *Nature* 260:804–5

149. Gitlin, D., Biasucci, A. 1969. Development of IgG, IgA, IgM, βIC, βIa, Cl₁ esterase inhibition, ceruloplasmin, transferin, haptoglobin, fibrinogen, plasminogen, orosomucoid, α2-macroglobulin and pre-albumin in the conceptus. *J. Clin. Invest.* 48:1433–66

150. Murgita, R. A., Tomasi, T. B. 1975. Suppression of the immune response by alpha-fetoprotein. I. Primary and secondary response. *J. Exp. Med.* 141:269–86

151. Murgita, R. A., Tomasi, T. B. 1975. Suppression of the immune response by alpha-fetoprotein. II. MLR and mitogen-induced lymphocyte transformation. *J. Exp. Med.* 141:440–52

152. Sheppard, H. W., Sell, S., Trefts, P., Bahu, R. 1977. Effects of alpha-fetoprotein on murine immune responses. I. Studies on mice. *J. Immunol.* 119:91–97

153. Sell, S., Sheppard, H. W., Poler, M. 1977. Effects of alpha-fetoprotein on murine immune response. II. Studies on rats. *J. Immunol.* 119:98–103

154. Littman, B. H., Alpert, E., Rocklin, R. E. 1977. Effect of purified alpha-fetoprotein on in vitro assays of cell-mediated immunity. *Cell. Immunol.* 30:35–42

155. Murgita, R. A., Goidl, E. A., Kontiainen, S., Wizzell, H. 1977. Alpha-fetoprotein induces suppressor T cells in vitro. *Nature* 267:257–59

156. Alpert, E., Dienstag, J. L., Sepersky, S., Littman, B. H., Rocklin, R. E. 1978. Immunosuppressive characteristics of human AFP: effect on tests of cell-mediated immunity and induction of human suppressor cells. *Immunol. Commun.* 7:163–85

157. von Schoultz, B. 1974. A quantitiative study of the pregnancy zone protein in the sera of pregnant and puerperal women. *Am. J. Obstet. Gynecol.* 119:792–97

158. Stimson, W. H. 1975. Studies on the immunosuppressive properties of a pregnancy-associated alpha-macro-globulin. *Clin. Exp. Immunol.* 25:199–206

159. McConnell, D. J., Loeb, J. N. 1974. Kallikrein inhibitory capacity of α2-macroglobulin subunits. *Proc. Exp. Biol. Med.* 147:891–96

160. Tunstall, A. M., James, K. 1975. The effect of human α-macroglobulin on the restoration of humoral responsiveness in x-irradiated mice. *Clin. Exp. Immunol.* 21:173–80

161. Cooperband, S. R., Bondevik, H., Schmid, K., Mannick, J. A. 1968. Transformation of human lymphocytes: inhibition by homologous alpha globulin. *Science* 159:1243–44

162. Gaugas, J. M. 1974. Glycoproteins in pregnancy serum which interact with concanavalin A and may suppress lymphocyte transformation. *Transplantation* 18:538–41

163. Bohn, H. 1971. Nachweis und charaklerisierung von Schwangerschafts—proteinen in der menschlichen placenta, sowie, ihre quantitative immunologische bestimmung im serum schwangerer frauen. *Arch. Gynaekol.* 210:440–57

164. von Schoultz, B., Stigbrand, T., Tarnvik, A. 1973. Inhibition of PHA-induced lymphocyte stimulation of the pregnancy zone protein. *FEBS Lett.* 38:23–26

165. Kasakura, S. 1971. A factor in maternal plasma during pregnancy which suppresses the reactivity of mixed leukocyte cultures. *J. Immunol.* 107:1296–1301

166. Stimson, W. H., Blackstock, J. C. 1976. Identification of an immunosuppressive factor in pregnancy serum. *Obstet. Gynecol.* 48:305–11

167. Petrucco, O. M., Seamark, R. F., Holmes, K., Forbes, I. J., Sijmons, R. G. 1976. Changes in lymphocyte function during pregnancy. *Br. J. Obstet. Gynecol.* 83:245–50

168. Breyere, E. J., Barrett, M. K. 1960. Tolerance in postpartum female mice induced by strain specific matings. *J. Natl. Cancer Inst.* 24:699–705

169. Breyere, E. J., Barrett, M. K. 1960. Prolonged survival of skin homografts in parous female mice. *J. Natl. Cancer Inst.* 25:1405–10

170. Kaliss, N., Dagg, N. K. 1964. Immune response engendered in mice by multiparity. *Transplantation* 2:416–25

171. Currie, G. A. 1970. The conceptus as an allograft: immunological reactivity of the mother. *Proc. R. Soc. Med.* 63:61–64

172. Jenkins, D. M., Hancock, K. W. 1972. Maternal unresponsiveness to paternal histocompatibility antigens in human pregnancy. *Transplantation* 13:618–19

173. Gatti, R. A., Svedmyr. E. A. J., Wigzell, H. 1974. Characterization of a serum inhibitor of MLC reactions. II. Molecular structure and dissociation of inhibition against responder and stimulator function. *Cell. Immunol.* 11:466–77

174. Gatti, R. A., Svedmyr, E. A. J., Leibold, W., Wigzell, H. 1975. Characterization of a serum inhibitor of MLC reactors. III. Specificity. *Cell. Immunol.* 15:432–51

175. Youtanankorn, V., Matangkasombut, P. 1973. Specific plasma factors blocking human maternal cell-mediated immune reaction to placental antigens. *Nature* 242:110–11

176. Pence, H., Petty, W. M., Rocklin, R. E. 1975. Suppression of maternal responsiveness to paternal antigens by maternal plasma. *J. Immunol.* 114:525–28

177. Revillard, J. P., Brochier, J., Robert, M., Bonneau, M., Traeger, J. 1976. Immunologic properties of placental eluates. *Transplant. Proc.* 8:275–79

178. Sengar, D. P. S., Opelz, G., Terrasaki, P. T. 1973. Suppression of mixed leukocyte response by plasma from hemodialysis patients. *Transplant. Proc.* 5:641–47

179. Riggio, R. R., Saal, S. D., Stengel, K. H., Rubin, A. L. 1976. Retroplacental serum factors and passive enhancement. *Transplant. Proc.* 8:281–85

180. Riggio, R. R., Saal, S. D., Cheigh, J. S., Kim, J. J., Stubenbord, W. 1., Stenzel, K. H., Rubin, A. L. 1978. Improved survival rates in presensitized recipients of kidney transplants by immunosuppression with maternal source gammaglobulin. *Lancet* 1:233–35

181. Voisin, G. A., Chaouat, G. 1974. Demonstration, nature and properties of maternal antibodies fixed on placenta and directed against paternal antigens. *J. Reprod. Fertil.* 21:89–103

182. Bonneau, M., Latour, M., Revillard, J. P., Robert, M., Traeger, J. 1973. Blocking antibodies eluted from human placenta. *Transplant. Proc.* 5:589–92

183. Soulillou, J. P., Carpenter, C. B., D'Apice, A. J. F., Strom, T. B. 1976. The role of non-classical Fc-receptor associated Ag-B antigens (Ia) in rat allograft enhancement. *J. Exp. Med.* 143:405–21

184. Chess, L., Evans, R., Humphreys, R. E., Strominger, J. L., Schlossman, S. F. 1976. Inhibition of antibody-dependent cellular cytotoxicity and Ig synthesis by antiserum prepared against a human B cell Ia-like molecule. *J. Exp. Med.* 144:113–22

185. Waldman, T. A., Broder, S. 1978. Suppressor cells in the regulation of the immune response. *Prog. Clin. Immunol.* 3:155–99

186. Cantor, H., Shen, F. W., Boyse, E. A. 1976. Separation of helper T cells from suppressor T cells expressing different Ly components. *J. Exp. Med.* 143:1391–1403

187. Moretta, L., Ferrarini, M., Cooper, M. D. 1978. Characterization of human T cell subpopulations as defined by specific receptors for immunoglobulins. *Contemp. Top. Immunobiol.* In press

188a. Rocklin, R. E., Rosenthal, A. S. 1977. Evidence that human leukocyte inhibitory factor (LIF) is an esterase. *J. Immunol.* 119:249–52

188b. Billington, W. D. 1964. Influence of immunological dissimilarity of mother and fetus on size of placenta in mice. *Nature* 202:317–18

189. Billington, W. D. 1965. The invasiveness of transplanted mouse trophoblast and the influence of immunological factors. *J. Reprod. Fertil.* 10:343–52

190. Boshier, D. P., Moriarty, K. M. 1970. Some effects on the conceptus of prior immunological sensitization of ewes to the sire. *J. Reprod. Fertil.* 21:495–500

191. Finkel, S. I., Lilly, F. 1971. Influence of histocompatibility between mother and fetus on placental size in mice. *Nature* 234:102–3

192. Hetherington, C. M. 1973. The absence of any effect of maternal-fetal incompatibility at the H-2 and H-3 loci on pregnancy in the mouse. *J. Reprod. Fertil.* 33:135–39

193. Clarke, A. G. 1969. Factors affecting the growth of trophoblast transplanted to the testis. *J. Reprod. Fertil.* 18:539–41

194. Koren, Z. Abrams, G., Behrman, S. G. 1968. The role of host factors in mouse trophoblastic tissue growth. *Am. J. Obstet. Gynecol.* 100:570–75

195. James, D. A. 1965. Effects of antigenic dissimilarity between mother and fetus on placental size in mice. *Nature* 205:613–14

196. Clarke, A. G. 1971. The effects of maternal pre-immunization on pregnancy in the mouse. *J. Reprod. Fertil.* 24:369–75

197. McLaren, A. 1975. Antigenic disparity—does it affect placental size, implantation, or population genetics? See Ref. 27, pp. 255–76

198. Beer, A. E., Billingham, R. E., Scott, J. R. 1975. Immunogenic aspects of implantation, placentation and fetoplacental growth rates. *Biol. Reprod.* 12: 176–89
199. Beer, A. E., Scott, J. R., Billingham, R. E. 1975. Histoincompatibility in maternal immunological status as determinants of fetal placental weight and litter size in rodents. *J. Exp. Med.* 142: 180–96
200. Breyere, E. J., Springer, W. W. 1969. Evidence of allograft rejection of the conceptus. *Transplant. Proc.* 1:71–75
201. Hetherington, C. M. 1971. The decidual cell reaction, placental weight, fetal weight, and placental morphology in the mouse. *J. Reprod. Fertil.* 25:417–24
202. Clarke, A. G., Hetherington, C. M. 1971. Effects of maternal preimmunization on the decidual cell reaction in mice. *Nature* 230:114–15
203. Terasaki, P. I., Mickey, M. R., Yamazaki, J. N. 1970. Maternal-fetal incompatibility. I. Incidence of HLA antibodies and possible association with congenital anomalies. *Transplantation* 9:538–43
204. Kitzmiller, J. L. 1977. Immunologic approaches to the study of preeclampsia. *Clin. Obstet. Gynecol.* 20:717–35
205. Stevenson, A. C., Davison, B. C., Say, B., Ustuoplu, S., Liya, D., Abul-Einen, M., Toppozada, H. K. 1971. Contribution of fetal/maternal incompatibility to etiology of pre-eclamptic toxemia. *Lancet* 2:1286–89
206. Scott, J. R., Beer, A. E., Stastny, P. 1976. Immunogenetic factors in preeclampsia and eclampsia. Erythrocyte, histocompatibility, and γ-dependent antigens. *J. Am. Med. Assoc.* 235:402–4

207. Bodmer, W. F. 1975. Discussion. See Ref. 27, p. 183.
208. Kreidl, A., Mandl, L. 1904. Uber den me bergang der immonhamolysine non der frucht auf die muher. *Weinklin. Wechscht.* 17:611
209. Schinkel, P. G., Ferguson, K. A. 1953. Skin transplantation in the fetal lamb. *Aust. J. Biol. Sci.* 6:533
210. Owen, J. J. Cooper, M. D., Raft, M. C. 1974. In vitro generation of B lymphocytes in mouse fetal liver, a mammalian "bursa equivalent." *Nature* 249:361–63
211. Silverstein, A. M. 1977. Ontogeny of the immune response: A perspective. In *Development of Host Defenses*, ed. M. D. Cooper, D. Dayton, pp. 1–10. New York: Raven
212. Zinkernagel, R. M., Callahan, G. N. Klein, J., Deunert, G. 1978. Cell surface changes in allogantigen activated T lymphocytes. *Nature* 271:251–53
213. Osoba, D. 1965. Immune reactivity in mice thymectomized soon after birth: normal responses after pregnancy. *Science* 147:298–99
214. Cooper, M. D., Dayton, D. H. eds. 1977. *Development of Host Defenses.* New York: Raven
215. Jones, W. R. 1976. Fetal and neonatal immunology. See Ref. 2, pp. 127–67
216. Linscott, W. D. 1970. Effect of cell surface antigen density on immunological enhancement. *Nature* 228:824–27
217. Bansal, S. C. 1974. Cytotoxicity and blocking factors in neoplasia. In *Progress in Immunology II,* ed. L. Brent, J. Holborow, pp. 394–97, Vol. 3. Amsterdam: North-Holland
218. Tung, K. 1974. Immune complexes in the renal glomerulus during normal pregnancy. *J. Immunol.* 112:186–200

Ann. Rev. Med. 1978. 29:231–83

IMMUNOTHERAPY ◆7279
FOR MALIGNANT DISEASE

James E. Goodnight, Jr., M.D., Ph.D. and Donald L. Morton, M.D.
Division of Oncology, Department of Surgery, University of California School of
Medicine, Los Angeles, California 90024; and the Department of Surgical Services,
Veterans Administration Hospital, Sepulveda, California 91343.

INTRODUCTION

Immunotherapy has been tested widely for the treatment of malignant disease
because of its potential for a highly selective systemic attack on tumor cells.
Unlike conventional treatment modalities that act directly on the cancer cell,
immunotherapy works by activating host defenses to control and destroy tumor
growth. Such an approach seems feasible, since host resistance appears to be
involved in survival from cancer. A dramatic example of this phenomenon is the
well-documented occurrence of spontaneous regression of human tumors (1).
Moreover, it has been found that tumors possess unique antigens not present in
normal tissues, and that these antigens elicit measurable immune responses in
the tumor host (2–7). Various means for stimulating these responses exist, and
these maneuvers clearly confer protection against tumor growth in experimental
animals. Above all, investigators are reporting that stimulation of host defenses
is beneficial for selected cancer patients. The hundreds of clinical trials recorded
in the International Registry of Tumor Immunology (8) are a measure of the
interest in immunotherapy for malignant disease.

In the early 1900s, success with immunization against infectious disease, plus
the observation that tumor transplants in animals were rejected, led investigators to think that patients might be immunized against cancer. However, they
failed to recognize that in outbred populations tumor transplants are rejected on
the basis of normal histocompatibility antigens. Thus, resistance specific for
tumors simply could not be demonstrated at that time. Nevertheless, attempts at
immunotherapy for cancer were reported (9). After Coley observed prolonged
regression of a neck sarcoma in a patient suffering from erysipelas, he tried
injecting mixtures of live and heat-killed bacteria into other patients with various
tumors (9). He reported some success with this treatment and the agents became
known as Coley's toxins. The interest declined, however, when these experiments could not be reproduced.

0066-4219/78/0401-0231$01.00
231

Solid experimental evidence for host immunity to tumors appeared in the 1950s. In careful transplantation experiments with methylcholanthrene (MCA)–induced sarcomas in inbred mice, specific, tumor-associated antigens were identified (2, 3). Members of the same inbred strain are so nearly genetically identical that they normally do not reject each others' tissues. Foley (2) showed that when an MCA sarcoma was transplanted to a recipient syngeneic to the donor, allowed to grow and then excised completely, the recipient became resistant to further challenges with that tumor. In the same system, Prehn & Main (3) demonstrated that skin grafts from the tumor donor would neither induce tumor resistance in the recipient nor be rejected, even if the recipient had been immunized to the tumor. Subsequently, Klein (10) showed that these MCA sarcomas were immunogenic in their host of origin. These findings established the existence of tumor-specific transplantation antigens and were critical to the development of tumor immunology.

Interest in immunotherapy for malignant disease was rekindled in the late 1960s when three reports of successful clinical immunotherapy appeared. In a series of patients in remission from acute lymphoblastic leukemia, Mathé and co-workers (11) found that duration of remission and survival could be markedly extended by immunostimulation with Bacillus Calmette-Guerin (BCG) inoculation and/or vaccination with allogeneic leukemia cells. Morton and his colleagues (12) observed that 90% of cutaneous metastases of malignant melanoma would regress following intralesional injection with BCG. Moreover, in 17% of these patients, uninjected nodules regressed concomitantly with injected lesions. A third report by Klein (13) indicated that the majority of superficial basal cell and squamous cell carcinomas of the skin would resolve if delayed cutaneous hypersensitivity was induced in the area by repeated applications of various chemicals.

This successful use of immunotherapy for malignant disease generated a wave of enthusiasm. For example, in the 10 year period from 1965 to 1975, the volume of publications per year on tumor immunology and immunotherapy increased from less than 200 to 18,000 papers (Figure 1). It seemed that a new era of cancer treatment had begun. However, this enthusiasm ignored the reality of experimental tumor systems, which had shown that the potency of immunotherapy was limited. Animals specifically sensitized to resist the growth of a particular tumor are still susceptible if the tumor challenge is large enough (i.e. greater than 10^7 cells). It has likewise become apparent in clinical studies that immunotherapy used alone is largely ineffective in achieving regression of established visceral malignancies. The number of tumor cells in humans that can be controlled by host defense mechanisms is approximately 10^8 (14). Measurable tumors contain many more cells than this. Recognition of this limitation has tempered enthusiasm for immunotherapy, and a more realistic attitude now prevails.

The mechanisms underlying immunotherapy are complex and far from understood. Nevertheless, specific tumor immunity is a legitimate biological phenomenon. In the transplantation experiments cited, specific, tumor-associated antigens have been identified (2, 3). Both serological and cell-mediated immune responses to these antigens can be demonstrated (4), and animals can be specifically sensitized to resist the growth of a particular tumor.

In addition, there are nonspecific mechanisms of host resistance to cancer. Macrophages activated by endotoxin or other stimuli can selectively identify and destroy neoplastic cells based on some means of recognition other than antigenic differences (15). Macrophages also can be specifically armed by T-lymphocytes to attack tumor cells (16). A combined specific effector mechanism exists whereby antitumor antibody provides the specificity, and a cytotoxic effector cell with a receptor for the immunoglobulin molecule attaches and completes the destruction of the tumor cell (17). Some of these investigations extend to human tumor-host interactions. However, much remains to be learned, particularly to what extent these mechanisms explain the observed

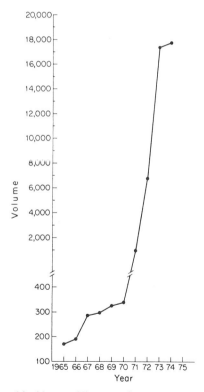

Figure 1.   The increased incidence of literature from 1965 to 1975. Note the sharp rise from a little over 300 to 1000 from 1970–71 (MEDLARS, National Library of Medicine).

responses to immunotherapy. This subject is beyond the scope of this review, but it has been thoroughly discussed in several excellent reviews (18–22).

Despite the limited potency of immunotherapy and the lack of knowledge of its basic mechanisms, there is compelling evidence from clinical trials to indicate that immunotherapy benefits selected cancer patients. Enough clinical experience with immunotherapy has been acquired to allow for preliminary conclusions. The purpose of this review is to put immunotherapy for malignant disease in perspective based on a careful examination of the majority of published clinical trials.

ELEMENTS OF IMMUNOTHERAPY

Immunotherapy may be categorized as nonspecific, active-specific, or passive. For nonspecific immunotherapy, agents such as BCG or *Corynebacterium parvum,* both potent stimulators of host resistance, are used to trigger antitumor responses. Active-specific immunotherapy elicits antitumor immune responses by vaccination with tumor cells or portions thereof. These vaccines may be modified in various ways to enhance their immunogenicity. For passive or adoptive immunotherapy, immune effectors from a specifically sensitized host are transferred to the cancer patient in an effort to provide specific antitumor reactivity.

Nonspecific Immune Therapy

BCG   BCG is an attentuated, live organism developed from a virulent strain of *Mycobacterium bovis* by Calmette and Guerin at the turn of the century (23). It has been used successfully throughout the world to immunize populations against tuberculosis. In addition, it is a potent stimulator of humoral and cellular immune responses (24). Most pertinent to this discussion is the fact that BCG inoculation of animals can induce resistance to tumor transplants and regression of some established tumors. This experimental work was recently reviewed by Bast and colleagues (18). Several factors are essential for successful BCG therapy in animal tumor models: (*a*) Tumor burden must be low. (*b*) The host must be immunocompetent. (*c*) Adequate amounts of BCG must be given. (*d*) BCG must be in close association with the tumor cells. (*e*) The tumor itself must be immunogenic. Similar observations have been made when BCG is used for human neoplasia.

The mechanisms underlying tumor regression following BCG injection are not completely understood. BCG does not appear to have a direct antitumor effect since tumor regression occurs only if the host raises an inflammatory response to the BCG. The most striking responses are seen following intralesional injection, which suggests that tumor destruction is a bystander effect of the hypersensitivity response to the BCG (12). However, Klein & Klein (25) performed an elegant experiment showing that immune responses are exquisitely specific for destruction of experimental tumors. They injected a mixture of tumor cells into an animal sensitized to only one of the tumor lines in the mixture. An inflammatory response resulted at the site of injection, and the line to which the animal was resistant was rejected. However, the other tumor line survived and grew out in the midst of the reaction.

There is no clear evidence that antibodies or specifically sensitized cells are responsible for tumor destruction following BCG injection, but specific antitumor responses do occur in this setting. It has been shown that the titer of antimelanoma antibody increases in melanoma patients treated with BCG (12). In a guinea pig hepatoma model, Hanna (26) also showed that antitumor antibody increased after BCG injection. Moreover, once the tumor regressed, the animal resisted late tumor challenges in sites distant from the original tumor, which indicates a systemic effect.

Side effects of BCG treatment are few when it is given by the Tine technique or with the Heaf gun, and usually consist of local inflammation, low-grade fever, malaise, and mild ulceration. With intralesional injection, more serious toxicities such as anaphylaxis, granulomatous hepatitis, systemic BCG infection, high fever and chills, or abscesses can occasionally occur (27). For these reasons, BCG should be administered only by personnel experienced in its use. BCG has been used widely in cancer therapy for local injection of accessible tumors, as adjuvant therapy for minimum residual disease, and in combination with chemotherapy for disseminated disease.

CORYNEBACTERIUM PARVUM   C. parvum is a gram-positive anaerobic organism, which, in contrast to BCG, is killed by physical or chemical means when used for immunotherapy. In animals, treatment with C. parvum inhibits the growth of tumor inoculations, and, at least for MCA sarcomas in mice, can cause regression of established tumor (28–30). Given intralesionally, C. parvum induces regression of cutaneous malignancies. C. parvum is maximally effective when injected into the regional lymph node drainage of the tumor (32).

C. parvum is a consistent macrophage stimulator, which may be the basis of its antitumor activity, since it can produce inhibition of tumor growth in animals depleted of T cells (31). Some of its effects depend on the route of administration. Given intravenously, C. parvum suppresses T cells, but given subcutaneously, it stimulates T-cell activity. It is an active potentiator of antibody production in response to a variety of antigens (32).

In man, C. parvum has been tested primarily as an adjuvant to chemotherapy for advanced malignant disease (33). Side effects from C. parvum therapy such as fever, chills, nausea, vomiting, and changes in blood pressure, are seen mainly with intravenous administration (34). Local inflammation results from subcutaneous administration.

LEVAMISOLE   Levamisole, a drug developed and used successfully as an antihelminthic, also acts to restore depressed immune responses. Renoux & Renoux (35) showed that mice treated with levamisole have increased resistance to *Brucella abortus* infection. In man, delayed cutaneous hypersensitivity responses are augmented by the drug (36). In addition, antibody responses to a variety of stimuli such as influenza are potentiated (37). Macrophage activity is increased after levamisole treatment as indicated by enhanced phagocytic activity (38).

Levamisole has been reported to be beneficial for several benign diseases. It helps clear aphthous stomatitis and warts. It gives symptomatic relief in systemic lupus, rheumatoid arthritis, and herpes simplex (32). Results of testing levamisole as an antitumor agent in animals have been inconsistent, although its use as a stimulant of host resistance suggests that it might be useful in treating malignancy. It has been tested in humans as an adjuvant to primary treatment for breast and lung carcinoma and initial results suggest benefit (39, 40). Side effects are low and are limited to mild GI distress and some fatigue, although some cases of agranulocytosis have been reported (41).

Active-Specific Immunotherapy

The primary goal of immunotherapy is to sharpen the specificity and augment the potency of immune responses that eradicate tumor cells. The most direct and specific way of achieving this goal is to stimulate the immune system with tumor antigens, in spite of their weak immunogenicity. The way in which an antigen is presented to the immune system influences the response. Altering the route of sensitization, the antigen dose, or the configuration of tumor antigens can result in a more effective antitumor response.

Alteration of the tumor cell surface may increase the immunogenicity of tumor antigens. The capacity of mouse leukemia cells to stimulate tumor transplantation resistance can be markedly increased by exposing the cells to neuraminidase, an enzyme obtained from *Vibrio cholera* (42). Neuraminidase cleaves sialic acid from cell surface glycoproteins, which may increase antigen exposure. Another method of increasing immunogenicity is to infect tumor cells with virus. The virus particles on the cell membrane may act as helper antigens, which in turn augment stimulation of the immune system (43). Lysates of virus-infected tumor cells have been used clinically to treat several kinds of cancer.

Intradermal injections of viable allogeneic tumor cells or tumor cell extracts are being used clinically to treat malignant melanoma, breast and lung cancer, soft-tissue sarcomas, and acute leukemia (44–47, 42). Animal experiments have shown that intradermal injection is a good route for sensitization. Moreover, since tumors of the same histologic type share common antigens, allogeneic tumor cells effectively stimulate tumor transplantation resistance (48). Because allogeneic cells are rejected on the basis of their normal histocompatibility antigens, the problem of tumor growth at the site of inoculation is eliminated. Clinical trials with viable allogeneic tumor vaccines have confirmed their safety and effectiveness. Immune responses can be augmented by mixing these tumor vaccines with immunostimulants such as complete Freund's adjuvant.

Passive Immunotherapy

Passive immunotherapy involves adoptive transfer of immune cells or antiserum with appropriate tumor specificity to the cancer patient. An alternative, the-oretical approach is the transfer of subcellular fractions of immune cells such as immune RNA or transfer factor to induce specific antitumor reactivity in the patient's own lymphocytes. This approach is logical insofar as the agent trans-ferred has activity against the tumor, and the recipient's immune system will accept and utilize it. However, logistical problems are involved in obtaining an adequate quantity of immunological agents with appropriate specificity and activity.

One precept of tumor immunology has been that of cell-mediated immunity as the primary effector function responsible for tumor destruction. For example, immunocompetent cells can be transferred from an inbred immunized animal to a nonimmunized animal to achieve tumor control. Control can be maintained as long as the cells persist. However, adoptively transferred allogeneic cells are eventually rejected, so that a continuous source of sensitized cells must be found. In humans, such a supply is usually unavailable, although one success has been achieved by transfer of blood from a patient who experienced a complete remission of melanoma (49). Another approach involves matching patients with the same tumor, sensitizing them to each other's tumor with subcutaneous transplants, and then exchanging their leukocytes. Response rates of 15–20% have been reported (50–52). This is at the price of some serious transfusion reactions, since allogeneic cells sensitize the patient to HL-A anti-gens. The use of immunocompetent cells from closely matched siblings is an alternative.

Passive transfer of antitumor antisera can induce tumor regression in some animal models (53). The antibody may be directly cytotoxic, or it may provide the specificity for cellular immune effectors with Fc receptors (17). Serotherapy is problematic though, because human sources of specific antitumor antisera for clinical use are often difficult to find, and heterologous antisera may cause serum sickness or anaphylaxis. Moreover, because antibodies occasionally can en-hance tumor growth, there is some risk to this method. Serotherapy has been tried in patients with Burkitt's lymphoma, malignant melanoma, and renal cell carcinoma on a limited basis, but no systematic, controlled, clinical trial has been reported (53).

Certain informational molecules obtained from sensitized lymphocytes have been shown to confer specific reactivity on unsensitized lymphocytes. The virgin cells become sensitized without exposure to the antigen. One such infor-mational agent is a low-molecular-weight, dialyzable substance known as trans-fer factor. Originally described by Lawrence a few years ago (54), this molecule transfers cell-mediated, but not humoral, responses to an antigen. Transfer factor has been used successfully to treat congenital immunodeficiency diseases such as Wiskott-Aldrich syndrome, ataxia-telangiectasia, and chronic mu-cocutaneous candidiasis. These advances led to limited clinical trials in cancer patients (55–57). A source of transfer factor with appropriate tumor specificity is a problem. Cohabitants of cancer patients have been used, and initial results suggest benefit, although these preliminary reports are largely anecdotal (57).

Mannick & Egdahl (58) showed that specific transplantation immunity could be transferred in rabbits using RNA extracted from sensitized lymphocytes. Pilch and co-workers (59) confirmed these observations, and extended them to antitumor responses. They showed that RNA extracted from lymphocytes of guinea pigs sensitized to a mouse tumor would confer specific antitumor reactivity on untreated mouse spleen cells. To clearly establish activity against specific tumor-associated antigens, they demonstrated the same phenomenon in a strain of inbred rats in which the tumor donor, effector cells, and RNA donor were syngeneic. This excluded any activity against normal histocompatibility antigens.

This demonstration of a xenogeneic immune RNA that would transfer specific reactivity was important for clinical trials, since it meant that appropriately sensitized animals could be used as a source of antihuman tumor-immune RNA. Immune RNA has virtually no toxicity, since lymphocytes cannot be instructed to attack "self"-antigens. Allergic reactions to the RNA are not a problem, since it is of low immunogenicity. Human lymphocytes exposed to immune RNA from sheep sensitized to a human tumor will destroy that tumor in vitro. Controls indicate that the activity is specific for the tumor and dependent upon exposure to the RNA. Initial clinical trials in humans with xenogeneic immune RNA recently were summarized by Ramming and colleagues (60).

CLASSIFICATION OF CLINICAL TRIALS

Although immunotherapy seems to be an important tool in the management of cancer, its full potential is unproven except for intralesional or topical treatment of accessible tumors. Its efficacy can be established only if published studies present an accurate and undistorted view. Results from clinical trials of immunotherapy vary considerably in their yield of information and reliability. The structure of clinical trials ranges from uncontrolled series to those in which patients are randomly assigned to treatment and control groups. Choice of controls, whether randomized, selected, historical, etc., affects the credibility of the data. Moreover, the conduct of clinical trials varies markedly in the number and selection of patients, the accuracy of diagnoses and staging, the period of follow-up, and the statistical treatment of results. The significance of a clinical trial depends on the clarity with which it excludes alternative explanations for its findings, which is in turn dependent upon the variables mentioned.

In this review, we attempt to classify clinical trials on the basis of how well each was able to show therapeutic benefit from immunotherapy for malignant disease. The trials are classified in order to evaluate and compare them as objectively as possible. In a review, the reader must necessarily view the subject through the eyes of the reviewer, which in turn introduces a major subjective influence. While a study may be highly interesting, it may have little in the way of substantive results. The conclusions presented in a particular study may reflect the bias of the reviewer, but the classification acts as a stimulus toward evaluating the studies in a uniform manner. The intent of the classification system is to give the reader some idea of the relative merit and significance of the clinical trials included in this review. The numbers assigned, listed in parenthesis after the trial, do not necessarily imply ranking, but rather serve to designate the category in which the study fell.

Type I studies were those that demonstrated that immunotherapy was an effective treatment for malignant disease on the basis of a frequent, clear-cut, and predictable response to the therapy. Studies in this category are mainly those limited to intralesional injection or topical treatment of accessible tumors. Confirmed studies were designated Type A, and unconfirmed studies were designated Type B. Additional criteria for inclusion in this category were: (a) Five or more patients must have shown clearly objective responses (greater than 50% reduction of tumor, lasting longer than one month). (b) The five or more responders must have represented 50% or more of the patients treated.

Type II studies were those that demonstrated therapeutic benefit based on a prospective, randomized, controlled trial. These studies had to have a definite therapeutic objective, an adequate number of patients, well-defined diagnoses and staging, and statistically significant results. In clinical trials, it is very difficult to control the myriad variables that influence results, and there may be unsuspected factors that introduce unintentional bias in the work. Random assignment of patients to treatment and control groups helps to balance these variables and ensure that prognostic factors are equal in the two groups.

Type III clinical trials were controlled but the assignment to treatment and control groups was not randomized. The key requirement for this category was the inclusion of data in the published results that allowed us to judge whether prognostic factors were equal in the treatment and control groups. With this proviso, studies with either simultaneous or sequential control groups were included in this category. Similar to Type II studies, the Type III studies had to have definite diagnoses and staging, and statistically valid results. The main evidence for therapeutic benefit from immunotherapy has come from Type I, II, or III studies. Only 20% of the studies reviewed fell into these classifications. The other classifications to be described suggest areas where immunotherapy may be beneficial, but they do not establish its value for treatment of malignant disease.

Type IV studies were controlled trials that demonstrated therapeutic benefit but the control group could not be fully evaluated from the data given. Most studies with historical controls fit into this category. It was difficult to judge whether prognostic factors were comparable in the earlier treatment groups.

Subtle changes in overall management can occur, besides the treatment being tested. Studies with simultaneous controls could be included here also, depending upon our assessment of the control group. Studies that compared treatment results to published series from other institutions were not considered controlled trials.

Type V studies were uncontrolled clinical trials that showed some therapeutic benefit (either complete tumor regressions or significant partial regressions), more than would be expected from spontaneous improvement. Studies were included in this category if two or more patients showed clearly objective responses (greater than 50% reduction in tumor, lasting longer than one month), and this result represented 15% or more of the patients tested.

Type VI studies were clinical trials in which therapeutic benefit could not be evaluated from the data given. This category included many studies that failed to show therapeutic benefit but were not designed to yield significant negative information. Examples include uncontrolled studies on small numbers of patients who had objective responses so infrequently as to be unevaluable. Controlled trials with either positive or negative results could be classified here for reasons such as an inappropriate control group, too few patients, or results that were not statistically significant. Examples include studies that were inadequately controlled for treatments other than the immunotherapy. Another group included here was uncontrolled trials testing adjuvant immunotherapy for control of microscopic residual disease. Since there was no measurable tumor, the end point was survival or duration of remission, and benefit in this situation cannot be evaluated in the absence of controls. In addition, several preliminary reports from well designed and well controlled studies were classified as Type VI if the data were inconclusive.

There were studies that clearly demonstrated that the method of immunotherapy being tested was of no therapeutic benefit. The criteria for evaluation of this group were essentially the same as for Type II studies except, in this instance, each produced significant negative results. These are designated as Type VII.

Our classification system is intended as a general guide. Obviously, the classifications are arbitrary, and not all readers would reach the same conclusions. However, every attempt was made to apply the criteria uniformly and to present a fair assessment of clinical investigation of immunotherapy for malignant disease.

CLINICAL TRIALS

Results from a large number of clinical trials of immunotherapy for malignant disease have been published. The effectiveness of this modality can best be appreciated by examination of the results obtained from treatment of the individual diseases. For this reason, the discussion of clinical trials has been arranged by site of disease.

Brain Tumors

The section on brain tumors (Table 1) is placed first in the discussion of clinical trials of immunotherapy for malignant disease strictly on an alphabetical basis. A priori, one would expect that immunotherapy for brain tumors is unlikely to be of benefit since the central nervous system seems to be an immunologically privileged site. Clinical trials, so far, have not invalidated this hypothesis. In 1969, Trouillas & Lapras (61) reported on the intrathecal injection of autologous, sensitized lymphocytes for control of glioblastoma multiforme (VI). The patients had pieces of tumor, removed at surgery, implanted subcutaneously. Their thoracic duct lymphocytes were then harvested and given intrathecally. Five patients were treated but no therapeutic benefit was demonstrated. Bloom and his colleagues (62) have been doing investigations of immunotherapy for glioblastoma since 1960. Their most recent report involved a randomized, prospective trial of 62 patients (VII). Both groups had surgical removal of tumor and irradiation. The immunotherapy patients were given intradermal, autologous tumor cells obtained from the surgical specimen. No therapeutic benefit was evident in patients receiving immunotherapy. All patients who received tumor cells were dead at 30 months, while of the 35 nonimmunotherapy patients, seven remained alive at that interval. Six of the seven patients died subsequently, and survival in the two groups showed no significant statistical difference. Thus far, there is no evidence of benefit from immunotherapy for malignant brain tumors.

Breast Carcinoma

In breast cancer, late recurrences of rapidly progressive disease are seen many years after primary treatment, which suggests that the disease was controlled by a suppressive mechanism in the interim. Moreover, the induction of local, delayed cutaneous hypersensitivity responses (DCH) in a chest wall recurrence of breast carcinoma, may cause it to regress. Such observations suggest that immunotherapy may be useful in the treatment of breast carcinoma. In addition to local control of skin metastases, immunotherapy has been used as an adjuvant to other treatments for control of both minimal residual disease and disseminated disease, as indicated in Table 2.

Intralesional injection of BCG has proved to be an effective means of control

Table 1   Brain tumors

Year	Investigator(s)	Ref.	Immunotherapy	Type of study
1969	Trouillas & Lapras	61	Intrathecal autologous sensitized lymphocytes	VI
1973	Bloom et al	62	Intradermal autologous tumor cells	VII

for skin metastases from breast carcinoma. Complete regression of tumor was observed in seven of eight patients by Smith and colleagues (63) (I-A), and in seven of 14 patients by Klein (64) (I-A). In all instances, the responders had or developed positive PPD skin tests. While this treatment produced a striking effect on the local disease, the response was limited to the treated lesion, and no determination of whether the treatment extended survival was reported. One report implied failure of intralesional BCG in this setting with only three of 20 patients showing a response (VI) (65). Whether this failure had to do with variations in the technique or the dose of BCG was not clear. Both of these variables plus the level of tumor burden are critical to the success of immunotherapy.

Other agents that induce DCH responses have been used successfully in the local treatment of chest wall recurrences of breast cancer. Nitrogen mustard injected intralesionally caused complete regression of treated lesions in five of six patients sensitized to the drug (I-B) (66). Tumor regression apparently was not a direct effect of the drug since unsensitized patients were not affected, and only 75% of patients could be sensitized. In another study, topical application of dinitrochlorobenzene (DNCB) to skin metastases in DNCB-sensitized patients caused complete regression of lesions in three of eight patients tested (V) (67). Intralesional injection of autologous lymphocytes stimulated with phytohemagglutinin (PHA) caused one complete regression and two partial responses in

Table 2   Breast carcinoma

Year	Investigator	Ref.	Immunotherapy	Type of study
Local treatment for skin metastases				
1971	Stjernsward & Levin	67	Topical DNCB	V
1972	Cheema & Hersh	68	Intralesional PHA-activated lymphocytes	V
1973	Smith et al	63	Intralesional BCG	I-A
1975	Garas et al	65	Intralesional BCG	VI
1975	Goldman	66	Intralesional nitrogen mustard	I-B
1976	Klein et al	64	Intralesional BCG	I-A
Adjuvant therapy for minimum residual disease				
1974	Anderson et al	70	Surgery—tumor autotransplant	VI
1976	Rojas et al	39	Radiation—levamisole	III
Treatment for disseminated disease				
1974	Oettgen et al	74	Transfer factor	VI
1975	Israel & Edelstein	33	C. parvum—chemotherapy	II
1976	Gutterman et al	73	Intradermal BCG—chemotherapy	III
1977	Pinsky et al	72	C. parvum—chemotherapy	VI

skin metastases of breast carcinoma (V) (68). In this study, injection of adjacent lesions with unstimulated lymphocytes or saline had no effect.

The importance of these observations of successful local immunotherapy is twofold. First, immunotherapy offers a useful alternative for obtaining local control of accessible, recurrent breast cancer; and second, its potential for stimulation of host resistance may improve systemic control of tumor.

As an adjuvant to other treatment, immunotherapy has been used to prevent or delay recurrence following primary treatment for breast cancer. Rather striking results were obtained in a series of patients with Stage III disease (UICC classification) treated with radiation therapy followed by immunotherapy with levamisole (III) (39). Forty-three patients were irradiated (4000 R), and then alternately assigned to levamisole (150 mg by mouth daily for three days every two weeks) or a placebo. Minimum follow-up was 21 months. In the levamisole groups, median time to recurrence was 25 months vs nine months for those taking a placebo. Patient survival rate in the levamisole group was 90% at 30 months, whereas only 35% of the placebo group were alive at this interval ($P < .01$). Control and treatment groups were apparently equal for age, menopausal status, child bearing, and extent of disease. However, the control group reported here did rather poorly compared to an overall 70% survival rate at 30 months for patients with Stage III disease reported by the American Joint Committee for Cancer Staging and End Results Reporting (AJCCS) (69). Survival rate in the placebo group was half that expected from the AJCCS statistics, which suggests that factors affecting prognosis were not equal in the control and treatment groups. However, the levamisole group survival rate was better than the AJCCS figures, indicating possible therapeutic benefit. The results of this study have not been confirmed, but a prospective randomized trial is in progress (39).

An adjuvant study in which irradiated, autologous, tumor implants were used following radical mastectomy for breast carcinoma has been reported (VI) (70). No therapeutic benefit could be established from this attempt to stimulate specific antitumor responses.

Adjuvant chemotherapy following mastectomy has been shown to reduce the recurrence of locally advanced breast carcinoma (71). The addition of immunostimulation to this regimen might give even better results. Studies are in progress to test this hypothesis (46).

The combination of immunotherapy and chemotherapy may improve treatment results for disseminated breast carcinoma. In a prospective, randomized trial, Israel & Edelstein (33) used subcutaneous *C. parvum* in addition to five-drug chemotherapy for 43 patients with metastatic breast carcinoma (II). A control group of 39 patients received only the chemotherapy. A statistically significant improvement in survival time was seen in the patients receiving combination chemo-immunotherapy with a median survival time of over 18 months, compared to less than 12 months for the control group ($P < .001$). More recently, Pinsky and colleagues (72) combined subcutaneous *C. parvum* with a four-drug regimen for disseminated breast carcinoma. Preliminary results from their randomized trial indicate that responders in the chemo-immunotherapy group survived significantly longer than the responders on chemotherapy alone (VI). However, the survival curves for the two groups as a whole are not significantly different. Final evaluation must await completion of the study.

In another study of disseminated breast carcinoma, Gutterman (73) compared the use of repeated intradermal BCG combined with three-drug chemotherapy to the use of chemotherapy alone (III). Forty-five patients in the chemo-immunotherapy group were compared to 44 historical controls. In the latter group, 23 patients died with a median survival time for the group of 14 months. Although the chemo-immunotherapy group was followed for only 12 months, just five patients had died, giving this group a projected median survival time of much longer than 14 months. Although this preliminary result appears significant, improvements in overall treatment might have influenced the results. Nevertheless, the test and control groups were comparable for age, menopausal status, disease-free interval, and prior therapy. All patients with disseminated disease were entered consecutively and treated in the same institution.

Results from these chemo-immunotherapy trials are promising, and indicate that potent drugs and immunostimulation may be effective in combination. The contribution of immunotherapy is dependent upon the capacity of the chemotherapy to reduce tumor burden significantly. For breast cancer, this is feasible and additional prospective, randomized trials to confirm these findings are needed.

Transfer factor has been tested as a method for treating disseminated breast carcinoma (VI) (74). After other treatments had failed, six patients were given transfer factor obtained from lymphocytes of healthy women. Only one patient responded. However, this was a patient with inflammatory breast carcinoma who showed an arrest of progression of disease for six months in the absence of any other treatment. Although no conclusions can be drawn from a single result, this response was quite interesting.

It is clear that conventional modalities are still the mainstay of treatment for breast carcinoma. However, it appears that immunotherapy may be of benefit at several points in the treatment of malignant breast disease, and its use merits additional study.

Colo-Rectal Carcinoma and Other Gastrointestinal Tumors

Survival figures for colo-rectal carcinoma treated by surgery alone have remained the same for many years. For a patient with Dukes' C colo-rectal carcinoma, the five-year survival expectancy with surgery alone is an average 32% (75). In an effort to improve these figures, primary surgical treatment has been combined with adjuvant irradiation and/or chemotherapy. An interim report of a clinical trial of adjuvant immunotherapy following surgery for Dukes' C colo-rectal carcinoma has appeared (IV) (76). The adjuvant therapy group (83 patients) was randomized to receive long-term 5-Fluorouracil (5-FU) plus intradermal BCG (50 patients), or long-term intradermal BCG only (33 patients).

These groups were compared to historical controls treated by surgery alone at the M. D. Anderson Hospital and Tumor Institute in Houston, Texas (73 patients). For both adjuvant groups, statistically significant increases in the disease-free interval and survival rate were noted over controls at a median follow-up of approximately 16 months. There was no significant difference between the two adjuvant groups. This was a preliminary report, and a much longer follow-up period will be required to determine if the actual incidence of recurrence is decreased or the absolute number of survivors increased. Because adjuvant therapy of any kind is unproven in colo-rectal disease, this study would be more convincing if a surgery-only control group was included in the prospective randomization.

According to Moertel and colleagues (77), the addition of immunotherapy to chemotherapy for advanced colo-rectal carcinoma has not increased the expected 20% objective response rate (VI). Methanol extractable residue of BCG (MER) was used for the immunotherapy in this study. In an earlier study, Moertel (78) noted response to MER injections alone in three of 36 patients with advanced GI malignancy (VI), but could not confirm the result in a subsequent study (VI) (79). In a trial reported by Engstrom and co-workers (80), the combination of 5-FU and BCG was compared to 5-FU alone for the treatment of advanced colo-rectal carcinoma (VI). Again, there was no difference in the objective response rates. So far, immunotherapy does not appear to be of benefit in this situation.

Griffen & Meeker (81) used passive immunotherapy to treat 32 patients who had advanced colo-rectal carcinoma (V). Patients were paired for cross transplantation of their tumors. The patients then exchanged leukocytes. Five objective responses (16%) were reported, which is a response rate consistent with this type of treatment for other tumors. No follow-up report has appeared.

Falk and colleagues (82) used intraperitoneally injected BCG plus oral BCG combined with chemotherapy for the treatment of advanced malignant tumors of the GI tract (VI). Results of this treatment are difficult to evaluate as the study was uncontrolled and variable treatment regimens were used. However, for patients with colon carcinoma metastatic to the liver, whose short life expectancy as a group has been well established, some benefit may have been gained from the treatment. For nine patients treated, median survival time was 12 months, and two patients were alive at 19 and 24 months. This protocol should be tested in a controlled trial.

The use of thymic humoral factor in GI malignancies has been reported by Turowski and colleagues (83). This study was uncontrolled, and, from the data given, therapeutic benefit could not be evaluated.

As indicated in Table 3, clear-cut benefit from immunotherapy for GI tumors remains to be demonstrated. Chemotherapy is relatively impotent for these tumors and immunotherapy has not been additive. Results from surgical treatment plus adjuvant immunotherapy are still very preliminary. Considerable improvement is needed in all phases of treatment for gastrointestinal malignancies.

Genitourinary Tumors

Intradermal BCG was given to a group of patients with disseminated carcinoma of the prostate in an effort to augment host resistance (VI) (84). No significant clinical benefit could be identified. Merrin and colleagues (85) reported the use of intratumoral injections of BCG in patients with advanced carcinoma of the prostate (VI). In some patients, this treatment did produce necrosis in the injected tumor, but no alteration in clinical course was noted. In both studies, the patients had large tumor burdens, which diminished the possibility for successful immunotherapy (Table 4).

For the treatment of recurrent superficial bladder cancer, Eidinger & Morales (86) tried intracavitary instillations of BCG (VI). Although this was a preliminary report, their data suggested a decrease in recurrence rate. This was a reasonable trial since local immunotherapy is effective for other types of accessible tumors.

Xenogeneic immune RNA has been used in the treatment of disseminated renal cell carcinoma (VI) (87). The immune RNA was obtained from sheep sensitized to human hypernephromas. No tumor regressions were seen in 20 patients treated, but seven patients showed an apparent arrest of progression of disease lasting a minimum of three months. A subgroup of eight patients, with pulmonary metastases only, seemed to be surviving longer that a similar group of historical controls, but the follow-up was short and the numbers small. Nine patients with advanced local disease removed at surgery were treated with immune RNA (87, 88). Each was at high risk for recurrence, but no recurrence was observed over a mean follow-up of 18 months. Therapeutic benefit in this setting must be demonstrated in a controlled trial, however.

Table 3 Colo-rectal carcinoma and GI tumors

Year	Investigator(s)	Ref.	Immunotherapy	Type of study
Adjuvant immunotherapy				
1976	Mavligit et al	76	BCG & 5-FU, Duke's C Colo-rectal cancer	VI
Mixed studies in advanced tumors				
1972	Griffen & Meeker	81	Tumor cell vaccine in advanced colon carcinoma	VI
1975	Moertel et al	78	MER injections	VI
1976	Falk et al	82	Oral and IP BCG in advanced GI tumors	VI
1976	Turowski et al	83	Thymic humoral factor in advanced GI tumors	VI
1976	O'Connell et al	79	MER injections	VI
1977	Engstrom et al	80	BCG, chemotherapy	VI
1977	Moertel et al	77	MER, BCG, chemotherapy	VI

Table 4   Genitourinary tumors

Year	Investigator(s)	Ref.	Carcinoma	Immunotherapy	Type of study
1973	Guinan et al	84	Metastatic prostate	Intratumor BCG	VI
1975	Merrin et al	85	Prostate	Intratumor BCG	VI
1976	Eidinger & Morales	86	Bladder	Intracavitary BCG	VI
1976	Skinner et al	88	Renal cell	Xenogeneic immune RNA	VI
1977	Ramming & deKernion	87	Renal cell	Xenogeneic immune RNA	VI

The role of immunotherapy for genitourinary tumors is as yet undetermined, but the studies identify important areas for further investigation.

Gynecological Cancers

A very interesting use of topical immunotherapy has been reported in post-hysterectomy patients with vaginal smears positive for malignant cells (I-B) (89). Positive cytological findings were documented on three repeat smears, then six patients with these findings were sensitized to DNCB. Once good DCH responses were obtained, an appropriate concentration of DNCB cream was carefully applied intravaginally, which produced an intense local reaction. Six weeks after treatment, repeat smears were all normal. In follow-up from 2 to 35 months (median, 21 months), all patients remained normal. The mechanism of response in these instances must be related to that for topical or intralesional immunotherapy of skin cancers and metastases. If the beneficial effects of the treatment can be confirmed in a larger number of patients, it should become a very useful therapy.

Immunotherapy by itself, or in combination with chemotherapy, has been tried for advanced gynecological cancer, but no clear evidence of effectiveness has appeared (Table 5). Tumor cell vaccines alone were apparently ineffective against established disease in one large study (VII) (90). A beneficial effect for advanced ovarian carcinoma using tumor cell vaccine combined with BCG has been claimed, but this result was based on one case with a short follow-up period (VI) (91). Uncontrolled trials combining chemotherapy and immunotherapy for various advanced gynecological tumors have shown some limited responses, but without control patients the contribution of immunotherapy cannot be determined (VI) (92, 93). Compared to patients treated with chemotherapy alone, patients with advanced ovarian carcinoma who received a combination of BCG, tumor cell vaccine, and chemotherapy had a significantly extended survival time, as reported by Hudson and colleagues (VI) (94). However, this was a small study based on historical controls with other variables besides immunotherapy existing between the test and control groups. These problems forestall any definitive conclusions, but this combination should be tested in a larger, more rigidly controlled trial.

Leukemia

ACUTE LYMPHOBLASTIC LEUKEMIA   A major stimulus to interest in immuno-therapy for malignant disease came from an early report by Mathé and co-workers (11), which showed that immunotherapy markedly prolonged remission and survival times in acute lymphoblastic leukemia (ALL) (II). Acute leukemia in remission was chosen as an appropriate clinical test of immunotherapy, because the low tumor burden offered a greater chance of success. Thirty patients with ALL in prolonged remission on chemotherapy had their drugs stopped. Ten of these patients were chosen randomly to receive no additional treatment, and all relapsed within five months. In contrast, 10 of 20 patients who were given immunotherapy that consisted of BCG and/or allogeneic leukemia cells remained in remission for more than 295 days. Seven of these patients have remained in remission for 7–12 years. Cures have probably been achieved since the treatment was stopped after five years (95).

Unfortunately, the usefulness of immunotherapy for ALL has not been estab-lished by subsequent studies, as seen in Table 6. One recent report by Otten (96) indicated that immunotherapy, consisting of BCG and allogeneic leukemia cells, was at least equal to chemotherapy in maintaining remission in ALL (II). Mathé and his group (97, 95) have continued to use immunotherapy for ALL and report a beneficial therapeutic effect. However, since the original report, they have not included a nonimmunotherapy control group in their studies. For this reason, and because chemotherapy is used whenever necessary to reinduce

Table 5 Gynecological cancers

Year	Investigator(s)	Ref.	Tumor type	Immunotherapy	Type of study
1962	Graham & Graham	90	Advanced gynecological tumors	Tumor cell vaccine	VII
1974	Imperato et al	91	Advanced ovarian carcinoma	Tumor cell vaccine and BCG	VI
1975	Guthrie & Way	89	Cytological vaginal carcinoma	Topical DNCB	I-B
1976	Pattillo	92	Advanced gynecological tumors	Tumor antigen vaccine, BCG, and chemotherapy	VI
1976	Hudson et al	94	Advanced ovarian carcinoma	Tumor cell vaccine, BCG, and chemotherapy	VI
1977	Rao et al	93	Advanced ovarian carcinoma	C. parvum chemotherapy	VI

remission in these studies, it is not possible to judge the therapeutic benefit gained from immunotherapy.

Two large, randomized, controlled studies have failed to show that BCG therapy is useful for maintaining chemotherapy-induced remissions of ALL (VII) (98, 99). Both studies compared repeated intradermal BCG treatment to chemotherapy for maintaining remission, and the latter treatment gave significantly better results. Results from BCG therapy were similar to no additional treatment. None of these studies reproduced the conditions of Mathé's original trial or that of Otten, because their immunotherapy consisted of BCG only and did not include allogeneic leukemia cells. From Mathé's view, treatments with BCG and BCG combined with leukemia cells were of equal efficacy. However, it may be that the contribution of specific-active stimulation by the leukemia cells is critical. In any case, chemotherapy for ALL has steadily improved, so it is unlikely that the conditions in Mathé's study will be reproduced (100). A recent report from the National Cancer Institute in which BCG and allogeneic leukemia cells were used in combination with current chemotherapy showed no advantage over the use of chemotherapy alone (VII) (101). There have been no other studies establishing therapeutic benefit from immunotherapy in ALL. They either have shown negative results (VI) (102, 103), or were too limited for definitive conclusions (VI) (104). At the present time, chemotherapy is the treatment of choice for ALL, and the role of immunotherapy is uncertain.

ACUTE MYELOGENOUS LEUKEMIA   Immunotherapy for the treatment of acute myelogenous leukemia (AML) has been more promising (Table 7). In a prospective randomized trial of patients in remission, Powles (105) reported that the

Table 6 Acute lymphocytic leukemia

Year	Investigator(s)	Ref.	Immunotherapy	Type of study
1968	Albo et al	125	Parental plasma, chemotherapy	VI
1969	Skurkovich et al	126	Reinfusion autologous cells and serum	IV
1969	Mathé et al	11	BCG, allogeneic leukemia cells	II
1971	Medical Research Council	98	BCG	VII
1972	Mathé et al	97	BCG, allogeneic leukemia cells	VI
1973	Leventhal et al	102	BCG, allogeneic leukemia cells, MTX, allogeneic leukemia cells	VI
1975	Ekert & Jose	104	BCG, chemotherapy	VI
1975	Heyn et al	99	BCG	VII
1975	Poplack et al	101	BCG, cells, chemotherapy	VII
1975	Sacks et al	103	RAJI cells, chemotherapy	VI
1976	Mathé et al	95	BCG, allogeneic leukemia cells	VI
1977	Otten	96	BCG, leukemia cells	II
1977	Kay	104a	BCG	VI

addition of immunotherapy with BCG and allogeneic leukemia cells to maintenance chemotherapy significantly prolonged survival time (II). Twenty-three patients receiving combined chemo-immunotherapy showed a median survival of 545 days compared to 303 days for patients receiving chemotherapy only ($P = .003$). Relapse rates and duration of remission were improved in the immunotherapy group, but were not significantly different from controls. In another prospective, randomized trial reported by Vogler & Chan (106), 41 patients with AML were given late consolidation chemotherapy, then randomly assigned to receive maintenance chemotherapy plus BCG or chemotherapy alone (II). There was a marked improvement in the duration of remission for 18 patients receiving chemo-immunotherapy: 39 weeks vs 26 weeks for the 23 control patients receiving drugs alone ($P = .002$).

Investigators from M. D. Anderson Hospital and Tumor Institute reported a trial of BCG therapy combined with chemotherapy for maintaining remission in patients with acute leukemia (IV) (107). The statistical treatment of the data and the controls in their initial report were criticized (108). However, they issued a revised report that maintained that there was improvement in the duration of remission for 14 AML patients treated with chemo-immunotherapy compared to 21 historical controls receiving chemotherapy only ($P = .04$) (109). Median survival time of those on chemotherapy alone was 78 weeks; for the group

Table 7   Acute myelogenous leukemia

Year	Investigator(s)	Ref.	Immunotherapy	Type of study
1973	Powles et al	105	BCG, leukemia cells, chemotherapy	II
1973	Freeman et al	114	BCG, leukemia cells	VI
1974	Vogler & Chan	106	BCG, chemotherapy	II
1974	Gutterman et al	107	BCG, chemotherapy	IV
1976	Powles	115	BCG, leukemia cells	VI
1976	Whiteside et al	110	BCG, leukemia cells, chemotherapy	VI
1976	Holland & Bekesi	42	Neuraminidase-treated cells, chemotherapy	VI
1977	Reizenstein et al	111	BCG, leukemia cells, chemotherapy	II
1977	Peto	112	BCG, leukemia cells, chemotherapy	VI
1977	Sauter et al	122	Viral oncolysate, chemotherapy	VII
1977	Whittaker & Slater	117	i.v. BCG, chemotherapy	VI
1977	Cuttner et al	118	MER, chemotherapy	VI
1977	Gee & Clarkson	120	Heptavalent pseudomonas vaccine, chemotherapy	VI
1977	McIntyre et al	121	Poly I:Poly C, chemotherapy	VII

receiving combined therapy, a median survival time had not been reached, but it appeared that it was going to be more than 98 weeks. In a small, uncontrolled trial, Whiteside and co-workers (110) indicated a marked improvement in survival time and duration of remission for patients receiving chemotherapy plus BCG and allogeneic cells (VI). Using similar chemo-immunotherapy in a prospective, randomized trial, Reizenstein and colleagues (111) from Sweden reported a doubling of median survival time from 10 to 20 months over chemotherapy alone ($P < .05$) (II). Thus, several studies indicate that immunotherapy used in combination with chemotherapy has improved the results of treatment for AML patients who can be brought into remission initially with drugs.

There have been two negative reports on the use of combined chemo-immunotherapy in maintaining remission in patients with AML. Peto (112), reporting for the British Medical Council, notes that BCG plus allogeneic blast cells do not add to remission or survival times over chemotherapy used alone (VI). Hewlitt and colleagues (113) used BCG in addition to known potent chemotherapy, and found that there was a slight trend in favor of the combined therapy, but it was not statistically significant (VII). Confirmation of therapeutic benefit from chemo-immunotherapy in AML must await additional trials, and is not yet the standard of care for this disease.

The use of BCG and allogeneic leukemia cells without chemotherapy as maintenance treatment for AML was reported initially by Freeman and co-workers (114) (VI). They also did frequent bone marrow studies, and with any increase in blast cells they started reinduction chemotherapy promptly. It was their impression that second and subsequent remissions were much easier to obtain than previously. In a later report, Powles (115) indicated that immunotherapy given without chemotherapy for maintenance gave similar results to the combined treatment in prolonging survival time (VI). Both of these reports were from uncontrolled trials however. M. D. Anderson Hospital and Tumor Institute has reported the use of BCG alone to maintain patients with adult acute leukemia in remission after the cessation of chemotherapy (VI) (73). Thirty-seven leukemia patients in remission on long-term drugs were given late, intensive, consolidation chemotherapy, and then the drugs were stopped. Thirty patients received BCG as ongoing treatment; seven received no additional treatment. Superior survival time and duration of remission were indicated for the BCG group, though, the result was compared to a group of historical controls who had not received the same chemotherapy. In fact, the same group of historical controls was used for comparison to show the benefit of late consolidation chemotherapy in another publication (VI) (116). The BCG data also compared favorably to the seven patients not receiving immunotherapy, but this was an extremely small group for comparison. Thus, the benefit of immunotherapy used alone in this setting remains unproven.

Holland & Bekesi (42) tried an innovative approach to immunotherapy for adult patients with AML (VI). The patients were brought into chemotherapy-induced remission, and then were given maintenance chemotherapy plus neuraminidase-treated allogeneic leukemia cells. A very small initial clinical trial suggested that this treatment enhanced the duration of remission and survival in patients with AML. A larger, prospective, randomized trial is in progress in which 24 patients have received maintenance drugs only, while a second group of 27 patients have been given maintenance drugs plus neuraminidase-treated leukemia cells (J. G. Bekesi, personal communication). In the chemotherapy-only group, 22 patients (92%) relapsed with a median duration of 33 weeks. In contrast, the combined chemo-immunotherapy group of 19 patients (70%) are still in remission, 11 for more than 75 weeks and five for more than three years. This appears very promising, but evaluation of therapeutic benefit must await completion and publication of the study.

Other immunotherapy treatments for AML have been tried with variable success. BCG given intravenously in combination with maintenance chemo-therapy for AML is reported to have an acceptable toxicity, and to yield a better survival than chemotherapy alone (VI) (117). MER combined with chemo-therapy is being tested for AML, but results are preliminary (VI) (118). Schwarzenberg (119) reported some years ago that adoptive transfer of leu-kocytes to AML patients failing on other treatments would induce complete remission, although these remissions were short-lived (V). Other treatments used in combination with chemotherapy, including virally treated leukemia cells, pseudomonas vaccine, and polynucleotides, have not shown therapeutic benefit (VII) (120–122). Thymic humoral factor has been used in the treatment of various hematologic malignancies, and is reported to give symptomatic im-provement, but the therapeutic benefit could not be evaluated from the data given (VI) (123).

OTHER LEUKEMIA STUDIES   Clinical trials of immunotherapy for leukemia that employed passive transfer of immune serum have been reported (Table 8). DeCarvalho (124) immunized horses (and a donkey) against human tumor and then used γ-globulin extracted from the equine serum to treat tumor patients (V). Fifteen patients with leukemia or lymphoma who had failed on other therapies were treated. He reported seven complete responses to the treatment, including two patients who had remissions of more than 12 and 29 months, respectively. This was a preliminary study, and no follow-up or confirmation has been published. Surprisingly, he reported relatively few side effects from this xenogeneic serum. In treating children with ALL, Albo and colleagues (125) used plasma from parents in addition to maintenance chemotherapy (VI), but there was no beneficial therapeutic response. Skurkovich and co-workers (126) reported that in children being treated with chemotherapy for ALL reinfusion of autologous cells and serum obtained early in remission and stored increased the duration of remission (IV). This result was in comparison to selected control patients receiving chemotherapy only. This was a small group of patients, and there has been no follow-up or confirmation.

Immunotherapy for chronic myelogenous leukemia (CML) has been at-tempted (IV) (127). Roswell Park Memorial Institute in Buffalo, New York reported a series of 15 patients with CML given BCG plus allogeneic cells in addition to maintenance chemotherapy. The cells were thought to be leukemia cells in culture, but later proved to be transformed lymphoblasts. These patients were compared to 28 selected historical controls from the same institution. The survival rate of the immunotherapy group appeared to be improved over the controls, 60% and 20% at five years, respectively ($P < 0.01$). However, this was a small number of patients with chronic disease receiving variable treatment over a long period of time. This combination should be tested in a larger randomized trial. Passive transfer of specifically cytotoxic serum to three patients with chronic lymphocytic leukemia (CLL) caused a drop in leukocyte counts and a reduction in lymph node size, but the response was variable and therapeutic benefit was not obvious (VI) (128).

Overall, the leukemia studies, particularly for AML, indicate that combination treatment with nonspecific and specific immunotherapy has merit and that specific stimulation with tumor cells may be necessary to the treatment. Moreover, it is apparent that immunostimulation works in combination with chemotherapy. That these results were obtained in patients in remission reinforces the concept that immunotherapy is best used when tumor burden is small. While several studies indicate that immunotherapy may help in the treatment of leukemia, the benefit has not been universal, and considerable testing in carefully controlled trials is necessary before its place in the treatment of hematologic malignancies can be determined.

Lymphomas

Burkitt's lymphoma clearly has tumor-associated antigens related to the Epstein-Barr virus (129). However, the results of immunotherapy for this disease have been disappointing (Table 9). A prospective, randomized study in which

Table 8 Other leukemia studies

Year	Investigator(s)	Ref.	Immunotherapy	Type of study
Chronic myelogenous leukemia				
1973	Sokal et al	127	BCG, lymphoid cells	IV
Chronic lymphocytic leukemia				
1968	Lazlo et al	128	Passive transfer of serum	VI
Mixed leukemia studies				
1962	DeCarvalho	124	Xenogeneic antileukemia serum	V
1966	Schwarzenberg et al	119	Adoptive transfer leukocytes	V
1976	Gutterman et al	73	BCG	VI
1976	Bodey et al	116	BCG	VI
1976	Aleksandrowicz & Skotnicki	123	Thymic humoral factor	VI
1977	Hewlett et al	113	BCG, chemotherapy	VII

BCG was given to patients with Burkitt's lymphoma in remission following chemotherapy showed no apparent therapeutic benefit (VII) (130). Relapse rate and duration of remission were the same in 21 immunotherapy patients and 19 control patients. Objective tumor regressions were reported in two patients with Burkitt's lymphoma treated with serum from patients in remission (VI) (131, 132). However, in a controlled study, Fass and colleagues (133) found no effect from the passive transfer of serum from patients in remission (VI), even though the serum had activity against Epstein-Barr virus antigens in vitro. An additional study of a single patient yielded a similar negative result (VI) (134).

Sokal and colleagues (135) reported a study of survival of lymphoma patients given a single BCG vaccination in addition to their conventional therapy (VI). Fifty patients with Stage IA or IIA were randomized to receive BCG vaccination or not. The relapse rate and duration of remission appeared better in the BCG-vaccinated group. While prognostic factors appeared similar in the two groups, there were a number of uncontrolled variables in the study, including various histologic diagnoses and other treatments. Given the number of variables, this study was too small to answer the question posed.

Preliminary results of a large, randomized, controlled trial that tested intradermal BCG added to standard chemotherapy for the treatment of non-Hodgkin's lymphoma have been reported by Jones & Salmon (136). The number of complete remissions achieved was not improved by BCG treatment, but there was a slight increase in the number of partial remissions obtained (not statistically significant). In the maintenance phase, the number of relapses was the same in the BCG group and the no-maintenance drug group. Thus, nonspecific immunotherapy does not appear to be additive in this setting.

In spite of the antigenicity of lymphomatous tumors and their apparent susceptibility to immune attack in transplantation systems, benefit from immunotherapy in clinical trials remains to be demonstrated. It is possible that the addition of active-specific immunostimulation would be helpful.

Lung Carcinoma

Several reports indicate that immunotherapy subsequent to primary treatment for early lung carcinoma is beneficial in reducing recurrences (Table 10). The

Table 9 Lymphoma

Year	Investigator(s)	Ref.	Immunotherapy	Type of study
1967	Burkitt	131	Passive transfer of serum	VI
1967	Ngu	132	Passive transfer of serum	VI
1970	Fass et al	133	Passive transfer of serum	VI
1970	Bluming & Serpick	134	Passive transfer of serum	VI
1974	Sokal et al	135	BCG vaccination, chemotherapy	VI
1976	Magrath & Ziegler	130	BCG	VII
1977	Jones & Salmon	136	Intradermal BCG, chemotherapy	VI

most dramatic of these was the study by McKneally and co-workers (137) of a series of patients with operable lung carcinoma who were randomized to receive either one postoperative dose of intrapleural BCG given via chest tube or no immunotherapy (II). Their study was based partly on the observation that patients who get empyema after operation for lung cancer seem to survive longer (138, 139). All patients with operable lung carcinoma were entered into their study, though oat cell carcinoma was excluded. Results in the group with Stage I disease were striking. At one year follow-up, 17 BCG-treated patients had no deaths and no recurrences. In contrast, 22 patients receiving no additional treatment had nine recurrences and five deaths at one year. This study has been continued, and at a median follow-up of 640 days, 26 of 28 BCG patients (93%) are free of disease compared to 22 of 33 nonimmunotherapy patients (67%) (P = .009) (140). Immunotherapy had very little effect in Stage II or Stage III disease. Thus, for early disease, this approach may be a major improvement in treatment.

Single-dose intradermal BCG following operation for lung carcinoma did not appear to be effective (VI) (141). Sixty BCG-treated patients were compared to a historical group of 60 patients who received surgery alone. There was a slight improvement in survival for the immunotherapy group, but it was not statistically significant. For successful immunotherapy in experimental tumor models, it is critical to get the immunostimulant into the regional lymphatics draining the tumor (18). This finding appears to be confirmed by the benefit from intrapleural BCG in McKneally's study compared to the failure of intradermal BCG in the same setting. However, McKneally was administering a larger dose of BCG than was given intradermally.

Table 10 Lung carcinoma

Year	Investigator(s)	Ref.	Immunotherapy	Type of study
Adjuvant immunotherapy following primary therapy				
1974	Edwards & Whitwell	141	Intradermal BCG, surgery	VI
1975	Amery et al	40	Levamisole, surgery	VI
1976	McKneally et al	137	Intrapleural BCG, surgery	II
1976	Pines	143	Intradermal BCG, radiation	II
1977	Stewart et al	145	Tumor antigen, chemotherapy, and surgery	II
1977	Takita et al	144	Neuraminidase-treated cells, ConA, CFA, and surgery	II
Treatment for disseminated disease				
1973	Alth et al	147	Tumor extract	VI
1975	Israel & Edelstein	33	*C. parvum,* chemotherapy	II
1976	Kimura et al	148	Strep OK-432, chemotherapy	VI
1977	Yamamura	155	Oil-attached cell-wall skeleton BCG	VI
1977	Dimitrov et al	146	*C. parvum,* chemotherapy	VI

A multicenter, prospective, randomized trial using levamisole as adjuvant therapy for resectable lung carcinoma has been reported (VI) (40). Oat cell carcinoma was excluded. The immunotherapy patients were given levamisole three days preoperatively, and 150 mg orally for three days every two weeks thereafter; the others were given a placebo. The published results of a one year follow-up showed a trend toward a decreased number of recurrences and increased survival time in favor of the levamisole group: 10 recurrences in 51 levamisole patients (20%) compared to 20 of 60 patients receiving a placebo (33%), but this difference is not statistically significant. It was interesting, however, that the recurrence rate in the levamisole group remained the same for both large and small primary tumors, while it increased markedly for larger tumors in the placebo group. In a more recent analysis of the data, Amery (142) noted that important differences were observed if the test and control groups were divided into patients weighing more or less than 70 kg. In the lighter patient group there were fewer recurrences or deaths, and this difference was highly significant when compared to patients receiving the placebo. In the heavier group, these differences did not exist. This finding suggests that immunopotentiation with levamisole is dose-related, and, in appropriate doses, it may be an effective adjuvant therapy. This must be demonstrated in an appropriately stratified trial however.

A group of patients with inoperable lung carcinoma confined to the chest was treated by irradiation followed by adjuvant immunotherapy (II) (143). The patients were randomized to receive postradiation BCG or no additional treatment. Minimum follow-up was two years. During the first year, 12 of 23 patients (52%) receiving no additional treatment died compared to five of 25 patients (20%) receiving BCG. The BCG group had a significantly better one year survival rate ($P < .02$), although after the first year of follow-up, survival rates in the two groups were similar. Patients receiving only palliative radiation were not entered in this group, but it was observed that they did not respond to BCG treatment. Those receiving a full course of radiation were apparently benefited initially by adjuvant immunotherapy.

A clinical trial of active-specific immunotherapy as an adjuvant to surgery and radiation for locally advanced lung carcinoma has been reported (VI) (44). All gross disease was removed surgically in 11 patients. If tumor remained in the bronchial stump or on the chest wall, radiation was given. By random selection, five patients received a vaccine of autologous tumor cells treated with concanavalin A suspended in Freund's adjuvant. The other six patients received no additional treatment until recurrence developed. Chemotherapy was used in both groups if recurrence appeared. Three of the five immunotherapy patients were alive with a median survival time for the group of 15 months at the time of the original study. All six patients in the control group died, with a median survival time of five months. An update of this study has been reported with 15 patients in each group (II) (144). In the immunotherapy group, seven patients are alive, the longest at 51 months, with a median survival time for the group of

34.8 months. In the control group, three patients are alive with the longest survivor at 26 months and a median survival for the group of 12.1 months. This difference in survival is statistically significant ($P < .05$).

Stewart and colleagues (145) have reported preliminary results from another study of patients with lung cancer who were treated with tumor antigen in complete Freund's adjuvant and chemotherapy following surgery (II). This was a prospective, randomized trial that compared adjuvant chemo-immunotherapy to chemotherapy alone. The data indicated an increase in survival time for the combined adjuvant therapy patients that was significantly better than for patients given chemotherapy alone ($P = .001$). Both the Takita and Stewart studies suggest benefit from adjuvant chemo-immunotherapy. However, relatively small numbers of patients were entered into the trials over a long period, which suggests some selection of patients and this may have influenced their findings.

Adjuvant immunotherapy for lung carcinoma is promising, especially for patients in the earlier stages of the disease. All studies of adjuvant treatment emphasize the need for a significant reduction of tumor burden before immunotherapy can be effective. Additional studies are warranted.

Immunotherapy has been used in the treatment of disseminated lung carcinoma. Israel & Edelstein (33) compared subcutaneous *C. parvum* combined with five-drug chemotherapy to chemotherapy alone in a prospective randomized trial (II). The median survival time for 75 patients receiving chemotherapy was only four months; in the chemo-immunotherapy group, 68 patients showed a median survival time of nine months, a significant improvement ($P < .001$). A similar increase in survival time was reported when combined chemo-immunotherapy was used for disseminated oat cell carcinoma. The immunotherapy group had a mean survival time of 9.1 months compared to five months for the control group ($P < .02$) (33). The benefit from *C. parvum* in this setting has not yet been confirmed by other investigators. Preliminary results from a prospective, randomized trial reported by Dimitrov and colleagues (146) showed no improvement in survival time (over chemotherapy alone) when patients received a combination of adriamycin and subcutaneous *C. parvum* for advanced lung carcinoma (VI). However, these are early results from a trial employing only single-agent chemotherapy.

A small, uncontrolled study using tumor cell extract as the sole treatment for disseminated lung carcinoma was reported by Alth and colleagues (147), but therapeutic effect appeared to be minimal (VI). A streptococcal agent, OK-432, was combined with chemotherapy for disseminated lung carcinoma by Kimura and co-workers (148) (VI). A slight increase in the median survival time was achieved in the treated group over a chemotherapy control group, but the data did not establish this as clearly beneficial. A group of patients with advanced lung carcinoma were given the oil-attached cell-wall skeleton of BCG in addition to conventional therapy (VI) (155). The 50% survival interval for patients with Stage III disease was 18 months, as opposed to seven months for patients treated by conventional therapy alone. Although this result was statistically significant, the latter group was comprised of historical controls, and it was not clear whether the conventional therapy in the treatment and the control group was comparable.

Despite the shortcomings of some clinical trials, it would appear that immunotherapy can be beneficial to patients with lung carcinoma. Immunotherapy must be combined with other agents that significantly reduce tumor burden. Additional randomized, controlled studies are needed, both for adjuvant treatment and for combination therapy for disseminated disease, if immunotherapy is to become an established treatment modality for lung carcinoma.

Malignant Melanoma

LOCAL IMMUNOTHERAPY   Results obtained in the treatment of malignant melanoma have been the major stimulus to the use of immunotherapy for other solid tumors. In immunocompetent patients, cutaneous metastases of malignant melanoma will consistently undergo complete regression following intralesional injection with BCG. This observation, originally reported by Morton and his colleagues (12), has been confirmed by numerous investigators (I-A) (156–160, 150–152, 63). Serial biopsies of injected lesions show an intense lymphocytic and mononuclear cell infiltrate and destruction of melanoma cells. Moreover, in 17% of patients receiving intralesional BCG, there is a concomitant regression of uninjected nodules (12, 156, 159, 151, 63). Approximately 20% of patients responding to this treatment remain free of disease over a long period; the longest is still living at ten years (153). However, most patients develop recurrent lesions and eventually die of metastatic melanoma. It is not known whether the intralesional treatment prolongs survival time in these patients. During the treatment of metastatic lesions with intralesional BCG, new lesions will develop in a significant number of patients. These may be treated as well. The treatment is ineffective in patients who remain anergic to both DNCB and PPD skin testing. If the tumor burden is large or visceral metastases are evident, local responses in the skin are less frequent. Clinically detectable visceral metastases very rarely regress concomitantly with skin lesions. However, for metastatic disease limited to the skin or for small subcutaneous nodules, the response to intralesional injection is consistent and may be considered a useful, alternative therapy. Occasional responses in distant nodal or visceral disease are seen, but not often enough to be clinically useful.

Other types of immunotherapy have been used successfully to control accessible metastases of malignant melanoma. The induction of local, delayed hypersensitivity responses to DNCB can be effective in eliminating cutaneous disease (I-B) (161, 162). Malek-Mansour (162) reported that skin metastases in five of seven patients with malignant melanoma completely regressed after DNCB treatment of the lesions (I-B). Two of these remained free of disease from one to three years.

Intralesional injection with smallpox vaccine (vaccinia virus) will destroy intradermal deposits of malignant melanoma (163–165). Hunter-Craig and his colleagues (165) reported that skin metastases regressed completely in six of ten patients following virus injection (I-B). Most of the patients had been followed less than ten months, but two were free of disease at 11 and 22 months after injection. Responders and nonresponders could not be separated on the basis of clinical findings. Responses were limited to the injected lesions, and subcutaneous or nodal disease did not respond. Side effects were those of smallpox vaccination. As another approach, mumps virus has been added to intralesional BCG injection, but it is not clear from the published data whether it augmented the response (VI) (166). Injection of mumps virus alone will cause regression of lesions (I-B) (152).

Intralesional injections of autochthonous lymphocytes stimulated with PHA-induced partial regressions of cutaneous melanoma, but did not eliminate the lesions (I-B) (68). Smith and his colleagues (63) reported that intralesional injection of transfer factor from persons sensitized to the patient's tumor caused regression of skin metastases of malignant melanoma (V). He noted one complete regression lasting more than two years. *C. parvum* has been injected into cutaneous metastases of malignant melanoma (V) (167). Six of 14 patients injected showed regression of lesions (three complete, three partial). There was no regression of noninjected lesions. Although some success has been achieved with all of these treatments, BCG has been the agent most tested and used for local immunotherapy of malignant melanoma (See Table 11).

ADJUVANT IMMUNOTHERAPY   Adjuvant immunotherapy may be effective for reducing the high risk of recurrence in certain patients following surgical treatment for malignant melanoma. Rationale for this form of therapy is suggested by several observations: (*a*) the concomitant regression of uninjected nodules in patients receiving intralesional BCG; (*b*) the increase in antimelanoma antibody after local immunotherapy; and (*c*) the prolonged survival time of patients treated with BCG for skin metastases who, based on the natural history of metastatic malignant melanoma, have a high likelihood of subclinical, visceral metastases as well.

A controlled trial using BCG as adjuvant therapy following surgery for malignant melanoma metastatic to the regional nodes was reported by Eilber and colleagues from UCLA (III) (45). Patients with Stage II disease treated by operation alone are known to have a 70% recurrence rate within two years, and 80% recur within five years. In Eilber's study, 126 patients entered after radical resection of regional nodes and histologic confirmation of stage of disease. Of these, 84 patients received immunotherapy consisting of weekly intradermal BCG (3×10^8 organisms by Tine technique) for 12–52 weeks, and then every two weeks thereafter for two years; 42 were treated by operation alone. The results were evaluated by life table analysis, and showed a marked improvement in the probability of patients remaining free of disease at two years postoperation. In the BCG-treated group, 64% of the patients were free of disease vs 36% in the group treated by operation alone ($P < .05$). In those who recurred, median time to recurrence in the BCG group was ten months, whereas for those treated by operation alone, the median time was four months. Whether the number of survivors will ultimately be greater with BCG therapy must await longer follow-up.

Immunotherapy was more effective in patients with a smaller tumor burden. Of patients receiving BCG for one lymph node (positive only on microscopic exam), 90% were disease-free at two years, while only 62% of those with a clinically palpable node remained free of disease on immunotherapy. In the surgery-only group, recurrence rate was the same for patients with microscopic or palpable nodal metastases, 36% and 32%, respectively. This study was not strictly randomized, but the immunotherapy and control groups were very similar, except for a larger number of patients over age 40 in the control group. A completely randomized, prospective trial using adjuvant immunotherapy for Stage II malignant melanoma is now in progress (167a).

Another controlled trial of adjuvant immunotherapy following operation for

Table 11 Malignant melanoma

Year	Investigator(s)	Ref.	Local immunotherapy for cutaneous or accessible disease	Type of study
1970	Morton et al	12	Intralesional BCG	I-A
1972	Nathanson et al	156	Intralesional BCG	I-A
1972	Seigler et al	157	Intralesional BCG	I-A
1973	Baker & Taub	158	Intralesional BCG	VI
1973	Pinsky et al	159	Intralesional BCG	I-A
1973	Smith et al	63	Intralesional BCG	V
1974	Grant et al	160	Intralesional BCG	I-A
1974	Lieberman et al	149	Intralesional BCG	V
1974	Morton et al	153	Intralesional BCG	I-A
1975	Israel et al	150	Intralesional BCG	I-A
1976	Karakousis et al	154	Intralesional BCG	VI
1976	Mastrangelo et al	151	Intralesional BCG	V
1976	Gerner & Moore	152	Intralesional BCG & PPD, mumps, Strep	I-B
1972	Klein & Holtermann	161	Topical DNCB	V
1973	Malek-Mansour	162	Topical & intralesional DNCB	I-B
1964	Burdick & Hawk	163	Intralesional vaccinia virus	VI
1966	Milton & Lane Brown	164	Intralesional vaccinia virus	V
1970	Hunter-Craig et al	165	Intralesional vaccinia virus	I-B
1973	Minton	166	Intralesional mumps virus, BCG	VI
1972	Cheema & Hersh	68	Intralesional activated lymphocytes	I-B
1973	Smith et al	63	Intralesional transfer factor	V
1975	Cunningham-Rundles et al	167	Intralesional C. parvum	V

malignant melanoma metastatic to the regional nodes has been reported from M. D. Anderson Hospital and Tumor Institute (IV) (73). An important difference, however, between this and the first study is that the UCLA group removed the lymph nodes prophylactically for staging, while at M. D. Anderson lymph node dissection was not done until the nodes were clinically positive. This means in this study immunotherapy was introduced later in the course of the disease in some patients. The treatment group was randomized to receive different doses of BCG. Results were compared to historical controls treated at M. D. Anderson by operation alone. This study showed that the number of recurrences was the same in the treatment and control groups, but those patients receiving high-dose BCG (6×10^8 viable organisms) had a longer disease-free interval and a longer survival ($P = .002$). Low-dose BCG (6×10^7 viable organisms) had essentially no effect on the course of the disease, which suggests a dose relation to immunostimulation. This dose dependence has been observed in experimental animal studies (18). A similar adjuvant study from Sloan-Kettering (New York) in which immunotherapy was introduced after resection of clinically involved regional nodes showed no difference in recurrence rate between treatment and control groups and no increase in survival rate in the immunotherapy group at two years follow-up (VII) (168). These investigators used a lower dose of BCG (4–6×10^7 organisms) however. Each of these studies suggest that the dose of BCG may be critical to the success of the treatment.

In the adjuvant study from M. D. Anderson, results showed no benefit from BCG therapy for patients with malignant melanoma of the head and neck (73). These investigators thought that their lack of success might be due to failure of the BCG to reach appropriate regional lymphatics of the head and neck. A report from UCLA indicated a trend in favor of BCG therapy for reducing the number of recurrences following surgery for head and neck melanoma, but this difference was not statistically significant (IV) (169). However, there was a significant increase in the disease-free interval (from four to 15 months) for immunotherapy patients over those treated by surgery alone ($P < .001$), and length of survival also was significantly increased ($P < .05$).

The potential usefulness of adjuvant immunotherapy for malignant melanoma makes it imperative that its efficacy be established with certainty. Evidence must come from well-conducted, prospective, randomized trials. The other adjuvant studies listed in Table 12 are either preliminary work, uncontrolled studies, or they compare results to historical controls obtained from other published series.

COMBINATION CHEMO-IMMUNOTHERAPY   For the treatment of disseminated malignant melanoma, nonspecific immunostimulation has been added to chemotherapy (Table 13). Gutterman and colleagues (179) reported a controlled trial using combined dimethyl-triazeno imidazole carboxamide (DTIC) and intradermal BCG vs DTIC alone (historical controls were treated by the same group of investigators at M. D. Anderson) (III). The overall response rate was 27%

Table 12   Malignant melanoma

Year	Investigator(s)	Ref.	Adjuvant immunotherapy following surgery	Type of study
1972	Bluming et al	170	Intradermal BCG	VI
1972	Ikonopisov	171	Tumor cells, intralesional BCG	VI
1973	Gutterman et al	172	Intradermal BCG	VI
1974	Morton et al	153	Intradermal BCG	VI
1975	Serrou et al	173	Tumor cells, intradermal BCG	VI
1975	MacGregor et al	174	Oral BCG	VI
1975	Thompson	175	Intradermal BCG	VI
1976	Karakousis et al	154	Intradermal BCG	VI
1976	Jewell et al	52	Exchange of tumors and leukocytes	VI
1976	Gutterman et al	73	Intradermal BCG	IV
1976	Eilber et al	45	Intradermal BCG	III
1976	Eilber et al	169	Intradermal BCG, head and neck	IV
1976	Gerner & Moore	152	Intradermal BCG, PPD, tumor cells	VI
1977	Cunningham et al	176	Intradermal BCG, DTIC	VI
1977	Pinsky et al	168	Intradermal BCG	VII
1977	Beretta	177	Intradermal BCG, DTIC	VI
1977	Spitler et al	178	Levamisole	VI

(6% complete responses) for combination therapy compared to 14% for DTIC alone. In patients without visceral metastases, the response rate was 55% with combination therapy vs 18% for drug only ($P = .025$). Overall, the duration of remission and length of survival was increased with chemo-immunotherapy over chemotherapy alone ($P = .05$). In another study a good response rate was obtained with DTIC and vincristine plus intradermal BCG and radiated allogeneic melanoma cells, but the data reported were preliminary and therapeutic benefit could not be evaluated (VI) (180).

Table 13   Malignant melanoma

Year	Investigator(s)	Ref.	Combination chemo-immunotherapy for disseminated disease	Type of study
1974	Gutterman et al	179	DTIC, intradermal BCG	III
1975	Currie & McElwain	180	DTIC, vincristine, BCG	VI
1975	Israel & Edelstein	33	Five-drug therapy, *C. parvum*	VI
1976	Gutterman et al	182	DTIC, MeCCNU, BCG	IV
1976	Newlands et al	181	DTIC, ICRF 159, BCG	VII
1977	Costanzi	183	Triple-drug chemotherapy, BCG	VII
1977	Mastrangelo et al	184	MeCCNU, vincristine, BCG	VII
1977	Presant et al	185	Cytoxan, DTIC, *C. parvum*	VII

A randomized, controlled trial comparing DTIC, 1,2-d:(3,5 dioxopiperazin-1-yl)propane (ICRF 159) plus intradermal BCG and radiated allogeneic melanoma cells has been reported (VII) (181). This study included patients with disseminated disease and those with only regional lymph node metastases. This latter group would be treated surgically in many centers. For disseminated disease, there was no statistically significant difference between chemo-immunotherapy and drugs alone. However, the number of patients in the trial was relatively small for detection of subtle differences. Investigators from M. D. Anderson Hospital and Tumor Institute reported that the addition of (1-(2-chloroethyl)-3-4-methylcyclohexyl)-1 nitrosourea (MeCCNU) to the DTIC-BCG combination gave results equal to the previous trial with DTIC-BCG, but no better (IV) (182).

A prospective, randomized trial comparing 1,3-bis(2-chloroethyl)-1-nitrosourea (BCNU), hydroxyurea, and DTIC with or without BCG to the DTIC-BCG combination has been reported (VII) (183). The response rate was better with the triple-drug therapy than with the DTIC-BCG combination; 28% vs 20%, respectively. Otherwise, survival rate was the same. The addition of BCG did not improve the results of triple-drug therapy. In a similar trial, the addition of BCG did not improve results obtained from MeCCNU and vincristine (VII) (184).

The addition of *C. parvum* to combination chemotherapy for patients with disseminated malignant melanoma has been reported to improve survival time (VI) (33). These results were from a nonrandomized trial, however. A recent prospective, randomized trial did not show benefit from intravenous *C. parvum* in this situation (185). Overall, the treatment for disseminated malignant melanoma is unsatisfactory. The role of immunotherapy given in combination with chemotherapy is uncertain, and the chemotherapy itself is relatively ineffective for this disease.

OTHER MELANOMA STUDIES   Passive immunotherapy has been used to treat malignant melanoma with some success (Table 14). Sumner & Foraker (49) transfused whole blood from a patient with malignant melanoma who had undergone complete spontaneous regression to two other melanoma patients (VI). One patient developed complete regression of his disease following transfusion. The adoptive transfer of specifically sensitized, immunocompetent cells has been tested extensively in clinical trials (186–188, 50, 52). The procedure involves matching patients with similar tumors, and then cross transplanting the tumor cells. Leukocyte transfusions are then exchanged between the partners. The overall response rate in patients with disseminated melanoma is about 20%. Nadler & Moore (50) reported two long-lasting complete regressions of melanoma in 86 patients (V). Krementz (51) reported responses in nine of 56 melanoma patients; three responses were complete for one year to over four years (V). Transfusion incompatibilities have been responsible for some patient deaths with this treatment modality.

Transfer factor has been tested for disseminated malignant melanoma in an effort to avoid some of the problems associated with exchange of intact cells. A recent report by Jewell and associates (52) indicated complete responses in three of nine patients receiving transfer factor from sensitized donors (V). In an earlier report, Spitler (189) reported one complete regression in four melanoma patients treated with transfer factor (VI). In the other studies with transfer factor, there was either no benefit or the therapeutic benefit could not be evaluated from the data given (190–192, 51). In another study (60), xenogeneic immune RNA was used for malignant melanoma, but was of limited benefit (VI). Fifteen patients with advanced melanoma showed no regressions in response to the treatment. Metastatic disease in some of the patients appeared to stabilize for a period of time but eventually progressed.

Active-specific immunotherapy consisting of tumor cell vaccines has not clearly shown benefit in the treatment of malignant melanoma (187, 193, 194). However, specific immunotherapy should be helpful since melanomas appear to have distinct, tumor-associated antigens, and immune responses to these antigens have been clearly demonstrated (7). Clinical trials of BCG combined with allogeneic tumor cell vaccine as an adjuvant to surgical resection of regional disease are in progress. Preliminary results show that patients receiving tumor cell vaccine increase their antimelanoma antibody titer more than those receiving BCG only or no additional treatment (K. Irie, personal communication,

Table 14 Malignant melanoma

Year	Investigator(s)	Ref.	Immunotherapy for established disease	Type of study
1960	Sumner & Foraker	49	Transfusion whole blood	VI
1969	Nadler & Moore	50	Exchange of tumors and leukocytes	V
1971	Curtis	186	Exchange of tumors and leukocytes	VI
1971	Krementz et al	187	Exchange of tumors and leukocytes	V
1973	Goodwin et al	188	Exchange of tumors and leukocytes	VI
1974	Krementz et al	51	Exchange of tumors and leukocytes	V
1976	Jewell et al	52	Exchange of tumors and leukocytes	V
1971	Krementz et al	187	Tumor cell vaccine	VI
1973	Seigler et al	193	Neuraminidase treated cells, BCG	VI
1974	Levy et al	194	Neuraminidase treated cells, BCG	VI
1971	Brandes et al	190	Transfer factor	VI
1972	Spitler et al	189	Transfer factor	VI
1973	Morse et al	191	Transfer factor	VI
1974	Krementz et al	51	Transfer factor	VI
1974	Price et al	192	Transfer factor	VI
1976	Jewell et al	52	Transfer factor	V
1977	Ramming et al	60	Xenogeneic immune RNA	VI
1972	Ghose et al	195	Chlorambucil-carrying antibody	VI
1973	Falk et al	196	Oral BCG	VI
1975	MacGregor et al	174	Oral BCG	VI

1977). The increase in antimelanoma antibody titer correlates very well with one year survival. Irrespective of the role of antibodies in controlling tumor, their presence indicates that specific responses may be important to the success of immunotherapy. It is possible that combinations of specific immunotherapy, nonspecific immunostimulation and potent drug therapy could improve the treatment of disseminated disease. At least, in certain situations, immunotherapy for malignant melanoma offers promise but much improvement and investigation are still needed.

Sarcomas

Osteosarcomas are aggressive tumors that cause death from pulmonary metastases, despite adequate surgical control of the primary tumor (Table 15). Sarcomas carry well-defined, tumor-associated antigens, and stimulate immune responses in their autochthonous hosts (197). An early report by Marcove and associates (198) suggested that active immunization with lysed sarcoma cells was helpful in prolonging the disease-free interval following surgery for osteosarcoma (VI). These were preliminary results, however, and the study was uncontrolled. In another adjuvant study reported by Marsh and co-workers (199), tumor removed at the time of amputation was transplanted to another patient with osteosarcoma (VI). The tumor-implant recipient's lymphocytes were then transfused to the tumor-implant donor. Preliminary data, again, were suggestive of benefit, but a follow-up report on 32 patients treated in this fashion

Table 15   Sarcomas

Year	Investigator(s)	Ref.	Tumor Type	Immunotherapy	Type of study
1971	Marcove et al	198	Osteosarcoma	Tumor cell vaccine	VI
1972	Marsh et al	199	Osteosarcoma	Exchange of tumor and lymphocytes	VI
1975	Neff & Enneking	200	Osteosarcoma	Exchange of tumor and lymphocytes	VII
1975	Eilber et al	201	Osteosarcoma	BCG, tumor cell vaccine	VII
1975	Levin et al	55	Osteosarcoma	Transfer factor	VI
1976	LoBuglio & Neidhart	56	Osteosarcoma	Transfer factor	VI
1976	Green et al	208	Osteosarcoma	Viral oncolysates	VI
1977	Ritts et al	203	Osteosarcoma	Transfer factor	VI
1970	Morton et al	205	Mixed	BCG, tumor cell vaccine	VI
1971	Morton et al	206	Mixed	BCG, tumor cell vaccine	VI
1973	LoBuglio et al	204	Alveolar soft part	Transfer factor	VI
1974	Gunnarson et al	209	Mixed	Chemotherapy, C. parvum	VI
1976	Townsend et al	47	Soft tissue	BCG, tumor cell vaccine	VI
1977	Sinkovics	207	Mixed	BCG, viral oncolysates, chemotherapy	VI

by Neff & Enneking (200) indicated that the number of recurrences and the length of disease-free interval were the same as in a group of historical controls treated by surgery alone (VII). A controlled trial of adjuvant immunotherapy consisting of BCG and allogeneic sarcoma cells following surgery for osteosarcoma was reported by Eilber and colleagues (201). In this study, adjuvant immunotherapy did not decrease recurrence or increase survival time, even in Stage I disease. As a group, these papers suggest that active immunization and/ or BCG as the only adjuvant to surgery do not help the osteosarcoma patients.

A report by Levin and colleagues (55) dealt with the use of transfer factor (TF) for osteosarcoma (VI). TF, obtained from the lymphocytes of relatives and household contacts, showed in vitro activity against the osteosarcoma patient's tumor. Six patients treated with TF after amputation for osteosarcoma (no metastases were noted at the time of surgery), were alive and free of disease 9–26 months after operation (median, 14 months). LoBuglio & Neidhart (56) reported an uncontrolled trial with five patients receiving TF as an adjunct to surgical resection for osteosarcoma (VI). Two patients recurred at 4 and 12 months; three were disease-free at 7, 8, and 12 months. For comparison, Eilber (201) reported a median recurrence time after operation of 3.1 months. This longer disease-free interval with TF is promising, but adjuvant studies cannot be evaluated in the absence of controls. A report from the Mayo Clinic suggested that there has been an improvement in survival from osteosarcoma unrelated to any therapeutic modality. This finding underscores the need for concomitant controls in testing any new agents (202). An interim report from a trial comparing TF with methotrexate, adriamycin, and vincristine given as adjuvant therapy following operation for osteosarcoma has appeared (VI) (203). No clear difference existed between the two groups at 20 months follow-up.

Osteosarcoma, even Stage I, has a dismal prognosis. These tumors grow so rapidly that the tumor burden from occult metastases may be too great even in the subclinical state for host resistance to have any effect. Potent cytoreductive therapy to lower tumor burden is essential with this type of cancer. Drugs with high activity against osteosarcoma are available, and, when given as adjuvant to surgical procedures, appear to reduce recurrences and increase survival time. Immunotherapy might be useful in maintaining remission in conjunction with the drugs or beyond the period of adjuvant chemotherapy. LoBuglio & Neidhart (56) mentioned two patients with metastatic disease whose tumors regressed on adriamycin and DTIC, and who remained in remission for 11 and 28 months on maintenance therapy with TF.

Immunotherapy has been used in the treatment of various soft-tissue sarcomas (VI) (205, 206, 47). Following surgical removal of the tumor, the patients in the latest study received either BCG plus allogeneic sarcoma cells or no additional treatment. Follow-up was two years. For Stages I and II disease, there were fewer recurrences in patients receiving immunotherapy. In this group, 61% of the patients remained free of disease vs 33% of those treated by operation alone. In those who recurred, the median disease-free interval was 12 months for the immunotherapy group, and six months for those treated by operation alone. These figures were not statistically significant, however. Immunotherapy did not benefit those with more advanced disease. Potent cytoreductive therapy is equally important for soft-tissue sarcomas. Adjuvant chemotherapy has come into use for soft-tissue sarcomas as well, and clinical trials combining immunotherapy with chemotherapy are in progress.

Immunotherapy has been used for the treatment of disseminated sarcomas. LoBuglio and associates (204) treated a patient with metastatic alveolar soft-part sarcoma with TF obtained from his twin brother (VI). The tumor did not progress during the period of treatment, although other factors also may have contributed to the remission. Israel & Edelstein (33) combined subcutaneous *C. parvum* with five-drug chemotherapy for treatment of disseminated, nonlymphomatous sarcomas in a randomized trial (II). Median survival time was longer by several months in the *C. parvum* chemo-immunotherapy group than in those receiving drugs alone ($P. < .03$). There have been no other studies to confirm this result. Sinkovics (207) recently noted (in a preliminary report) that the addition of viral oncolysate to BCG and chemotherapy for the treatment of disseminated sarcomas improved the response rate (VI). The use of viral oncolysates alone had no effect in 12 patients with disseminated osteosarcoma (VI) (208).

The marked antigenicity of sarcomas, combined with the ready demonstration of immune responses to tumor in sarcoma patients, suggests that immunotherapy should be helpful. However, such a role has yet to be defined.

Skin Carcinoma

Klein (13, 210) reported that skin cancers could be eradicated with local immunotherapy, and provided part of the stimulus for the current interest in immunotherapy for malignant disease (Table 16). He described the induction of local DCH responses by various agents to eliminate a high percentage of treated lesions. This included patients with multiple, superficial, basal cell carcinomas, squamous cell carcinomas in situ, premalignant keratoses, and leukoplakia. Elimination of these lesions was accomplished without systemic toxicity or damage to normal skin.

Table 16 Carcinoma of the Skin

Year	Investigator(s)	Ref.	Immunotherapy	Type of study
1968	Klein	13	Topical TEIB or DNCB	I-A
1969	Klein	210	Topical TEIB or DNCB	I-A
1970	Williams & Klein	212	Topical 5-FU	I-A
1971	Stjernsward & Levin	67	Topical DNCB	I-A
1973	Levis et al	211	Topical DNCB	I-A
1976	Raaf et al	213	Topical DNCB and 5-FU	VI
1976	Klein et al	64	Various topical and intralesional agents	I-A

For the treatment of basal cell carcinomas, Klein sensitized five patients to TEIB (2,3,5-triethylene imino-1,4-benzoquinone). TEIB was then applied topically to multiple, superficial basal cell carcinomas. He reported a 95% success rate for these lesions (I-A) (13, 210). This claim was supported by a description of a dramatic result in a single patient with 140 lesions. The individual response rate in other patients, or the number of individual lesions treated, was not described, so expectations for individual patients were not clear. Levis and colleagues (211) reported a much lower success rate for treatment of basal cell carcinomas (I-A). They used DNCB topically to treat five patients with 113 lesions, and found that only 32% of the lesions completely regressed. An additional 29% showed partial regression. Another patient, not included in their data, had uncountable lesions but obtained a good response to DNCB treatment. Individual response rates for complete regression varied from 22 to 70% of the lesions. They were treating both superficial and nodular basal cell disease, and the response was equal for both, but nodular lesions measuring greater than 5 mm did not respond. Stjernsward & Levin (67) reported that at least one basal cell carcinoma regressed completely in eight of nine patients treated with topical DNCB (I-A). They observed, however, that not all lesions responded, and they did not give the actual number of lesions treated or the overall response rate. For comparison, Williams & Klein (212) have reported that topical 5-flourouracil (5-FU) produced resolution of 56% of nodular basal cell carcinomas (I-A). This result is inferior to surgical excision. Thus, for patients with multiple lesions that are not suitable for conventional therapy, local immunotherapy may be tried. However, for single or large lesions, excision is the treatment of choice.

Klein (13, 210) has used topical immunotherapy for treating superficial squamous cell carcinomas in patients with xeroderma pigmentosum and arsenical dermatitis (I-A). Again, he reports a high success rate (90%) in eradicating these lesions. Seven patients with xeroderma pigmentosum and six patients with arsenical dermatitis were treated with either topical TEIB or DNCB. No analysis of the data or breakdown for individual patients was given. He observed that this high success rate was limited to superficial lesions. Deeper or recurrent lesions responded less well, although benefit could be obtained by the addition of topical 5-FU. Topical 5-FU alone reportedly eliminated 80% of superficial squamous cell carcinomas (I-A) (212). However, this treatment also had a lower success rate for deeper lesions. In xeroderma pigmentosum, the appearance of new lesions seemed to decrease with topical immunotherapy. Raaf and colleagues (213) reported a single case in which topical DNCB was combined with topical 5-FU for treating a large, squamous cell carcinoma resulting from arsenic exposure (VI). This lesion was refractory to DNCB alone, but regressed completely with both agents. In this patient, 60 smaller lesions regressed completely with topical DNCB alone. Klein, too, advocates the combined treatment.

According to Klein, certain types of premalignant skin lesions can be eliminated by topical immunotherapy. This treatment caused 95% of multiple solar keratoses in 18 patients to completely resolve (13, 210). Arsenical keratoses were refractory to treatment, however, and did not respond. In 14 patients with leukoplakia, good initial responses could be obtained, but the lesions recurred in four to six weeks. Repeated treatment reduced the incidence of recurrence, but Klein gave no data on individual patients.

Thus, for malignant and premalignant lesions of the skin, high success rates have been reported for topical immunotherapy. However, the published reports have emphasized the dramatic successes, and given little data on which to base expectations for individual patients. The study by Levis and colleagues is an exception. Nevertheless, topical immunotherapy appears to be a useful tool for treating superficial skin malignancies and is well worth a trial when conventional treatment is not suitable.

Miscellaneous Advanced Cancers

In clinical trials where immunotherapeutic agents have been tested against a variety of advanced cancers, the results generally have not been striking. However, many of these studies (Table 17) represent interesting techniques or concepts, and some good responses have been obtained. When nonspecific immunostimulation with BCG was added to chemotherapy, Villasor (214) re-

Table 17 Miscellaneous advanced cancers

Year	Investigator(s)	Ref.	Immunotherapy	Type of study
Nonspecific immunostimulation				
1965	Villasor	214	BCG, chemotherapy	VI
1974	Asada	215	Mumps virus	VI
1975	Israel & Edelstein	216	C. parvum	V
Active specific immunostimulation				
1964	Aswaq et al	217	Autologous tumor cell vaccine, complete Freund's adjuvant (CFA)	VI
1967	Czajkowski et al	219	Autologous tumor coupled with rabbit γ-globulin	VI
1969	Cunningham et al	220	Autologous tumor coupled with rabbit γ-globulin	VI
1970	Hughes et al	218	Tumor extract, CFA	VI
1972	Humphrey et al	221	Tumor homogenate	V
1977	Wallack et al	222	Vaccinia tumor cell oncolysate	V
Passive transfer immunotherapy				
1960	Finney et al	223	IM and intralesional injections plasma fractions	VI
1963	Woodruff & Nolan	224	Adoptive transfer spleen cells	VI
1967	Andrews et al	225	Exchange of tumors and TD lymphocytes	VI
1972	Yonemoto & Terasaki	226	Thoracic duct lymphocytes	V
1973	Symes & Riddell	227	Intra-arterial pig lymph node cells	V
1976	Vetto et al	57	Transfer factor	V
1976	Frenster	228	PHA-activated autologous lymphocytes	VI

ported increased responses and survival rates over chemotherapy alone for advanced disease (VI). However, his data were not statistically significant. Asada (215) claimed very good results for advanced cancer using mumps virus inoculation (VI). The criteria for good response and the role of the mumps virus, apart from other treatments the patient received, were unclear, however.

Israel & Edelstein (216) treated advanced cancers that were refractory to other treatments with intravenous *C. parvum* (V). They obtained nine partial responses of 50% or greater in 33 patients. Length of response could not be evaluated because chemotherapy then was resumed in these patients. However, response was better than expected from nonspecific immunostimulation in the presence of established tumor.

Another group of studies dealt with active-specific immunostimulation for the treatment of advanced cancer. Aswaq and colleagues (217) administered autologous tumor cells in complete Freund's adjuvant, but obtained no objective responses (VI). Hughes and colleages (218) used a similar procedure and reported a 10% response rate in 21 patients with advanced disease (VI). Czajkowski and colleages (219) coupled autologous tumor cells to rabbit γ-globulin in an effort to increase immunogenicity of the cells. They reported two objective responses in 14 patients after administration of this vaccine (VI). With the same treatment, Cunningham and co-workers (220) obtained only one response in 35 patients (VI). Humphrey and colleagues (221 reported a 23% response rate in 96 patients following administration of tumor homogenate (V). Data regarding the extent or length of these responses were not given. Wallack and associates (222) used an autochthonous tumor cell vaccine lysed by vaccinia virus in 13 patients with various advanced cancers (V). They noted two short-term responses. In general, active-specific immunostimulation as the sole therapy for advanced malignant disease is of limited value.

The passive transfer of immunotherapeutic agents has been used to treat advanced disease. An early study by Finney and colleagues (223) tested intramuscular and intralesional injections of autologous plasma fractions (VI), but these were of limited benefit. The adoptive transfer of spleen cells from unrelated donors to patients with advanced cancer elicited no objective responses, as reported by Woodruff & Nolan (VI) (224). Andrews and colleagues (225) transferred tumors between patients with similar disease and then exchanged thoracic duct lymphocytes obtained from the partner (VI). They obtained no response in four patients. Yonemoto & Terasaki (226) administered thoracic duct lymphocytes obtained from HL-A–matched siblings to tumor patients (V). They reported two objective responses in six patients. An interesting technique was described by Symes & Riddell (227) in which pigs were sensitized to human tumors, then the pig lymphocytes were given to the tumor patient via the arterial distribution of the tumor (V). They obtained four objective responses in 14 patients. Vetto and colleagues (57) used transfer factor obtained from the cells of household contacts of tumor patients to treat advanced disease (V). Six objective responses were obtained in 35 patients; three of these responses were complete. Reinfusion of PHA-stimulated, autologous lymphocytes caused regression of pulmonary metastases in three of five patients with widespread metastatic tumor (VI) (228). However, metastases in other locations progressed and all of the patients succumbed to their disease.

While these studies represent unique approaches to the treatment of advanced tumors, they are logistically very difficult. Immunotherapy is of limited potency in dealing with advanced disease, and as the only treatment against established tumor, these approaches have been of low yield. However, they suggest possibilities that may be of value in combination with other treatment.

SUMMARY AND CONCLUSIONS

The bulk of clinical evidence indicates that immunotherapy is not a panacea for malignant disease, but then neither are other treatments now available. Because of its limited potency, immunotherapy is unlikely to become the primary treatment for any neoplasm except for those tumors accessible to topical or intralesional therapy. Immunotherapy depends on stimulation or augmentation of host defenses, which an established tumor has already overcome. Immunotherapy potentially can restore host defenses to a state that might have prevented the tumor in the first place, but it is not reasonable to expect more. The host has a capacity to deal with a limited number of cancer cells, but against gross established disease its defenses are limited.

Other treatments for cancer have limitations as well. Operation and radiation can control local disease, but fail to achieve cure because of microscopic systemic spread. Chemotherapy is potent and systemic in its effects, but kills tumor cells by first-order kinetics and may fail to eliminate the last tumor cell. Very little residual tumor is required to produce recurrence and death from most cancers. All of these treatment modalities have toxicities that occasion restraint in their use. Recognition of these limitations has resulted in a multimodality approach to cancer therapy, and in this setting a treatment that could selectively attack a small volume of tumor cells on a systemic basis would be very useful. The question at hand is whether immunotherapy can fill this role.

The most successful use of immunotherapy for malignant disease has been the intralesional injection of various agents to induce local DCH responses. Excellent control of local disease has been obtained in skin cancers and cutaneous metastases of malignant melanoma and breast carcinoma. However, it is not clear that this treatment improves survival, except for those long-term survivors who obtained dramatic control of regional malignant melanoma with BCG injections. Unfortunately, most patients go on to die of their disease. Whether there is destruction of systemic micrometastases, hence improved survival time following intralesional injection, has great import for the role of immunotherapy in cancer management. In experimental animals, intralesional injection of certain tumors confers systemic protection against subsequent tumor inocula (26). Following injection of melanoma in humans, there is a rise in antimelanoma antibody titer, and in some cases concomitant regression of uninjected lesions (12). This result indicates development of systemic resistance to tumor, but whether long-term control ensues is unanswered in human studies.

A direct extension of the question of improved survival time following intralesional injection is whether immunotherapy can be used to control microscopic residual disease following primary treatment for neoplasia. This is potentially the most useful area for immunotherapy, and there are several good, controlled studies outlined in this review that have shown benefit from such an approach. The most promising of these is the intrapleural injection of BCG following resection for early lung carcinoma (137, 140). Similary, repeated intradermal BCG treatment may benefit melanoma patients following resection of regional lymph node disease (45, 73). Levamisole seemed to help patients following radiation for advanced breast carcinoma and may have helped some patients after resection for lung carcinoma (39, 40). These studies are unconfirmed, but there are enough positive reports to lend credence to the hypothesis that immunotherapy results in systemic control of disease. It clearly warrants further investigation. A logical extension of adjuvant immunotherapy is to inject accessible tumors prior to surgical resection. This is currently under investigation for malignant melanoma and lung carcinoma.

Immunotherapy has been given in combination with chemotherapy for advanced malignant disease in an effort to increase the response and survival rates. For advanced breast cancer, both BCG and *C. parvum* have been added to chemotherapy with reportedly beneficial results (33, 73). As yet, these reports are unconfirmed, but no negative studies have appeared. In some controlled trials for acute myelogenous leukemia, the addition of immunotherapy to maintenance chemotherapy reportedly improves duration of remission and survival, but others have obtained negative results in the same setting. For disseminated melanoma, some investigators have claimed benefit for BCG added to chemotherapy, but there are several negative reports. The addition of MER or BCG to chemotherapy clearly does not improve results for advanced colon carcinoma. Overall, it seems that if chemotherapy produces a good response, which implies a marked lowering of tumor burden, immunotherapy seems to be additive. Otherwise, no effect is gained from the immunotherapy.

As the sole treatment for established tumors, immunotherapy plays a limited role. It may be considered if other alternatives have been exhausted. Some procedures have produced a few dramatic responses. A good example is cross transplantation of tumor and leukocyte exchange in patients with advanced melanoma. This has a fairly consistent response rate of about 15–20%, and has resulted in a few long-term regressions. This procedure involves the risk of severe transfusion reactions, however. These procedures are logistically difficult, potentially toxic, and help relatively few patients. However, these investigations do indicate that immunotherapy is not totally without effect against established disease.

In combination with other treatment modalities, immunotherapy appears to be effective against several types of human cancer, if the other modalities are able to reduce tumor burden to a low level. Any treatment that substantially lowers tumor burden is immunotherapy in the sense that it gives host defense mechanisms the opportunity to gain control of the disease. Immunotherapy is still an experimental treatment for cancer. However, there are enough good results from the clinical trials covered in this review to warrant continued investigation. There are many results, which, if confirmed in subsequent investigation, offer considerable benefit to selected patients.

There is much to be learned about the practical application of immunotherapy. The optimal dose and timing, as well as the route of administration, for most immunotherapeutic agents have not been fully determined. The short-term side effects have been documented, but long-term toxicities still must be defined. Enhancement of tumor growth has been seen in animal studies, and, while not conclusively demonstrated in humans, it is a potential problem. The brain is an immunologically privileged site and is where recurrence often appears. All of these problems have yet to be solved.

It would be helpful if these problems could be resolved in animal models. However, certain discrepancies exist between animal models and human cancer (229). Experimental animals are usually young, healthy, inbred adults. In contrast, the human tumor host is frequently very young or very old, and the population is genetically diverse. Experimental tumors are usually artificially induced, have a short latent period, rapid growth, and a relatively high immunogenicity. By comparison, human tumors arise spontaneously, have a long latent period, relatively slow growth, and a low immunogenicity. Animal models that more closely approximate the variability and unpredictability of human cancer must be developed. Because of the desperate nature of the disease, clinical investigators have been unwilling to wait for the development of these animal models before using a modality that is potentially beneficial for the cancer patient. At present, the well-conducted, carefully controlled, clinical trial is the major investigative tool for immunotherapy of human malignant disease.

Can the potency of immunotherapy be increased? The answer can only come from a full understanding of the mechanisms of tumor immunity and host defense against cancer. A variety of effector cells, and in some cases antibody, show activity against tumors in various assays. Knowing which effectors are the most important in vivo for tumor destruction, how they work, and what stimulates their production, might allow selective stimulation and augmentation of the most desirable response. Factors such as soluble tumor antigens and antigen-antibody complexes have been shown to retard host resistance to tumors. Finding ways to eliminate these adverse activities may result in a stronger antitumor response.

The development of accurate monitors of the effects of immunotherapy is an absolute necessity. As it stands now, the measure of effectiveness of immunotherapy in most situations is the maintenance of a disease-free state or increased survival time. Some patients do not benefit from the treatment or do not need it. There is a need for a test to identify the effects of immunotherapy, so that therapy that is not benefiting patients could be stopped or changed to an alternate form. Good monitoring would allow more rapid progress. An important side benefit from this research could be the ability to detect and follow early tumor growth.

Immunotherapy almost certainly has not reached its full potential, and many improvements are feasible. The results of these initial years of clinical investigation suggest that immunotherapy will have a role in the treatment of malignant disease. We are as Shakespeare's soothsayer described himself: "In nature's infinite book of secrecy, a little I can read." We only partially perceive the complex events involved in host resistance to cancer. Assuredly, progress will come as we learn to read more.

ACKNOWLEDGMENTS

This study was supported by USPHS grants CA12582, CA09010 awarded by the National Cancer Institute, DHEW: and the Medical Research Service of the Veterans Administration.

Literature Cited

1. Everson, T. C., Cole, W. H. 1966. *Spontaneous Regression of Cancer,* Philadelphia: Saunders
2. Foley, E. J. 1953. Antigenic properties of methylcholanthrene-induced tumors in mice of the strain of origin. *Cancer Res.* 13:835–37
3. Prehn, R. T., Main, J. M. 1957. Immunity to Methylcholanthrene-induced sarcomas. *J. Natl. Cancer Inst.* 18:769–78
4. Old, L. J., Boyse, E. A., Clark, D. A., Carswell, E. A. 1962. Antigenic properties of chemically-induced tumors. *Ann. NY Acad. Sci.* 101:80–106
5. Klein, G., Clifford, P., Klein, E., Stjernsward, J. 1966. Search for tumor-specific immune reactions in Burkitt lymphoma patients by the membrane immunoflourescence reaction. *Proc. Natl. Acad. Sci. USA* 55:1628–35
6. Hellstrom, I., Hellstrom, K. E., Pierce, G. E., Bill, A. H. 1968. Demonstration of cell bound and humoral immunity against neuroblastoma cells. *Proc. Natl. Acad. Sci. USA* 60:1231–38
7. Morton, D. L., Malmgren, R. A., Holmes, E. C., Ketcham, A. S. 1968. Demonstration of antibodies against human malignant melanoma by immunofluorescence. *Surgery* 64:233–40
8. Windhorst, D. 1976. The International Registry of Tumor Immunotherapy. *Med. Clin. North Am.* 60:641–48
9. Nauts, H. C., Fowler, G. A., Bogatko, F. H. 1953. A review of the influence of bacterial infection and of bacterial products (Coley's toxins) on malignant tumours in man. *Acta Med. Scand.* S276:1–103
10. Klein, G., Sjogren, H. O., Klein, E., Hellstrom, K. E. 1960. Demonstration of resistance against methylcholanthrene-induced sarcomas in the primary autochthonous host. *Cancer Res.* 20:1561–72
11. Mathe, G., Amiel, J. L., Schwarzenberg, L., Schneider, M., Cattan, A., Schlumberger, J. R., Hayat, M., De Vassal, F. 1969. Active immunotherapy for acute lymphoblastic leukemia. *Lancet* 1:697–99
12. Morton, D. L., Eilber, F. R., Malmgren, R. A., Wood, W. C. 1970. Immunological factors which influence response to immunotherapy in malignant melanoma. *Surgery* 68:158–64
13. Klein, E. 1968. Tumors of the skin. X. Immunotherapy of cutaneous and mucosal neoplasms. *NY State J. Med.* 68:900–11
14. Southam, C. M. 1967. Evidence for cancer-specific antigens in man. *Prog. Exp. Tumor Res.* 9:1–39
15. Hibbs, J. B., Lambert, L. J., Remington, J. S. 1972. Possible role of macrophage mediated nonspecific cytotoxicity in tumour resistance. *Nature New Biol.* 235:48–50
16. Alexander, P. 1976. The functions of the macrophage in malignant disease. *Ann. Rev. Med.* 27:207–24
17. Perlmann, P., Perlmann, H., Wigzell, H. 1972. Lymphocyte-mediated cytotoxicity *in vitro:* induction and inhibition by humoral antibodies and nature of effector cells. *Transplant Rev.* 13:91–116
18. Bast, R. C., Zbar, B., Borsos, T., Rapp, H. J. 1974. BCG and cancer (first of two parts). *N. Engl. J. Med.* 290:1413–20
19. Bast, R. C., Zbar, B., Borsos, T.,

Rapp, H. J. 1974. BCG and cancer (second of two parts). *N. Engl. J. Med.* 290:1458–69

20. Pilch, Y. H., Meyers, G. H. Jr., Sparks, F. C., Golub, S. H. 1975. In *Current Problems in Surgery,* ed. M. M. Ravitch, pp. 1–46, Chicago: Yearb. Med.

21. Golub, S. H. 1975. In *Cancer–A Comprehensive Treatise,* ed. F. F. Becker, Vol. 4, pp. 259–300. New York: Plenum

22. Zbar, B., Ribi, E., Kelly, M., Granger, D., Evans, C., Rapp, H. J. 1976. Immunologic approaches to the treatment of human cancer based on a guinea pig model. *Cancer Immunol. Immunother.* 1:127–37

23. Calmette, A. 1936. In *L'Infection Bacillaire et al Tuberculose Chez l'Homme et Chez l'Animaux,* p. 752. Paris: Masson

24. Nathanson, L., 1974. Use of BCG in the treatment of human neoplasms: a review. *Semin. Oncol.* 1:337–50

25. Klein, E., Klein, G. 1972. Specificity of homograft rejection *in vivo* assessed by inoculation of artificially mixed compatible and incompatible tumor cells. *Cell. Immunol.* 5:201–8

26. Hanna, M. G. Jr. 1974. Immunologic aspects of BCG mediated regression of established tumors and metastases in guinea pigs. *Semin. Oncol.* 1:319–35

27. Sparks, F. C., Silverstein, M. J., Hunt, J. S., Haskell, C. M., Pilch, Y. H., Morton, D. L. 1973. Complications of BCG immunotherapy in patients with cancer. *N. Engl. J. Med.* 289:827–30

28. Halpern, B. M., Biozzi, G., Stiffel, C., Mouton, D. 1966. Inhibition of tumor growth by administration of killed *Corynebacterium parvum.* *Nature New Biol.* 212:853–54

29. Woodruff, M. F. A., Boak, J. L. 1966. Inhibitory effect of injection of *Corynebacterium parvum* on the growth of tumour transplants in isogenic hosts. *Br. J. Cancer* 20:345–55

30. Milas, L., Hunter, N., Basic, I., Withers, H. R. 1974. Complete regressions of an established murine fibrosarcoma induced by systemic application of *Corynebacterium granulosum. Cancer Res.* 34:2470–75

31. Woodruff, M. F. A., Dunbar, N., Ghaffar, A. 1973. The growth of tumors in T-cell deprived mice and their response to treatment with *Corynebacterium parvum. Proc. R. Soc. London Ser. B.* 184:97–102

32. Oettgen, H. F., Pinsky, C. M., Delmonte, L. 1976. Treatment of cancer with immunomodulators. *Med. Clin. North Am.* 60:511–37

33. Israel, L., Edelstein, R. 1975. In *Immunological Aspects of Neoplasia,* pp. 485–504. Baltimore: Williams & Wilkins

34. Fisher, B., Rubin, H., Sartiano, G., Ennis, L., Wolmark, N. 1976. Observations following *Corynebacterium parvum* administration to patients with advanced malignancy: a phase I study. *Cancer* 38:119–30

35. Renoux, G., Renoux, M. 1973. Stimulation of anti-Brucella vaccination in mice by tetramisole, a phenylimidothiazole salt. *Infect. Immun.* 8:544–48

36. Tripodi, D., Parks, L. C., Brugmans, J. 1973. Drug-induced restoration of cutaneous delayed hypersensitivity in anergic patients with cancer. *N. Engl. J. Med.* 289:354–57

37. Brugmans, J., Schuermans, V., De Cock, W., Theinpont, D., Janssen, P., Verhaegen, H., Van Nimmen, L., Louwagie, A. C., Steven, E. 1973. Restoration of host defense mechanisms in man by levamisole. *Life Sci.* 13:1499–1504

38. Hoebeke, J., Franchi, G. 1973. Influence of tetramisole and its optical isomers on the mononuclear phagtocytic system. Effect on carbon clearance in mice. *J. Reticuloendothel. Soc.* 14:317–23

39. Rojas, A. F., Feierstein, J. N., Mickiewicz, E., Glait, H., Olivari, A. J. 1976. Levamisole in advanced human breast cancer. *Lancet* 1:211–15

40. Amery, W., Swierenga, J., Gooszen, H. C., Vanderschueren, R. G., Cosermans, J., Louwagie, A., Stam, J., Veldhuizen, R. W., Lopes Cordozo, E. 1975. Immunopotentiation with levamisole in resectable bronchogenic carcinoma: a double-blind controlled trial. *Br. Med. J.* 3:461–64

41. Ruuskanen, O., Remes, M., Makela, A. L., Isomaki, H., Toivanen, A. 1976. Levamisole and agranulocytosis. *Lancet* 2:958–59

42. Holland, J. F., Bekesi, J. G. 1976. Immunotherapy of human leukemia with neuraminidase-modified cells. *Med. Clin. North Am.* 60:539–49

43. Gillette, R. W., Boone, C. W. 1976. Augmented immunogenicity of tumor cell membranes produced by surface budding viruses: parameters of optimal immunization. *Int. J. Cancer* 18:216–22

44. Takita, H., Brugarolas, A. 1973. Adjuvant immunotherapy for bronchogenic carcinoma: preliminary results. *Cancer Chemother. Rep. Part 3* 4:293–98

45. Eilber, F. R., Morton, D. L., Holmes, E. C., Sparks, F. C., Ramming, K. P. 1976. Adjuvant immunotherapy with BCG in treatment of regional lymph node metastases from malignant melanoma. *N. Engl. J. Med.* 294:237–40

46. Sparks, F. C., Wile, A. G., Ramming, K. P., Silver, H. K. B., Wolk, R. W., Morton, D. L. 1976. Immunology and adjuvant chemoimmunotherapy of breast cancer. *Arch. Surg.* 111:1057–62

47. Townsend, C. M. Jr., Eilber, F. R., Morton, D. L. 1976. Skeletal and soft tissue sarcomas: treatment with adjuvant immunotherapy. *J. Am. Med. Assoc.* 236:2187–89

48. Morton, D. L. 1973. Horizons in tumor immunology.*Surgery* 74:69–79

49. Sumner, W. C., Foraker, A. G. 1960. Spontaneous regression of human melanoma: clinical and experimental studies. *Cancer* 13:79–81

50. Nadler, S. H., Moore, G. E. 1969. Immunotherapy of malignant disease. *Arch. Surg.* 99:376–81

51. Krementz, E. T., Mansell, P. W. A., Hornung, M. O., Samuels, M. S., Sutherland, C. A., Benes, E. N. 1974. Immunotherapy of malignant disease: the use of viable sensitized lymphocytes or transfer factor prepared from sensitized lymphocytes. *Cancer* 33:394–401

52. Jewell, W. R., Thomas, J. H., Sterchi, J. M., Morse, P. A., Humphrey, L. J. 1976. Critical analysis of treatment of stage II and stage III melanoma patients with immunotherapy. *Ann. Surg.* 183:543–49

53. Wright, P. W., Hellstrom, K. E., Hellstrom, I., Bernstein, I. D. 1976. Serotherapy of malignant disease. *Med. Clin. North Am.* 60:607–22

54. Lawrence, H. S., 1969. Transfer factor. *Adv. Immunol.* 11:195–266

55. Levin, A. S., Byers, V. S., Fudenberg, H. H., Wybran, J., Hackett, A. J., Johnston, J. O., Spitler, L. E. 1975. Osteogenic sarcoma: immunologic parameters before and during immunotherapy with tumor-specific transfer factor. *J. Clin. Invest.* 55:487–99

56. LoBuglio, A. F., Neidhart, J. A. 1976. Transfer factor: a potential agent for cancer therapy. *Med. Clin. North Am.* 60:585–90

57. Vetto, R. M., Burger, D. R., Nolte, J. E., Vandenbark, A. A., Baker, H. W. 1976. Transfer factor therapy in patients with cancer. *Cancer* 37:90–97

58. Mannick, J. A., Egdahl, R. H. 1962. Transformation of nonimmune lymph node cells to state of transplantation immunity by RNA: a preliminary report. *Ann. Surg.* 156:356–66

59. Pilch, Y. H., Fritze, D., Kern, D. 1976. Immune RNA in the immunotherapy of cancer. *Med. Clin. North Am.* 60:567–83

60. Ramming, K. P., deKernion, J. B., Pilch, Y. H. 1977. In *Handbook of Cancer and Immunology,* ed. H. Waters, Washington: Smithsonian Inst. Press. In press

61. Trouillas, P., Lapras, C. 1969. Cellular immunotherapy of cerebral neurospongioma. *J. Med. Lyon* 1172:1269–91

62. Bloom, H. J. G., Peckham, M. J., Richardson, A. E., Alexander, P. A., Payne, P. M. 1973. Glioblastoma multiforme: A controlled trial to assess the value of specific active immunotherapy in patients treated by radical surgery and radiotherapy. *Br. J. Cancer* 27:253–67

63. Smith, G. V., Morse, P. A., Deraps, G. D., Raju, S., Hardy, J. D. 1973. Immunotherapy of patients with cancer. *Surgery* 74:59–68

64. Klein, E., Holtermann, O., Milgrom, H., Case, R. W., Klein, D., Rosner, D., Djerassi, I. 1976. Immunotherapy for accessible tumors utilizing delayed hypersensitivity reactions and separated components of the immune system. *Med. Clin. North Am.* 60:389–418

65. Garas, J., Besbeas, S., Papamatheakis, J., Gropas, G., Maragoudakis, S., Katsenis, A.,

Kiparissiadis, P., Konstadakos, P., Georgaka, A. 1975. Attempt with immunotherapy to control metastatic skin nodules from breast cancer by BCG. *Panminerva Med.* 17:193–95

66. Goldman, L. I. 1975. Immunotherapy of solid tumors. I. Preliminary studies with nitrogen mustard for nonspecific immunopotentiation in human cancer. *J. Surg. Res.* 18: 513–21

67. Stjernsward, J., Levin, A. 1971. Delayed hypersensitivity-induced regression of human neoplasms. *Cancer* 28: 628–40

68. Cheema, A. R., Hersh, E. M. 1972. Local tumor immunotherapy with *in vitro* autochthonous lymphocytes. *Cancer* 29:982–86

69. Copeland, M., ed. 1973. *Clinical staging system for carcinoma of the breast.* Chicago: Am. J. Comm. Cancer Staging End Results Rep., September

70. Anderson, J. M., Kelly, F., Wood, S. E., Halnan, K. E. 1974. Stimulatory immunotherapy in mammary cancer. *Br. J. Surg.* 61:778–84

71. Bonadonna, G., Brusamolino, E., Valagussa, P., Rossi, A., Brugnatelli, L., Brambilla, C., De Lena, M., Tancini, G., Bajetta, E., Musumeci, R., Veronesi, U. 1976. Combination chemotherapy as an adjuvant treatment in operable breast cancer. *N. Engl. J. Med.* 294:405–10

72. Pinsky, C. M., DeJager, R. L., Kaufman, R. J., Mike, V., Hansen, J. A., Oettgen, H. F., Krakoff, I. H. 1977. In *Immunotherapy of Cancer: Present Status of Trials in Man,* ed. W. D. Terry, D. Windhorst, New York: Raven. In press

73. Gutterman, J. U., Mavligit, G. M., Burgess, M. A., Cardenas, J. O., Blumenschein, G. R., Gottlieb, J. A., McBride, C. M., McCredie, K. B., Bodey, G. P., Rodriguez, V., Freireich, E. J., Hersh, E. M. 1976. Immunotherapy of breast cancer, malignant melanoma, and acute leukemia with BCG: prolongation of disease-free interval and survival. *Cancer Immunol. Immunother.* 1:99–107

74. Oettgen, H. F., Old, L. J., Farrow, J. H., Valentine, F. T., Lawrence, H. S., Thomas, L. 1974. Effects of dialyzable transfer factor in patients with breast cancer. *Proc. Natl.*

Acad. Sci. USA 71:2319–23

75. Storer, E. H., Lockwood, R. A. 1969. In *Principles of Surgery,* ed. S. I. Schwartz, p. 958. New York: McGraw-Hill

76. Mavligit, G. M., Burgess, M. A., Seibert, G. B., Jubert, A. V., McBride, C. M., Gehan, E. A., Gutterman, J. U., Khankhanian, N., Speer, J. F., Martin, R. C., Copeland, E. M., Hersh, E. M. 1976. Prolongation of postoperative disease-free interval and survival in human colorectal cancer by BCG or BCG plus 5-fluorouracil. *Lancet* 1:871–75

77. Moertel, C. G., O'Connell, M. J., Ritts, R. E. Jr., Schutt, A. J., Reitemeier, R. J., Hahn, R. G., Frytak, S. K. 1977. See Ref. 72

78. Moertel, C. G., Ritts, R. E. Jr., Schutt, A. J., Hahn, R. G. 1975. Clinical studies of methanol extraction residue fraction of Bacillus Calmette-Guerin as an immunostimulant in patients with advanced cancer. *Cancer Res.* 35:3075–83

79. O'Connell, M. J., Ritts, R. E. Jr., Moertel, C. G. 1976. Immunological assessment of MER and placebo in advanced cancer: a double blind study. *Proc. Am. Assoc. Cancer Res.* 17:214

80. Engstrom, P. F., Paul, A. R., Catalano, R. B., Mastrangelo, M. J., Creech, R. H. 1977. See Ref. 72

81. Griffen, W. O. Jr., Meeker, W. R. 1972. Colon carcinoma and immunologic phenomena. *Surg. Clin. North Am.* 52:839–45

82. Falk, R. E., MacGregor, A. B., Landi, S., Ambus, U., Langer, B. 1976. Immunostimulation with intraperitoneally administered Bacillus Calmette Guerin for advanced malignant tumors of the gastrointestinal tract. *Surg. Gynecol. Obstet.* 142:363–68

83. Turowski, G., Cybulski, L., Politowski, M., Turaszwili, T., Zubel, M. 1976. First trials of immunopotentiation by thymus extract (TFX) in surgical patients with malignant disease. *Acta Med. Pol.* 17:19–39

84. Guinan, P., Bush, I. M., John, T., Sadoughi, N., Ablin, R. J. 1973. BCG immunotherapy in carcinoma of the prostate. *Lancet* 2:443–44

85. Merrin, C., Han, T., Klein, E., Wajsman, Z., Murphy, G. P. 1975. Immunotherapy of prostatic car-

cinoma with Bacillus Calmette Guerin. *Cancer Chemother. Rep.* 59:157–63

86. Eidinger, D., Morales, A. 1976. Treatment of superficial bladder cancer in man. *Ann. NY Acad. Sci.* 277:239–40

87. Ramming, K. P., deKernion, J. B. 1977. Immune RNA therapy for renal cell carcinoma: survival and immunologic monitoring. *Ann. Surg.* In press

88. Skinner, D. G., deKernion, J. B., Brower, P. A., Ramming, K. P., Pilch, Y. H. 1976. Advanced renal cell carcinoma: treatment with xenogeneic immune ribonucleic acid and appropriate surgical resection. *J. Urol.* 115:246–50

89. Guthrie, D., Way, S. 1975. Immunotherapy of nonclinical vaginal cancer. *Lancet* 2:1242–43

90. Graham, J. B., Graham, R. M. 1962. Autogenous vaccine in cancer patients. *Surg. Gynecol. Obstet.* 114:1–4

91. Imperato, S., Rossi, R., Ermiglia, G., De Marini, M., Cassolino, A. 1974. Active specific and non-specific immunotherapy with immunological monitoring in late stage ovarian cancers. *Acta Eur. Fertil.* 5:25–39

92. Pattillo, R. A. 1976. Immunotherapy and chemotherapy of gynecologic cancers. *Am. J. Obstet. Gynecol.* 124:808–17

93. Rao, B., Wanebo, H. J., Ochoa, M., Lewis, J. L., Oettgen, H. F. 1977. Intravenous *corynebacterium parvum*: an adjunct to chemotherapy for resistant advanced ovarian carcinoma. *Cancer* 39:514–26

94. Hudson, C. N., McHardy, J. E., Curling, O. M., English, P. E., Levin, L., Poulton, T. A., Crowther, M., Leighton, M. 1976. Active specific immunotherapy for ovarian cancer. *Lancet* 2:877–79

95. Mathé, G., Schwarzenberg, L., De Vassal, F., Delgado, M. 1976. Immunotherapy for acute lymphoid leukemia. *Lancet* 1:143–44

96. Otten, J. 1977. See Ref. 72

97. Mathé, G., Pouillart, P., Schwarzenberg, L., Amiel, J. L., Schneider, M., Hayat, M., De Vassal, F., Jasmin, C., Rosenfeld, C., Weiner, R., Rappaport, H. 1972. Attempts at immunotherapy of 100 patients with acute lymphoid leukemia: some factors influencing results. *Natl. Can-*

cer Inst. Monogr. 35:361–71

98. Medical Research Council. 1971. Treatment of acute lymphoblastic leukaemia: comparison of immunotherapy (BCG), intermittent methotrexate, and no therapy after a five-month intensive cytotoxic regimen (Concord trial). *Br. Med. J.* 4:189–94

99. Heyn, R. M., Joo, P., Karon, M., Nesbit, M., Shore, N., Breslow, N., Weiner, J., Reed, A., Hammond, D. 1975. BCG in the treatment of acute lymphocytic leukemia. *Blood* 46:431–42

100. Pinkel, D., Simone, J., Hustu, H. O., Rhomes, J. A. A. 1972. Nine years' experience with "total therapy" of childhood acute lymphocytic leukemia. *Pediatrics* 50:246–51

101. Poplack, D. G., Graw, R. G., Pomeroy, T. C., Henderson, E. S., Leventhal, B. G. 1975. Chemotherapy (CT) vs. chemotherapy and immunotherapy (CT + IMT) in childhood acute lymphatic leukemia (ALL). *Proc. Am. Soc. Clin. Oncol.* 16:230

102. Leventhal, B. G., LePourhiet, A., Halterman, R. H., Henderson, E. S., Herberman, R. B. 1973. Immunotherapy in previously treated acute lymphatic leukemia. *Natl. Cancer Inst. Monogr.* 39:177–87

103. Sacks, K. L., Olweny, C., Mann, D. L., Simon, R., Johnson, G. E., Poplack, D. G., Leventhal, B. G. 1975. A clinical trial of chemotherapy and RAJI immunotherapy in advanced acute lymphatic leukemia. *Cancer Res.* 35:3715–20

104. Ekert, H., Jose, D. G. 1975. Chemotherapy and BCG in acute lymphocytic leukemia. *Lancet* 2:713–14

104a. Kay, H. 1977. See Ref. 72

105. Powles, R. L., Crowther, D., Bateman, C. J. T., Beard, M. E. J., McElwain, T. J., Russel, J., Lister, T. A., Whitehouse, J. M. A., Wrigley, P. F. M., Pike, M., Alexander, P., Hamilton-Fairley, G. 1973. Immunotherapy for acute myelogenous leukemia. *Br. J. Cancer* 28:365–76

106. Vogler, W. R., Chan, Y. K. 1974. Prolonging remission in myeloblastic leukemia by tice strain Bacillus Calmette Guerin. *Lancet* 2:128–31

107. Gutterman, J. U., Rodriguez, V.,

Mavligit, G. M., Burgess, M. A., Gehan, E., Hersh, E. M., McCredie, K. B., Reed, R., Smith, T., Bodey, G. P., Freireich, E. J. 1974. Chemoimmunotherapy of adult acute leukaemia: prolongation of remission in myeloblastic leukaemia with BCG. *Lancet* 2:1405–9

108. Peto, R., Galton, D. A. G. 1975. Chemoimmunotherapy of adult acute leukaemia. *Lancet* 1:454

109. Gutterman, J. U., Hersh, E. M., Gehan, E. A., Freireich, E. J. 1975. Chemoimmunotherapy of adult acute leukaemia. *Lancet* 1:454–55

110. Whiteside, M. G., Cauchi, M. N., Paton, C. Stone, J. 1976. Chemoimmunotherapy for maintenance in acute myeloblastic leukemia. *Cancer* 38:1581–86

111. Reizenstein, P., Brenning, G., Engstedt, L., Franzen, S., Gahrton, G., Gullbring, B., Holm, G., Hocker, P., Hoglund, S., Hornsten, P., Jameson, S., Killander, A., Killander, D., Klein, E., Lantz, B., Lindemalm, C., Lockner, D., Lonnqvist, B., Mellstedt, H., Palmblad, J., Pauli, C., Skarberg, K. O., Uden, A. M., Vanky, F., Wadman, B. 1977. See Ref. 72

112. Peto, R. 1977. See Ref. 72

113. Hewlett, J. S., Balcerzak, S., Gutterman, J. 1977. See Ref. 72

114. Freeman, C. B., Harris, R. G., Colin, G., Leyland, M. J., MaCiver, J. E., Delamore, I. W. 1973. Active immunotherapy used alone for the maintenance of patients with acute myeloid leukaemia. *Br. Med. J.* 4:571–73

115. Powles, R. L. 1976. Immunologic maneuvers in the management of acute leukemia. *Med. Clin. North Am.* 60:463–72

116. Bodey, G. P., Freireich, E. J., Gehan, E. A., McCredie, K. B., Rodriguez, V., Gutterman, J. U., Burgess, M. A. 1976. Late intensification therapy for acute leukemia in remission. Chemotherapy and immunotherapy. *J. Am. Med. Assoc.* 235:1021–25

117. Whittaker, J. A., Slater, A. J. 1977. See Ref. 72

118. Cuttner, J., Glidewell, O., Holland, J. F. 1977. See Ref. 72

119. Schwarzenberg, L., Mathé, G., Schneider, M., Amiel, J. L., Cattan, A., Schlumberger, J. R. 1966. Attempted adoptive immunotherapy of acute leukaemia by leucocyte

transfusions. *Lancet* 2:365–68

120. Gee, T. S., Clarkson, B. D. 1977. See Ref. 72

121. McIntyre, O. R., Rai, K., Glidewell, O., Holland, J. F. 1977. See Ref. 72

122. Sauter, C., Cavalli, F., Lindenmann, J., Gmur, J., Berchtold, W., Alberto, P., Obrecht, P., Senn, H. J. 1977. See Ref. 72

123. Aleksandrowicz, V., Skotnicki, A. B. 1976. The role of the thymus and thymic humoral factors in immunotherapy of aplastic and proliferation disease of the hemopoietic system. *Acta Med. Pol.* 17:1–17

124. DeCarvalho, S. 1963. Preliminary experimentation with specific immunotherapy of neoplastic disease in man. I. Immediate effects of hyperimmune equine gamma globulins. *Cancer* 16:306–30

125. Albo, V., Hartmann, J. R., Krevit, M. 1968. Fresh plasma as an adjuvant to the chemotherapy of previously treated children with ALL. *Proc. Am. Assoc. Clin. Res.* 9:2

126. Skurkovich, S. V., Makhonova, L. A., Reznichenko, F. M., Chervonskiy, G. I. 1969. Treatment of children with acute leukemia by passive cyclin immunization with autoplasma and autoleukocytes operated during the remission period. *Blood* 33:186–97

127. Sokal, J. E., Aungst, C. W., Grace, J. T. Jr. 1973. Immunotherapy in well-controlled chronic myelocytic leukemia. *NY State J. Med.* 73:1180–85

128. Laszlo, J., Buckley, C. I. III, Amos, D. B. 1968. Infusion of isologous immune plasma in chronic lymphocytic leukemia. *Blood* 31:104–10

129. Klein, G. 1975. The Epstein-Barr virus and neoplasia. *N. Engl. J. Med.* 293:1353–57

130. Magrath, I. T., Ziegler, J. L. 1976. Failure of BCG immunostimulation to affect the clinical course of Burkitt's lymphoma. *Br. Med. J.* 1:615–18

131. Burkitt, D. 1967. In *Treatment of Burkitt's Tumour*, ed. J. H. Burchenal, D. Burkitt, p. 197. New York: Springer-Verlag

132. Ngu, V. A. 1967. See Ref. 131, p. 204

133. Fass, L., Herberman, R. B., Ziegler, J., Morrow, R. H. Jr. 1970. Evaluation of the effect of remission

plasma on untreated patients with Burkitt's lymphoma. *J. Natl. Cancer Inst.* 44:145–49

134. Bluming, A. Z., Serpick, A. A. 1970. Treatment of recurrent Burkitt's tumor with autologous remission plasma. *Oncology* 24:304–12

135. Sokal, J. E., Aungst, C. W., Snyderman, M. 1974. Delay in progression of malignant lymphoma after BCG vaccination. *N. Engl. J. Med.* 291:1226–30

136. Jones, S. E., Salmon, S. E., eds. 1977. *Adjuvant Therapy of Cancer*, pp. 549–56. Amsterdam: North-Holland

137. McKneally, M. F., Maver, C., Kausel, H. W. 1976. Regional immunotherapy of lung cancer with intrapleural BCG. *Lancet* 1:377–79

138. Takita, H. 1970. Effect of postoperative empyema on survival of patients with bronchogenic carcinoma. *J. Thorac. Cardiovasc. Surg.* 59:642–44

139. Ruckdeschel, J. C., Codish, S. D., Stranahan, A., McKneally, M. F. 1972. Postoperative empyema improves survival in lung cancer: documentation and analysis of a natural experiment. *N. Engl. J. Med.* 287:1013–17

140. McKneally, M. F., Maver, C. M., Kausel, H. W. 1977. Intrapleural BCG stimulation in lung cancer. *Lancet* 1:593

141. Edwards, F. R., Whitwell, F. 1974. Use of BCG as an immunostimulant in the surgical treatment of carcinoma of the lung. *Thorax* 29:654–58

142. Amery, W. K. 1977. See Ref. 72

143. Pines, A. 1976. A 5 year controlled study of BCG and radiotherapy for inoperable lung cancer. *Lancet* 1:380–81

144. Takita, H., Takada, M., Minowada, J., Han, T., Edgerton, F. 1977. See Ref. 72

145. Stewart, T. H. M., Hollinshead, A. C., Harris, J. E., Raman, S. 1977. See Ref. 72

146. Dimitrov, N. V., Conroy, J., Suhrland, L. G., Singh, T., Teitlebaum, H. 1977. See Ref. 72

147. Alth, G., Denck, H., Fischer, M., Karrer, K., Kokron, O., Korizek, E., Micksche, M., Ogris, E., Reider, C., Titscher, R., Wrba, H. 1973. Aspects of the immunologic treatment of lung cancer. *Cancer Chemother. Rep. Part. 3*, 4:271–74

148. Kimura, I., Ohnoshi, T., Yasuhara,

S., Sugiyama, M., Urabe, Y., Fujii, M., Machida, K. I. 1976. Immuno-chemotherapy in human lung cancer using the streptococcal agent OK-432. *Cancer* 37:2201–3

149. Lieberman, R., Spitler, L. E., Wybran, J., Fudenberg, H. H., Levinson, D., Epstein, W. 1974. Clinical and immunologic evaluation in patients with metastatic malignant melanoma (cutaneous only) treated with intralesional BCG therapy. *Clin. Res.* 22:130A

150. Israel, L., Depierrre, A., Edelstein, R., Cros-Decan, J., Maury, P. 1975. Effect of intranodular BCG in 22 melanoma patients. *Panminerva Med.* 17:187–88

151. Mastrangelo, M. J., Sulit, H. L., Prehn, L. M., Bornstein, R. S., Yarbro, J. W., Prehn, R. T. 1976. Intralesional BCG in the treatment of metastatic malignant melanoma. *Cancer* 37:684–92

152. Gerner, R. E., Moore, G. E. 1976. Feasibility study of active immunotherapy in patients with solid tumors. *Cancer* 38:131–43

153. Morton, D. L., Eilber, F. R., Holmes, E. C., Hunt, J. S., Ketcham, A. S., Silverstein, M. J., Sparks, F. C. 1974. BCG immunotherapy of malignant melanoma: summary of a seven-year experience. *Ann. Surg.* 180:635–43

154. Karakousis, C. P., Douglass, H. O. Jr., Yeracaris, P. M., Holyoke, E. D. 1976. BCG immunotherapy in patients with malignant melanoma. *Arch. Surg.* 111:716–18

155. Yamamura, Y. 1977. See Ref. 72

156. Nathanson, L. 1972. Regression of intradermal malignant melanoma after intralesional injection of *Mycobacterium bovis* strain BCG. *Cancer Chemother. Rep.* 56:659–65

157. Seigler, H. F., Shingleton, W. W., Metzgar, R. S., Buckley, C. E., Bergoc, P. M., Miller, D. S., Fetter, B. G., Phaup, M. D. 1972. Nonspecific and specific immunotherapy in patients with melanoma. *Surgery* 72:162–74

158. Baker, M. A., Taub, R. N. 1973. BCG in malignant melanoma. *Lancet* 1:1117–18

159. Pinsky, C. M., Hirshaut, Y., Oettgen, H. F. 1973. Treatment of malignant melanoma by intratumoral injection of BCG. *Natl. Cancer Inst. Monogr.* 39:225–28

160. Grant, R. M., Cochran, A. J., Hoyle, D., Mackie, R., Murray,

E. L., Ross, C. 1974. Results of administering BCG to patients with melanoma. *Lancet* 2:1096-1100

161. Klein, E., Holtermann, O. A. 1972. Immunotherapeutic approaches to the management of neoplasms. *Natl. Cancer Inst. Monogr.* 35:379-91

162. Malek-Mansour, S. 1973. Remission of melanoma with DNCB treatment. *Lancet* 27:503-4

163. Burdick, K. H., Hawk, W. A. 1961. Vitiligo in a case of vaccinia virus-treated melanoma. *Cancer* 17:708-12

164. Milton, G. W., Lane Brown, M. M. 1966. The limited role of attenuated smallpox virus in the management of advanced malignant melanoma. *Aust. NZ J. Surg.* 35:286-90

165. Hunter-Craig, I., Newton, K. A., Westburg, G., Lacey, B. W. 1970. Use of vaccinia virus in the treatment of metastatic malignant melanoma. *Br. Med. J.* 2:512-15

166. Minton, J. P. 1973. Mumps virus and BCG vaccine in metastatic melanoma. *Arch. Surg.* 106:503-6

167. Cunningham-Rundles, W. F., Hirshaut, Y., Pinsky, C. M., Oettgen, H. F. 1975. Phase I trial of intralesional *Corynebacterium parvum*. *Clin. Res.* 23:337A

167a. Morton, D. L., Eilber, F. R., Holmes, E. C., Townsend, C. M., Mirra, J., Weisenburger, T. 1977. Adjuvant therapy in melanomas and sarcomas. See Ref. 136, pp. 391-97

168. Pinsky, C. M., Hirshaut, Y., Wanebo, H. J., Fortner, J., Mike, V., Schottenfeld, D., Oettgen, H. F. 1977. See Ref. 72

169. Eilber, F. R., Townsend, C. M. Jr., Morton, D. L. 1976. Results of BCG adjuvant immunotherapy for melanoma of the head and neck. *Am. J. Surg.* 132:476-79

170. Bluming, A. Z., Vogel, C. L., Ziegler, J. L., Mody, N., Kamya, G. 1972. Immunological effects of BCG in malignant melanoma: two modes of administration compared. *Ann. Intern. Med.* 76:405-11

171. Ikonopisov, R. L. 1972. The rationale of immunostimulation procedures in the therapeutic approach to malignant melanoma of the skin. *Tumori* 58:121-27

172. Gutterman, J. U., McBride, C. M., Freireich, E. J., Mavligit, G. M., Frei, E. III, Hersh, E. M. 1973. Active immunotherapy with BCG for recurrent malignant melanoma.

Lancet 1:1208-12

173. Serrou, B., DuBois, J. B., Meiss, L., Romieu, C. 1975. Local active immunotherapy for malignant melanoma. *Panminerva Med.* 17:182-86

174. MacGregor, A. B., Falk, R. E., Landi, S., Ambus, U., Langer, B. 1975. Oral bacillus Calmette Guerin immunostimulation in malignant melanoma. *Surg. Gynecol. Obstet.* 141:747-54

175. Thompson, R. B. 1975. Active immunotherapy with BCG for melanoma. *Panminerva Med.* 17:189-92

176. Cunningham, T. J., Schoenfeld, D., Wolters, J., Nathanson, L., Cohen, M., Patterson, B. 1977. See Ref. 72

177. Beretta, G. 1977. See Ref. 72

178. Spitler, L. E. Sagebiel, R., Wong, P., Malm, T., Chase, R., Gonzalez, R. 1977. See Ref. 72

179. Gutterman, J. U., Mavligit, G. M., Gottlieb, J. A., Burgess, M. A., McBride, C. E., Einhorn, L., Freireich, E. J., Hersh, E. M. 1974. Chemoimmunotherapy of disseminated malignant melanoma with dimethyl-triazeno imidazole carboxamide and bacillus Calmette-Guerin. *N. Engl. J. Med.* 291:592-96

180. Currie, G. A., McElwain, T. J. 1975. Active immunotherapy as an adjunct to chemotherapy in the treatment of disseminated malignant melanoma: a pilot study. *Br. J. Cancer* 31:143-56

181. Newlands, E. S., Oon, C. J., Roberts, J. T., Elliott, P., Mould, R. F., Topham, C., Madden, F. J. F., Newton, K. A., Westburg, G. 1976. Clinical trial of combination chemotherapy and specific active immunotherapy in disseminated melanoma. *Br. J. Cancer* 34:174-79

182. Gutterman, J. U., Mavligit, G. M., Reed, R., Burgess, M. A., Gottlieb, J., Hersh, E. M. 1976. Bacillus Calmette Guerin immunotherapy in combination with DTIC (NSC-45388) for the treatment of malignant melanoma. *Cancer Treat. Rep.* 60:177-82

183. Costanzi, J. J. 1977. See Ref. 72

184. Mastrangelo, M. J., Bellet, R. E., Berd, D. 1977. See Ref. 72

185. Presant, C. A., Bartolucci, A., Smalley, R., Vogler, W. R. 1977. See Ref. 72

186. Curtis, J. E. 1971. Adoptive immunotherapy in the treatment of advanced malignant melanoma. *Proc. Am. Assoc. Clin. Res.* 12:52

187. Krementz, E. T., Samuels, M. S., Wallace, J. H., Benes, E. N. 1971. Clinical experiences in immunotherapy of cancer. *Surg. Gynecol. Obstet.* 133:209–17

188. Goodwin, D. P., Hornung, M. O., Krementz, E. T. 1973. Extraction and use of melanoma-associated protein for immunotherapy. *Oncology* 27:258–65

189. Spitler, L. E., Levin, A. S., Blois, M. S., Epstein, W., Fudenberg, H. H., Hellstrom, I., Hellstrom, K. E. 1972. Lymphocyte responses to tumor-specific antigens in patients with malignant melanoma and results of transfer factor therapy. *J. Clin. Invest.* 51:92

190. Brandes, L. J., Galton, D. A. G., Wiltshaw, E. 1971. New approach to immunotherapy of melanoma. *Lancet* 2:293–5

191. Morse, P. A. Jr., Deraps, G. D., Smith, G. V., Raju, S., Hardy, J. D. 1973. Transfer factor therapy of human cancer. *Clin. Res.* 21:71

192. Price, F. B., Hewlett, J. S., Deodhar, S. D., Barna, B. 1974. The therapy of malignant melanoma with transfer factor. *Cleveland Clin. Q.* 41:1–4

193. Seigler, H. F., Shingleton, W. W., Metzgar, R S., Buckley, C. E., Bergoc, P. M. 1973. Immunotherapy in patients with melanoma. *Ann. Surg.* 178:352–9

194. Levy, N. L., Seigler, H. F., Shingleton, W. W. 1974. A multiphase immunotherapy regimen for human melanoma: clinical and laboratory results. *Cancer* 34:1548–57

195. Ghose, T., Norvell, S. T., Guclu, A., Cameron, D., Bodurtha, A., MacDonald, A. S. 1972. Immunochemotherapy of cancer with chloramubucil-carrying antibody. *Br. Med. J.* 3:495–99

196. Falk, R. E., Mann, P., Langer, B. 1973. Cell-mediated immunity to human tumours. *Arch. Surg.* 107:261–65

197. Morton, D. L., Malmgren, R. A. 1968. Human osteosarcomas: immunologic evidence suggesting an associated infectious agent. *Science* 102:1279–81

198. Marcove, R. C., Southam, C. M., Levin, A., Mike, V., Huvos, A. 1971. A clinical trial of autogenous vaccine in osteogenic sarcoma in patients under the age of twenty-five. *Surg. Forum* 22:434–35

199. Marsh, B., Flynn, L., Enneking, W. J. 1972. Immunologic aspects of osteosarcoma and their application to therapy. *J. Bone Jt. Surg.* 54A:1367–97

200. Neff, J. R., Enneking, W. F. 1975. Adoptive immunotherapy in primary osteosarcoma. *J. Bone Jt. Surg.* 57 A:145–48

201. Eilber, F. R., Townsend, C. M.Jr., Morton, D. L. 1975. Osteosarcoma: results of treatment employing adjuvant immunotherapy. *Clin. Orthop. Relat. Res.* 111:94–100

202. Taylor, W. F., Ivins, J. C., Dahlin, D. C., Pritchard, D. J. 1977. See Ref. 72

203. Ritts, R. E. Jr., Pritchard, D. J., Gilchrist, G. S., Ivins, J. C., Taylor, W. F. 1977. See Ref. 72

204. LoBuglio, A. F., Neidhart, J. A., Hilberg, R. W., Metz, E. N., Balcerzak, S. P. 1973. The effect of transfer factor therapy on tumor immunity in alveolar soft part sarcoma. *Cell. Immunol.* 7:159–65

205. Morton, D. L., Eilber, F. R., Joseph, W. L., Wood, W. C., Trahan, E., Ketcham, A. S. 1970. Immunological factors in human sarcomas and melanomas: a rational basis for immunotherapy. *Ann. Surg.* 172:740–49

206. Morton, D. L., Holmes, E. C., Eilber, F. R., Wood, W. C. 1971. Immunological aspects of neoplasia: a rational basis for immunotherapy. *Ann. Intern. Med.* 74:587–604

207. Sinkovics, J. G. 1977. Immunotherapy with viral oncolysates for sarcoma. *J. Am. Med. Assoc.* 237:869

208. Green, A. A., Pratt, C., Webster, R. G., Smith, K. 1976. Immunotherapy of osteosarcoma patients with virus-modified tumor cells. *Ann. NY Acad. Sci.* 277:396–410

209. Gunnarson, A., McKhann, C. F., Simmons, R. L., Grage, T. B. 1974. Metastatic sarcoma: combined surgical and immunotherapeutic approach: neuraminidase treated tumor cells as tumor vaccine. *Minn. Med.* 57:558–61

210. Klein, E. 1969. Hypersensitivity reactions at tumor sites. *Cancer Res.* 29:2351–62

211. Levis, W. R., Kraemer, K. H., Klinger, W. G., Peck, G. L., Terry, W. D. 1973. Topical immunotherapy of basal cell car-

cinomas with dinitrochlorobenzene. *Cancer Res.* 33:3036–42
212. Williams, A. C., Klein, E. 1970. Experiences with local chemotherapy and immunotherapy in premalignant and malignant skin lesions. *Cancer* 25:450–62
213. Raaf, J. H., Krown, S. E., Pinsky, C. M., Cunningham-Rundles, W., Safai, B., Ottegen, H. F. 1976. Treatment of Bowen's disease with topical dinitrochlorobenzene and 5-fluorouracil. *Cancer* 37:1633–42
214. Villasor, R. P. 1965. The clinical use of BCG vaccine in stimulating host resistance to cancer. *J. Philipp. Med. Assoc.* 41:619–32
215. Asada, T. 1974. Treatment of human cancer with mumps virus. *Cancer* 34:1907–28
216. Israel, L., Edelstein, R. 1975. A phase II study of daily intravenous corynebacterium in 33 disseminated cancers. *Proc. Am. Assoc. Cancer Res.* 16:67
217. Aswaq, M., Richards, V., McFadden, S. 1964. Immunologic response to autologous cancer vaccine. *Arch. Surg.* 89:485–87
218. Hughes, L. E., Kearney, R., Tully, M. 1970. A study in clinical cancer immunotherapy. *Cancer* 26:269–78
219. Czajkowski, N. P., Rosenblatt, M., Wolf, P. L., Vasquez, J. 1967. A new method of active immunization to autologous human tumour tissue. *Lancet* 2:905–9
220. Cunningham, T. J., Olson, K. B., Laffin, R., Horton, J., Sullivan, J. 1969. Treatment of advanced cancer with active immunization. *Cancer* 24:932–37
221. Humphrey, L. J., Boehm, B., Jewell, W. R., Boehm, O. R. 1972. Immunologic response of cancer pa-

tients modified by immunization with tumor vaccine. *Ann. Surg.* 176:554–58
222. Wallack, M. K., Steplewski, Z., Koprowski, H., Rosato, E., George, J., Hulihan, B., Johnson, J. 1977. A new approach in specific active immunotherapy. *Cancer* 39:560–64
223. Finney, J. W., Byers, E. H., Wilson, R. H. 1960. Studies in tumor autoimmunity. *Cancer Res.* 20:351–56
224. Woodruff, M. F. A., Nolan, B. 1963. Preliminary observations on treatment of advanced cancer by injection of allogeneic spleen cells. *Lancet* 2:426–29
225. Andrews, G. A., Congdon, C. C., Edwards, C. L., Gengozian, N., Nelson, B., Vodopick, H. 1967. Preliminary trials of clinical immunotherapy. *Cancer Res.* 27:2535–41
226. Yonemoto, R. H., Terasaki, P. I. 1972. Cancer immunotherapy with HLA compatible thoracic duct lymphocyte transplantation. *Cancer* 30:1438–43
227. Symes, M. O., Riddell, A. G. 1973. The use of immunized pig lymph node cells in the treatment of patients with advanced malignant disease. *Br. J. Surg.* 60:176–80
228. Frenster, J. H. 1976. Phytohemagglutinin-activated autochthonous lymphocytes for systemic immunotherapy of human neoplasms. *Ann. NY Acad. Sci.* 277:45–50
229. Bartlett, G. L., Kreider, J. W., Purnell, D. M. 1976. Immunotherapy of cancer in animals: models or muddles? *J. Natl. Cancer Inst.* 56:207–10

Ann. Rev. Med. 1979. 30:17–24

HAIRY CELL LEUKEMIA ♦7303

Raul C. Braylan, M.D.

Department of Pathology, University of Florida College of Medicine,
Gainesville, Florida 32610

Jerome S. Burke, M.D.

Department of Pathology, Stanford University Medical Center,
Stanford, California 94305

INTRODUCTION

Hairy cell leukemia, or leukemic reticuloendotheliosis, is a chronic leukemia that has received increased attention in recent years. Much of the
current vogue in the recognition of this disease may be due to the employ-
ment of the term "hairy cell," first used by Schrek & Donnelly (1) to
describe the villous cytoplasmic projections of the leukemic cells as viewed
under phase microscopy. Because of the curious nature of the hairy cell,
there has been considerable interest in attempting to define the cytogenesis,
natural history, and factors necessary for accurate diagnosis and effective
therapy of this disease.

CLINICAL AND LABORATORY FEATURES

Although termed "leukemia," paradoxically the majority of patients with
hairy cell leukemia are aleukemic and present with pancytopenia and clinical hypersplenism (2–6). The disease tends to affect males aged 50–60, and
is relatively less frequent in females. Initial symptoms such as fatigue,
lassitude, infections, bruising, or abdominal fullness are related to the pancytopenia or enlarged spleen. Many patients are, in fact, asymptomatic and
the disease is only discovered on routine hematologic survey or physical
examination. The most striking physical finding is an enlarged, frequently
massive spleen (2–6). Lymphadenopathy is distinctly uncommon; hepato-
megaly generally is moderate.

0066-4219/79/0401-0017$01.00

17

Blood studies usually reveal a normochromic normocytic anemia, thrombocytopenia, and leukopenia averaging 2–3 X 10^3 white blood cells/mm^3 with a relative lymphocytosis (2–7). Overt leukemia with white blood cell counts greater than 10 X 10^3/mm^3 is rare at presentation (2–4, 7). Hairy cells frequently are difficult to recognize in peripheral blood smears (Figure 1) and are commonly misdiagnosed as "atypical" lymphocytes (7). In some cases no hairy cells can be identified in the blood. If hairy cells are observed or suspected, the tartrate-resistant acid phosphatase reaction (TRAP) is a useful cytochemical test to confirm the diagnosis (8). It should be realized that the TRAP, which marks for isoenzyme 5, is not completely specific and the intensity of positivity may be extremely variable (9). In rare cases the reaction may be negative (2, 3). Bone marrow aspirates generally result in dry taps (2, 3, 7, 9) but in our experience marrow biopsy is one of the most reliable diagnostic procedures.

The results of other clinical and laboratory studies have not been consistently abnormal. Except for one reported case of monoclonal gammopathy (10), immunoelectrophoretic studies are essentially unremarkable (2, 4). Serum muramidase levels are generally normal or slightly depressed (2, 3), and chromosomal analysis has not been fruitful except for one recent study reporting loss of Y chromosomes in 2 of 20 patients studied (11). Investigation of platelet aggregation revealed some functional abnormalities (12, 13),

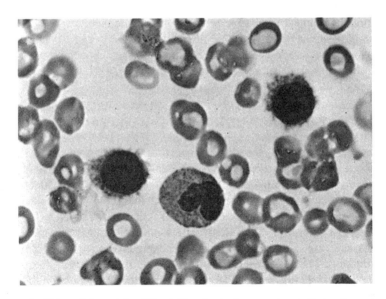

Figure 1   Hairy cells in peripheral blood. Note the size in comparison to the band granulocyte (X 1200).

but intrinsic red cell defects have not been described. Red cell survival studies using ^{51}Cr show increased sequestration of erythrocytes in the spleen (2, 3) and quantitative scanning reveals that the splenic red cell volume is generally increased, particularly in comparison to myelo- and lymphoproliferative disorders with similar splenomegaly (14).

PATHOLOGY

Bone marrow and spleen are usually heavily involved by the leukemic cells and are the most common tissues available to the pathologist for diagnosis. Liver and lymph nodes may also be of diagnostic value. The marrow may be partially or completely replaced (7). In tissue sections the hairy cells appear homogeneous and bland without mitoses or large nucleoli, and are characterized by a distinct water-clear zone of cytoplasm around the cell nuclei that imparts a halo appearance (Figure 2). This is in contrast to the lack of visible cytoplasm and close apposition of nuclei in chronic lymphocytic leukemia, most often confused with hairy cells in biopsies (7, 15). Marrow reticulin is often increased, which may account for the frequency

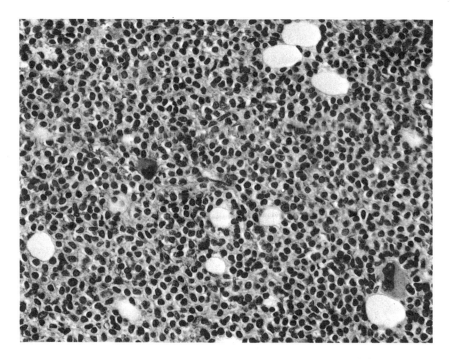

Figure 2   Bone marrow infiltrated by hairy cell leukemia with the characteristic clear zones around the nuclei. Residual megakaryocytes are present (X 300).

of poor yields on aspiration (6, 7, 15). Imprint smears are a useful adjunct to the biopsy, particularly when coupled with staining for TRAP (16). As in the bone marrow, the splenic histology of hairy cell leukemia is distinctive (2, 6, 17); the splenic red pulp, cords, and sinuses are diffusely infiltrated by a uniform population of monotonous-appearing hairy cells resulting in reduction in the size of the white pulp (2). Blood-filled spaces of variable size in the red pulp (blood "lakes") are often seen (17), which perhaps provides a morphologic explanation for the increased erythrocyte pooling (14). In addition to hairy cells and erythrocytes, histochemical studies of the spleen reveal increased numbers of macrophages in the pulp cords (18), which supports the ultrastructural observation of leukoerythrophagocytosis by splenic macrophages (19). The increased phagocytic activity of apparently normal macrophages may account, at least in part, for the hypersplenic syndrome in hairy cell leukemia. Transmission electron microscopic studies may also be of value in the diagnosis of this disease since in many instances the leukemic cells contain a characteristic cytoplasmic ribosomal-lamellar complex (20, 21). Although these complexes are frequently observed in hairy cell leukemia, they are not pathognomonic and have been described in other disorders (22).

THERAPY AND PROGNOSIS

Infection secondary to pancytopenia is the primary complication in hairy cell leukemia (4, 5, 23). The majority of studies indicate that splenectomy is the treatment of choice in hairy cell leukemia (2, 3, 5). However, the indication for splenectomy will depend upon the degree of pancytopenia and splenomegaly. For most patients splenectomy usually results in restoration of normal hemtologic parameters and/or sufficient clinical improvement to ameliorate the symptomatology. One series, however, reported either failure or only a partial reversion of the pancytopenia in some 40% of patients (3); these patients had a median survival approximately five times less than patients who responded completely to splenic removal. Nonetheless, the overall survival at five years in hairy cell leukemia is approximately 50% (2) and survivals over ten years have been recorded (2, 5). All patients with hairy cell leukemia, regardless of response to splenectomy, have persistent bone marrow involvement (7). It is possible that patients who do not respond to splenectomy have more severe marrow involvement, hence the impairment of marrow granulocyte reserve and leukocyte production (24). This is significant since the majority of patients with hairy cell leukemia who fail after splenectomy succumb to infectious complications (3, 5). In particular there has been recent indication of a curiously increased incidence of mycobacterial infections (3, 25), which may be related to the monocytopenia reported in this disorder (26). The danger of infection adds a cautionary note to the use of chemotherapeutic agents in hairy cell leukemia. With few exceptions (3, 27), cytotoxic agents or steroids have not been beneficial either as initial therapy or following splenectomy. On the contrary, aggressive chemotherapy, generally employed because of a misdiagnosis of acute leukemia or lymphoma, often leads to dire consequences in the patient with hairy cell leukemia (2, 5). The failure of chemotherapy in controlling this disease may be related to the fact that hairy cells have a low proliferative capacity as has been shown by thymidine incorporation and flow cytometry (18). At present, no effective treatment is known for patients not responding to splenectomy. However, recent attempts to remove circulating hairy cells by leukapheresis in leukemic patients have met with some success (28, 29). Controlled prospective studies will be necessary to assess therapeutic alternatives for patients with progressive or late stage disease.

THE NATURE OF THE HAIRY CELL

The origin of the neoplastic cells of hairy cell leukemia is still highly controversial. Multiple cytochemical, structural, and functional techniques that define normal hematopoietic elements have been applied to hairy cells to characterize their nature, but no consistent results have been obtained (12, 18, 20, 30–39). Most studies suggested either a monocytic origin (35–37) or a B lymphocytic derivation (31, 32, 34, 38), and a few investigators consider that hairy cells may be B lymphocytes with phagocytic properties (12, 33, 39), or hybrid cells (30), or unique elements that are not detected in normal conditions (18). Hairy cells do not have high phagocytic capacity, although in vitro they have a limited ability to ingest particles or microorganisms (12, 18, 20, 33, 36, 39). Most observers found receptors for the Fc fragment of IgG (18, 30, 33, 35–37) on hairy cells but the detection of complement receptors varied widely (18). Structurally, hairy cells display ample surface ridges and ruffles (Figure 3) (18) that account for their "hairy" appearance. This complex surface may also contribute to their large electronic size as detected by Coulter analysis (18). The peculiar ruffled surface of hairy cells as observed by scanning microscopy may be seen in normal monocytes but it is not a feature of freshly isolated normal or neoplastic lymphocytes (18). In most reported instances, hairy cells demonstrated surface-associated immunoglobulins (SIg) (12, 18, 30–34, 36), which suggests a B cell lineage. Some observations indicate that at least in part the SIg may have been extrinsically bound to the cells and not an actual cell product (18, 33, 38). However, several studies demonstrated restriction of the SIg to a single light-chain determinant (12, 18, 30), and a few observations indicated the presence of cytoplasmic immunoglobulin (30, 34) and even immunoglobulin synthesis in hairy cells (12, 32, 34, 39), which would

conclusively demonstrate their B lymphocytic origin. Moreover, monoclonal serum immunoglobulin elevation in hairy cell leukemia has been
reported (10). It must be emphasized, however, that these results have not
been universally confirmed. The presence or synthesis of immunoglobulins
in hairy cell populations has not always been observed (18, 40) and the
finding of a serum paraprotein in hairy cell leukemia is an exceedingly rare
event (2, 4). These differences in results may be due to a lack of standardized
methods to assay the different functional characteristics of hairy cells. It is
also reasonable to assume that these cells, although morphologically and
cytochemically homogeneous, vary in their expression of such characteristics. However, an important source of discrepancy may result from the lack
of strict diagnostic criteria to define hairy cell leukemia. There is evidence
that some of the clinical and hematological criteria that are used to diagnose
hairy cell leukemia may be seen in disorders that differ histologically and
biologically from conventional hairy cell leukemia. That is, typical B cell
lymphoproliferative disorders with a monoclonal serum paraprotein and
with cells containing cytoplasmic immunoglobulins may present with
splenomegaly, pancytopenia, and TRAP-positive hairy cells (40, 41). Obviously, these findings raise questions about the validity of some functional
studies in hairy cell leukemia and stress the necessity of reliable and uniform
criteria for defining and diagnosing this disease.

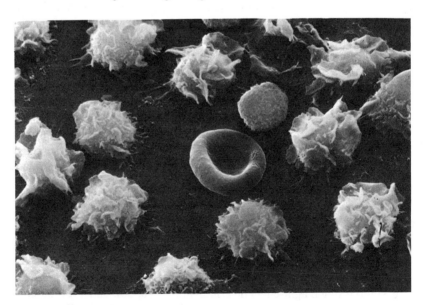

Figure 3   Hairy cells as observed by scanning electron microscopy. Note the ample surface
ruffles. An erythrocyte is seen in the middle of the field (X 3700).

Literature Cited

1. Schrek, R., Donnelly, W. J. 1966. "Hairy" cells in blood in lymphoreticular neoplastic disease and "flagellated" cells of normal lymph notes. *Blood* 27:199–211
2. Burke, J. S., Byrne, G. E. Jr., Rappaport, H. 1974. Hairy cell leukemia (Leukemic reticuloendotheliosis). I. A clinical pathologic study of 21 patients. *Cancer* 33:1399–1410
3. Catovsky, D. 1977. Hairy-cell leukaemia and prolymphocytic leukaemia. *Clin. Haematol.* 6:245–68
4. Flandrin, G., Daniel, M. T., Fourcade, M., Chelloul, N. 1973. Leucemie a "tricholeucocyte" (hairy cell leukemia). Etude clinique et cytologique de 55 observations. *Nouv. Rev. Fr. Hematol.* 13:609–40
5. Katayama, I., Finkel, H. E. 1974. Leukemic reticuloendotheliosis. A clinicopathologic study with review of literature. *Am. J. Med.* 57:115–26
6. Naeim, F., Smith, G. S. 1974. Leukemic reticuloendotheliosis. *Cancer* 34:1813–21
7. Burke, J. S. 1978. The value of the bone marrow biopsy in the diagnosis of hairy cell leukemia. *Am. J. Clin. Pathol.* In press
8. Yam, L. T., Li, C. Y., Lam, K. W. 1971. Tartrate-resistant acid phosphatase isoenzyme in the reticulum cells of leukemic reticuloendotheliosis. *N. Engl. J. Med.* 284:357–60
9. Katayama, I., Yang, J. P. S. 1977. Reassessment of a cytochemical test for differential diagnosis of leukemic reticuloendotheliosis. *Am. J. Clin. Pathol.* 68:268–72
10. Golde, D. W., Saxon, A., Stevens, R. H. 1977. Macroglobulinemia and hairy cell leukemia. *N. Engl. J. Med.* 296:92–93
11. Golomb, H. M., Lindgren, V., Rowley, J. D. 1978. Chromosome abnormalities in patients with hairy cell leukemia. *Cancer* 41:1374–80
12. Golomb, H. M., Vardiman, J., Sweet, D. L. Jr., Simon, D., Variakojis, D. 1978. Hairy cell leukaemia: Evidence for the existance of a spectrum of functional characteristics. *Br. J. Haematol.* 38:161–70
13. Levin, P. H., Katayama, I. 1975. The platelet in leukemic reticuloendotheliosis. Functional and morphological evidence of a qualitative disorder. *Cancer* 36:1353–58
14. Lewis, S. M., Catovsky, D., Hows, J. M., Ardalan, B. 1977. Splenic red cell

pooling in hairy cell leukaemia. *Br. J. Haematol.* 35:351–57
15. Vykoupil, K. F., Thiele, J., Georgii, A. 1976. Hairy cell leukemia. Bone marrow findings in 24 patients. *Virchows Arch. A* 370:273–89
16. Krause, J. R., Srodes, C., Lee, R. E. 1977. Use of the bone marrow imprint in the diagnosis of leukemic reticuloendotheliosis ("hairy cell leukemia"). *Am. J. Clin. Pathol.* 68:368–71
17. Nanba, K., Soban, E. J., Bowling, M. C., Berard, C. W. 1977. Splenic pseudosinuses and hepatic angiomatous lesions. Distinctive features of hairy cell leukemia. *Am. J. Clin. Pathol.* 67:415–26
18. Braylan, R. C., Jaffe, E. S., Triche, T. J., Nanba, K., Fowlkes, B. J., Metzger, H., Frank, M. M., Dolan, M. S., Yee, C. L., Green, I., Berard, C. W. 1978. Structural and functional properties of the "hairy" cells of leukemic reticuloendotheliosis. *Cancer* 41:210–27
19. Burke, J. S., Mackay, B., Rappaport, H. 1976. Hairy cell leukemia (Leukemic reticuloendotheliosis). II. Ultrastructure of the spleen. *Cancer* 37:2267–74
20. Daniel, M. T., Flandrin, G. 1974. Fine structure of abnormal cells in hairy cell (tricholeukocytic) leukemia, with special reference to their in vitro phagocytic capacity. *Lab. Invest.* 30:1–8
21. Katayama, I., Schneider, G. B. 1977. Further ultrastructural characteristics of hairy cells of leukemic reticuloendotheliosis. *Am. J. Pathol.* 86:163–82
22. Brunning, R. D., Parkin, J. 1975. Ribosome-lamella complexes in neoplastic hematopoietic cells. *Am. J. Pathol.* 79:565–78
23. Bouza, E., Burgaleta, C., Golde, D. W. 1978. Infections in hairy-cell leukemia. *Blood* 51:851–59
24. Yam, L. T., Chaudhry, A. A., Janckila, A. J. 1977. Impaired marrow granulocyte reserve and leukocyte mobilization in leukemic reticuloendotheliosis. *Ann. Intern. Med.* 87:444–46
25. Marie, J. P., Degos, L., Flandrin, G. 1977. Hairy-cell leukemia and tuberculosis. (Letter.) *N. Engl. J. Med.* 297:1354
26. Seshadri, R. S., Brown, E. J., Zipursky, A. 1976. Leukemic reticuloendotheliosis. A failure of monocyte production. *N. Engl. J. Med.* 295:181–84
27. Davies, T. E., Waterbury, L., Abeloff, M., Burke, P. J. 1976. Leukemic reticuloendotheliosis: Report of a case with prolonged remission following in-

24   BRAYLAN & BURKE

28. Keitt, A. S., Weiner, R. S. 1978. Therapeutic leukapheresis in hairy cell leukemia. *Clin. Res.* 26:52A (Abstr.)
29. Moore, J. O., Fay, J., Logue, G. L. 1977. Hairy cell leukemia: Proliferative potential and treatment with intensive leukopheresis. *Blood* 50:156 (Abstr.)
30. Burns, G. F., Nash, A. A., Worman, C. P., Barker, C. R., Hayhoe, F. G. J. 1977. A human leukaemic cell expressing hybrid membrane phenotypes. *Nature* 268:243–45
31. Catovsky, D., Pettit, J. E., Galetto, J., Okos, A., Galton, D. A. G. 1974. The B-lymphocyte nature of the hairy cell of leukaemic reticuloendotheliosis. *Br. J. Haematol.* 26:29–37
32. Debusscher, L., Bernheim, J. L., Collard-Ronge, E., Govaerts, A., Hooghe, R., Lejeune, F. J., Zeicher, M., Stryckmans, P. A. 1975. Hairy cell leukemia: Functional, immunologic, kinetic, and ultrastructural characterization. *Blood* 46:495–507
33. Fu, S. M., Winchester, R. J., Rai, K. R., Kunkel, H. G. 1974. Hairy cell leukemia: Proliferation of a cell with phagocytic and B-lymphocyte properties. *Scand. J. Immunol.* 3:847–51
34. Golde, D. W., Stevens, R. H., Quan, S. G., Saxon, A. 1977. Immunoglobulin

synthesis in hairy cell leukaemia. *Br. J. Haematol.* 35:359–65
35. Jaffe, E. S., Shevach, E. M., Frank, M. M., Green, I. 1974. Leukemic reticuloendotheliosis: Presence of a receptor for cytophilic antibody. *Am. J. Med.* 57:108–14
36. King, G. W., Hurtubise, P. E., Sagone, A. L. Jr., LoBuglio, A. F., Metz, E. N. 1975. Leukemic reticuloendotheliosis. A study of the origin of the malignant cell. *Am. J. Med.* 59:411–16
37. Scheinberg, M., Brenner, A. I., Sullivan, A. L., Cathcart, E. S., Katayama, I. 1976. The heterogeneity of leukemic reticuloendotheliosis, "hairy cell leukemia." Evidence for its monocytic origin. *Cancer* 37:1302–7
38. Stein, H., Kaiserling, E. 1974. Surface immunoglobulins and lymphocyte-specific surface antigens on leukaemic reticuloendotheliosis cells. *Clin. Exp. Immunol.* 18:63–71
39. Utsinger, P. D., Yount, W. J., Fuller, C. R., Logue, M. J., Orringer, E. P. 1977. Hairy cell leukemia: B-lymphocyte and phagocytic properties. *Blood* 49:19–27
40. Neiman, R. S., Sullivan, A., Jaffe, R. 1978. Malignant lymphoma simulating leukemic reticuloendotheliosis. *Cancer.* In press
41. Katayama, I. 1977. Hairy cell leukemia. (Letter.) *N. Engl. J. Med.* 296:881

AUTHOR INDEX

(Names appearing in capital letters indicate authors of chapters in this volume.)

438   AUTHOR INDEX

Bateman, C. J. T., 393, 394
Battaglia, F. C., 358
Batzing, B. L., 182
Bauer, H., 205
Baughn, R. E., 267, 268
Bayley, H., 93, 99, 102, 111, 114, 116, 125, 137
Beal, D., 41
Beale, D., 3, 5
Bear, H. D., 274
Beard, M. E. J., 393, 394
Beaufils, H., 326
Beck, D., 359
Becka, L. N., 9
Becker, E. L., 39
Becker, K. E., 51
Becker, L. A., 43
Becker, M. J., 84
Beer, A. E., 347, 349-51, 356, 357, 362-64
Behrman, S. G., 363
Bekesi, J. G., 380, 394, 395
Bell, G. I., 229
Bellet, R. E., 406, 407
Benacerraf, B., 164, 170, 231, 241-44, 247, 251, 285, 298, 301, 306
Benes, E. N., 381, 407, 408
Benisek, W. F., 101, 108
Bennett, D., 206, 347
Bennett, J. C., 43
Bennett, V., 67
Bennich, H. (H.), 43, 48
Bennink, J. R., 247
Bentwich, Z., 223, 229
Bentzel, C., 333
Berard, C. W., 432-34
Berchtold, W., 394, 396
Bercovici, T., 111, 128
Berd, D., 406, 407
Beretta, G., 406
Berger, J., 325, 326
Berggard, I., 35
Bergman, C., 104
Bergoc, P. M., 402, 408
Bergstein, J. M., 336, 337
Bergstrom, S., 347
Berken, A., 170
Berlin, R. D., 256, 267, 268, 277, 288, 289
Bernard, E. F., 336
Bernard, O., 347
Berney, M., 285
Bernheim, J. L., 433
Bernstein, I. D., 381
Bernstein, I. L., 340
Bernstein, J. M., 164, 171
Besbeas, S., 386
Bessis, M., 170, 171
Betuel, H., 355, 360
Bhalla, D. K., 223, 224
Bhan, A. K., 334, 335, 337
Bhisey, A. N., 261-64, 282

Bianco, A. R., 268, 269
Bianco, C., 227, 228, 272, 273, 275, 277, 279, 280, 283, 288, 289
Biasucci, A., 359
Biddison, W. E., 247
Biedler, J. L., 204
Bienenstock, J., 226
Bill, A. H., 375
Billingham, R. E., 347, 349-51, 356, 357, 362, 363
Billington, W. D., 347-50, 352, 363
Bina-Stein, M., 148
Bing, D. H., 73, 80
Biozzi, G., 379
Birchmeier, W., 67
Bishop, J. M., 204
Bispink, L., 113, 134, 142
Bisson, R., 113, 143
Bjaring, B., 200
Black, J. L., 106
Blackman, L., 264, 265, 268
Blackstock, J. C., 360
Blake, J. T., 256, 286, 289
Blanden, R. V., 243, 244, 246, 248, 250
Blant, E. R., 133
Blaustein, A., 224
Blecher, M., 106, 141, 268, 269
Bloch, K. E., 92
Blois, M. S., 408
Bloom, B. R., 246, 250, 268-72, 276, 289
Bloom, H. J. G., 385
Blostein, R., 63
Bloth, B., 43
Bluestone, R., 309
Blumenschein, G. R., 386, 388, 395, 405, 406, 416
Blumenthal, R., 82
Bluming, A. Z., 398, 406
Blusse van Oud Alblas, A., 305
Boak, J. L., 379
Bobrow, M., 305
Bode, W., 9, 12, 25
Bodey, G. P., 386, 388, 394, 395, 397, 405, 406, 416
Bodmer, J. (G.), 302, 303, 305
Bodmer, W. (F.), 241, 242, 244, 247, 248, 302, 303, 305, 349, 364
Bodurtha, A., 408
Boehm, B., 413, 414
Boehm, O. R., 413, 414
Boehmer, H. von, 244, 245, 247, 249, 251
Bogatko, F. H., 375
Bohn, H., 360
Bolognesi, D. P., 185
Bonadonna, G., 387
Bondevik, H., 360
Bonnard, G. D., 355

Bonneau, M., 355, 360-62
Bonsen, P. P. M., 78
Bonventre, P. F., 267, 268, 277, 288
Boone, C. W., 380
Boos, W., 109
Border, J. R., 164
Border, W. A., 336, 337, 340
Borland, R., 350
Bornstein, R. S., 402
Borsos, T., 46, 378, 405
Borthistile, B. K., 271
Boshier, D. P., 363
Boulware, T., 264
Bourgois, A., 43
Bourne, F. J., 233
Bourne, H. R., 105
Bouza, E., 432
Bowling, M. C., 432
Bowyer, D. E., 79, 80
Boyd, A. E. III, 106
Boyse, E. A., 178-82, 184-88, 190, 192-97, 200, 201, 204, 206, 297, 362, 375, 377
Bradbury, S., 349
Braendstrup, O., 286, 289
Brahim, F., 228
Brambell, F. W. R., 352
Brambilla, C., 387
Bramwell, M. E., 348
Brand, L., 92
Branden, C., 92
Brandes, L. J., 408
Brandolin, G., 109
Brandt, P. W., 104
Branton, D., 59, 66, 67
Brawn, J., 355, 360
BRAYLAN, R. C., 429-36; 432-34
Bregman, M. D., 108, 129, 130, 132, 141
Brennan, J. C., 333, 334
Brenner, A. I., 433
Brenning, G., 394, 395
Brentjens, J. R., 332, 333
Breslow, N., 393
Breslow, R., 117
Bretscher, M. S., 63
Breuer, W., 109
Breuiller, M., 356
Breyere, E. J., 360, 363
Bridges, A. J., 115
Bright, S., 243
Brissie, N. T., 258
Brochier, J., 355, 360, 361
Brock, D. J. H., 92
Broder, S., 362
Brodie, S. E., 256, 277
Brons, N. H. C., 223
Bronson, P. M., 159, 161, 164
Brooks, R. E., 336
Brovet, J. C., 49
Brower, P. A., 391

440   AUTHOR INDEX

AUTHOR INDEX 441

Dietrich, F. M., 228
Dimitriu, A., 160, 165
Dimitrov, N. V., 399, 401
Dirksen, E. R., 283
Dixon, F. J., 325, 332-36
Djerassi, I., 386, 411
Dodd, G. H., 110
Dodsen, M., 353
Dofuku, R., 204
Doherty, P. C., 241-44, 246-48, 300
Doi, B. S., 340
Dolan, M. S., 432-34
Donnelly, W. J., 429
Dorf, M. E., 251
Dorhout Mees, E. J., 328
Dorrington, K. J., 11, 43, 44, 269-72
DosReis, G. A., 282, 283
Doughty, R. W., 354
DOUGLAS, S. D., 255-95; 223, 229, 256, 258, 264, 265, 269, 270, 272, 276, 277, 279-81, 288
Douglass, H. O. Jr., 406
Dourmashkin, R. R., 73, 79, 80
Douthwaite, R. M., 350
Douzou, P., 92
Downey, H., 225
Drath, D., 256, 275, 279
Dray, S., 353
Dreyer, W. J., 40
Dreyfuss, G., 133
Drinker, C. K., 225
Drysdale, J. W., 359
DuBois, J. B., 406
Dubois, J. M., 104
Dudovi, F. J., 147
Dugas, H., 92
Dukor, P., 39, 79, 227, 228
Dulbecco, R., 156, 162
Dumonde, D. C., 165
Dunbar, N., 379
Dunlop, M. B. C., 246
Dupont, B., 302, 307, 354
Dutton, R. C., 158, 160
Dvorak, H. F., 279
Dvorkin, B., 358
Dwek, R. A., 45
Dy, M., 160, 165
Dyke, K. V., 276

E

Eberle, A., 107
Eckstein, B., 356
Eddleston, A. L. W. F., 269, 289
Edebo, L. B., 160
Ededin, M., 352
Edelman, G. M., 35, 40, 41, 143, 347, 352

Edelman, I. S., 107
Edelson, P. J., 264-68, 277, 279, 283, 284, 288, 289
Edelstein, R., 379, 386, 387, 399, 401, 402, 406, 407, 411, 413, 414, 416
Eden, A., 279, 280
Edgerton, F., 399, 400
Edidin, M., 59, 66, 317
Edmundson, A. B., 5, 7, 9, 11, 13, 28, 32, 40
Edwards, C. L., 413, 414
Edwards, F. R., 399
Edwards, R. G., 348, 351
Eernisse, J. G., 302, 352
Egan, J. D., 336, 337, 340
Egdahl, R. H., 382
Eggens, J. H., 226
Eggers, H. J., 201
Ehlenberger, A. G., 272
Ehrenberg, E., 47
Eidels, L., 49
Eidinger, D., 391
Eilber, F. R., 376, 378-80, 402-6, 410, 415, 416
Einhorn, L., 405, 406
Einstein, A., 169
Eisen, H. N., 156, 162
Ekert, H., 393
Elder, J. H., 145-47
Elgsaeter, A., 66
Ellerson, J. R., 11, 43
Elliott, P., 406, 407
Ellner, S. J., 256, 286, 289
Elsbach, P., 261
Elson, J., 347-49
Elwood, C. M., 333, 336, 337
Ely, K. R., 5, 7, 9, 11, 13, 28, 32, 40
Elzenga-Claasen, I., 256, 281
Embling, P., 233
Ende, E., 156
Enders, A. C., 348
Engel, J., 46
Engelman, D. M., 92
English, P. E., 391, 392
Engstedt, L., 394, 395
Engstrom, P. F., 389, 390
Enneking, W. F., 409, 410
Ennis, L., 379
Epp, O., 9, 11, 12, 25, 27, 29, 44
Epstein, R., 245
Epstein, W., 408
Erbs, C., 264-66, 279, 289
Erecinska, M., 112, 113, 143
Erickson, R. P., 346
Erlanger, B. F., 333
Ermiglia, G., 391, 392
Ernster, L., 110
Escher, E., 107, 108
Essex, M., 205

Estren, S., 224
Evans, C., 378
Evans, D. J., 325
Evans, R., 256, 287, 289, 362
Everson, G., 257
Everson, T. C., 375

F

Faarup, P., 340
Fahey, J. L., 241, 248
Faiers, A. B., 43
Fainter, L. K., 226
Fairbanks, B., 61
Falk, R. E., 44, 389, 390, 406, 408
Farley, R. A., 109
Farnham, A. E., 275, 276
Farr, A. G., 234
Farrow, J. H., 388
Fasold, H., 109
Fass, L., 398
Faulk, W. P., 350, 352, 362
Fausch, M. D., 7, 13
Fauve, R. M., 347
Fay, J., 433
Fearon, D. T., 273
Febres, F., 356
Fehlhammer, H., 9, 12, 25
Feierstein, J. N., 380, 387, 416
Feinstein, A., 3, 5, 41, 49
Feiring, A., 117
Feldman, D., 107
Feldman, J. D., 278, 288, 332
Fellous, M., 346
Fenn, W. O., 157, 279
Fenner, F., 246
Ferber, E., 51
Ferguson, J. J. Jr., 101
Ferguson, K. A., 364
Fernandes, G., 280
Fernandez, L. A., 282
Fernando, N. V. P., 222
Ferrara, G. B., 306
Ferrarini, M., 362
Ferre, F., 356
Ferris, B., 259, 261
Fessel, W. J., 309
Festenstein, H., 243, 273, 274
Fett, J. W., 13
Fetter, B. F., 402
Fewtrell, C., 51
Fichtelius, K. E., 226
Field, M. E., 225
Finch, J. T., 92
Findlay, J. B. C., 111
Fink, A. L., 92
Finkel, H. E., 429, 430, 432, 433
Finkel, S. I., 363
Finlayson, G., 326
Finn, F., 94, 116

452 AUTHOR INDEX

456 AUTHOR INDEX

SUBJECT INDEX

458   SUBJECT INDEX

B

Bacillus Calmette-Guérin
  (BCG), 259–60, 376–79
breast cancer and, 385–86
gastrointestinal tumors and,
  388–89
genitourinary tumors and,
  390–91
gynecological cancers and,
  391
leukemia and, 392–97
lung cancer and, 399–400
lymphomas and, 398
malignant melanoma and,
  402–9
sarcomas and, 410–11
Bacitracin
phagocytosis and, 166
Bacteria
contact angles of
  antibiotics and, 165
Fc-mediated phagocytosis of,
  271–72
leukocytic engulfment of
  interfacial tensions and,
  157
nonopsonized
  phagocytosis and contact
  angles of, 161–62
Bacteriorhodopsin
chemical cross-linking and,
  143
reactivated ATPase of, 112
B cells, 49–50, 212, 223–24
antibodies
  testing for, 306–7
antibody secretion of
  T cells inducing, 214–16
distribution in tissues,
  227–28
germinal centers and, 230–31
hairy cells and, 433–34
macrophage binding of, 278
migration patterns of,
  228–29, 232
in pregnancy, 353
as receptors, 43
in spleen, 225
Bahçet's disease
HLA-B5 and, 311
Bence-Jones protein
structure of, 13
Bisalkylimidates, 128, 145
Blastocyst
immunoglobulins coating,
  347
Blastogenesis, 235
Bone marrow
hairy cell leukemia
  infiltration of, 431
Brain tumors
immunotherapy for, 385

Breast cancer
HLA system and, 314
immunotherapy for, 385–88
levamisole and, 380
Brucella abortus
phagocytosis of, 161
Burkitt's lymphoma
HLA system and, 314
immunotherapy for, 397–98
serotherapy for, 381

C

Calcitonin
macrophage plasma
  membrane and, 264–65
microphage plasma
  membrane receptors for,
  268–69
Calcium
erythrocyte membrane and,
  67
cAMP
macrophage plasma
  membrane and, 264
photoaffinity analog of, 133
in photoaffinity labeling
  studies, 101
receptor
  photoaffinity labeling of,
  138
Cancer
see specific type
Candida albicans
Hageman factor and, 164
Candidiasis
chronic mucocutaneous, 381
Carbenes
for photoaffinity labeling,
  116–17
N-Carboxymethylhistidine
formation of, 95–96
O-Carboxymethylserine
production of, 95
O-Carboxymethyltyrosine
formation of, 95
Cardiolipin
liposome susceptibility to
  antibody-complement
  and, 73
Celiac disease
HLA system and, 313
Cell-mediated immunity, 84–85
intracellular parasites and,
  245–47
macrophage activation and,
  165
MHC and, 243–47
Cell-mediated lysis, 72–82
Cell-mediated tubulointerstitial
  disease, 337–39
Cell-surface antigens
of mouse leukemia

in vitro analysis of,
  179–206
of the TL system, 194–204
cGMP
in photoaffinity labeling
  studies, 101
Chloromycetin
phagocytosis and, 166
Chlorpromazine
Con A vacuolation and, 284
Cholesterol
liposomal immunogenicity
  and, 83
liposomes and, 76
macrophage plasma
  membrane, 260–61
Chromatin
cross-linking and, 148–49
Chymotrypsin
diazoacetyl, 93–96
Cis interactions
antigen-antibody interactions
  and, 44–45
in Fab New, 19
in immunoglobulin
  molecules, 7–8, 12
Cleft lip
HLA system and, 315
Colchicine
macrophage migration and,
  282
macrophages and, 263–64
Coley's toxins, 375
Colitis
ulcerative
  HLA system and, 243, 313
Colo-rectal cancer
immunotherapy for, 388–89
Complement
activation, 39
antibody-mediated, 49
IgM and, 46–47
lipids as targets for, 73
opsonization by, 163
tubulointerstitial, 333
Concanavalin A
macrophage interaction of,
  166
monovalent dimers of
  preparation of, 143
photoreactive derivative of,
  130–31
pinocytosis enhanced by,
  277, 283–84
Conception
maternal exposure to
  antigens related to,
  346–52
Corticosteroids
macrophages and, 358
Corticosterone
photoaffinity labeling of,
  134